Biostatistics for Oral Healthcare

Biostatistics for Oral Healthcare

Jay S. Kim, Ph.D.

Loma Linda University
School of Dentistry
Loma Linda, California 92350

Ronald J. Dailey, Ph.D.

Loma Linda University
School of Dentistry
Loma Linda, California 92350

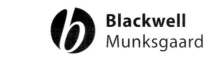

Blackwell
Munksgaard

Jay S. Kim, Ph.D., is Professor of Biostatistics at Loma Linda University, CA. A specialist in this area, he has been teaching biostatistics since 1977 to students in public health, medical school, and dental school. Currently his primary responsibility is teaching biostatistics courses to dental hygiene students, pre-doctoral dental students and students in advanced dental education. He also collaborates with the faculty and students on a variety of research projects.

Ronald J. Dailey, Ph.D., M.A., is the Associate Dean for Academic Affairs at Loma Linda University School of Dentistry. He has taught dental, dental hygiene and college students for the past 32 years.

© 2008 by Blackwell Munksgaard,
a Blackwell Publishing Company

Editorial Offices:
Blackwell Publishing Professional,
2121 State Avenue, Ames, Iowa 50014-8300, USA
Tel: +1 515 292 0140
9600 Garsington Road, Oxford OX4 2DQ
Tel: 01865 776868

Blackwell Publishing Asia Pty Ltd,
550 Swanston Street, Carlton South,
Victoria 3053, Australia
Tel: +61 (0)3 9347 0300

Blackwell Wissenschafts Verlag,
Kurfürstendamm 57, 10707 Berlin, Germany
Tel: +49 (0)30 32 79 060

First published 2008 by Blackwell Munksgaard, a Blackwell Publishing Company

Library of Congress Cataloging-in-Publication Data

Kim, Jay S.
   Biostatistics for oral healthcare / Jay S. Kim, Ronald J. Dailey. – 1st ed.
      p. ; cm.
   Includes bibliographical references and index.
   ISBN-13: 978-0-8138-2818-3 (alk. paper)
   ISBN-10: 0-8138-2818-X (alk. paper)
   1. Dentistry–Statistical methods.   2. Biometry.   I. Dailey, Ronald.   II. Title.
   [DNLM: 1. Biometry–methods.   2. Dentistry.   WA 950 K49b 2008]
   RK52.45.K46 2008
   617.60072–dc22

                                        2007027800

978-0-8138-2818-3

Set in 10/12pt Times by Aptara Inc., New Delhi, India
Printed and bound in by C.O.S. Printers PTE LTD

For further information on
Blackwell Publishing, visit our website:
www.blackwellpublishing.com

Disclaimer
The contents of this work are intended to further general scientific research, understanding, and discussion only and are not intended and should not be relied upon as recommending or promoting a specific method, diagnosis, or treatment by practitioners for any particular patient. The publisher and the author make no representations or warranties with respect to the accuracy or completeness of the contents of this work and specifically disclaim all warranties, including without limitation any implied warranties of fitness for a particular purpose. In view of ongoing research, equipment modifications, changes in governmental regulations, and the constant flow of information relating to the use of medicines, equipment, and devices, the reader is urged to review and evaluate the information provided in the package insert or instructions for each medicine, equipment, or device for, among other things, any changes in the instructions or indication of usage and for added warnings and precautions. Readers should consult with a specialist where appropriate. The fact that an organization or Website is referred to in this work as a citation and/or a potential source of further information does not mean that the author or the publisher endorses the information the organization or Website may provide or recommendations it may make. Further, readers should be aware that Internet Websites listed in this work may have changed or disappeared between when this work was written and when it is read. No warranty may be created or extended by any promotional statements for this work. Neither the publisher nor the author shall be liable for any damages arising herefrom.

The last digit is the print number: 9 8 7 6 5 4 3 2

Contents

Preface

Like many projects, this project started out to meet a need: we were teaching classes of dental hygiene, dental and post graduate dentists and could not find a textbook in statistics designed with the dental health professional in mind. So, we started to write a brief syllabus. We realized that most dentists will not become researchers, however, all will become consumers of research and will need to understand the inferential statistical principles behind the professional journals they read.

The goal of *Biostatistics for Oral Healthcare* is to give the reader a conceptual understanding of the basic statistical procedures used in the health sciences. Emphasis is given to the rationales, applications, and interpretations of the most commonly used statistical techniques rather than on their mathematical, computational, and theoretical aspects.

Achieving an effective level of communication in a technical book is always a difficult challenge. If written at too low a level, a book will not really explain many important points and risks insulting intelligent readers as well as boring them. However, if written at too advanced a level, then a book may have difficulty finding an audience. We have tried to write at a fairly elementary level, but have not hesitated to discuss certain advanced ideas. And we have gone rather deeply into a number of important concepts and methods.

DESCRIPTIVE STATISTICS

The content of Chapters 1 through 5 includes the basic concepts of statistics and covers descriptive statistics. Included are discussions of the rationale for learning and using statistics, mathematical concepts and guidelines for studying statistical concepts (Chapter 1); organizing and graphing data (Chapter 2); describing distributions, measures

of central tendency, and measures of variation (Chapter 3); random variables including both discrete and continuous (Chapter 4); and the three most useful distributions in the health sciences: binomial distribution, Poisson distribution and normal distribution.

INFERENTIAL STATISTICS

The discussion of inferential statistics begins in Chapter 6 where the recurring question of sufficient sample size is addressed. Chapters 7 through 9 covers how to determine appropriate sample size for a population and compute confidence intervals as well as hypothesis testing and estimation for one-sample and two-sample cases for the mean and other statistics. Chapter 10 describes hypothesis testing for categorical data.

ADVANCED TOPICS

We began the text with a review of basic mathematical and statistical concepts and we end the text with some of the more sophisticated statistical concepts and procedures. We include discussions of one-way and two-way analysis of variance as well as a description of parametric statistical methods used for data analysis. And finally, we discuss nonparametric statistics and survival analysis that are particularly useful in dental and medical clinical trials.

It is our sincere hope that the conceptual approach of this book will prove to be a valuable guide for dental health professionals in basic introductory courses as well as more advanced graduate level courses. We hope that we have been successful in providing an integrated overview of the most useful analytical techniques that students and practitioners are bound to encounter in their future studies, research activities and most importantly, as consumers of evidence based dentistry.

We are grateful to Mr. J. Tanzman for his assistance in preparing the probability tables included in the Appendix. Thanks are also due to the students who took statistics courses in which the original manuscript was used as a textbook; their contributions to shaping this book can not be overstressed. Finally, it is a great pleasure to acknowledge Dr. Martha Nunn for her support and encouragement. Table H in the Appendix is her idea.

J. S. Kim, Ph.D.
R. J. Dailey, Ph.D.
Loma Linda, California

Chapter 1

Introduction

1.1 WHAT IS BIOSTATISTICS?

Statistics is a field of mathematical sciences that deals with data. Biostatistics is a branch of statistics that emphasizes the statistical applications in the biomedical and health sciences. It is concerned with making decisions under uncertainties that occur when the data are subjected to variation. Some of the sources of variation are known and can be controlled, whereas some other sources are not known and cannot be controlled. Human beings vary in many aspects. There exist inherent differences among all of us in our physiology, biochemistry, anatomy, environment, lifestyles, pathogenesis, and responses to various dental and medical treatments. The word *statistics* is used both to refer to a set of data and to a field of study.

Advancing technology has enabled us to collect and safeguard a wide variety of data with minimal effort, from patients' demographic information to treatment regimens. Nowadays it is not uncommon for clinics, small or large, to have an efficient and impressive database management system that handles massive amounts of patient records. Clinicians, researchers, and other health sciences professionals are constantly collecting data on a daily basis. It is difficult to make sense of this confusing and chaotic array of raw data by visual inspections alone. The data must be processed in meaningful and systematic ways to uncover the hidden clues. Processing the data typically involves organizing them in tables and in clinically useful forms, displaying the information in charts and graphs, and analyzing their meaning, all in the presence of variability. The methods of statistical analysis are powerful tools for drawing the conclusions that are eventually applied to diagnosis, prognosis, and treatment plans for patients.

The following are some examples in which biostatistics is applied to answering questions raised by researchers in the field of health sciences.

1. In dental sciences, gingival recession represents a significant concern for patients and a therapeutic problem for clinicians. A clinical study was conducted to evaluate and compare the effects of a guided tissue regeneration procedure and connective tissue graft in the treatment of gingival recession defects.
2. Dental researchers conducted a study to evaluate relevant variables that may assist in identifying orthodontic patients with signs and symptoms associated with sleep apnea and to estimate the proportion of potential sleep apnea patients whose ages range from 8 to 15 years.
3. Candidiasis is a common infection among the immunocompromised patients. The most causative agent is *Candida albicans*, which is a fungus that produces chlamydospores. *C. albicans* can be harbored in the bristles of a toothbrush and possibly reinfect the patient during treatment. A study was conducted to determine the effectiveness of the three most popular mouthrinses against *C. albicans* that is harbored in the bristles of a toothbrush.
4. The medical research on attention deficit hyperactivity disorder (ADHD) is based almost exclusively on male subjects. Do boys have greater chances of being diagnosed as having ADHD than do girls? Is the prevalence rate of ADHD among boys higher than that among girls?
5. Coronary angioplasty and thrombolytic therapy (dissolving an aggregation of blood factors) are well-known treatments for acute myocardial infarction. What are the long-term effects of the two treatments, and how do they compare?

Most of the scientific investigations typically go through several steps.

1. Formulation of the research problem
2. Identification of key variables
3. Statistical design of an experiment

4. Collection of data
5. Statistical analysis of the data
6. Interpretation of the analytical results

Vast amounts of resources, time, and energy are being dedicated by health sciences professionals in the pursuit of research projects such as those described in the examples above. Statistics is an absolutely indispensable tool, providing the techniques that allow researchers to draw objective scientific conclusions.

1.2 WHY DO I NEED STATISTICS?

Students raise the question, "Why do I need statistics?" as often as many people say, "I hate going to the dentist." Unfortunately, many students have had an unpleasant experience in mathematics and statistics while in school. These individuals are as likely to dislike statistics as patients are to dislike dental procedures after a bad experience with a previous dental treatment.

Students who are pursuing a professional degree in the fields of health sciences, such as dentistry, dental hygiene, medicine, nursing, pharmacy, physical therapy, and public health, are often required to take at least one statistics course as part of the graduation requirements. An important part of students' training is to develop an ability to critically read the literature in their specialty areas. The amount of statistics used in journal articles in biomedical and health sciences can easily intimidate readers who lack a background in statistics. The dental and medical journal articles, for example, contain *results* and *conclusions* sections in which statistical methods used in the research are described. Health science professionals read journals to keep abreast of the current research findings and advances. They must understand statistics sufficiently to read the literature critically, assessing the adequacy of the research and interpreting the results and conclusions correctly so that they may properly implement the new discoveries in diagnosis and treatment. As reported by Dawson-Saunders and Trapp [1], many published scientific articles have shortcomings in study design and analysis.

A part of statistics is observing events that occur: birth, death due to a heart attack, emergence of premolar teeth, lifetime of a ceramic implant, spread of influenza in a community, amount of an increase in anterior-posterior knee laxity by exercises, and so on. Biostatistics is an essential tool in advancing health sciences research. It helps assess treatment effects, compare different treatment options, understand how treatments interact, and evaluate many life and death situations in medical sciences. Statistical rigor is necessary to be an educated researcher or clinician who can shun the overgeneralization, objectively criticize, and appreciate the research results published in the literature.

Learning should be fun. The study of statistics can be fun. Statistics is not "sadistics." It is an interesting subject. In fact, it is a fascinating field. Sir William Osler was quoted as saying that "medicine is a science of uncertainty and an art of probability." It is no wonder that in dental schools and medical schools, as well as other post-graduate health science professional schools, statistics is an integral part of the curriculum.

1.3 HOW MUCH MATHEMATICS DO I NEED?

Some students come to statistics classes with mathematics anxiety. This book is not intended to entice students and train them to become expert statisticians. The use of mathematics throughout the book is minimal; no more than high school or college level algebra is required. However, it is fair to say that with greater knowledge of mathematics, the reader can obtain much deeper insights into and understanding of statistics.

To dispel anxiety and fear of mathematics, plain English is used as much as possible to provide motivation, explain the concepts, and discuss the examples. However, the readers may feel bombarded with statistical terms and notation. Readers should not let this discourage them from studying statistics. Statistical terms in this book are clearly defined. Definitions and notation are the language by which statistical methods and results are communicated among the users of statistics.

1.4 HOW DO I STUDY STATISTICS?

Statistics books cannot be read like English, history, psychology, and sociology books, or like magazine articles. You must be prepared to read slowly and carefully and with great concentration and thought. Do not hesitate to go back and review the material discussed in the previous sections. Statistics is unique in that the concept being introduced in the current section is often the foundation for the concepts to be introduced in the following sections. It is a good idea to frequently review the materials to gain deeper insight and enhance your understanding.

It is not necessary to memorize the formulas in the book. Memorization and regurgitation will not help you learn statistics. Instead of spending time memorizing the formulas, strive to understand the basic concepts. Think of a few relevant examples in your discipline where the concepts can be applied. Throughout the study of this book, ask yourself a couple of questions: What is the intuition behind the concept? How could I explain the formula to my brother in the sixth grade so that he can understand? These questions will force you to think intuitively and rigorously.

1.5 REFERENCE

1. Dawson-Saunders, Beth, and Trapp, Robert G. *Basic & Clinical Biostatistics*. Second Edition. Appleton & Lange. 1994.

Chapter 2

Summarizing Data and Clinical Trials

2.1 RAW DATA AND BASIC TERMINOLOGY

In most cases, the biomedical and health sciences data consist of observations of certain characteristics of individual subjects, experimental animals, chemical, microbiological, or physical phenomena in laboratories, or observations of patients' responses to treatment. For example, the typical characteristics of individual subjects (sample units) are sex, age, blood pressure, status of oral hygiene, gingival index, probing depth, number of decayed, missing, and filled (DMF) teeth, mercury concentration in amalgam, level of pain, bonding strength of an orthodontic material, cholesterol level, percentage of smokers with obsessive-compulsive disorder, or prevalence rate of HIV positive people in a community. Whenever an experiment or a clinical trial is conducted, measurements are taken and observations are made. Researchers and clinicians collect data in many different forms. Some data are numeric, such as height (5′6″, 6′2″, etc.), systolic blood pressure (112 mm Hg, 138 mm Hg, etc.), and some are non-numeric, such as sex (female, male) and the patient's level of pain (no pain, moderate pain, severe pain). To adequately discuss and describe the data, we must define a few terms that will be used repeatedly throughout the book.

Definition 2.1.1. A **variable** is any characteristic of an object that can be measured or categorized. An object can be a patient, a laboratory animal, a periapical lesion, or dental or medical equipment. If a variable can assume a number of different values such that any particular value is obtained purely by chance, it is called a **random variable**. A random variable is usually denoted by an upper-case letter of the alphabet, X, Y, or Z.

Example 2.1.1. The following variables describe characteristics of a patient:

- Sex
- Age
- Smoking habits
- Quigley-Hein plaque index
- Heartbeat
- Amount of post-surgery pain
- Saliva flow rate
- Hair color
- Waiting time in a clinic
- Glucose level in diabetics

Raw data are reported in different forms. Some may be in the form of letters.

Sex	Status of Oral Hygiene	Level of Post-Surgery Pain
F = female M = male	P = poor F = fair G = good	N = no pain M = mild pain S = severe pain E = extremely severe pain

And some data are in numeric values.

Subject No.	Age (yrs.)	BP (mm Hg)	Pocket Depth (mm)	Cholesterol (mg/dl)
1	56	121/76	6.0	167
2	43	142/95	5.5	180
—	—	—	—	—
—	—	—	—	—
115	68	175/124	6.5	243

Note: BP, blood pressure.

The characteristics of individual subjects to be measured are determined by the researcher's study goals. For each characteristic there might be a few different ways to represent the measurements. For example, a clinician who is interested in the oral health of dental patients has selected tooth mobility as a variable (characteristic) to follow. Tooth mobility can be measured either by the precise distance in millimeters that the tooth can be moved, or it can be categorized as class I, class II, or class III. In another case, the ambient temperature may be the variable, which can be recorded in a specific numeric value, such as 71.3° F, or it can be classified as being cold, warm, or hot.

Definition 2.1.2. The collection of all elements of interest having one or more common characteristics is called a **population**. The elements can be individual subjects, objects, or events.

Example 2.1.2. Some examples of population are

- the entire group of endodontists listed in the directory of the California Dental Association;
- students enrolled in dental schools or medical schools in the United States in fall 2007;
- collection of heads and tails obtained as a result of an endless coin-tossing experiment;
- American children who have an early childhood caries problem;
- patients who contracted endocarditis as a result of dental treatments;
- vitamin tablets from a production batch; and
- all patients with schizophrenia.

The population that contains an infinite number of elements is called an **infinite population**, and the population that contains a finite number of elements is called a **finite population**.

Definition 2.1.3. The numeric value or label used to represent an element in the population is called an **observation**, or **measurement**. These two terms will be used synonymously.

Example 2.1.3. Information contained in five patient charts from a periodontal office is summarized in Table 2.1.1. Three observations, sex, age, and pocket depth, were made for each of the five patients.

Variables are classified as either qualitative or quantitative.

Definition 2.1.4. A **qualitative variable** is a characteristic of people or objects that cannot be naturally expressed in a numeric value.

Table 2.1.1. Periodontal data on pocket depth (mm).

Patient No.	Sex	Age	PD
1	M	38	4.5
2	F	63	6.0
3	F	57	5.0
4	M	23	3.5
5	F	72	7.0

Note: PD, pocket depth.

Example 2.1.4. Examples of a qualitative variable are

- sex (female, male);
- hair color (brown, dark, red, . . .);
- cause of tooth extraction (advanced periodontal disease, caries, pulp disease, impacted teeth, accidents, . . .);
- orthodontic facial type (brachyfacial, dolichofacial, mesofacial);
- specialty area in dentistry (endodontics, orthodontics, pediatric dentistry, periodontics, implants, prosthodontics, . . .);
- type of treatment;
- level of oral hygiene (poor, fair, good); and
- cause of herpes zoster.

Definition 2.1.5. A **quantitative variable** is a characteristic of people or objects that can be naturally expressed in a numeric value.

Example 2.1.5. Examples of a quantitative variable are

- age
- height
- weight
- blood pressure
- attachment level
- caloric intake
- gingival exudate
- serum cholesterol level
- survival time of implants

- DAT and MCAT scores
- bone loss affected by periodontitis
- success rate of cardiac bypass surgery
- fluoride concentration in drinking water
- remission period of lung cancer patients

Quantitative variables take on numeric values, and therefore basic arithmetic operations can be performed, such as adding, dividing, and averaging the measurements. However, the same arithmetic operations do not make sense for qualitative variables. These will be discussed further in

Chapter 3. Random variables are classified into two categories according to the number of different values that they can assume: discrete or continuous.

Definition 2.1.6. A **discrete variable** is a random variable that can take on a finite number of values or a countably infinite number (as many as there are whole numbers) of values.

Example 2.1.6. The following variables are discrete:

- The number of DMF teeth. It can be any one of the 33 numbers, 0, 1, 2, 3, . . . , 32.
- The size of a family.
- The number of erupted permanent teeth.
- The number of patients with no dental or medical insurance.
- The number of patients with osseous disease.
- The number of ankylosis patients treated at L.A. county hospital.

Definition 2.1.7. A **continuous variable** is a random variable that can take on a range of values on a continuum; that is, its range is uncountably infinite.

Example 2.1.7. Continuous variables are

- treatment time
- temperature
- pocket depth
- amount of new bone growth
- diastolic blood pressure
- concentration level of anesthesia
- torque value on tightening an implant abutment
- blood supply in a live tissue
- acidity level in saliva
- force required to extract a tooth
- amount of blood loss during a surgical procedure

The actual measurements of continuous variables are necessarily discrete due to the limitations in the measuring instrument. For example, the thermometer is calibrated in 1°, speedometer in 1 mile per hour, and the pocket depth probe in 0.5 mm. As a result, our measurement of continuous variables is always approximate. On the other hand the discrete variables are always measured exactly. The number of amalgam fillings is 4, and the number of patients scheduled for surgery on Monday is 7, but the pocket depth 4.5 mm can be any length between 4.45 mm and 4.55 mm. Many discrete variables can be treated as continuous variables for all practical purposes. The number of colony-forming units (CFUs) in a dental waterline sample may be recorded as 260,000, 260,001, 260,002, . . . , where the discrete values approximate the continuous scale.

2.2 THE LEVELS OF MEASUREMENTS

Statistical data arise whenever observations are made or measurements are recorded. The collection of the raw data is one of the key steps to scientific investigations. Researchers in health sciences collect data in many different forms. Some are labels, such as whether the carving skills of the applicants to dental schools are unacceptable, acceptable, or good. Some are in numerical form, such as the class ranking of the third-year dental students. The numerical data can convey different meanings. The student ranked number one in the class is not necessarily 10 times better than the student ranked number 10. However, an orthodontist who typically earns $500,000 a year from her practice makes twice as much as an orthodontist whose income from his practice is $250,000 per year. We treat the numbers differently because they represent different levels of measurement. In statistics, it is convenient to arrange the data into four mutually exclusive categories according to the type of measurement scale: nominal, ordinal, interval, and ratio. These measurement scales were introduced by Stevens [1] and will be discussed next.

Definition 2.2.1. A **nominal measurement scale** represents the simplest type of data, in which the values are in unordered categories. Sex (F, M) and blood type (type A, type B, type AB, type O) are examples of nominal measurement scale.

The categories in a nominal measurement scale have no quantitative relationship to each other. Statisticians use numbers to identify the categories, for example, 0 for females and 1 for males. The numbers are simply alternative labels. We could just as well have assigned 0 for males and 1 for females, or 2 for females and 5 for males. Similarly, we may assign the numbers 1, 2, 3, and

4 to record blood types, 1 = type A, 2 = type B, 3 = type AB, and 4 = type O. Any four distinct numbers could be used to represent the blood types. Although the attributes are labeled with numbers instead of words, the order and magnitude of the numbers do not have any meaning at all. The numbers in a nominal measurement scale can be added, subtracted, divided, averaged, and so on, but the resulting numbers tell us nothing about the categories and their relationships with each other. For example, $2 + 5 = 7$ and $(5 + 2)/2 = 3.5$, but neither 7 nor 3.5 renders any meaningful relationship to any characteristic of females or males. It is important for us to understand that numbers are used for the sake of convenience and that the numerical values allow us to perform the data analysis.

Example 2.2.1. Examples of nominal scale are presented.

- Yes/no response on a survey questionnaire
- Implant coatings
- Type of sedation
- Type of filling material in root canal (gutta-percha, calcium hydroxide, eugenol, silver, . . .)
- Marital status
- Specialty area in medicine
- Religious faith
- Edema (angioneurotic, cardiac, dependent, periorbital, pitting, and glottis)

Definition 2.2.2. In the **ordinal measurement scale**, the categories can be ordered or ranked. The amount of the difference between any two categories, though they can be ordered, is not quantified.

Post-surgery pain can be classified according to its severity; 0 represents no pain, 1 is mild pain, 2 is moderate pain, 3 is severe pain, and 4 is extremely severe pain. There exists a natural ordering among the categories; severe pain represents more serious pain than mild pain. The magnitude of these numbers is still immaterial. We could have assigned 1 = extremely severe pain, 2 = severe pain, 3 = moderate pain, 4 = mild pain, and 5 = no pain, instead of 0, 1, 2, 3, and 4. The difference between no pain and mild pain is not necessarily the same as the difference between moderate pain and severe pain, even though both pairs of categories are

numerically one unit apart. Consequently, most of the arithmetic operations do not make much sense in an ordinal measurement scale, as they do not in a nominal scale.

The numbers assigned indicate rank or order but not magnitude or difference in magnitude among categories. Precise measurement of differences in the ordinal scale does not exist. For example, the competency of dentists or physicians can be ranked as poor, average, good, or superior. When dentists are classified as superior, a large variation exists among those in the same category.

Example 2.2.2. Here are some examples of ordinal measurement scales.

- Löe-Silness gingival index
- Tooth mobility
- Miller classification of root exposure
- Pulp status (normal, mildly necrotic, moderately necrotic, severely necrotic)
- Curvature of the root (pronounced curvature, slight curvature, straight)
- Letter grade
- Difficulty of the national board exam (easy, moderately difficult, very difficult, . . .)
- Disease state of a cancer (stage 1, stage 2, . . .)

The third level of measurement scale is called the interval measurement scale.

Definition 2.2.3. In the **interval measurement scale** observations can be ordered, and precise differences between units of measure exist. However, there is no meaningful absolute zero.

Temperature is an example of the interval scale. Suppose the room temperature readings have been recorded: $40°$ F, $45°$ F, $80°$ F, and $85°$ F. We can express $80°$ F $> 40°$ F ($80°$ F is warmer than $40°$ F), and $45°$ F $< 85°$ F ($45°$ F is colder than $85°$ F). We can also write $45°$ F $- 40°$ F $= 85°$ F $- 80°$ F $= 5°$ F. The temperature differences are equal in the sense that it requires the same amount of heat energy to raise the room temperature from $40°$ F to $45°$ F as it does from $80°$ F to $85°$ F. However, it may not be correct to say that $80°$ F is twice as warm as $40°$ F, even though $80°$ F $= 40°$ F $\times 2$. Both Celsius and Fahrenheit have artificial zero degrees. In other words, the temperature $0°$ in Celsius or in Fahrenheit does not mean the total absence of temperature. The unique feature of the interval measurement scale is the absence of meaningful absolute zero.

Example 2.2.3. The examples of the interval measurement scale are not as common as other levels of measurement.

- IQ score representing the level of intelligence. IQ score 0 is not indicative of no intelligence.
- Statistics knowledge represented by a statistics test score. The test score zero does not necessarily mean that the individual has zero knowledge in statistics.

The highest level of measurement is called the ratio measurement scale.

Definition 2.2.4. The **ratio measurement scale** possesses the same properties of the interval scale, and there exists a true zero.

Most of the measurement scales in health sciences are ratio scales: weight in pounds, patient's waiting time in a dental office, temperature on the Kelvin scale, and age. Zero waiting time means the patient did not have to wait. The ratio measurement scale allows us to perform all arithmetic operations on the numbers, and the resulting numerical values do have sensible meaning. As we mentioned earlier, the amount of knowledge represented by a statistics test score is on an interval measurement scale. On the other hand, the test score that represents the number of the correct answers is on a ratio scale. The test score 0 indicates that there are zero correct answers; a true absolute zero exists. The test score of 99 means that an individual has three times as many correct answers as an individual who scored 33 on the test.

Example 2.2.4. The examples of the ratio measurement scale are presented.

- Treatment cost
- Saliva flow rate
- Length of root canal
- Attachment loss
- Diastema
- Intercondylar distance
- Systolic blood pressure
- Amount of new bone growth
- Amount of radiation exposure
- Implant abutment height
- O_2 concentration in the nasal cannula
- Sugar concentration in blood

If the temperature is expressed as cold, warm, and hot, an interval variable becomes an ordinal variable. A health maintenance organization administrator might want to express treatment cost as low, average, and high; then a ratio variable becomes an ordinal variable. In general, interval and ratio measurement scales contain more information than do nominal and ordinal scales. Nominal and ordinal data are encountered more frequently in behavioral and social sciences than in health sciences or engineering. The distinction among the four levels of measurement is important. As we shall see later, the nature of a set of data will suggest the use of particular statistical techniques.

2.3 FREQUENCY DISTRIBUTIONS

In the previous sections, we learned how to classify various types of statistical data. In this section we study the basic statistical techniques that are useful in describing and summarizing the data. Though it is extremely rare, one might collect data for the entire population. When population data are available, there are no uncertainties regarding the characteristics of the population; all of the pertinent statistical questions concerning the population are directly answered by observation or calculation. In most of the practical situations, however, the data represent a sample of measurements taken from a population of interest. The statistical techniques in this book are discussed under the assumption that the sample data, not population data, are availble.

2.3.1 Frequency Tables

The first step in summarizing data is to organize the data in some meaningful fashion. The most convenient and commonly used method is a **frequency distribution**, in which raw data are organized in table form by class and frequency. For nominal and ordinal data, a frequency distribution consists of categories and the number of observations that correspond to each category. Table 2.3.1. displays a set of nominal data of prosthodontic services provided at a large dental clinic during the period of 1991–1998 [2].

Table 2.3.1. The number of gold crowns and metal ceramic crowns provided during 1991–1998.

Type of Crown	Number of Crowns
Gold crown	843
Metal ceramic crown	972

A survey was taken to assess job satisfaction in dental hygiene [3]. Table 2.3.2. presents a set of ordinal data of 179 responses to one of the questions in the survey questionnaire, "If you were to increase appointment length, could you provide better quality care for your patients?" There are five choices for the individual's response: strongly disagree, disagree, neutral, agree, and strongly agree. Since there are five choices, a typical frequency distribution would have five categories as shown in Table 2.3.2. It is not necessary that a frequency distribution for the ordinal data should have all of the categories. Sometimes researchers would prefer combining two adjacent categories. For example, combine "strongly disagree" and "disagree," and combine "agree" and "strongly agree." The combined data would have three categories: **disagree** (67 individuals), **neutral** (49 individuals), and **agree** (63 individuals).

It has been speculated that a possible cause for root canal failure is the persistence of bacteria that have colonized dentinal tubules. To reduce this risk and time-consuming endodontic therapy, new equipment and materials are constantly being introduced. A study was conducted to evaluate the effect of disinfection of dentinal tubules by intracanal laser irradiation using an in vitro model. The following data represent the count of bacterial (*Enterococcus faecalis*) colonies found in the samples after they had been treated by the neodymium: yttrium-aluminum-garnet (Nd: YAG) laser [4].

It is clear that we must do more than a simple display of raw data as in Table 2.3.3 if we

Table 2.3.2. Responses to a survey question: If you were to increase appointment time, you could provide better quality care for your patients.

Response Category	Number of Individuals
Strongly disagree	24
Disagree	43
Neutral	49
Agree	33
Strongly agree	30

Table 2.3.3. Count of bacterial colonies.

280	284	172	176	304	200	254	299	190	396
272	196	408	400	184	410	325	206	380	476
236	275	308	188	184	346	210	448	396	304
300	300	200	365	330	220	160	416	184	192
360	272	185	390	250	412	424	172	304	296
120	366	335	180	304	356	440	200	300	588
280	320	500	438	346	213	412	306	320	418
295	282	354	315	196	380	287	207	396	302
306	275	272	358	304	364	286	386	385	301

want to make some useful sense out of them. Rearrangement of the data in ascending order enables us to learn more about the count of the bacterial colonies. It is easy to see from Table 2.3.4 the smallest count is 120, and the largest count is 588. There are several counts that are tied, for example, five samples have the same count of 304 bacterial colonies. The data in Table 2.3.4, even in ordered form, are still too unwieldy. To present raw data, discrete or continuous, in the form of a frequency distribution, we must divide the range of the measurements in the data into a number of non-overlapping intervals (or classes). The intervals need not have the same width, but typically they are constructed to have equal width. This will make it easier to make comparisons among different classes. If one class has a larger width, then we may get a distorted view of the data. Bearing in mind that we wish to summarize the data, having too many intervals is not much improvement over the raw data. If we have too few intervals, a great deal of information will be lost.

So, how many intervals should we have? Some authors [5] suggest that there should be 10–20 intervals. Of course, a set of data containing a small number of measurements should have only a few intervals, whereas a set of data containing

Table 2.3.4. Count of bacterial colonies arranged in ascending order.

120	160	172	172	176	180	184	184	184	185
188	190	192	196	196	200	200	200	206	207
210	213	220	236	250	254	272	272	272	275
275	280	280	282	284	286	287	295	296	299
300	300	300	301	302	304	304	304	304	304
306	306	308	315	320	320	325	330	335	346
346	354	356	358	360	364	365	366	380	380
385	386	390	396	396	396	400	408	410	412
412	416	418	424	438	440	448	476	500	588

thousands of measurements over a wide range of values may need more than 20 intervals. The number of observations in the data and the range of values influence the determination as to how many intervals and how wide the intervals should be. In general, we suggest that one should have the number of intervals approximately equal to the square root of the number of observations. Let n denote the total number of measurements or data points. The number of intervals $= \sqrt{n}$. Since $\sqrt{90} \simeq 9.49$, for the bacterial colony data in Table 2.3.3, we will need about 9 or 10 intervals to construct a frequency distribution. The symbol "$\simeq$" means approximately equal. Once the number of intervals has been selected, the interval width can be determined by dividing the range by the number of intervals.

$$\text{Width of the interval} = \frac{\text{Range of data}}{\text{Number of intervals}}.$$

Constructing a frequency distribution uses the following steps:

Step 1. Select the number of non-overlapping intervals.

Step 2. Select a starting point for the lowest class limit. This can be the smallest value in the data or any convenient number less than the smallest observed value.

Step 3. Determine the upper and lower limits for each interval.

Step 4. Count the number of observations in the data that fall within each interval.

The results are then presented as in Table 2.3.5 for the bacterial colony data. Table 2.3.5 shows how the data are distributed across the 10 non-overlapping intervals, with relatively few observations at the end of the range (412.5–612.5), and a large part of the measurements falling around the value 300. The intervals must be non-overlapping so that the observations can be placed in only one class. The upper and lower limits for the intervals

have a fraction 0.5 that no other measurements in the data have. All the observations in Table 2.3.3 are in whole numbers. Thus, an advantage of a selection of such limits is that we can avoid having measurements fall on the boundary between two adjacent intervals. We could, of course, select the limits without the fraction 0.5: The first interval can be [112, 162), instead of (112.5, 162.5), and the second interval can be [162, 212), instead of (162.5, 212.5). With the intervals so defined, if an observation has a value 162, we place it in the next interval [162, 212). An observation with a value 212 will be placed in the third interval. Another advantage of having the fraction 0.5 in the class limits is that this eliminates a gap between the intervals. There should be enough intervals to accommodate the entire data. In other words, the intervals must be exhaustive. The width of an interval is obtained by subtracting the lower limit from the upper limit. In Table 2.3.5, the width of an interval is $162.5 - 112.5 = 50.0$. The data presented in Table 2.3.5 is known as **grouped data** because each class contains a collection of measurements.

We said above that the intervals should have an equal width, but one exception occurs when a distribution is open-ended with no specific beginning or ending values. Examples of this are often seen in age-related data as shown in Table 2.3.6. The frequency distribution for age is open-ended for the first and last classes. The frequency distribution is an effective organization of data, but certain information is inevitably lost. We can't tell from Table 2.3.5 precisely what those five measurements are in the third interval (212.5, 262.5). All we know is that there are five observations between 212.5 and 262.5. The guidelines discussed in this section should be followed when one is constructing a frequency distribution. As we have noticed, several different frequency tables can be constructed for the same data. All are correct, just different, because of a different starting point for

Table 2.3.5. Frequency table for bacterial colony data.

Interval	Frequency	Interval	Frequency
112.5–162.5	2	362.5–412.5	16
162.5–212.5	19	412.5–462.5	6
212.5–262.5	5	462.5–512.5	2
262.5–312.5	27	512.5–562.5	0
312.5–362.5	12	562.5–612.5	1

Table 2.3.6. Restorative patients by age.

Age	No. of Restorative Patients	Age	No. of Restorative Patients
30 or younger	16	51–60	37
31–40	24	61–70	41
41–50	23	71 or older	33

the first interval, a different number of classes, or a different width for intervals. In summary, a frequency distribution

1. is a meaningful, intelligible way to organize data.
2. enables the reader to make comparisons among classes.
3. enables the reader to have a crude impression of the shape of the distribution.

2.3.2 Relative Frequency

To facilitate the interpretation of a frequency distribution, it is often helpful to express the frequency for each interval as a proportion or a percentage of the total number of observations. A **relative frequency distribution** shows the proportion of the total number of measurements associated with each interval. A proportion is obtained by dividing the absolute frequency for a particular interval by the total number of measurements. A relative frequency distribution for bacterial colony data is presented in Table 2.3.7. The numbers in the parentheses are the corresponding percent values. The relative frequency for the class (162.5, 212.5) is $\frac{19}{90} \simeq 0.21$, or $\left(\frac{19}{90}\right) \times 100\% \simeq 21.0\%$. The figures shown in the tables are rounded off to the nearest 100th. Relative frequencies are useful for comparing different sets of data containing an unequal number of observations. Table 2.3.7 displays the absolute, relative, and cumulative relative frequencies. The cumulative relative frequency for an interval is the proportion of the total number

of measurements that have a value less than the upper limit of the interval. The cumulative relative frequency is computed by adding all the previous relative frequencies and the relative frequency for the specified interval. For example, the cumulative relative frequency for the interval (262.5, 312.5) is the sum, $0.02 + 0.21 + 0.06 + 0.30 = 0.59$, or 59%. This means that 59% of the total number of measurements is less than 312.5. The cumulative relative frequency is also useful for comparing different sets of data with an unequal number of observations.

Example 2.3.1. At a large clinic, 112 patient charts were selected at random; the systolic blood pressure of each patient was recorded. Using the blood pressure data presented in Table 2.3.8, construct a frequency distribution, including relative frequency and cumulative relative frequency.

Solution

i. We need to determine the number of nonoverlapping intervals. There are 112 observations in the data set, and $\sqrt{112} \simeq 10.58$. Therefore, we choose to have 11 intervals.
ii. For the selection of the interval width, notice that the smallest systolic blood pressure measurement is 96, and the largest measurement is 179. Therefore,

$$\text{Width of the interval} = \frac{\text{Range of data}}{\text{Number of intervals}}$$
$$= \frac{179 - 96}{11} \simeq 7.55.$$

Given this information, it would seem reasonable to have the interval width of 8. We also choose

Table 2.3.7. A relative frequency distribution for bacterial colony data.

Interval	Frequency	Relative Frequency (%)	Cumulative Relative Frequency (%)
112.5–162.5	2	2	2
162.5–212.5	19	21	23
212.5–262.5	5	6	29
262.5–312.5	27	30	59
312.5–362.5	12	13	72
362.5–412.5	16	18	90
412.5–462.5	6	7	97
462.5–512.5	2	2	99
512.5–562.5	0	0	99
562.5–612.5	1	1	100
Total	90	100	

Table 2.3.8. Systolic blood pressure (mm Hg) of 112 patients.

116	130	134	158	138	98	130	170	120	104	125	136	160	126
140	110	116	108	138	104	125	120	130	120	128	123	110	140
124	110	140	120	130	145	144	140	140	145	117	120	120	138
110	130	118	120	120	125	135	140	118	130	132	162	133	112
110	122	120	152	110	160	112	150	122	158	110	118	115	133
122	112	145	128	140	120	110	105	110	105	145	112	124	122
120	140	110	120	150	129	179	118	108	110	144	125	123	117
120	118	120	131	96	127	130	131	112	138	126	162	110	130

to have 92.5 as a starting point, which becomes the lower limit of the first interval. Any other reasonable value that is less than the smallest observed value would do just as well as a starting point. Once we determine the number of intervals, the interval width, and the starting point, we can construct a frequency distribution displayed in Table 2.3.9.

2.4 GRAPHS

Although a frequency distribution is an effective way to organize and present data, graphs can convey the same information more directly. Because of their nature, qualitative data are usually displayed in bar graphs and pie charts, whereas quantitative data are usually displayed in histograms, box-whisker plots, and stem and leaf plots. Graphs can aid us in uncovering trends or patterns hidden in data, and thus they are indispensible. They help us visualize data. Graphs make data look "alive." There are many graphing techniques. Books have been written devoted to graphs

[6, 7]. Our discussions in this section are limited to the most useful graphs for research and clinical data in health sciences.

2.4.1 Bar Graphs

In a **bar graph** categories into which observations are tallied appear on the abscissa (X-axis) and the corresponding frequencies on the ordinate (Y-axis). The height of a vertical bar represents the number of observations that fall into a category (or a class). When two sets of data with an unequal number of observations are being compared, the height of a vertical bar should represent proportions or percentages. A bar graph in Figure 2.4.1 displays how an estimated 120,000 deaths each year from hospital errors compare with the top five leading causes of accidental death in the United States [8].

Table 2.4.1 summarizes a survey conducted to find out how many cases of seizures have occurred in dental offices [9]. Since the number of respondents is not the same for the specialty areas in

Table 2.3.9. Frequency distribution for the SBP data.

Interval	Frequency	Relative Frequency (%)	Cumulative Relative Frequency (%)
92.5–100.5	2	1.79	1.79
100.5–108.5	6	5.36	7.15
108.5–116.5	20	17.86	25.01
116.5–124.5	29	25.89	50.90
124.5–132.5	21	18.75	69.65
132.5–140.5	17	15.18	84.83
140.5–148.5	6	5.36	90.19
148.5–156.5	3	2.68	92.87
156.5–164.5	6	5.36	98.23
164.5–172.5	1	0.89	99.12
172.5–180.5	1	0.89	100.01*
Total	112	100.01*	

Note: *The total sum exceeds 100% due to the round-off errors.
SBP, systolic blood pressure.

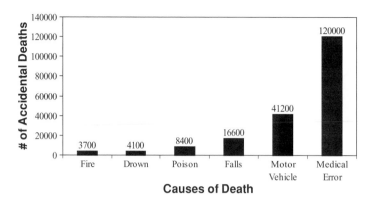

Figure 2.4.1 Accidental deaths (Source: National Safety Council, 1998).

Table 2.4.1. The number of seizures in dental offices.

Specialty Area	Number of Respondents	Seizures Occurred	Percent of Seizures
General dentistry	719	212	29.5%
Endodontics	60	35	58.3%
Oral surgery	88	33	37.5%
Orthodontics	89	17	19.1%
Periodontics	70	25	35.7%
Prosthodontics	41	11	26.8%
Others	232	69	29.7%

dentistry, the height of the vertical bars should represent the percentages as shown in Figure 2.4.2.

2.4.2 Pie Charts

Categorical data are often presented graphically as a **pie chart**, which simply is a circle divided into pie-shaped pieces that are proportional in size to the corresponding frequencies or percentages as illustrated in Figure 2.4.3. The variable for pie charts can be nominal or ordinal measurement scale. To

construct a pie chart, the frequency for each category is converted into a percentage. Then, because a complete circle corresponds to 360 degrees, the central angles of the pieces are obtained by multiplying the percentages by 3.6.

2.4.3 Line Graph

A **line graph** is used to illustrate the relationship between two variables. Each point on the graph represents a pair of values, one on the X-axis and the other on the Y-axis. For each value on the X-axis there is a unique corresponding observation on the Y-axis. Once the points are plotted on the XY plane, the adjacent points are connected by straight lines. It is fairly common with line graphs that the scale along the X-axis represents time. This allows us to trace and compare the changes in quantity along the Y-axis over any specified time period. Figure 2.4.4 presents a line graph that represents the data on the number of lifetime births per Japanese woman for each decade between 1930 and 2000.

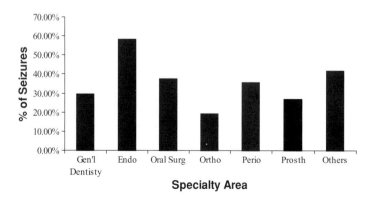

Figure 2.4.2 Seizure incidents in dental offices.

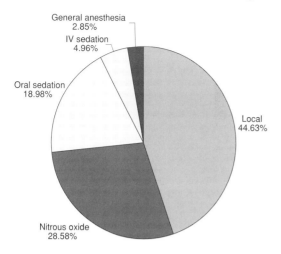

General anesthesia 2.85%

IV sedation 4.96%

Oral sedation 18.98%

Local 44.63%

Nitrous oxide 28.58%

Figure 2.4.3 Type of anesthesia used in dental offices.

piled a database of specific prosthodontic treatments provided at Loma Linda University School of Dentistry during the period of 1991–1998. One of the prosthodontic treatments of their interest was fixed partial dentures (FPD), subclassified by number of units involved and by gold or metal ceramic constituent materials. Figure 2.4.5 contains two lines for comparison; the bottom line for the gold and the top line for the metal-ceramic fixed partial dentures. We can trace and compare the chronological changes in the number of FPDs preferred by the patients over a specific time period during 1991–1998. We can plot more than two observations along the Y-axis for a given value on the X-axis to compare different groups. Multiple lines are then constructed by connecting the adjacent points by straight lines.

The line graph in Figure 2.4.4 clearly displays the trends in the number of births per woman in Japan since the decade of the 1930s. The rate has been declining steadily except for a break between 1960 and 1970. Japan has experienced a precipitous drop in the birth rate between 1950 and 1960. The lifetime births per woman in Japan in 2000 is less than one-third of that in 1930. The line graph tells us that since 1980, the birth rate in Japan has fallen below replacement level of 1.7–1.8 births per woman. If the current birth rate stays the same, Japanese population will continue to shrink.

We can have two or more groups of data with respect to a given variable displayed in the same line graph. Loo, Cha, and Huang [2] have com-

2.4.4 Histograms

Figure 2.4.6 displays a bar graph for the systolic blood pressure data of $n = 112$ patients in Table 2.3.9. A **histogram** is similar in appearance and construction to a bar graph except it is used with interval or ratio variables. That is, a histogram is used for quantitative variables rather than qualitative variables. The values of the variable are grouped into intervals of equal width. Like a bar graph, rectangles are drawn above each interval, and the height of the rectangle represents the number of observations in the interval. To stress the

Figure 2.4.4 Lifetime births per Japanese woman. (Source: Japan's National Institute of Population and Social Security Research).

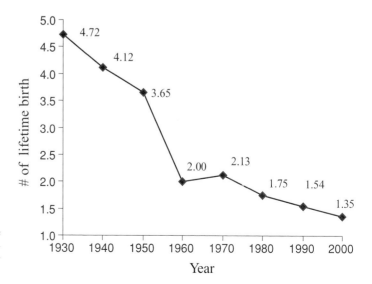

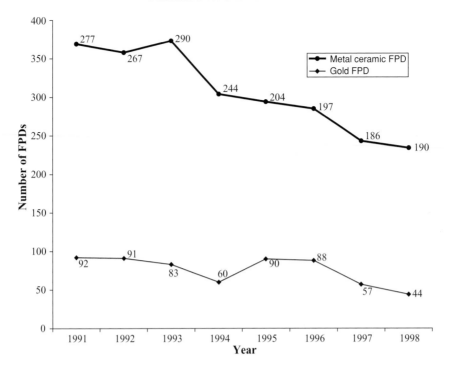

Figure 2.4.5 Gold and metal ceramic fixed partial dentures.

continuous, quantitative nature of the class intervals, the bars of adjacent class intervals in a histogram should touch with no space between the bars, as can be seen in Figure 2.4.6. The class intervals for the systolic blood pressure are represented along the X-axis (horizontal axis), and frequency is represented along the Y-axis (vertical axis). Either frequency or relative frequency can be represented along the Y-axis. The relative frequency for each class interval is shown in Table 2.3.9 as well. Notice in Table 2.3.8 that 47 of the 112 blood pressure measurements, which amounts to about 42%, end in zero. This suggests that those persons who recorded the blood pressure values may have

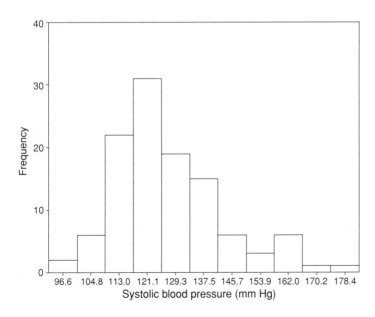

Figure 2.4.6 Histogram: Systolic blood pressure with 11 class intervals.

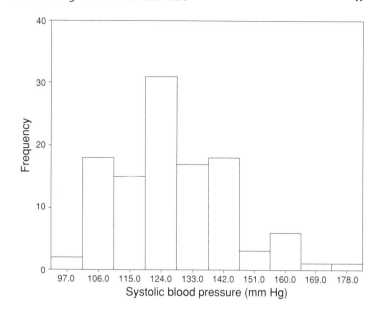

Figure 2.4.7 Histogram: Systolic blood pressure with 10 class intervals.

had a strong preference for the numbers ending in zero.

A histogram is one of the most widely used graphing techniques that enables us to understand the data. The histogram in Figure 2.4.6 has 11 class intervals, with the first interval starting at 92.5 mm Hg. We can construct an alternative histogram with 10 class intervals, instead of 11 class intervals, to see the effect of our choice. The width of the 10 intervals in Figure 2.4.7 is 9 mm Hg. The starting point of the two histograms is the same, both starting at 92.5. Notice that these two histograms have a rather different shape even though they are created from the same data and their starting points are precisely the same. The only minor difference between them is that one has 11 intervals and the other 10 intervals. To further explore the effects of our choices, readers are encouraged to construct yet another histogram that has 11 class intervals, but the graph starts at 94.5 mm Hg. Starting the graph 2 units to the right of the starting point of the original graph produces a figure that looks different. In general, histograms are sensitive to choices we make in the number of class intervals and the starting point of the graph. As we make different choices, we may see dramatically different histograms that may give us different impressions about the same set of data.

The following are a few general comments about histograms:

- Histograms serve as a quick and easy check of the shape of a distribution of the data.
- The construction of the graphs is subjective.
- The shape of the histograms depends on the width and the number of class intervals.
- Histograms could be misleading.
- Histograms display grouped data. Individual measurements are not shown in the graphs.
- Histograms can adequately handle data sets that are widely dispersed.

Example 2.4.1. A group of food scientists selected 639 random samples of commercially available pickles and their volume was measured in cubic centimeters. Four technicians who measured the volume of individual pickle samples had been instructed to round off the measurements to the nearest 5 or 10. Therefore, the actual measurements of 806.5 cm^3 and 948.7 cm^3 were recorded as 805 cm^3 and 950 cm^3 so that all of the recorded data points end in 0 or 5. We have learned in Section 2.1 that the volume is a continuous variable. Figure 2.4.8 shows the histogram for these pickle data with 22 class intervals. Nothing appears to be out of ordinary about this histogram. However, a histogram for the same data constructed with 50 class intervals, presented in Figure 2.4.9, shows a fascinating shape. Low bars are sandwiched between high bars. The height discrepancy between the low and high bars is remarkable. It is highly

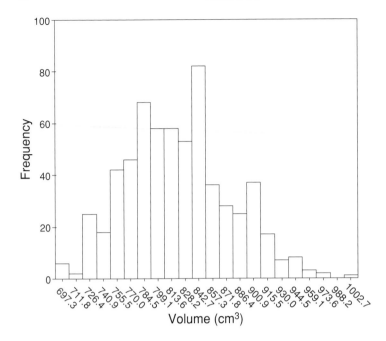

Figure 2.4.8 Histogram for pickle data with 22 class intervals.

unusual for a continuous variable to behave as such. A careful examination of the data set indicated that only 19.7% of the measurements end in 5, and a lopsided 80.3% of the measurements end in 0. Consequently, the class intervals containing the measurements ending in 5 tend to have much lower frequency. Figure 2.4.9 revealed that most likely the technicians have made round-off

errors. They may have preferred to round off the measurements to the nearest 10 when they should have rounded off to the nearest 5.

Solution

1. As we have seen in the above examples, we can use one data set to construct a variety of different histograms that might have different

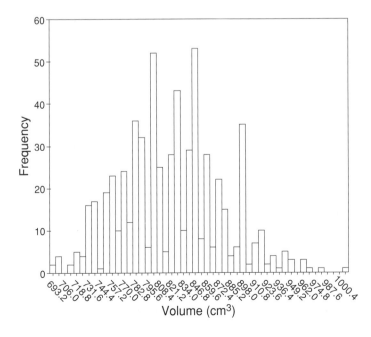

Figure 2.4.9 Histogram for pickle data with 50 class intervals.

appearances. The subjective nature of the histogram suggests that we must be cautious about how we use histograms and not be enamored with their use.

2. Histograms should not be constructed with open class intervals. When the width of the class intervals is not equal, special care should be exercised.

2.4.5 Stem and Leaf Plots

Suppose we have a discrete quantitative random variable, such as the number of fixed prostheses present, or a continuous random variable, such as the amount of epithelial attachment loss suffered by a patient. The first task in understanding the data is to obtain a basic idea of the distribution of the random variable, that is, to determine the general shape of the distribution, how widely the measurements are spread, and whether or not the measurements have a distinct pattern. The **stem and leaf plot** is a method of organizing data that uses part of the data as the "stem" and part of the data as the "leaves" to form groups. In stem and leaf plots measurements are grouped in such a way that individual observed values are retained while the shape of the distribution is shown. The stem and leaf plot consists of a series of numbers in a column, called the stem, with the remaining trailing digits in the rows, called the leaves. The stem is the major part of the observed values.

Figure 2.4.10 presents a stem and leaf plot of the systolic blood pressure data in Table 2.3.8. The first column shows the frequency for each leaf. The first row in the plot indicates that there are two observations, which are 96 and 98. The third row indicates that there are four observations, which are 105, 105, 108, and 108. In the stem and leaf plot, the first one or two digits form the stems and the last digits of the observed values constitute the leaves. In a sense a stem and leaf plot is an extension of a histogram. An important advantage of a stem and leaf plot over a histogram is that the plot provides all the information contained in a histogram while preserving the value of the individual observations.

Example 2.4.2. The bone height of 17 implant patients was measured in millimeters. The total of 49 measurements of their bone height was recorded.

Frequency	Stem	Leaf
2	9.	68
2	10.	44
4	10.	5588
17	11.	00000000000022222
10	11.	5667788888
22	12.	0000000000000022223344
10	12.	5555667889
14	13.	00000000112334
6	13.	568888
10	14.	0000000044
4	14.	5555
3	15.	002
2	15.	88
0	16.	0022
1	17.	0
1	17.	9

Figure 2.4.10 Stem and leaf plot for the blood pressure data in Table 2.3.8.

The number of implants placed in each patient varied from 1 to 6.

The integer part of these measurements, 2, 3, 4, 5, 6, 7, 8, 9, 10, 11, and 12 will serve as stems and row labels. The number appearing after the decimal point will be represented as a leaf on the corresponding stem. The entire data set in Table 2.4.2 is displayed in Figure 2.4.11. Some statisticians like to have a vertical line drawn to the right of the column of stems as shown in the figure, or some simply put dots (·) after the stems.

Frequency	Stem	Leaf
1	2	4
4	3	0222
17	4	00000000888888888
2	5	66
7	6	0000044
6	7	222222
6	8	000008
3	9	066
1	10	0
1	11	2
1	12	0

Figure 2.4.11 Stem and leaf plot of the bone height data.

Table 2.4.2. Bone height (mm) of implant patients.

4.0	5.6	7.2	8.0	7.2	9.6	6.0	3.0	4.0	9.0	4.0	4.8	3.2
6.0	6.0	4.0	7.2	7.2	4.8	6.4	6.0	8.0	12.0	5.6	4.8	8.0
10.0	8.0	7.2	2.4	4.8	4.0	4.8	4.8	3.2	4.8	8.0	8.8	4.0
4.8	3.2	4.0	9.6	6.4	7.2	11.2	4.8	6.0	4.0			

The steps for constructing a stem and leaf plot can be summarized as follows:

1. Separate each value of the measurement into a stem component and a leaf component. The stem component consists of the number formed by all but the rightmost digit of the value. For example, the stem of the value 76.8 is 76 and the leaf is 8. For the value 45.6, the stem is 45 and the leaf is 6.
2. Write the smallest stem in the data set at the top of the plot, the second smallest stem below the first stem, and so on. The largest stem is placed at the bottom of the plot. Alternatively, the largest stem can be placed at the top of the plot and the smallest stem at the bottom.
3. For each measurement in the data, find the corresponding stem and write the leaf to the right of the vertical line or period. It is convenient, although it is not necessary, to write the leaves in ascending order, that is, the smallest first and the largest at the end of the row.

We note that the leaf component for a stem and leaf plot can have more than one digit. Suppose that a data point for the mercury concentration in an amalgam sample is 87.42%. The leaf can consist of a two-digit number, 42. A stem and leaf plot can be constructed rather quickly and easily. No decisions are needed on the number of class intervals or the width of the class intervals. It is easy to determine the median and the range of the data from the plot. As mentioned above, unlike a histogram, it provides an overview of the distribution while retaining the individual observed values.

2.5 CLINICAL TRIALS AND DESIGNS

Perusing journal articles in biomedical and health sciences areas, one cannot help but be overwhelmed by an impressive array of new discoveries in treatments and new developments in materials and equipment in dentistry and medicine.

All advances require proper clinical and scientific scrutiny to ensure the efficacy and safety of patients before new methods are allowed to be used in patient treatment. One cannot emphasize enough the importance of maintaining high standards of research in the clinical trials of new drugs and treatment methods. The proper use of statistical methods is critical in all phases of clinical trials. This section is intended to familiarize the readers with several statistical terms that are used whenever a clinical trial or an experiment is undertaken. An experimental study that involves human subjects is called a clinical trial. A typical experiment in health sciences includes an **experimental group** (or treatment group), a **negative control group**, and a **positive control group**. The purpose of control groups is to set up a direct comparison with the experimental group.

Definition 2.5.1.

- A **negative control group** is synonymous with most people's idea of a control. The subject's response is observed in an untreated group or a **placebo** group.
- A **positive control group** is a treatment group that shows the subjects are capable of response. Positive control in general is equally important but for some reason is less frequently practiced.

Positive control is also known as **active control**. We note that if there is no significant difference between the groups, we may not know if either treatment was effective, detection was not sensitive, treatment was inadequate, compliance with the treatment was inadequate, or there was heterogeneity in those subjects receiving treatments.

A company called Wellness, Inc. was about to introduce a new mouthrinse product for the prevention of gingivitis. The product was tentatively named Oral-Fresh. To study the effectiveness of the product the investigators recruited 210 patients who met the inclusion criteria. These subjects were randomly assigned to each of the three treatment groups: Oral-Fresh, placebo, and peridex. Each

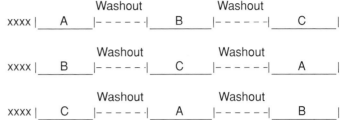

Figure 2.5.1 Crossover designs with 2 and 3 treatments.

treatment group contained 70 subjects. Specific instructions were given to the subjects regarding the use of the treatments, such as the amount of mouthrinse and the rinsing time, to control the experiment. The subject's compliance with the products was carefully monitored. To assess the effectiveness of the mouthrinse, the gingival index of each patient was measured at the baseline and at the 3-month time point. In this study, placebo and peridex were used as negative and positive control groups, respectively. The trial can be conducted as a single-blind or a double-blind.

Definition 2.5.2.

Single-blind study. Only the participating subjects are blinded with regard to whether they are treatment or control subjects.

Double-blind study. Neither the subjects nor the investigators evaluating the outcome variables know whether or not the subjects received treatment.

Parallel groups design. The simplest and most widely used design for clinical trials is the **parallel groups design** (also called parallel design). In a parallel design, subjects are randomly assigned to receive only one of the treatments, without considering their prognostic variables. Although it is simple and easy to apply, the parallel design allows subjects to receive only one of the treatments, with the object of studying differences between the treatments.

Crossover design. The design in which subjects receive all of the treatments sequentially in

time is known as a **crossover design**. In a crossover design, each subject receives two or more different treatments. The simplest case is when there are only two treatments (see Figure 2.5.1). In this design each subject receives both treatments; half the subjects are randomly selected to receive treatment **A** first and then, after a suitably chosen period of time, called washout period, cross over to treatment **B**. The washout period is necessary to prevent the carryover effect of the first treatment persisting into the time period of the second treatment. The washout period must be long enough to remove the carryover effect.

The main advantages of the crossover design are that the subjects act as their own control and that the treatments are compared within subjects. In a crossover design with two treatments, for example, each subject provides two measurements: one for treatment A and one for treatment B. The difference between these two measurements will eliminate any subject effect from the comparisons. In fact, this is the purpose of the crossover design: to eliminate treatment effects arising from differences among the subjects.

For the clinical trial with three treatments, there are three groups of subjects. At the beginning of the trial, the groups are randomly assigned to one of the three treatments (see Figure 2.5.1). For example, the second treatment group is initially assigned to B, and after the washout period, is assigned (or crossed over) to C. After another washout period, the group is now assigned to A, as shown in

Figure 2.5.1. Some disadvantages of the crossover design are the carryover effects, withdrawal of subjects from the study before the next treatment, and the amount of time it takes to complete the study. For further discussions on design and analysis of crossover trials, the readers are referred to specialized textbooks such as Pocock [10] and Senn [11].

2.6 CONFOUNDING VARIABLES

A bulk of clinical studies and research projects in biomedical and health sciences involve comparing the means, proportions, variances, or survival times between two treatment groups and the relationship between two variables. In these studies, the investigators tend to assume that the only difference between the two groups is the treatment itself. However, the two groups can vary in many different ways: one group might have better oral hygiene, a much higher cholesterol level, or the control group might have a serious bone resorption problem at the start of the study. Under these circumstances, it is difficult to know whether the difference detected is due to the treatment or to the differences in oral hygiene, cholesterol level, or bone resorption.

The statistical results are said to be **confounded** when the results can have more than one explanation. For example, in a study to examine the relationship between the percent of gray hair on the heads of adults and the risk of myocardial infarction, both the percent of gray hair and the risk of myocardial infarction increase as age increases [12, 13]. The **confounding variable** is an extraneous variable that is associated both with the outcome variable and treatment or risk factor.

Example 2.6.1. In a study to investigate the relationship between coronary heart disease (CHD) and physical exercise, smoking habit is a confounding variable. Past research has established that smoking is a serious risk factor for CHD. Individuals who smoke are much less likely to exercise and exhibit lower levels of health consciousness [14].

Example 2.6.2. A study by Jovanovic et al. [15] showed that smoking is the most important etiological factor in the development of oral squamous

cell carcinoma. It has been suggested that alcohol is one of the major causes of squamous cell carcinoma [16], and alcohol consumption is known to be closely related to smoking. Therefore, in this study, alcohol is a confounding variable.

There may be more than one confounding variable in a study. For example, in a study designed to determine if an association exists between cigarette smoking and signs of periodontal disease [17], age, sex, plaque, and calculus can be confounding variables. Good studies are designed to minimize the influence of confounding variables. For valid results and conclusions to be obtained, confounding variables must be controlled. For example, in Example 2.6.1 smokers and non-smokers should be grouped separately to determine the relationship between CHD and exercise.

2.7 EXERCISES

1 Make a list of at least five variables in dentistry or medicine.

2 Find at least five examples of population in health sciences.

3 For the following dental variables, indicate if the measurement is qualitative or quantitative. For quantitative variables, indicate whether they are discrete or continuous.
   a. Patient status
   b. Color of gingiva
   c. Length of a crown
   d. Root resorption
   e. Number of amalgam fillings
   f. Pulse rate
   g. Orthognathic jaw classification
   h. Sensitivity of tooth
   i. Treatment time
   j. Number of patients without medical insurance
   k. Golf score
   l. Anxiety level
   m. Type of mucosa
   n. Mercury concentration in amalgam
   o. Size of periradicular lesion
   p. Shear strength of a bonding material

4 Classify measures of the following according to the level of measurement scale.

a. Amount of new bone growth
b. Tooth mobility
c. Bone graft type
d. Drilling temperature
e. Soft tissue thickness
f. Interfacial width
g. Type of surgical approach
h. Occlusal force measured in millipascals
j. Type of filling material in root canal
k. Degree of curvature of a root
l. Level of complexity in a surgical procedure
m. Type of drug used in general anesthesia
n. Amount of epithelial growth
o. Shape of alveolar ridge
p. Number of roots obturated
q. Bite force

5 What do scores of 0 and 100 on the national board exam mean? Discuss them in terms of the statistical concepts you have learned in this chapter.

6 Eke, Braswell, and Fritz [18] concluded that the microbiota associated with the progression of experimental peri-implantitis and periodontitis induced concurrently in partially edentulous mouths are similar by comparing the relative proportions of microbial groups. Identify the measurement scale of the variables (relative proportions) used in their study.

7 The most recent study conducted by the Association of American Medical Colleges [19] on medical school diversity among the U.S. medical school graduates in 1998–99 showed that 65.8% are White, 18.2% Asian/Pacific Islander, 7.7% Black, 6.7% Hispanic, 0.9% American Indian, and 0.7% unknown. Construct an appropriate graph to compare the six categories.

8 The impact of moving was measured in an asthma study to compare the asthma prevalence in children who remained on the primitive island of Tokelau with children who moved to the developed island of New Zealand [20]. Using the data in the table below, construct an appropriate graph.

	Tokelau	New Zealand
Definite asthma	1.3 %	6.9 %
Probable asthma	9.8	18.4
Total asthma	11.0	25.0

9 The following are two of the most popular weight-loss programs; one is American Heart Association eating plan and the other Dean Ornish heart disease reversal diet. Construct an appropriate chart or charts to compare the two diet programs.

	Total Daily Diet (%)		
	Carbohydrates	Fat	Protein
AHA	55	30	15
Dean Ornish	70	10	30

10 The findings by Nielson Media Research indicates that advertisers are not afraid to spend money on Super Bowl ads. The companies say that the exposure during the Super Bowl justifies the expense. What type of a graph would you use to illustrate the trend in ad fees on TV during the Super Bowl games?

Price of a 30-second Super Bowl ad, adjusted for inflation. (in millions)

Year	1995	1996	1996	1998	1999	2000	2001
Price	$1.1	1.2	1.3	1.4	1.7	2.1	2.3

11 What are the advantages and disadvantages of grouped and ungrouped frequency distributions?

12 Roll a die 30 times and construct a frequency table showing the number of times each die face occurred.

13 Sölerling et al. [21] studied 169 mother-child pairs in a 2-year investigation exploring whether the mothers' xylitol consumption could be used to prevent mother-child transmission of *Mutans streptococci* (MS). The 106 mothers in xylitol group were requested to chew xylitol-sweetened gum at least 2 or 3 times a day, starting 3 months after delivery. In the two control groups, the 30 mothers received chlorhexidine, and 33 mothers received fluoride varnish treatments at 6, 12, and 18 months after delivery. At 2 years of age, 9.7% of the children in the xylitol, 28.6% in the chlorhexidine, and 48.5% in the fluoride varnish group showed a detectable level of MS. Construct a graph to present their research results.

14 The systolic blood pressure data is arranged by sex. There are 38 female patients and 36 male patients in the data set. (a) Draw two separate histograms. (b) Construct a stem and leaf for each group to compare the two groups.

Female							
116	158	98	125	136	126	140	117
110	116	108	125	120	123	140	125
110	140	145	120	138	118	120	118
125	135	140	118	130	120	118	122
120	96	127	130	131	138		
Male							
130	134	138	130	170	120	104	123
160	138	104	120	130	128	110	144
124	140	120	130	145	144	140	110
117	120	110	130	120	132	162	108
133	112	131	112				

15 Pemphigus vulgaris (PV) is a potentially life-threatening illness that manifests itself initially in the mouth in the majority of patients. Sirois et al. [22] reported the following 42 clinical cases of oral PV evaluated and diagnosed by dentists. Discuss how you would graphically present the nominal data.

Location of Lesion	No. of Patients with Oral PV
Buccal mucosa	18
Gingiva	13
Multiple sites	6
Tongue	2
Palate	3
Floor of mouth	0
Skin	0

16 The ages of 54 patients treated by a general dentist during the first week in June are listed below. Construct a stem and leaf to display the shape of the age distribution.

66	81	42	34	85	23	18	67	55	59	62	40	42	53	52	54	64	57
9	26	54	73	69	48	54	55	33	40	46	62	54	43	47	44	42	18
70	47	41	35	31	61	29	22	19	8	67	58	29	26	54	72	37	41

17 To group data on the number of DMF teeth reported by a project team of dental researchers, Dr. Smith uses the classes 0–5, 6–11, 12–16, 18–24, and 24–32. Explain where difficulties might arise with his classes.

18 As of 1999, there are an estimated $800,000$ to $900,000$ people living with HIV or AIDS in the United States. Centers for Disease Control and Prevention [23] estimated the annual new HIV infections by race is the following: 26% White, 54% Black, 19% Hispanic, and 1% others. How would you present the data to make comparisons between the races?

2.8 REFERENCES

1. Stevens, S. On the theory of scales of measurements. *Science*, 1946; 103:667–680.
2. Loo, C., Cha, S., and Huang, J. Trends of Prosthodontic Procedures in Loma Linda University School of Dentistry from 1991 to 1998. Dental students project presentation. Loma Linda University. 2000.
3. Anderson, K., Dennis, S., and Thielen, M. Appointment Length? How This Relates to Job Satisfaction in Dental Hygiene. Dental hygiene students project presentation. Loma Linda University. 2001.
4. Cecchini, S. Disinfection of dentin by intracanal laser irradiation: An in vitro model (Master's thesis). Loma Linda University. 2000.
5. Kirk, R. E. *Statistics: An Introduction*. Fourth edition. Harcourt Brace.1999.
6. Cleveland, W. S. *Visualizing Data*. Hobart Press, Summit, New Jersey.1993.
7. Tukey, J. *Exploratory Data Analysis*, Addison-Wesley, 1977.
8. National Safety Council website. Available at www.nsc.org. Accessed March,1998.
9. Ayre, J., Mashni, M., and Wuerch, R. Seizures in Dental Offices. Dental students project presentation. Loma Linda University. 1999.
10. Pocock, S. J. *Clinical Trials: A Practical Approach*. John Wiley & Sons.1983.
11. Senn, S. *Cross-over Trails in Clinical Research*. John Wiley & Sons. 1993.
12. Mattila, K. J., Nieminen, M.S., Valtonen, V.V, et al. Association between dental health and acute myocardial infarction. *British Medical Journal*. 1989: 298, 779–781.
13. Mattila, K. J. Infections and coronary heart disease (dissertation). Helsinki: University of Helsinki, Finland. 1990.
14. Näslund, G. K., Frédrikson, M., Hellenius, M., and de Faire, U. Effect of diet and physical exercise intervention

programmes on coronary heart disease risk in smoking and non-smoking men in Sweden. *J. Epidemiol Community Health.* 1996: 50, 131–136.

15. Jovanovic, A., Schulten, E. A., Kostense, P. J., Snow, G. B., van der Waal, I. Tobacco and alcohol related to the anatomical site of oral squamous cell carcinoma. *J. Oral Pathol Med.* 1993: 22, 459–462.

16. Hsu, T. C., Furlong, C., and Spitz, M. R. Ethyl alcohol as a cocarcinogen with special reference to the aerodigestive tract: a cytogenetic study. *Anticancer Res.* 1991: 11, 1097–1102.

17. Stoltenberg, J. L., et al. Association Between Cigarette Smoking, Bacterial Pathogens, and Periodontal Status. *J Periodontol.* 1993: 64, 1225–1230.

18. Eke, P. I., Braswell, L. D., and Fritz, M. E. Microbiota Associated with Experimental Peri-Implantitis and Periodontitis in Adult Macaca mulatta Monkeys. *J. of Periodontology:* 1998, 69, 190–194.

19. *Handbook of Academic Medicine.* Washington, DC: Association of American Medical Colleges. 2004.

20. Leadbitter, P., Pearce, N., Cheng, S., et al. Relationship between fetal growth and the development of asthma and atopy in children. *Thorax.* 1999; 54: 905–910.

21. Sölderling, E., Isokangas, P., Pienihäkkinen, K., and Tenovuo, J. Influence of Maternal Xylitol Consumption on Acquisition of Mutans Streptococci by Infants. *J. Dent. Res.* 2000; 79, 882–887.

22. Sirois, D., Leigh, J. E., and Sollecito, T. P. Oral Pemphigus Vulgaris Preceding Cutaneous Lesions. *JADA.* 2000: 131, 1156–1160.

23. Centers for Disease Control website. Available at www.cdc.gov. Accessed May, 2000.

Chapter 3

Measures of Central Tendency, Dispersion, and Skewness

3.1 INTRODUCTION

In the preceding chapter we studied frequency distributions and graphs to visually summarize and display data. These techniques allow us to obtain useful information from raw data. However, it is desirable to further describe certain characteristics of data using quantitative measures. It is often necessary to summarize data by means of a couple of numbers that are descriptive of the entire data. The statistical measures that describe such characteristics as the center or middle of the data are called **measures of location** or **measures of central tendency (or central location)**. The term central tendency refers to the value on which a distribution tends to center. In the next several sections, we present six different measures of location: mean, weighted mean, median, mode, geometric mean, and harmonic mean. Descriptions of grouped data, percentiles and quartiles are also presented.

The most widely used measure of location is *average*. However, a company that manufactures surgical latex gloves will not be able to stay in business very long if it makes only average-sized gloves. The measures of central tendency are not enough to describe the data adequately. In addition to knowing the average, we must know how the data are dispersed, or spread. The measures that determine the level of dispersion are called **measures of dispersion**, or **measures of variation**. Typical measures of dispersion are range, variance, and standard deviation. These measures of variation will be discussed in the later part of the chapter. In particular, the last few sections present the **box plot**, which is an extremely useful technique for exploratory data analysis, and the concepts of **coefficient of variation** and **skewness**.

3.2 MEAN

The most frequently used measure of central tendency is an **arithmetic mean** or simply a **mean**. The mean, commonly known as the average, is the sum of n measurements divided by n. In terms of describing data, people usually think of average. Average is an interesting concept. Paraphrasing Feinsilbur and Meed [1], while very few of the dental and medical students want to be an average student, all of them are interested in the average score on the national board exam. The average number of children American families have is 2.3. But no family we know actually has 2.3 children. Some families have 2 children, and some 3 children. But never 2.3 children.

Because we need to compute the mean for a set of data arising from many different situations, it would be most convenient to have a general formula that is always applicable. The **sample size**, or the number of observations in a sample, is denoted by the letter n. If the letter X represents the variable, the n values of the sample data are represented by $X_1, X_2, \ldots, X_n$. In general, X_j indicates the jth measurement in a data set. We can write:

$$\text{Sample mean} = \frac{X_1 + X_2 + \cdots + X_n}{n}.$$

This formula will encompass any number of measurements in a set of any sample data. It will be further simplified by using symbols $\overline{X}$ and $\sum$.

The following two symbols will be used repeatedly throughout the book:

1. $\overline{X}$ is the symbol for **sample mean**, read as "X bar."
2. $\sum$ is capital *sigma*, a Greek letter, and $\sum X_i$ stands for the sum of X_i's.

Using the above notation, we write the sample mean as:

$$\overline{X} = \frac{X_1 + X_2 + \cdots + X_n}{n} = \frac{\sum_{i=1}^{n} X_i}{n}.$$

In statistics, it is customary to denote the characteristics of samples by uppercase English letters and the characteristics of populations by lowercase Greek letters. The mean of a sample is denoted by $\overline{X}$, and the mean of a population is denoted by μ, the Greek letter mu (pronounced "mew").

Suppose that a surgeon examined five patients with intraoral swelling. She measured the diameter of the swelling and reported the following measurements: 5.5, 7.0, 4.5, 8.5, and 10 mm. The sample mean of the data can be written as:

$$\overline{X} = \frac{\sum_{i=1}^{5} X_i}{5} = \frac{X_1 + X_2 + \cdots + X_5}{5} = 7.1.$$

Some people prefer to write the sample mean, $\overline{X} = \frac{1}{n} \sum_{i=1}^{n} X_i$, instead of $\frac{\sum_{i=1}^{n} X_i}{n}$. By multiplying both sides of the equation $\overline{X} = \frac{1}{n} \sum_{i=1}^{n} X_i$ by n, we get $\sum_{i=1}^{n} X_i = n \cdot \overline{X}$. For non-negative data, no individual value can exceed n times the average. To illustrate this fact, let us consider an example.

Example 3.2.1. Suppose the mean annual income of four orthodontists is $225,000. Would it be possible for any one of them to have an annual income of $950,000?

Solution. $\sum_{i=1}^{n} X_i = (4) \cdot (225,000) = 900,000$. Since the total sum is $900,000, it is not possible for any one of them to have reported an annual income of $950,000.

Example 3.2.2. Chewing tobacco has high levels of sugars and the users typically keep it in their mouth a few hours at a time. Therefore, it may be cariogenic. A sample of 6 chewing tobacco users and 8 non-users, all of whom are non-smokers, are compared with respect to the number of decayed or filled teeth (DFT; see Table 3.2.1). Two samples are involved in this example; one sample of 6 subjects from a population of chewing tobacco users and another sample of 8 from a population of non-users. The random variables of interest are X and Y. X is the random variable representing the number of DFT for the chewing tobacco users, and Y is the random variable representing the number

Table 3.2.1. Number of DFT.

Chew Tobacco	Non-users	Chew Tobacco	Non-users
16	4	12	1
19	6	17	6
15	3		5
20	6		7

of DFT for the non-users. The two sample means, $\overline{X}$ and $\overline{Y}$ are

$$\overline{X} = \frac{X_1 + X_2 + \cdots + X_6}{6}$$
$$= \frac{16 + 19 + 15 + 20 + 12 + 17}{6} = 16.5.$$
$$\overline{Y} = \frac{Y_1 + Y_2 + \cdots + Y_8}{8}$$
$$= \frac{4 + 6 + 3 + 6 + 1 + 6 + 5 + 7}{8} = 4.75.$$

Suppose a mistake had been made and the number of DFT for the third subject in the non-users group was recorded as 31, instead of 3. Then the sample mean would be: $\overline{Y} = (4 + 6 + 31 + 6 + 1 + 6 + 5 + 7)/8 = 8.25$. The mean number of DFT has increased by 3.50, from 4.75 to 8.25. The impact of one large value on the mean is quite dramatic. Similarly, one extremely small value might decrease the mean by an inordinately large amount. In other words, a mean is rather sensitive to extremely small or extremely large values. This is not a desirable feature for a measure of location. However, the mean is simple to calculate; it can be calculated for any set of numerical data. There is one and only one mean for any quantitative data set. It possesses many other desirable statistical properties that will be discussed in later chapters. It is no accident that the mean is popular as a measure of central tendency for both discrete and continuous observations. Is the mean appropriate to describe the central location for either nominal or ordinal data we discussed in Section 2.2? Let's consider the following two cases.

Case 1. Orthodontists use three facial types to classify a patient's facial shape:
1. Brachyfacial
2. Dolichofacial
3. Mesofacial

Case 2. Periodontists use the following scale to categorize a patient's periodontal disease state:

1. None   2. Mild   3. Moderate
4. Severe   5. Extremely severe

The variable for the facial type in case 1 is nominal. The numbers assigned to the three different facial types are labels for convenience. Thus, the average facial type of 2.1 has no meaning at all. We could have easily assigned $0 = $ Brachy, $1 = $ Dolicho, and $2 = $ Meso. Similarly, for the ordinal variable in case 2, we could have labeled the categories $0 = $ none, $1 = $ mild, $3 = $ moderate, $5 = $ severe, and $7 = $ extremely severe. The average score of 3.85 for the periodontal disease state is meaningless. There is an exception to this rule, however. In the case of a dichotomous variable where two possible outcomes are represented by 0 and 1, the mean of the observations is equal to the proportion of 1's in the data. For example, $0 = $ female and $1 = $ male. Or $0 = $ no periapical abscess, and $1 = $ periapical abscess. Suppose Dr. Johnson examines 12 patients and finds that 9 have no evidence of periapical abscess and 3 have periapical abscess as shown in Table 3.2.2. The average is

$$\overline{X} = \frac{0+0+0+0+0+0+0+1+0+1+0+1}{12}$$
$$= 0.25.$$

The proportion of the patients who have the periapical abscess is 25%, which is equal to the mean of the data. However, if we labeled $1 = $ no periapical abscess and $2 = $ periapical abscess, the average

Table 3.2.2. Periapical abscess data.

Subject No.	Periapical Abscess (X)	Sex (Y)
1	0	0
2	0	0
3	0	1
4	0	1
5	0	1
6	0	1
7	0	0
8	1	0
9	0	0
10	1	1
11	0	0
12	1	1

of the data

$$\overline{X} = \frac{1+1+1+1+1+1+1+2+1+2+1+2}{12}$$
$$= 1.25$$

has no meaning. The mean of the dichotomous variable is equal to the proportion of the male patients in the sample. That is:

$$\overline{Y} = \frac{0+0+1+1+1+1+0+0+0+1+0+1}{12}$$
$$= 0.5.$$

This means that the 50% of the patients in Dr. Johnson's sample are males. However, if we had labeled $1 = $ female and $2 = $ male, the mean

$$\overline{Y} = \frac{1+1+2+2+2+2+1+1+1+2+1+2}{12}$$
$$= 1.5$$

would have no meaning. The average score becomes meaningful only when two possible outcomes of a dichotomous variable are represented by 0 and 1.

Have you noticed that the mean is always between the smallest and the largest observations of a data set? This fact should become intuitively clear once we describe a physical interpretation of the mean. Suppose we have a data set consisting of pocket depth measurements of 5 patients, 10, 5, 7, 12, and 6 mm. The mean of the data is $\overline{X} = (10 + 5 + 7 + 12 + 6)/5 = 8$. Imagine a stick that has a uniform mass from one end to the other. Suppose we put a marker on the stick that corresponds to every measurement in the data set. The minimum value of the data will be marked at the left end of the stick, and the maximum value of the data will be marked at the right end of the stick. The intermediary values will be appropriately scaled and marked along the stick as shown in Figure 3.2.1. If we tie an equal weight, say 1/5 oz., to each of the five markers, the point at which the stick can be balanced on the edge of a knife corresponds to the mean of the data.

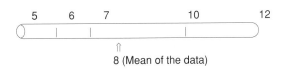

Figure 3.2.1 The balancing point of the stick is the mean of the data.

From the above physical interpretation of the mean, it should be clear that the mean must be located somewhere between the minimum and maximum observations in the data. It cannot be smaller than the minimum value, nor can it be larger than the maximum value.

Next we will discuss some properties of the mean. Suppose $X_1, X_2, \ldots, X_n$ are n observations and c is any given constant. Then the mean of $X_1 \pm c, X_2 \pm c, \ldots, X_n \pm c$ is the same as adding or subtracting the constant from the mean of the observations, that is, $\overline{X} \pm c$. Similarly, the mean of $c \cdot X_1, c \cdot X_2, \ldots, c \cdot X_n$ or the mean of X_1/c, $X_2/c, \ldots, X_n/c$ $(c \neq 0)$ is the same as multiplying or dividing the mean $\overline{X}$ by c, that is, $c \cdot \overline{X}$ or $\overline{X}/c$. This fact is stated below.

1. $\dfrac{(X_1 \pm c) + (X_2 \pm c) + \cdots + (X_n \pm c)}{n}$

$= \dfrac{\sum_{i=1}^{n}(X_i \pm c)}{n}$

$= \overline{X} \pm c$, for any constant c.

2. $\dfrac{cX_1 + cX_2 + \cdots + cX_n c}{n}$

$= \dfrac{\sum_{i=1}^{n} cX_i}{n} = c\overline{X}.$

3. $\dfrac{X_1/c + X_2/c + \cdots + X_n/c}{n} = \dfrac{\sum_{i=1}^{n} X_i/c}{n}$

$= \overline{X}/c, \quad (c \neq 0).$

4. $\dfrac{\sum_{i=1}^{n}(c_1 X_i \pm c_2)}{n} = c_1 \overline{X} \pm c_2.$

Example 3.2.3. (i) Dr. Lee is a clinic lab instructor. He has 8 third-year dental students under his supervision. The mid-term exam scores of the 8 students were $68, 88, 79, 94, 70, 84, 85$, and 72. The mean score is $(68 + 88 + 79 + 94 + 70 + 84 + 85 + 72)/8 = 80.0$. However, Dr. Lee decided to reward all of the students with 5 bonus points for their commitment and dedication to their clinical work. Given the constant $c = 5$, using property 1 above, we can easily calculate the mean of the 8 students after adding 5 bonus points; $\overline{X} + c = 80 + 5 = 85$.

(ii) The weight of 5 oral surgery patients was measured in kilograms; $87, 67, 104, 97, 47$. The average weight is $(87 + 67 + 104 + 97 + 47)/5 = 80.4$ (kg). Suppose we want to present the average weight in pounds. Because 1 kg. is approximately equal to 2.2 pounds, we need to multiply each measurement by 2.2 to convert it to pounds and then calculate the mean. By using the above property 2, the average weight in pounds can be obtained by simply multiplying $c = 2.2$ to $\overline{X} = 80.4$. That is, $c\overline{X} = (2.2) \cdot 80.4 = 176.88$.

Strictly speaking, the word *mean*, which is also known as *expected value*, is not an alternative for the word *average*. The word *mean* pertains to the population, and the word *average* pertains to the sample. They have different interpretations. In this book, the distinction between the two words is not made, unless there is a danger of causing confusion.

3.3 WEIGHTED MEAN

Suppose your statistics instructor indicated that the homework accounts for 10%, the mid-term examination accounts for 30%, and the final examination accounts for 60% of the grade for Statistics 101. A student named John Elmo scored 60 on the homework, 75 on the mid-term examination, and 93 on the final examination. How would you calculate John's average score for the course? Would it be correct to calculate his average for the course as $\overline{X} = \dfrac{60 + 75 + 93}{3} = 76.0$? According to your instructor's grading policy, the final examination is six times as important as the homework, and twice as important as the mid-term examination performance. We would be making a serious error if we overlooked the fact that the scores in the data do not have equal importance.

In order to properly reflect the relative importance of the observations, it is necessary to assign them weights and then calculate a **weighted mean**. Let $X_1, X_2, \ldots, X_n$ be n measurements, and their relative importance be expressed by a corresponding set of numbers $w_1, w_2, \ldots, w_n$. The weight w_1 is assigned to X_1, the weight w_2 to $X_2, \cdots$, and the weight w_n to X_n. It is required that the sum of the weights is 1.0. That is,

$$\sum_{i=1}^{n} w_i = w_1 + w_2 + \cdots + w_n = 1.0.$$

Definition 3.3.1. A weighted mean (or weighted average) is given by

$$\overline{X}_w = w_1 X_1 + w_2 X_2 + \cdots + w_n X_n$$
$$= \sum_{i=1}^{n} w_i X_i, \quad \text{where } \sum_{i=1}^{n} w_i = 1.0.$$

Example 3.3.1. John Elmo's scores are given by $X_1 = 60$ (homework), $X_2 = 75$ (mid-term examination), and $X_3 = 93$ (final examination). The corresponding weights are $w_1 = 0.10$, $w_2 = 0.30$, and $w_3 = 0.60$. The sum of the weights is $w_1 + w_2 + w_3 = 0.10 + 0.30 + 0.60 = 1.0$. So John's weighted mean score is

$$\overline{X}_w = \sum_{i=1}^{3} w_i X_i = (0.10)(60)$$
$$+ (0.30)(75) + (0.60)(93) = 84.3.$$

Example 3.3.2. A survey was conducted in four cities in California by the California Dental Association to determine what percent of dentists and physicians have a solo practice. It was found

Location	Solo Practice (%)
Los Angeles (X_1)	24
Sacramento (X_2)	53
San Diego (X_3)	47
San Francisco (X_4)	28

The arithmetic mean is

$$\overline{X} = \frac{24 + 53 + 47 + 28}{4} = 38.0.$$

Out of the four cities surveyed, 38% of the dentists and physicians on the average have a solo practice. But does the survey correctly represent the average percent of the solo practices in the four cities? There are many more dentists and physicians practicing in Los Angeles than in Sacramento. Therefore, the degree of importance to reflect the number of dentists and physicians in each city must be considered. Let's assume, for the sake of argument, that of 2,526 dentists and physicians in Los Angeles, 606 have solo practices, 184 of 348 in Sacramento, 228 of 486 in San Diego, and 522 of 1,866 in San Francisco have solo practices. The total number of dentists and physicians in these cities is $2,526 + 348 + 486 + 1,866 = 5,226$. The proportion of dentists and physicians

in each city is

$$\text{Los Angeles: } w_1 = \frac{2526}{5226} \simeq 0.48$$
$$\text{Sacramento: } w_2 = \frac{348}{5226} \simeq 0.07$$
$$\text{San Diego: } w_3 = \frac{486}{5226} \simeq 0.09$$
$$\text{San Francisco: } w_4 = \frac{1866}{5226} \simeq 0.36.$$

These proportions will define the weights to be assigned to the four cities. We can now calculate the weighted mean

$$\overline{X}_w = \sum_{i=1}^{4} w_i X_i = (0.48)(24) + (0.07)(53)$$
$$+ (0.09)(47) + (0.36)(28) = 29.54.$$

The weighted mean of the percent of solo practices in the four cities is 29.54%. To ensure the accuracy of the weight calculations, it is a good practice to check if the sum of the weights is indeed $0.48 + 0.07 + 0.09 + 0.36 = 1.00$.

The arithmetic mean we discussed in Section 3.2 can be expressed

$$\overline{X} = \frac{1}{n} \sum_{i=1}^{n} X_i = \frac{1}{n}(X_1 + X_2 + \cdots + X_n)$$
$$= \frac{1}{n} X_1 + \frac{1}{n} X_2 + \cdots + \frac{1}{n} X_n.$$

From the above expression, it is easy to notice that the arithmetic mean is a special case of a weighted mean, where the weights are all equal to $\frac{1}{n}$. In other words, $w_1 = w_2 = \cdots = w_n = \frac{1}{n}$. A physical interpretation of the weighted mean can be made similar to the one we did for the mean discussed in Section 3.2. The only difference is that, instead of tying the equal weights, different weights $w_1, w_2, \ldots, w_n$ are tied to each of the corresponding markers on the stick. The weighted mean for a data set is the point where the stick is balanced.

3.4 MEDIAN

To avoid the possibility of being misled by a few extremely small or extremely large observations, we alternatively describe the center of a data set with a statistical measure other than the arithmetic mean. An alternative measure of central location, which is almost as popular as the arithmetic mean, is the **median** or the **sample median**. Suppose there are n observations in a set of data. To find the median, all n observations must be arranged in ascending order. Then the median is defined as follows.

Definition 3.4.1. Let $X_1, X_2, \cdots, X_n$ be a sample of n observations arranged in ascending order. The sample **median** is the middle observation if n is odd. If n is even, the sample median is the average of the two middle observations.

Another way to describe the median is: if n is odd, the $\left(\dfrac{n+1}{2}\right)^{\text{th}}$ largest observation is the median. If n is even, the average of $\left(\dfrac{n}{2}\right)^{\text{th}}$ and $\left(\dfrac{n}{2}+1\right)^{\text{th}}$ largest observations is the median. For a sample with an odd number of observations, there is always a unique central value. If a data set has five measurements, the third largest is the central value in the sense that two measurements are smaller and two measurements are larger. For a sample with an even number of observations, there is no unique central value. If a data set has four measurements, the two middle observations (the second and the third largest) must be averaged.

Example 3.4.1. A retrospective study was done by an orthodontist to quantify changes resulting from quad helix expansion therapy (used primarily to expand the maxillary dental arch) using the patient records following completion of active orthodontic treatment. Dr. Bee selected seven dolichofacial patients and measured their maxillary intermolar distance in millimeters. His observations were: 47.4, 42.2, 49.0, 47.6, 48.5, 45.8, 41.4.

To find the median of the data, we must first arrange the observations in ascending order: 41.4, 42.2, 45.8, 47.4, 47.6, 48.5, 49.0. Because there is an odd number ($n = 7$) of observations in the sample, the sample median is $\left(\dfrac{n+1}{2}\right)^{\text{th}} = \left(\dfrac{7+1}{2}\right)^{\text{th}} = 4^{\text{th}}$ largest one. Therefore, 47.4 is the median. We can arrange the

data in descending order. The same argument will be applied to determine the median.

Example 3.4.2. As baby boomers age, a healthy, attractive smile becomes important to their appearance. Nothing conveys good health like aesthetically pleasing teeth. It has been reported that tooth whitening has grown significantly in popularity and continues to have a major impact on the practice of dentistry [2]. Six baby boomers were asked how much they would be willing to spend on teeth whitening done by dentists. Their responses in dollars ($) are arranged in ascending order: 200, 250, 300, 350, 375, 425. Since there is an even number ($n = 6$) of observations, the median is the average of the two middle values. The third and fourth largest values are the two middle values. Then the median is given by $\dfrac{300 + 350}{2} = 325$. The three smallest of the six observations are less than the median 325, and the three largest are greater than the median 325.

In general, we say that $\overline{X}_M$ is the median of a data set if one half of the observations in the data are less than or equal to $\overline{X}_M$, and one half of the observations in the data are greater than or equal to $\overline{X}_M$.

Suppose in Example 3.4.2, the patient's response was 650, instead of 425. How would this affect the median? Replacing 425 by 650, the observations are arranged in ascending order: 200, 250, 300, 350, 375, 650. We see that the median still is the average of the two middle values, $(300 + 350)/2 = 325$. Similarly, if we had 50 in place of 200 in the sample, it would not change the median at all. The median remains the same. What would happen to the mean? This is left to the readers to think about. What we have observed here is that, unlike the arithmetic mean, the median is insensitive to very large or very small values but sensitive only to the number of observations in the sample. Hence, if we are studying an income variable or housing price where some extremely large values pull the mean away from the center of the data, the median has an advantage as a measure of central location because it stays in the middle of the data, unaffected by extremely large values. Income and housing data are generally known as right-skewed. The discussion on skewness is presented in Section 3.16. The median can be used not only with quantitative data, but also with qualitative ordinal data that can be ranked, for example, the amount of calculus on teeth (none, slight, moderate, heavy). The median can be used to describe the "middle" that is the most common among the measurements.

3.5 MODE

Another measure used to describe the center of a data set is the **mode**, the observation that occurs most frequently and occurs more than once. An advantage of the mode is that no calculation is involved. It can be determined simply by counting the frequencies. The mode is the only measure of central tendency that can be used for qualitative variables, such as facial type, anesthetic injection (inferior alveolar, infiltration, posterior superior alveolar, mandibular block), ethnic background of patients, and blood type. Even for quantitative variables that are inherently discrete, such as family size, the number of visits to dental office, and the number of pregnancies, the mode is sometimes a more meaningful measure of central tendency than the mean or the median. It makes more sense to say that the most typical American family size is 4, or typical American women have 2 pregnancies in their lifetime, rather than that the average American family size is 3.8 or that American women have 1.9 pregnancies on the average. A disadvantage is that a data set may have several modes or no mode at all if no values occur more than once.

Example 3.5.1. A group of patients was being screened for a clinical trial to determine if a heightened intake of confectionery sugars over a short period of time caused an increased level of *Streptococcus mutans* bacteria on the overall dentition. Gingival index (GI) of the patients was one of the variables the dental scientists observed.

Subject No.	GI	Subject No.	GI	Subject No.	GI
1	2	7	0	13	0
2	1	8	0	14	2
3	0	9	2	15	1
4	1	10	1	16	1
5	3	11	1	17	3
6	1	12	2	18	1

From the above gingival index data the following frequency table can be constructed. It is easy to see that the mode is 1.

Gingival Index	Frequency
0	4
1	8
2	4
3	2

Example 3.5.2. Dental fear has been shown to be one of the leading factors in avoiding dental treatment. Many dentalphobic patients would rather risk severe oral pain and discomfort than seek dental care. Fear may cause various negative physiological responses such as faster heart rate, increased respiratory rate, perspiration, tense muscles, and nausea. Even moderate levels of anxiety may produce significant iatrogenic consequences in medically compromised patients [3]. To assess the effect of dental fear, patients' pulse rate was taken while they were sitting in the dental chair. Their pulse rates were 92, 88, 90, 94, 92, 86, 95, 94, 93, 92, 82, 90, 96, 94, 92, 89, 94. There are 4 patients with a pulse rate of 92, and another 4 with 94. Both 92 and 94 are the most frequently occurring values. Therefore, there are two modes, one at 92 and the other at 94.

Example 3.5.3. It is well-known that tricyclic antidepressants and antihypertensives may influence salivary flow. Decreased salivary flow diminishes the natural cleansing of the oral cavity, thus increasing the incidence of periodontal disease and caries. To explore what effects ascorbic acid levels in saliva might have on periodontal disease and caries, a periodontist took 30 salivary samples from his patients and measured their ascorbic acid levels, which are shown in Table 3.5.1.

A simple calculation shows that the mean ascorbic acid level is $\overline{X} = 0.216$. Two middle values are the 15th and 16th largest ones, both of which are 0.22. Thus, the median is $\overline{X}_M = 0.22$. Ascorbic acid level of 0.10 is observed most frequently in the table. So the mode of the data set is 0.10: mean $= 0.216$, median $= 0.22$, and mode $= 0.10$. Both the mean and median are located in the "middle" of the data, but the mode of 0.10 is located far to the left of the middle. In the case of the ascorbic acid data in Table 3.5.1, the mean and the median are much better measures of location than the mode.

Table 3.5.1. Ascorbic acid level (mg%) in 30 salivary samples.

0.11	0.14	0.21	0.25	0.10	0.26	0.36	0.22	0.17	0.13
0.33	0.13	0.10	0.21	0.23	0.31	0.19	0.33	0.22	0.28
0.24	0.28	0.37	0.10	0.15	0.31	0.29	0.12	0.08	0.26

In fact, the mode, in this example, will be misleading as a measure of central location. A data set that has one mode is called **unimodal**. Sometimes data sets can have more than one mode, as in Example 3.5.2, where there are two modes. A data set that has two modes is called **bimodal**. In the real world it is much more common for data to have one mode than to have two or more modes.

3.6 GEOMETRIC MEAN

The change in growth of bacterial colonies over time is proportional to the number of colonies that were present at a previous time. Roughly speaking, the rate of growth is multiplicative, not additive. For example, on the first day, the count of the bacterial colonies is 100, on the second day it is 10, 000, on the third day it is 1, 000, 000, and so on. Propagation of a certain infectious disease in a population is another such example. During a flu epidemic, 80 cases were reported to the county public health department in the first week, 160 cases in the second week, 320 cases in the third week, and 640 cases in the fourth week. The arithmetic mean would not be appropriate as a measure of central tendency in these situations because of the effects of extremely large values. Some people may consider the median, but another measure that is appropriately used is the **geometric mean**.

Definition 3.6.1. The sample geometric mean of n non-negative observations, $X_1, X_2, \cdots, X_n$, in a sample is defined by the nth root of the product:

$$\overline{X}_G = \sqrt[n]{X_1 \cdot X_2 \cdots X_n} = (X_1 \cdot X_2 \cdots X_n)^{\frac{1}{n}}.$$

Because the nth root is involved in the calculation, all of the measurements must be non-negative. If there are any negative measurements in a data set, the geometric mean cannot be used.

Example 3.6.1. (a) The geometric mean of two values 4 and 16 is $\sqrt{(4)(16)} = 8.0$.

(b) The geometric mean of three measurements 2, 8, and 256 is $\sqrt[3]{(2)(8)(256)} = 16.0$.

Example 3.6.2. The American Dental Association has been concerned about the passage of oral microbes into dental water lines. It mandates that bacterial count in the dental unit water lines be reduced to 200 colony-forming units per milliliter (cfu/ml). The current standard considers water to be safe for human consumption when it contains a maximum of 500 cfu/ml. A test was conducted to determine the efficacy of microfilters using tap water in reducing the bacterial counts in dental unit water lines. The water samples were taken at 24-, 48-, and 72-hour intervals, and the samples were then inoculated on agar plates and incubated at 37°C for 48 hours. The count of bacterial colonies at 24 hours was 2, at 48 hours was 34, and at 72 hours was 226. The most appropriate measure of central location of this type of data is the geometric mean. The geometric mean of the bacterial counts at the three time points is

$$\overline{X}_G = \sqrt[3]{(2)(34)(226)} = 24.862.$$

The geometric mean is used primarily in averaging ratios, growth rates, percents, concentrations of one chemical substance to another, and economic indices. Readers, who are interested in further exploring the geometric mean, are referred to Forthofer and Lee [4].

3.7 HARMONIC MEAN

Suppose your dentist's office is 10 miles away from your home. On the way to his office the traffic was light and you were able to drive 60 miles per hour. However, on the return trip the traffic was heavy and you drove 30 miles per hour. What was the average speed of your round trip? Was it 45 mph $\left(\dfrac{60 + 30}{2} = 45.0 \right)$? Most of us have seen this kind of problem in algebra textbooks. Because you have traveled the total of 20 miles in 30 minutes, the correct average speed is 40 mph. This average is known as the **harmonic mean**.

Definition 3.7.1. The harmonic mean of n observations, $X_1, X_2, \cdots, X_n$, is given by the reciprocal of the arithmetic mean of the reciprocals of the n observations. That is,

$$\overline{X}_H = \frac{1}{\frac{1}{n}\left(\sum_{i=1}^{n}\frac{1}{X_i}\right)}$$

Example 3.7.1. In the above discussion, the two measurements are $X_1 = 60$ mph, and $X_2 = 30$ mph. The harmonic mean of these two values is

$$\overline{X}_H = \frac{1}{\frac{1}{2}\left(\frac{1}{60}+\frac{1}{30}\right)} = \frac{2}{\left(\frac{1}{60}+\frac{1}{30}\right)}$$
$$= \frac{2}{\left(\frac{1}{60}+\frac{2}{60}\right)} = \frac{120}{3} = 40.$$

Example 3.7.2. An experiment was performed in a biomaterials laboratory with three types of composite materials. For the experiment $480 worth of composite A was purchased at $30 per package, $480 worth of composite B at $40 per package, and $480 worth of composite C at $32 per package. The average cost per package is given by the harmonic mean:

$$\overline{X}_H = \frac{1}{\frac{1}{3}\left(\frac{1}{30}+\frac{1}{40}+\frac{1}{32}\right)} = 33.488.$$

The average cost per package is about $33.50.

In addition to what we have discussed, there are other measures of central location. For example, the **midrange** is sometimes used. The midrange is simply the average of the smallest and the largest observations. Think of it as the midpoint between two values; one is the minimum and the other is the maximum. It is simple to calculate but very sensitive to the minimum and maximum values in a sample. The midrange is given by

$$\text{Midrange} = \frac{X_{\text{Minimum}} + X_{\text{Maximum}}}{2}.$$

Example 3.7.3. Irreversible pulpitis is characterized by pain that is spontaneous and lingers for some time after the removal of stimulus. Dr. Bonds treated nine patients with irreversible pulpitis, and measured the amount of time in seconds that pain lingered after the stimulus removal. Here are her data: 35, 45, 20, 65, 5, 25, 30, 35, 15. The minimum is 5 and the maximum is 65. The midrange of the data is $\dfrac{5+65}{2} = 35.0$.

3.8 MEAN AND MEDIAN OF GROUPED DATA

We have seen in the previous chapter that a grouped data set loses some information. The exact value of each observation in the grouped data is lost; we only know how many measurements there are in each class. Dental and medical researchers sometimes report their experimental observations as grouped data in the form of a frequency distribution [5, 6, and 7]. Even if the values of individual measurements are not available, we still might be interested in obtaining a numerical summary of the data. To determine the mean, we can get a good approximation by assigning a midpoint of the class interval to all those observations that fall into the same class. For example, the anesthetic activity of articaine with epinephrine has been demonstrated to be comparable to that of other anesthetic combinations, including lidocaine with epinephrine [8]. Malamed et al. [8] present the results of a clinical investigation consisting of three studies designed to compare the safety and efficacy of 4% articaine with epinephrine (Treatment A, 1:100, 000) with that of 2% lidocaine with epinephrine (Treatment B, 1:100, 000). Their patient demographics is presented in Table 3.8.1.

For the subjects treated with 2% lidocaine with epinephrine, 20 patients are in the age group 4–12, 396 are in 13–64 age group, 23 in 65–74 age group, and 4 in 75–80 age group. To

Table 3.8.1. Patient demographics.

Age	No. of Treated Subjects with A 1:100,000	No. of Treated Subjects with B 1:100,000
4–12	50	20
13–64	778	396
65–74	43	23
75–80	11	4

determine the mean age of the patients from the grouped data, the midpoint of the class interval must be calculated by adding the class limits and dividing it by 2. The midpoint of the first age group 4–12 is $(4 + 12)/2 = 8.0$. The midpoints of the second, third, and fourth age groups are $(13 + 64)/2 = 38.5$, $(65 + 74)/2 = 69.5$, and $(75 + 80)/2 = 77.5$. It is assumed that all 20 patients in the first group are equal to 8.0, all 396 in the second group are equal to 38.5, all 23 in the third group are equal to 69.5, and all 4 in the fourth group are equal to 77.5 years old. A total of $20 + 396 + 23 + 4 = 443$ patients are assigned to this particular treatment. Thus the mean age is given by

$$\overline{X} = \frac{(20)(8.0) + (396)(38.5) + (23)(69.5) + (4)(77.5)}{443}$$
$$= 39.085.$$

The above calculation shows the average age of the 443 patients is about 39.1 years. This procedure is usually quite satisfactory because the errors being introduced in the calculation will tend to "average out." A general formula will be presented to calculate the mean of a grouped data.

Definition 3.8.1. Suppose there are k class intervals. Let $X_1, X_2, \cdots, X_k$ be the midpoint of the intervals, and $f_1, f_2, \cdots, f_k$ be the corresponding frequencies. Then the total number of observations is the sum of the frequencies, $\sum_{i=1}^{k} f_i = N$, and the mean is given by the expression

$$\overline{X} = \frac{(f_1)(X_1) + (f_2)(X_2) + \cdots + (f_k)(X_k)}{\sum_{i=1}^{k} f_i}$$
$$= \frac{\sum_{i=1}^{k} f_i X_i}{\sum_{i=1}^{k} f_i}$$

In the example we discussed above, the midpoints of the intervals are $X_1 = 8.0$, $X_2 = 38.5$, $X_3 = 69.5$, and $X_4 = 77.5$, and their corresponding frequencies are $f_1 = 20$, $f_2 = 396$, $f_3 = 23$, and $f_4 = 4$. The total number of observations is the sum of the frequencies,

$$\sum_{i=1}^{4} f_i = 20 + 396 + 23 + 4 = 443.$$

Example 3.8.1. Two of the most important clinical parameters for the prognosis of a periodontically involved tooth are attachment loss and mo-

Table 3.8.2. Attachment loss of 51 patients.

Attachment loss (mm)	No. of subjects
$0 \leq X < 2$	14
$2 \leq X < 4$	16
$4 \leq X < 6$	12
$6 \leq X < 8$	7
$8 \leq X < 10$	2

bility. A pool of patient subjects was screened for a clinical trial to evaluate the effects on natural extrinsic dental stain from the use of a dentifrice containing 0.5% calcium peroxide, 1500 ppm sodium monofluorophosphate in a precipitated calcium carbonate base. The amount of attachment loss was one of the inclusion-exclusion criteria. Table 3.8.2 presents the attachment loss of 51 patients examined by the dental researchers for the study. Let X denote the random variable representing the amount of attachment loss in millimeters. The class defined by $2 \leq X < 4$ includes the patient subjects whose attachment loss is greater than or equal to 2 mm but less than 4 mm.

The midpoints of the class intervals are $X_1 = 1.0$, $X_2 = 3.0$, $X_3 = 5.0$, $X_4 = 7.0$, and $X_5 = 9.0$. The corresponding frequencies are $f_1 = 14$, $f_2 = 16$, $f_3 = 12$, $f_4 = 7$, and $f_5 = 2$. So the mean of the grouped data is obtained by

$$\overline{X} = \frac{\sum_{i=1}^{k} f_i X_i}{\sum_{i=1}^{k} f_i}$$
$$= \frac{(14)(1.0) + (16)(3.0) + (12)(5.0) + (7)(7.0) + (2)(9.0)}{51}$$
$$= 3.7059.$$

The mean attachment loss of these 51 patients is approximately 3.7 mm.

A natural question in our minds at this time is how can we find the **median from a grouped data set**. The median of a set of grouped data is found essentially in the same manner as the grouped mean. Recall that the median of a distribution is the midpoint such that half of the data lies below and the other half lies above. If we knew the values of attachment loss of the 51 patients in Table 3.8.2, the 26th largest observation will be the median. There are 14 observations in the first class and 16 observations in the second class; therefore, the 26th largest observation falls in the second class.

To determine the median, we must first count $26 - 14 = 12$ more observations beyond the 14 that fall in the previous class. Assuming that 16 observations in the class are evenly spaced, we add 12/16 of the width of the class interval to the left-hand limit of the second class. That is, $2 + (12/16) \cdot 2 = 3.5$. Thus, 3.5 mm is the median of the grouped data in the Table 3.8.2. We will now summarize this in the following definition.

Definition 3.8.2. Let L be the left-hand limit of the class into which the median falls, d be the width of the class interval, f be the frequency of the class, and k be the number of observations we need in the class to reach the median. Then the general formula is

$$\overline{X}_M = L + \frac{k}{f} d.$$

Example 3.8.2. Let us find the median age of the grouped data in Table 3.8.1 for the patients treated with 2% lidocaine with epinephrine. There are 443 patients. The midpoint, the 222nd largest observation, falls in the second class, which contains 396 patients. The left-hand limit of the second class is $L = 13$, $d = 64 - 13 = 51$, $f = 396$, and $k = 222 - 20 = 202$. Using the formula we can easily obtain the median:

$$\overline{X}_M = L + \frac{k}{f} d = 13 + \frac{202}{396}(51) = 39.015.$$

The median age of the patients in the grouped data is about 39.0.

3.9 MEAN OF TWO OR MORE MEANS

Sometimes researchers report a data set that is a collection of averages of two or more observations. To present the results of the experiment they may want to produce descriptive statistics, including the mean. Suppose we have three sections of Statistics 101. The average score of the final examination is $\overline{X}_A = 71$ for section A, $\overline{X}_B = 85$ for section B, and $\overline{X}_C = 78$ for section C. Is the mean

of the three sections

$$\overline{X} = \frac{\overline{X}_A + \overline{X}_B + \overline{X}_C}{3} = \frac{71 + 85 + 78}{3} = 78.0?$$

If the class size of the three sections is the same, then $\overline{X} = 78.0$ is the correct mean. But if section A has 48 students, section B has 24 students, and section C has 29 students, we must weigh the three means according to their class size. Section A with 48 students should be given twice the weight that is given to Section B with only 24 students. That is,

$$\overline{X}_W = \frac{(48)\overline{X}_A + (24)\overline{X}_B + (29)\overline{X}_C}{48 + 24 + 29}$$

$$= \frac{(48)71 + (24)85 + (29)78}{101} = 76.337.$$

Definition 3.9.1. Let $n_1, n_2, \cdots, n_k$ be the sample sizes of k samples, and $\overline{X}_1, \overline{X}_2, \cdots, \overline{X}_k$ be the respective means of the k samples. Then the mean of the k means is given by the following weighted mean:

$$\overline{X}_W = \frac{n_1 \overline{X}_1 + n_2 \overline{X}_2 + \cdots + n_k \overline{X}_k}{n_1 + n_2 + \cdots + n_k}.$$

Example 3.9.1. Post and core buildups represent an important preprosthetic procedure prior to the restoration of an endodontically treated tooth. The dental practitioners are faced with the dilemma of selecting from an ever-increasing variety of materials, techniques, and designs related to the procedure. To provide guidelines, a dental scientist selected five different types of direct post-core systems cemented into extracted human cuspid teeth, and their peak load (kilograms) was measured using an Instron universal testing machine. The mean peak load of these five types of direct post-core systems and their sample sizes are [9] $\overline{X}_1 = 101.99$, $\overline{X}_2 = 94.78$, $\overline{X}_3 = 99.09$, $\overline{X}_4 = 128.76$, $\overline{X}_5 = 76.47$, and $n_1 = 7, n_2 = 6, n_3 = 6, n_4 = 7, n_5 = 14$. Then the mean peak load of these five means is

$$\overline{X}_W = \frac{n_1 \overline{X}_1 + n_2 \overline{X}_2 + \cdots + n_k \overline{X}_k}{n_1 + n_2 + \cdots + n_k}$$

$$= \frac{(7)(101.99) + (6)(94.78) + (6)(99.09) + (7)(128.76) + (14)(76.47)}{7 + 6 + 6 + 7 + 14} = 96.226.$$

The weighted mean, thus obtained, is the same as the grand mean of all 40 observations pooled together.

In the following we summarize important properties of four widely used measures of location.

Mean:

- Most widely used and dependent on the value of every observation
- Balance point of a distribution
- Not appropriate for qualitative data
- Sensitive to extreme values
- Inappropriate for highly skewed data

Weighted Mean:

- Reflects relative importance of observations
- Useful to find the grand mean of k means

Median:

- Insensitive to extreme values
- Sensitive to the sample size
- Widely used for highly skewed distributions
- Appropriate for ordinal variables

Mode:

- Most typical value in the data
- Only measure appropriate for nominal data
- More appropriate than mean or median for quantitative variables that are inherently discrete

In this chapter we have discussed measures of central tendency. However, no two patients respond precisely the same way to a given treatment, and no two dentists or physicians treat their patients exactly the same way. This is due to variation. Variation in all aspects of health sciences is inevitable. Let us consider an example. The initial development of gingivitis is directly dependent on the accumulation of the supragingival plaque. To evaluate the plaque control that eludes many patients, investigators randomly selected 7 dental students and 7 medical students. From each of the 14 subjects, using a cotton pellet a plaque sample was taken from the smooth surface of their right maxillary molar area. After 24 hours of incubation, the samples were observed for bacterial colony growth, represented by the amount of colony-forming units (cfu) as follows:

Medical students:
   30, 150, 250, 280, 310, 410, 530

Dental students:
   230, 260, 265, 280, 295, 300, 330

The mean for each of the above two data sets is 280. The CFU measurements for the 7 medical students vary much more than those for the dental students, but the means for the two groups are the same. It would be totally inappropriate for anyone to conclude that the plaque condition of these two groups are about the same because the means are the same. This illustrates the fact that the mean alone is not enough to accurately describe the data. The measures of central tendency we discussed so far represent points on which a distribution tends to center or concentrate. The measures of central location convey important information about data, but they do not tell us anything about the variability or dispersion of observations. Many measures of variability have been proposed to represent the spread of observations around some central location. We will discuss most useful measures of variability in health sciences: range, percentiles, interquartile range, variance, standard deviation, and coefficient of variation.

3.10 RANGE

The simplest measure of variability is the **range** (or **sample range**), which is the distance between the largest and smallest observations. Let the range be denoted by R, and $X_1, X_2, \cdots, X_n$ be n observations. Then the range is given by

$$R = X_{\max} - X_{\min}.$$

From the data in Section 3.9, the range of the medical students is $R = 530 - 30 = 500$, and the range of the dental students is $R = 330 - 230 = 100$. The range is easy to calculate, but it depends on only two extremes, the smallest and the largest, ignoring all of the intermediary values. That is, the range does not reflect the dispersion of the values between the two extreme observations. This is the main shortcoming of the range. All three cases below have the same range since they have the common extreme observations, regardless of the values between them.

Case 1: 30, 150, 250, 280, 310, 410, 530
Case 2: 30, 30, 30, 30, 30, 30, 530
Case 3: 30, 530, 530, 530, 530, 530, 530

Range has the following disadvantages:

1. The sampling stability (variability from one sample to the next) of the range is very poor.
2. It depends on the sample size. The more samples we have, the more likely we are to observe greater extreme values. Therefore, the larger range will likely be observed as we increase the sample size.
3. It is very sensitive to the two extreme values and ignores the rest of the observations.
4. It is not meaningful for unordered qualitative data.

3.11 PERCENTILES AND INTERQUARTILE RANGE

A measure of variability that is better than the range would use more information from data by including more than the two extreme observations and would not depend on the sample size. Percentiles and quartiles are intended to divide data into 100 parts and 4 parts, respectively.

Definition 3.11.1. The **percentile point**, or simply **percentile**, is a point below which a specified percent of observations lie. The percentile is denoted by $p_\%$; the 95th percentile is denoted by p_{95}. Some prefer to write a fraction in the subscript as $p_{0.95}$.

The percentiles are not the same as percents. If a dental student has scored 82 of a possible 100 on the National Board Examination Part II, then he has obtained a percentage score of 82. But it does not indicate the position of his score relative to the scores obtained by the dental students who took the same board exam. His score could be the highest, lowest or somewhere in between. On the other hand, if his score of 82 corresponds to 90th

percentile, he has performed better than 90% of all the dental students who took the exam at the same time he did.

Example 3.11.1. Composite resins are widely used for esthetic restorations in anterior teeth. An ideal composite restoration possesses such properties as color matched with existing dentition, wear resistant, unabrasive to natural teeth, easy to repair, and color stable. The success of composite resin restorations depends primarily on color stability over time. To test the color stability of a composite currently used widely in dentistry, the total of 56 specimens of the composite resin was prepared in uniform dimension. These specimens were then exposed to a staining medium for a duration of 24 hours at 39°C. Coffee was used as the staining medium. The L value of each specimen was measured by a Minolta chromameter for color change after 24-hour immersion. The L value quantifies metric lightness on the scale of 0 to 100. The higher the L value, the lighter the color of the specimen. Table 3.11.1 displays the L value data for color stability of the composite resin.

Using the data in Table 3.11.1, we construct a percentile graph as shown in Figure 3.11.1. Percentile graphs are the same as the graphs constructed based on the cumulative relative frequency discussed in Section 2.3.

From the percentile graph, we can find the approximate percentile ranks corresponding to given L values and vice versa. For example, to find the percentile rank of an L value of 61.85, find 61.85 on the X-axis and draw a vertical line to the graph. Then draw a horizontal line to the Y-axis. Note that the horizontal line intersects the Y-axis at 80. The L value of 61.85 corresponds to approximately the 80th percentile. To find an L value corresponding to the 40th percentile, first draw a horizontal line to the graph and then a vertical line to the X-axis. The vertical line intersects the X-axis at about 59.80.

Table 3.11.1. L value data for color stability of a composite resin [10].

54.59	58.70	62.58	61.24	59.43	55.85	54.81	59.82
61.25	61.15	59.96	56.22	59.72	61.59	60.77	60.38
53.52	61.34	61.48	61.91	60.47	55.36	54.47	53.59
62.29	62.63	60.50	55.08	51.84	61.77	63.40	59.64
54.40	55.71	62.47	63.23	55.97	55.21	53.47	61.49
63.34	62.50	59.35	60.76	56.06	59.87	62.47	58.64
59.64	60.05	58.10	62.81	61.34	58.63	59.88	61.63

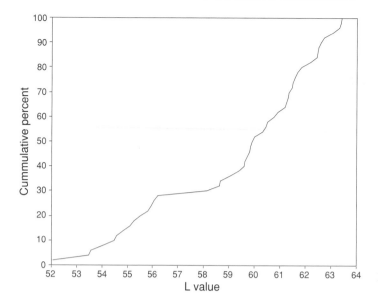

Figure 3.11.1 Percentile graph for stainability of composite resin data.

Thus, the 40th percentile corresponds to an L value of approximately 59.80.

The percentile graph is a convenient tool to find values and their corresponding percentiles. The use of these graphs yields only approximation, however. There is a mathematical method to compute percentiles for data. The percentile corresponding to a given observation, X, is given by the formula

Percentile
$= \dfrac{(\text{Number of observations less than } X) + 0.5}{\text{Total number of observations in data}}$
$\times 100\%.$

Example 3.11.2. There are 14 dentists and physicians in a clinic. The number of hours they spent in patient contact during the first week in June are 42, 30, 25, 28, 8, 40, 32, 28, 36, 44, 15, 40, 41, 38. To find the percentile rank of 36 hours, first arrange the data in ascending order: 8, 15, 25, 28, 28, 30, 32, 36, 38, 40, 40, 41, 42, 44. Because there are 7 observations below the data value of 36, substitution in the formula yields,

$$\text{Percentile} = \frac{7 + 0.5}{14} \times 100\% \simeq 53.57.$$

The value of 36 hours corresponds to approximately the 54th percentile. Conversely, to find the observed value corresponding to a given

percentile, we can use the formula

$$k = \frac{n \cdot p_\%}{100}, \quad \text{the } k \text{ indicates the } k^{\text{th}} \text{ largest observation.}$$

If k is not an integer, round it up to the next integer.

Example 3.11.3. Endodontic rotary files, which are made of nickel titanium, are being tested for their reliability. For this study 12 rotary files and 12 endodontists were selected at random, and each file was used by an endodontist. The endodontists were asked to record the number of uses of the files before they became unusable due to breakage or deformity. The data is given by 6, 3, 12, 23, 2, 6, 18, 11, 9, 5, 9, 8.

(i) To find the value corresponding to the 75th percentile, rearrange the observations in ascending order: 2, 3, 5, 6, 6, 8, 9, 9, 11, 12, 18, 23. Then substitute in the above formula

$$k = \frac{12 \cdot 75}{100} = 9.$$

Since $k = 9$, the midpoint between the 9th and 10th largest observations, that is, the midpoint between 11 and 12, corresponds to the 75th percentile. In this case, 11.5 is the 75th percentile.

(ii) To find the value corresponding to the 40th percentile, compute $k = \dfrac{12 \cdot 40}{100} = 4.8$. Since $k = 4.8$ is not an integer, round it up to the next whole number. Then $k = 5$. The midpoint between the

5th and 6th largest observations is $\dfrac{6+8}{2} = 7$, and the value 7 corresponds to the 40th percentile.

Percentiles are intended to divide data into 100 parts. The remainder of this section is devoted to quartiles, which divide data into approximately four equal parts. The range as a measure of variability has a major deficiency because it is sensitive to two extreme values (which two values?). It is desirable to have a measure of dispersion that is not easily influenced by a few extreme values. **Interquartile range** is such a measure. The 25th, 50th, and 75th percentiles are known as 1st, 2nd, and 3rd quartiles, and denoted by Q_1, Q_2, and Q_3. Using the percentile notation, $Q_1 = p_{25}$, $Q_2 = p_{50}$, and $Q_3 = p_{75}$.

Definition 3.11.2. The **sample interquartile range** (IQR) is the distance between Q_1 and Q_3.

$$IQR = Q_3 - Q_1.$$

The interquartile range contains about 50% of the data. If the *IQR* is large, then the data tend to be widely dispersed. On the other hand, if the *IQR* is small, then the data tend to be concentrated around the center of the distribution. For the data in Example 3.11.2, the Q_1 can be computed as follows. First, $k = \dfrac{12 \cdot 25}{100} = 3$. So the Q_1 is the midpoint between the 3rd and 4th largest values; $\dfrac{5+6}{2} = 5.5$. The IQR is now given as $IQR = Q_3 - Q_1 = 11.5 - 5.5 = 6$. As an exploratory data analysis, one should scrutinize data for extremely small or extremely large observations.

Definition 3.11.3. Outlier observations (or simply, outliers) are extremely small and extremely large observations compared to the rest of the values in the data.

There are several statistical methods to check for outliers. One method that uses the *IQR* is described:

Step 1. Multiply the *IQR* by 1.5, $(1.5) \cdot IQR$.
Step 2. Subtract $(1.5)IQR$ from the Q_1, and add to the Q_3 to form an interval

$$[Q_1 - (1.5) \cdot IQR, \ Q_3 + (1.5) \cdot IQR].$$

Step 3. Any data points that fall outside this interval are considered outliers.

Example 3.11.4. In Example 3.11.3, $Q_1 = 5.5$, $Q_3 = 11.5$, and $IQR = 6$. The lower limit of the interval is $5.5 - (1.5) \cdot 6 = -3.5$, and the upper limit is $11.5 + (1.5) \cdot 6 = 20.5$. The largest observation 23 lies outside the interval, and hence, it can be considered an outlier. Note that the lower limit is -3.5, a negative value, even though the observed values for the number of uses cannot fall below zero. In a case such as this, the realistic lower limit is in fact zero.

Data often contain outliers. Outliers can occur due to a variety of reasons: an inaccurate instrument, mishandling of experimental units, measurement errors, or recording errors such as incorrectly typed values or misplacement of a decimal point. The observations may have been made about a subject who does not meet research criteria; for example, a research study on hypertension may have included a patient with low blood pressure, due to experimenters' oversight. An outlier can also be a legitimate observation that occurred purely by chance.

If we can explain how and why the outliers occurred, they should be deleted from the data. Suppose a periodontist is collecting data on the periodontal attachment level of patients with acute periodontitis. A value of 75 mm for the attachment level is clearly an error. Unless we can be certain that a decimal point is missing and the correct value is 7.5 mm, this particular outlier observation should be thrown out.

3.12 BOX-WHISKER PLOT

We have learned in Chapter 2 that graphs are very effective ways to summarize and present data. A type of graph that gives a visual representation of location, variability, and outliers is the box-whisker plot, or simply called the box plot. The box plot involves basically only a few values: the lowest value, the first quartile, median, the third quartile, and the largest value. Figure 3.12.1 displays the box plot for the endodontic file data in Example 3.11.3.

The bottom line of the box, in the middle of the graph, represents the first quartile (Q_1), and

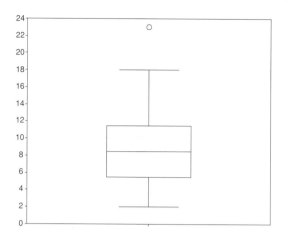

Figure 3.12.1 Box-whisker plot for endodontic file data.

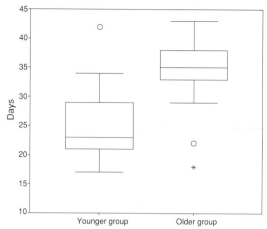

Figure 3.12.2 Box plot for two groups for time required to splint avulsed tooth.

the top line of the box represents the third quartile (Q_3). The horizontal line going through the middle of the box describes the median (Q_2). Therefore, the middle 50% of the data values lie within the box. The shorter the height of the box, the heavier the concentration of the middle 50% of the data around the median; the taller the height of the box, the greater the dispersion of the middle 50% of the data about the median. In fact, the height of the box is the interquartile range, $IQR = Q_3 - Q_1$. The two lines projecting out from the bottom and top sides of the box are called whiskers. The bottom whisker extends to the smallest value within $Q_1 - (1.5) \cdot IQR$, and the top whisker extends to the largest value within $Q_3 + (1.5) \cdot IQR$. The small circle (○) above the top whisker indicates the outlier. Notice that the bottom whisker is shorter than the top whisker. This means the three smallest observations (2, 3, and 5) in the first quartile are much less spread out than the two observations (12 and 18) that fall between Q_3 point and $Q_3 +$ (1.5) $\cdot IQR$.

Example 3.12.1. The table below shows the length of time required to splint an avulsed tooth with alveolar fracture for patients 18 years old or younger and for those older than 18 years.

The box plots are especially useful for comparing two or more sets of data. Figure 3.12.2 above displays the data in Table 3.12.1. The younger group has one outlier that falls above the limit, $Q_3 + (1.5) \cdot IQR$, and the older group has two outliers that fall below the limit, $Q_1 - (1.5) \cdot IQR$. One of the outliers in the box plot is indicated by a star (∗), which means it is an outlier observation that lies below $Q_1 - (3.0) \cdot IQR$. The outliers that lie above $Q_3 + (3.0) \cdot IQR$ are also indicated by ∗. These are referred to as extreme outliers. It is easy to see that the first quartile, median, and third quartile for the younger group are smaller than those for the older group. The IQR of the younger group is much larger than that of the older group. Further discussions on the box-whisker plots and their applications can be found in Tukey [11].

Table 3.12.1. The length of time required to splint an avulsed tooth.

Subject No.	Age ≤ 18	Age > 18	Subject No.	Age ≤ 18	Age > 18	Subject No.	Age ≤ 18	Age > 18
1	24	35	8	29	35	15	21	36
2	17	29	9	21	37	16	20	43
3	33	38	10	20	35	17	22	18
4	30	35	11	23	34	18	32	30
5	22	33	12	21	38	19	24	
6	28	37	13	23	42	20	42	
7	19	39	14	34	22	21	26	

3.13 VARIANCE AND STANDARD DEVIATION

The variability in the sample is measured to understand the level of dispersion that exists in the population. The most popular and frequently used measures of variability are the **variance** and the **standard deviation** (SD). Unlike the range and the interquartile range, these two measures of dispersion use all of the observations in a data set. The measures of central location—mean, median, and mode—do not reflect the variability of data at all. Intuitively, we want a statistic that is small when the observations are closely bunched around the mean and large when they are spread out.

In the Figure 3.13.1, the data values in (b) are more dispersed than those in (a). We therefore might attempt to calculate the sum of the deviations of individual observations from the mean $\overline{X}$, $\sum_{i=1}^{n}(X_i - \overline{X})$ in order to quantify the variability. The problem with this measure is that, regardless of the observed values, whether they are closely clustered around $\overline{X}$ or not, it can be shown mathematically that the sum of the deviations is always equal to zero:

$$\sum_{i=1}^{n}(X_i - \overline{X}) = 0.$$

From Figure 3.13.1, it should be clear that the observations less than $\overline{X}$ will yield negative deviations, and those larger than $\overline{X}$ will yield positive deviations. Their respective sums will cancel each other out, thereby resulting in the zero sum. The sum, $\sum_{i=1}^{n}(X_i - \overline{X})$, will always be zero for any data set. To avoid this, we might consider the distance between the individual observations and the mean, that is, to consider the absolute values, $|X_i - \overline{X}|$. Although nothing is wrong with a measure of variability based on the absolute

values, it does not possess any desirable statistical properties.

An alternative approach to consider is the square of the deviations from the mean that are non-negative. Hence, we will make use of the sum of the squared deviations, $\sum_{i=1}^{n}(X_i - \overline{X})^2$. Suppose we have two samples, each taken from the same population, one with $n = 8$, and the other with $n = 800$. The sample with $n = 800$ will naturally have a larger value of $\sum_{i=1}^{n}(X_i - \overline{X})^2$ than the sample with $n = 8$. To ensure that the sample size does not influence the measure of dispersion, a logical approach is to work with the arithmetic mean of the squared deviations,

$$\frac{\sum_{i=1}^{n}(X_i - \overline{X})^2}{n}.$$

This measure is quite intuitive. It possesses some desirable statistical properties, which are not discussed in this book, and it is preferred by many statisticians (see [12] and [13]). However, it tends to underestimate the population variance, σ^2. We will modify the above formula by dividing the sum by $(n - 1)$, instead of n. This modified version gives an unbiased estimate of the population variance and will be used throughout the book as the measure of variability.

Definition 3.13.1. Let n be the sample size and $X_1, X_2, \ldots, X_n$ be the n observations. The sample variance of the data, denoted by S^2, is defined by

$$S^2 = \frac{\sum_{i=1}^{n}(X_i - \overline{X})^2}{n - 1}, \quad (n \geq 2).$$

Example 3.13.1. A clinic director believes quality care begins from the moment the patient walks into his office. He has learned from the patient satisfaction survey that one of the areas where improvement should be made is the waiting time in the lobby. He asked his assistant to randomly select one patient a day and carefully observe the waiting time of the patient. The waiting time data for this week, Monday through Saturday, is 35, 23, 10, 40, 28, 21 (minutes). What is the variance of his patients' waiting time?

Solution. First, we need to compute the mean, $\overline{X}$
$$= \frac{35 + 23 + 10 + 40 + 28 + 21}{6} = \frac{157}{6} = 26.167.$$

(a)

(b)

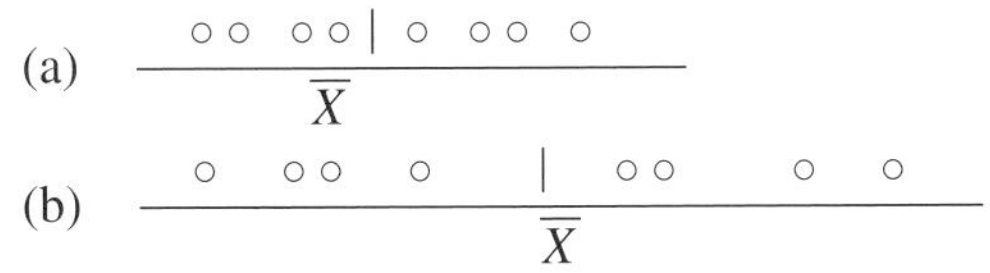

Figure 3.13.1 Comparison of dispersion for two cases.

The variance in waiting time is given by

$$S^2 = \frac{\sum_{i=1}^{n}(X_i - \overline{X})^2}{n-1}$$

$$= \frac{(35 - 26.2)^2 + (23 - 26.2)^2 + (10 - 26.2)^2 + (40 - 26.2)^2 + (28 - 26.2)^2 + (21 - 26.2)^2}{6 - 1}$$

$$= 114.17$$

This example involves only six observations, but a variance computation involving a large number of observations can be quite tedious. A shortcut formula that is equivalent to the one given in Example 3.13.1 is

$$S^2 = \frac{\sum_{i=1}^{n} X_i^2 - n(\overline{X})^2}{n-1}, \quad (n \geq 2).$$

In many practical situations the mean would contain a round-off error. If, for example, we have rounded off the mean to the nearest tenth, each term $(X_i - \overline{X})^2$ in the sample variance formula $S^2 = \sum_{i=1}^{n}(X_i - \overline{X})^2/(n-1)$ would have some rounding error. The shortcut formula would contain an error but not as great an error as the sample variance formula. An alternative formula circumvents this problem and also is more convenient to use:

$$S^2 = \frac{\sum_{i=1}^{n} X_i^2 - \frac{\left(\sum_{i=1}^{n} X_i\right)^2}{n}}{n-1}, \quad (n \geq 2).$$

We will now present some useful properties of the variance. You may wonder how addition and subtraction of a constant or the changes in the units affect the variance. Suppose $X_1, X_2, \ldots, X_n$ are n observations. Addition (or subtraction) of a constant c to each of the n observations will **shift** or **translate** all the observations by exactly c units to the right (or to the left), leaving the variability among the observations intact. See Figure 3.13.2.

Now let's think about the effect of multiplying each observation by the same constant c. If $c > 1$, then the multiplication will make the data values spread out more, and thus, the variance of the data will be larger. On the other hand, if $0 < c < 1$, the

multiplication will bring the observations closer together, and therefore the variance will be smaller. Let S_X^2 denote the sample variance of n observations, $X_1, X_2, \ldots, X_n$, and $S_{X \pm c}^2$ be the sample variance of $X_1 \pm c, X_2 \pm c, \ldots, X_n \pm c$. Let S_{cX}^2 be the sample variance of $cX_1, cX_2, \ldots, cX_n$, and $S_{aX \pm b}^2$ be the sample variance of $aX_1 \pm b, aX_2 \pm b, \cdots, aX_n \pm b$. Then the following relations hold:

1. $S_X^2 = S_{X \pm c}^2$ for any given constant c

2. $S_{cX}^2 = c^2 S_X^2$ for a constant $c > 0$

3. $S_{aX \pm b}^2 = a^2 S_X^2 \ (a > 0)$

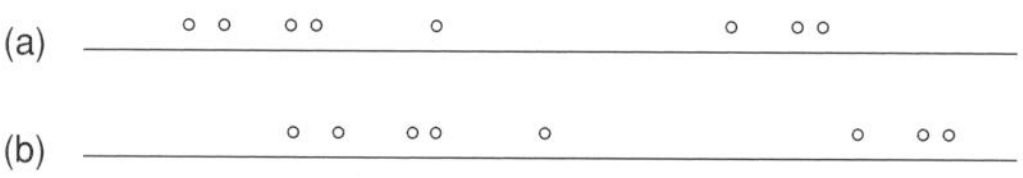

Example 3.13.2. A study was performed to evaluate the strength of a certain prefabricated post for post-and-core buildups in endodontically treated teeth. Seven canines of similar length were treated endodontically and prepared with standardized drill bits to receive the respective posts. A composite base resin was used for the buildup. The length of the teeth was approximately 18 mm, and 4 mm of gutta-percha was left in the apex. The posts were sandblasted and cemented with composite cement. The following fracture load data were collected after thermocycling the tooth samples and tested under load using an Instron machine at 45 degrees: 109.73, 44.83, 42.86, 57.43, 74.23, 95.88, 48.04 kg [14]. The mean and variance are:

$$\overline{X} = 67.57, \text{ and } S^2 = \frac{\sum_{i=1}^{n}(X_i - \overline{X})^2}{n-1} = 705.87.$$

(i) Suppose the Instron machine was not calibrated properly, and the correct measurement of the fracture load should be 1.5 kg higher. After revising the data by adding 1.5 kg to each of the seven observations, what would be the variance? By the above property 1, the variance of the original fracture data and the variance of the revised data

$$(109.73 + 1.5, 44.83 + 1.5, 42.86 + 1.5, 57.43$$
$$+ 1.5, 74.23 + 1.5, 95.88 + 1.5, 48.04 + 1.5)$$

(a) ───── o o o o   o   o   o o ─────

(b) ───── o o o o   o   o   o o ─────

Figure 3.13.2 Observations in (a) and (b) have the same variance.

should be the same. That is, $S_X^2 = S_{X \pm 1.5}^2 = 705.87$, where $c = 1.5$.

(ii) If the fracture data were converted to pounds by multiplying the measurements in kilograms by 2.2 (1.0 kg = 2.2 pounds), what would the variance of the converted data be? Using property 2, we see that the variance of the converted data is

$$S_{2.2 \cdot X}^2 = (2.2)^2 S_X^2 = (2.2)^2 \cdot (705.87)$$
$$= 3416.41 \quad (c = 2.2).$$

Sample variances are no longer in the same units of measurement as the original data. The observations on the fracture load were measured in kilograms, and thus the unit of the sample variance would be squared kilograms. To compensate for the fact that the deviations from the mean were squared, the positive square root of the sample variance is taken; this is known as the sample SD of a data set. Both the SD and the mean are expressed in the same unit of measurement as the original data. Primarily for this reason, the SD is the most widely used measure of variability.

Definition 3.13.2. The sample SD, denoted by S, is defined by

$$\sqrt{S^2} = S = \sqrt{\frac{\sum_{i=1}^{n} \left(X_i - \overline{X} \right)^2}{n-1}}.$$

To avoid rounding off errors, which was discussed previously, we may use the alternative formula to calculate the SD as given by

$$\sqrt{S^2} = S = \sqrt{\frac{\sum_{i=1}^{n} X_i^2 - \frac{\left(\sum_{i=1}^{n} X_i \right)^2}{n}}{n-1}}.$$

The SD of the fracture load data in Example 3.13.2 is $S = \sqrt{705.87} = 26.568$ (kg).

The corresponding properties for SD can be stated:

1. $S_X = S_{X \pm c}$ for any given constant c.
2. $S_{cX} = c \cdot S_X$ for a constant $c > 0$.
3. $S_{aX \pm b} = a \cdot S_X$ $(a > 0)$.

Like the variance, SD is not affected by the

translation of the observations by $c = 1.5$:

$$S_X = S_{X \pm 1.5} = \sqrt{705.87} = 26.568 \quad (c = 1.5).$$

If the observations change in scale by a factor of c, the variance changes by a factor of c^2, but the SD changes by a factor of $\sqrt{c^2} = c$.

$$S_{2.2 \cdot X} = (2.2) \cdot S_X = (2.2) \cdot (26.568)$$
$$= 58.450 \quad (c = 2.2).$$

Example 3.13.3. Five maxillary premolar teeth are in jar 1, and three maxillary premolar teeth are in jar 2. The width of each tooth in these jars is measured from distal surface to mesial surface. The three teeth in jar 2 have identical width, equal to the average width of the five teeth in jar 1. If the three teeth in jar 2 are combined with those in jar 1, would the standard deviation of the widths of the combined sample of eight teeth be larger than that of the original five teeth in jar 1?

Solution. Let $X_1, X_2, \cdots, X_5$ be the width of the five premolar teeth in jar 1, and let $\overline{X}$ be their mean. Let Y_1, Y_2, and Y_3 be the width of the three premolar teeth in jar 2. From the given description, we have $Y_1 = Y_2 = Y_3 = \overline{X}$. The mean width of the combined eight teeth is:

$$\frac{(X_1 + X_2 + \cdots + X_5 + Y_1 + Y_2 + Y_3)}{8}$$
$$= \frac{(X_1 + X_2 + \cdots + X_5 + \overline{X} + \overline{X} + \overline{X})}{8}$$
$$= \frac{(X_1 + X_2 + \cdots + X_5 + 3 \cdot \overline{X})}{8}$$
$$= \frac{X_1 + X_2 + \cdots + X_5 + 3 \cdot \left(\frac{X_1 + X_2 + \cdots + X_5}{5} \right)}{8}.$$

Multiplying both the numerator and the denominator of the above expression by 5, we get:

$$\frac{5(X_1 + X_2 + \cdots + X_5) + 3 \cdot (X_1 + X_2 + \cdots + X_5)}{5 \cdot 8}$$
$$= \frac{8(X_1 + X_2 + \cdots + X_5)}{40}$$
$$= \frac{X_1 + X_2 + \cdots + X_5}{5} = \overline{X}.$$

The mean width of the combined eight teeth is the same as that of the original five teeth in jar 1. The variance of the width of the original five teeth in jar 1 is:

$$S_O^2 = \frac{(X_1 - \overline{X})^2 + (X_2 - \overline{X})^2 + (X_3 - \overline{X})^2 + (X_4 - \overline{X})^2 + (X_5 - \overline{X})^2}{5 - 1}.$$

The variance of the widths of the combined teeth is:

$$S_C^2 = \frac{(X_1 - \overline{X})^2 + \cdots + (X_5 - \overline{X})^2 + (Y_1 - \overline{X})^2 + \cdots + (Y_3 - \overline{X})^2}{8 - 1}$$

$$= \frac{(X_1 - \overline{X})^2 + \cdots + (X_5 - \overline{X})^2 + 0 + 0 + 0}{7}, \quad \text{since } Y_1 = Y_2 = Y_3 = \overline{X},$$

$$= \frac{(X_1 - \overline{X})^2 + (X_2 - \overline{X})^2 + (X_3 - \overline{X})^2 + (X_4 - \overline{X})^2 + (X_5 - \overline{X})^2}{7}.$$

Numerators in S_O^2 and S_C^2 are the same but the denominator in the expression S_C^2 is larger than that in S_O^2, therefore, the variance of the widths in a combined sample is smaller.

The following table summarize a few symbols that will be used repeatedly throughout the text. It is customary to denote the population variance and standard deviation by σ^2 and σ (sigma, the Greek letter).

Parameter	Sample	Population
Mean	$\overline{X}$	μ
Variance	S^2	σ^2
Standard deviation	S	σ

3.14 COEFFICIENT OF VARIATION

Although the SD is the most widely used measure of variability, one disadvantage is that it depends on the unit of measurement. The **coefficient of variation** is a measure used to compare the variability among two or more sets of data representing different quantities with different units of measurement. For instance, the strength of two types of prefabricated posts, carbon fiber post (CFP) and polyethylene fiber-reinforced post (PFRP), on endodontically treated teeth are being studied. The sample mean and the sample SD of the fracture load for CFP are $\overline{X}_A = 67.57$ kg and $S_A = 26.57$ kg, and those for PFRP are $\overline{X}_B = 132.55$ lbs and $S_B = 36.19$ lbs, respectively. It does not make much sense to compare these two SDs directly because they are reported in different units of measure. The coefficient of variation is

what we need in this situation to measure relative variations.

Definition 3.14.1. The coefficient of variation (CV) is given by

$$CV = \frac{S}{\overline{X}} \cdot 100\%, \quad \text{or} \quad CV = \frac{\sigma}{\mu} \cdot 100\%.$$

The CV expresses the SD as a percent of the arithmetic mean of what is being measured. The CV is also useful in comparing the dispersions of two or more distributions with markedly different means, even if they are all in the same measuring unit. For example, the CV of the fracture load for carbon fiber posts and polyethylene fiber-reinforced posts are

$$CV_A = \frac{26.57}{67.57} \cdot 100\% = 39.3\%,$$

and

$$CV_B = \frac{36.19}{132.55} \cdot 100\% = 27.3\%.$$

This indicates that the measurements of polyethylene fiber-reinforced posts is less dispersed and more precise.

Example 3.14.1. Consider the following two sets of data.

Data $1 = \{0, 5, 10\}$, and Data $2 = \{70, 80, 90\}$.

Data 1 represents the quiz scores of three students on the scale of 0 to 10, and data 2 represents the final exam scores of three students on the scale of 0 to 100. Calculations show that $\overline{X}_1 = 5.0$, $S_1 = 5.0$, $\overline{X}_2 = 80.0$, and $S_2 = 10.0$. These two data sets have markedly different means. The SD $S_2 = 10.0$, of data 2 is twice the standard deviation,

$S_1 = 5.0$, of data 1. However, their CVs are

$$CV_1 = \frac{5.0}{5.0} \cdot 100\% = 100\%$$

and

$$CV_2 = \frac{10.0}{80.0} \cdot 100\% = 12.5\%.$$

Thus, the dispersion of data 1 relative to its mean is about eight times larger than the dispersion of data 2 relative to its mean.

Example 3.14.2. Accurate preoperative evaluation of bone quality is essential to assist the clinician with the treatment-planning stages of implant therapy. The long-term clinical success of dental implants is reportedly influenced by both the quality and quantity of available bone. There are two competing techniques that enable us to measure alveolar bone density within the edentulous areas of jaws: quantitative computerized tomography (QCT) and cone-beam computed tomography (CBCT). Both techniques were used to evaluate the bone density of 10 partially or completely edentulous human cadaver heads [15]. Measurements taken using QCT were represented in milligrams per cubic centimeter, and those by using CBCT were represented in percents. Suppose that the researchers reported the mean and the SD of QCT and CBCT as $\overline{X}_Q = 4.53$, $S_Q = 2.28$, $\overline{X}_C = 78.5$, and $S_C = 24.3$. Because the units of measurement are different, the coefficient of variation should be used to compare the dispersion of the measurements done by the two methods. The CV of QCT and CBCT are:

$$\frac{S_Q}{\overline{X}_Q} = \frac{2.28}{4.53} \cdot 100\% = 50.3\%,$$

and

$$\frac{S_C}{\overline{X}_C} = \frac{24.3}{78.5} \cdot 100\% = 31.0\%.$$

Measurements of bone density samples done using CBCT are less dispersed and therefore, more precise than QCT.

Whenever experimental researchers collect data as part of their scientific investigation, they should be aware of several criteria briefly described here.

- Validity: The relationship between what it is supposed to measure and what it actually does measure.

- Accuracy: Refers to how close the measurement is to the true value.
- Precision: Refers to how close repeated measurements are to each other.
- Unbiasedness: Refers to the measurements that are free of systematic errors.
- Reliability: Refers to the extent to which the measurements can be replicated.

Detailed discussions on these criteria can be found in Brunette [16]. Precision of measurements is directly related to the variance and the SD. If the precision level is low, the SD is high. If the precision level is high, the SD is low. Let's consider an example.

Example 3.14.3. A health maintenance organization operates four laboratories located in different areas in Southern California. In an attempt to assess the quality of the performance of the laboratories, the Quality Assurance Department prepared identical samples of mouthrinse, and sent six samples to each of the laboratories. Alcohol has generally been used in mouthrinses for its antiseptic properties. For alcohol to be an effective antimicrobial agent, the concentration needs to be between 50% and 70% [17]. The mouthrinse samples sent to the laboratories contain 60% alcohol. The laboratories were required to analyze the samples and report the amount of alcohol in the mouthrinse samples. Figure 3.14.1 displays the alcohol content in the samples each laboratory has analyzed.

1. Lab A has the largest variation and therefore the lowest precision level. Except for one sample, the analytical results are either far below or far above the true value, indicating that the performance of Lab A is not accurate.
2. With all six measurements close to the true value of 60% alcohol content, the performance of Lab B is the most accurate. The precision level is second best because all the measurements are close to each other. The overall performance of Lab B is the best of the four laboratories.
3. The performance of Lab C is the second best (why?).
4. Lab D is the most precise, with all six measurements closer to each other than the other three laboratories. But the accuracy of Lab D is the worst. Not knowing the true value, such laboratories can be misled into believing that the quality of their performance is very good

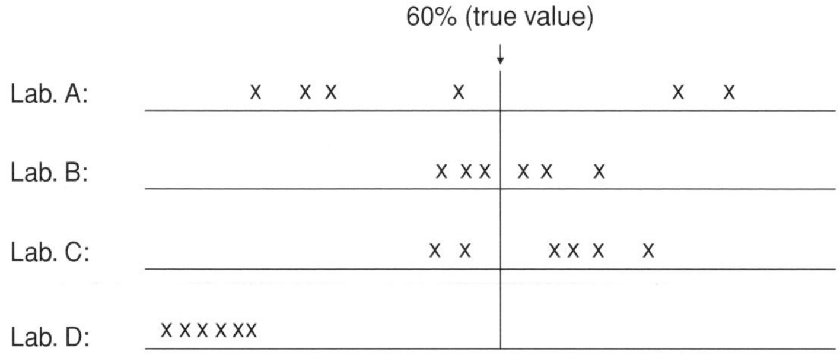

60% (true value)

Figure 3.14.1　Analytical results of alcohol contents by four laboratories.

because of the high precision level of the analytical results. This is a classic case of "precision of inaccuracy." However, once the problem of inaccuracy is recognized, it is relatively easy for Lab D to improve its performance by calibration of its analytical instruments. Generally speaking, it is more difficult and takes greater effort to enhance the precision than the accuracy.

3.15 VARIANCE OF GROUPED DATA

In Section 3.8 we discussed the mean and median of grouped data. Our next interest is a measure of dispersion of the grouped data. In particular, we are interested in calculating the variance and the SD. Using the same notation as in Section 3.8, let $X_1, X_2, \cdots, X_k$ be the midpoint of the intervals, and $f_1, f_2, \cdots, f_k$ be the corresponding frequencies. The variance and the SD of grouped data are given by

$$S^2 = \frac{\sum_{i=1}^{k}(X_i - \overline{X})^2 f_i}{\left\{\sum_{i=1}^{k} f_i\right\} - 1}$$

and

$$S = \sqrt{\frac{\sum_{i=1}^{k}(X_i - \overline{X})^2 f_i}{\left\{\sum_{i=1}^{k} f_i\right\} - 1}}.$$

The variance and SD of the grouped data presented in Table 3.8.2 are as follows: the midpoints of the intervals are $X_1 = 1.0$, $X_2 = 3.0$, $X_3 = 5.0$, $X_4 = 7.0$, $X_5 = 9.0$; the corresponding frequencies are $f_1 = 14$, $f_2 = 16$, $f_3 = 12$, $f_4 = 7$, $f_5 = 2$, $\sum_{i=1}^{5} f_i = 51$; and the mean of the grouped data is $\overline{X} = 3.71$. By the below formula 13.15.1.

3.16 SKEWNESS

Some important characteristics of a distribution that can be observed from histograms, stem and leaf plots, or box plots are the symmetry and shape of the distribution. Data are said to be **symmetrically distributed** if the half of the distribution below the median matches the distribution above the median. In other words, the relative position of the data points on both sides of the median will match. The distribution of standardized test scores and blood pressure data are known to be symmetric. Of course, a distribution could be asymmetric or skewed.

Definition 3.16.1. A distribution that has a long "tail" to the right is said to be **skewed to right**, or right-skewed (or **positively skewed**), and a distribution that has a long "tail" to the left is said to

$$S^2 = \frac{\sum_{i=1}^{k}(X_i - \overline{X})^2 f_i}{\left\{\sum_{i=1}^{k} f_i\right\} - 1}$$

$$= \frac{(1.0 - 3.71)^2 \cdot 14 + (3.0 - 3.71)^2 \cdot 16 + (5.0 - 3.71)^2 \cdot 12 + (7.0 - 3.71)^2 \cdot 7 + (9.0 - 3.71)^2 \cdot 2}{51 - 1}$$

$$= 5.2518 \text{ (mm)}^2,$$

and

$$S = \sqrt{5.2518 \text{ (mm)}^2} = 2.2917 \text{ mm}. \tag{3.15.1}$$

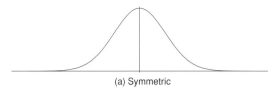

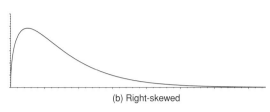

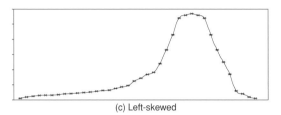

Figure 3.16.1 Symmetric, right- and left-skewed distributions.

be **skewed to left**, or left-skewed (or **negatively skewed**).

If a distribution is skewed to right, the observations above the median will tend to be farther from the median, and the right end of the distribution may contain extreme values. On the other hand, if a distribution is skewed to left, then the observations below the median will tend to be farther from the median, and there may be extreme values in the left side of the distribution.

In many samples, the relationship between the sample mean and the sample median can aid us in determining the symmetry of a distribution. For a symmetric distribution, the sample mean and the sample median are approximately the same. For a right-skewed distribution, the mean tends to be larger than the median as it gets pulled to the right

Table 3.16.1. Mean and median price of houses sold in 2001.

City	n	Median ($)	Mean ($)
Chino Hills	1, 172	259, 000	269, 000
Diamond Bar	957	258, 000	311, 000
Hacienda Heights	580	263, 000	365, 000
Rowland Heights	513	242, 000	300, 000
Walnut	411	325, 000	354, 000

Source: Southern California Realtors Association.

by extreme values on the right end of the tail. For a left-skewed distribution, the mean tends to be smaller than the median as it gets pulled to the left by extreme values on the left end of the tail. Income distribution and housing market are known to be right-skewed. Age at which patients need complete dentures and the incidence of an oral carcinoma related to age are examples of the left-skewed distribution. The lifetime of crowns is also known to be left-skewed. Very few crowns fail within 5 years, but a vast majority of the crowns last more than 10 years. Figure 3.16.1 displays symmetric, right-skewed, and left-skewed distributions.

In case of a symmetric unimodal distribution, mean, median, and mode will coincide. In case of a symmetric bimodal distribution as shown in Figure 3.16.2, mean and median are equal, but the two modes do not coincide with mean and median. For right-skewed distributions, the mean will tend to be larger than the median, and for left-skewed distributions, the mean will tend to be smaller than the median, as can be seen in Figure 3.16.1. Table 3.16.1 presents the mean and the median price of the houses sold in five communities in Southern California during the year 2001. In all five communities, the median price of the house is lower than the average because the distribution of the housing price is right-skewed.

The box plots discussed earlier can give us a rough idea about the skewness of data. For instance, if the lower whisker is longer than the upper

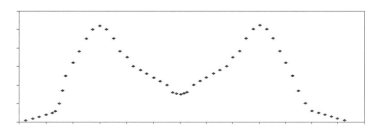

Figure 3.16.2 A symmetric bimodal distribution.

whisker, then the data are likely to be left-skewed. On the other hand if the upper whisker is longer than the lower whisker, then the data are likely to be right-skewed. If a distribution is moderately skewed, then the following crude relationship between mean, median, and mode holds:

$$(\text{Mean} - \text{Mode}) \simeq 3(\text{Mean} - \text{Median}).$$

The most widely used skewness index is stated.

$$SK = \frac{\sum_{i=1}^{n}(X_i - \overline{X})^3}{\left[\sum_{i=1}^{n}(X_i - \overline{X})^2\right]^{3/2}}$$

If a distribution is symmetric, $SK = 0$; if it is right-skewed (or positively skewed), $SK > 0$; and if it is left-skewed (negatively skewed), $SK < 0$. A distribution with the skewness index $SK = 1.122$ is more skewed to right than a distribution with $SK = 0.768$. Similarly, a distribution with the skewness index $SK = -0.948$ is more skewed to left than a distribution with $SK = -0.375$.

Example 3.16.1. Ten subjects were chosen to study the length of time an adult rinses with a mouthwash in relation to the manufacturer's recommended rinsing time. The random variable X_i represents the length of time in seconds the ith subject has rinsed.

Subject No.	X_i	$(X_i - \overline{X})$	$(X_i - \overline{X})^2$	$(X_i - \overline{X})^3$
1	15	−11.5	132.25	−1520.875
2	34	7.5	56.25	421.875
3	33	6.5	42.25	274.625
4	10	−16.5	272.25	−4492.125
5	32	5.5	30.25	166.375
6	30	3.5	12.25	42.875
7	35	8.5	72.25	614.125
8	32	5.5	30.25	166.375
9	18	−8.5	72.25	−614.125
10	26	−0.5	0.25	−0.125

From the data we can compute $\overline{X} = 26.5$, $\sum_{i=1}^{10}(X_i - \overline{X})^2 = 720.5$, $\sum_{i=1}^{10}(X_i - \overline{X})^3 = -4941.0$, $SK = \frac{-4941.0}{(720.5)^{3/2}} = -0.2555$. The above data are skewed to the left. Note that a mirror image of the data would be skewed to the right and its skewness index would be, $SK = 0.2555$.

3.17 EXERCISES

1   Explain what these mean.
 a. X_i b. $\overline{X}$ c. $\sum_{j=1}^{4} X_j$ d. μ

2   Peri-Gel is an antimicrobial gel that is designed to treat chronic adult periodontitis. For the pilot study to test the effectiveness of Peri-Gel, 11 patients with chronic adult periodontitis were selected. These patients have been instructed to use Peri-Gel for 3 months by applying it deeply into their periodontal pockets. Dr. Brown, a periodontist, reported the amount of pocket depth reduction in his patient subjects. What is the mean reduction in pocket depth?

0.4, 1.2, 0.6, 1.0, 0.5, 0.6, 1.1, 1.4, 0.8, 0.7, 0.6 (mm)

3   In Example 3.2.2, if you took another sample of six chewing tobacco users, and another sample of eight non-users, do you expect to get sample means that are different from those in the example? If so, then why?

4   Suppose that a mistake had been committed in Example 3.2.2 by recording 28 DMFT instead of 15 for the third subject in the chewing tobacco group. Find the error this would cause in computing the mean DMFT.

5   (a) If the average DAT score of 12 first year dental students is 17, how many of them could have scored 22 or higher? (b) If the average MCAT score of 7 first year medical students is 33, how many of them could have scored 39 or higher?

6   There are three brands of periapical dental film. The price of brand A is $6.45 per package, $7.25 per package for brand B, and $5.98 for brand C. Riverside Dental Clinic purchased 150 packages during the last year, of which 20% are brand A, 30% brand B, and 50% brand C. What is the average cost of periapical dental film per package Riverside Dental Clinic has paid for?

7   What is the median of two measurements 85.3 and 89.5?

8   An orthodontic resident took a sample of four brachyfacial patients who have not started orthodontic treatment. To monitor the effect of quad helix expansion therapy, she measured their maxillary intermolar distance in millimeter. What is the median distance if the measurements are

39.5, 44.5, 42.0, 39.0? Calculate the mean and compare it to the median.

9 Twenty-four children in Mrs. Maruo's kindergarten class underwent a dental examination at the end of the school year. The number of carious teeth each child has is presented below. What is the median number of carious teeth the children in Mrs. Maruo's class have? What is the mode?

3	5	3	2	0	0	7	5
1	6	2	2	8	4	2	2
4	4	3	6	7	0	1	8

10 Twenty-six dental residents are enrolled in a biostatistics course. Their ages are 32, 29, 27, 31, 47, 39, 29, 28, 37, 32, 29, 30, 33, 30, 29, 28, 28, 32, 28, 28, 31, 29, 32, 28, 29, 34. Find the mode.

11 In an orthodontic clinic 21 patients were treated in 1 week. The patient charts show the following information about facial type. Is the mode an appropriate measure of location for the data? If so, find the mode.

Patient ID	Facial Type	Patient ID	Facial Type
1	Dolicho	12	Brachy
2	Brachy	13	Dolicho
3	Brachy	14	Meso
4	Meso	15	Meso
5	Meso	16	Meso
6	Dolicho	17	Dolicho
7	Meso	18	Brachy
8	Meso	19	Dolicho
9	Meso	20	Meso
10	Dolicho	21	Dolicho
11	Meso		

12 During a thorough periodontal examination the mesio-, mid-, and distobuccal sites, as well as the corresponding lingual and palatal sites, are routinely checked. Most periodontists sweep the probe continuously through the sulcus to get a better feel for the pocket depths as a whole. A periodontist reported pocket depths (mm) of his 15 patients as follows. Find the mode. Is the data bimodal?

1.5	3.5	7.0	4.0	5.5	2.0	3.5	8.5
5.5	9.0	3.5	4.0	5.5	2.0	1.0	

13 Find the geometric mean of 0.4, 1.2, 28.8, and 312.0.

14 The relationship between the arithmetic mean and the geometric mean is $\overline{X_G} \leq \overline{X}$. That is, given a set of non-negative observations, the arithmetic mean is always at least as large as the geometric mean. When do you think they are equal?

15 Dr. Johnson is an experienced, long-term investor. He understands that the stock market will always fluctuate. His investment strategy is to purchase the stocks when they are down to keep his average purchase price lower. In each of the four previous months this year he bought $10,000 worth of a denture care company's stocks. In January he bought them at $200 per share, in February at $125 per share, in March at $100 per share, and in April at $80 per share. What is his average purchase price per share of this denture care company's stocks? Verify that the harmonic mean is $112.68.

16 Acute chest syndrome, which is an acute pulmonic process in patients with sickle cell disease, is a common major clinical problem associated with the disease. Fifty-eight patients whose ages ranging from 1 to 12 have been admitted to the Loma Linda Community Hospital Pediatric Ward during a 1-year period. Laboratory profiles showed their hemoglobin ranged between 4.2 gm/dl and 12.0 gm/dl. Suppose the hemoglobin data were presented as follows. Compute the mean of the hemoglobin level from the table.

Hemoglobin (gm/dl)	No. of Patients
$3.0 < X \leq 6.0$	16
$6.0 < X \leq 9.0$	26
$9.0 < X \leq 12.0$	17

17 Calculate the mean of the bacterial colony data from Table 2.3.4. and from Table 2.3.6 in Section 2.3.1, and compare the two means.

18 Calculate the median of the hemoglobin data in Exercise 16.

19 To evaluate the caries-detecting ability of the practicing dentists, a sample of 10 dentists with at least 5 years of practice experience was selected. Each dentist was shown a set of panoramic and periapical radiographs chosen from patient records. Correct detection of caries by the subjects after viewing the radiographs is represented in percent (%): 27.8, 65.4, 17.5, 29.6, 22.0, 26.0, 38.0, 34.5, 28.6, 42.8. What is the midrange of the caries-detecting ability? Compare the midrange with other measures of central location.

20 Fracture resistance of four endodontic post systems under chewing conditions was measured in kilograms. Suppose the mean and the sample size of each endodontic post system is given as $\overline{Y}_1 = 93.1$, $n_1 = 5$, $\overline{Y}_2 = 79.6$, $n_2 = 7$, $\overline{Y}_3 = 82.2$, $n_3 = 10$, and $\overline{Y}_4 = 71.4$, $n_4 = 9$. What is the average of these four means of the fracture resistance?

21 Find an example in dentistry or medicine where (a) the median is a more appropriate location measure than the mean, and (b) the mode is a more appropriate location measure than the mean.

22 Twenty patients have been recruited for a clinical trial to assess the efficacy of a newly designed toothpaste. To establish a baseline gingival index for the research study, each patient subject was examined and their gingival index was measured at 20 sites, 10 each from maxillary and mandibular molars. The experimenters reported individual subject's average gingival index as follows: 2.3, 1.4, 3.1, 2.6, 0.5, 1.4, 0.2, 3.6, 1.8, 3.3, 2.6, 0.1, 1.8, 3.8, 2.1, 2.6, 3.4, 2.7, 2.0, 1.3. Find the range. What is the mode? Would you report the range with the mode to describe the data?

23 From Figure 3.11.1, find the 90th percentile rank. What is the percentile rank corresponding to the L value of 59.50?

24 The mid-term exam scores of 21 dental residents in Biostatistics 101 are shown below. Compute the percentile corresponding to a score of 93.

88	91	78	93	98	95	82	68	87	72	64
90	80	70	87	76	40	89	96	95	78	

25 From the data in Exercise 24, find the values corresponding to the 25th and the 75th percentiles.

26 Using the data in Table 3.11.1, find the quartiles, interquartile range, and detect outliers.

27 Which one of the measures of central tendency is most influenced by extreme values in a skewed distribution?

a. Mean b. Mode c. Median d. 95th percentile.

28 Patients' pocket depth data is shown below. Find the interquartile range, and identify outliers if any:

4.5	3.0	5.5	7.0	2.5	1.0	8.5	13.0	6.0	1.5	6.5
5.5	3.0	4.0	4.5	6.0	5.5	2.5	2.0	3.0	5.0	4.0

29 A manufacturer of a mouthrinse product recommends that the users should keep their product in the mouth for 30 to 45 seconds after brushing teeth to get the maximum benefit. As a class project, hygiene students took a sample of 20 female and 22 male dental students who are regular users of mouthrinse products to determine if they follow the manufacturer's recommendation, and to find out if sex is a factor in compliance. The amount of time the subjects kept the mouthrinse in their mouth in seconds is as follows.

Females	35	42	30	45	53	28	33	34	35	40
	38	46	50	30	45	35	40	55	38	43
Males	26	15	35	40	25	38	28	38	35	30	25
	20	18	22	20	30	26	34	16	24	27	30

a. Find the quartiles and the interquartile range for each group separately.
b. Find the quartiles and the interquartile range for both groups combined.
c. Identify the outliers for each group, if there are any.
d. Construct the box plots for the two groups and compare them.

30 Hearing impairment as an occupational hazard affects a large spectrum of vocations across the world. From airport employees to rock concert musicians, many people suffer from job-related noise pollution. The habitual use of high-frequency ultrasonic scalers can potentially contribute to tinnitus and hearing impairment among dental professionals. To assess the level of their exposure to high-frequency ultrasonic scalers, a sample of 38 dental hygienists and dentists was taken. Below are the number of hours in a typical week that they are exposed to the ultrasonic scalers. Find the sample variance and the sample SD. Find also the interquartile range.

12	18	25	6	28	14	5	10	15	20	22	15	12
6	25	12	4	8	24	4	18	16	15	20	5	6
20	22	7	2	5	12	8	8	10	5	10	9

31 From the data in Exercise 29, (a) compute the SD after subtracting 2 from each observation. (b) What is the SD of the data if you were to divide the observations by 4? Would you expect the standard deviation to get smaller or larger than that for the original data?

32 A dental researcher has collected the following data to compare the strength of two types of bonding materials, Brand A and Brand B.
a. Compute mean, variance, and SD for each brand.
b. What are their CV?

Brand A (kg)		Brand B (kg)	
43.5	60.5	57.6	39.8
58.5	55.7	40.8	47.8
42.7	46.7	66.4	55.2
48.4			

33 The mouthrinses, along with their contained alcohol percentages, include essential oils, cetylpyridinium chloride, and chlorhexidine glycol. Ten samples of mouthrinses were sent to three laboratories for their analysis of the contents: Lab A analyzed the samples for essential oils and reported their measurements in percentages (%), Lab B for cetylpyridinium chloride and reported in milligrams per cubic centimeter, and Lab C for chlorhexidine glycol and reported in percentages (%). Calculate the mean and SD of each lab data, and discuss how you would compare their variabilities.

Lab A (%)	58.6	65.4	76.0	60.7	53.3	45.8	62.1	74.6	51.8	59.2
Lab B (mg/cc)	5.0	4.4	5.3	5.0	3.8	5.5	4.7	3.8	4.0	5.2
Lab C (%)	12.3	11.6	13.0	12.9	10.4	13.8	11.3	10.7	11.7	12.9

34 As a class project, a group of hygiene students took a survey with practicing dental hygienists to assess the level of their compensation in Riverside County. Twenty-eight hygienists participated in the study. Their weekly pay is presented below. Calculate the skewness index and discuss the skewness of the data. Is it right-skewed or left-skewed?

1,445,	1,540,	1,300,	1,450,	1,275,	1,450,	1,400
1,660,	1,700,	1,380,	1,215,	1,675,	1,220,	1,380

35 The lifetime of implants placed in 76 grafted maxillary sinuses is shown. The lifetimes are in months. What are the variance and the SD of the grouped implant lifetime data?

Lifetime (month)	Frequency	Lifetime (month)	Frequency
0–9	4	40–49	11
10–19	7	50–59	14
20–29	3	60–69	16
30–39	8	70–79	13

3.18 REFERENCES

1. Feinsilber, M., and Meed, W. *American Averages*. Bantam Doubleday Dell. New York, 1980.
2. Golstein, R. E., and Garber, D. A. *Complete Dental Bleaching*. Illinois, Quintessence Publishing Co., Inc. 1995.
3. Hanratty, B., Hong, E., and Yong, G. Anxiety Reduction Through Modification of Dental Handpiece Noise as Perceived by the Dental Patient. Loma Linda University student project. 2000.
4. Forthofer, R. N., and Lee, E. S. *Introduction to Biostatistics: A Guide to Design, Analysis, and Discovery*. Academic Press. 1995.
5. Heilman, J. R., Kiritsy, M. C., Levy, S. M., and Wefel, J. S. Assessing Fluoride Levels of Carbonated Soft Drinks. *JADA*: 1995,130, 1593–1599.
6. Schuller, A. A., Thomsen, I. O., and Holst, D. Adjusting Estimates of Alveolar Bone Loss for Missing Observations: Developing and Testing a General Model. *J. Dent. Res.*: 1999. 78, 661–666.
7. Wennstrom, J. L., Serino, G., Lindhe, J., Eneroth, L., and Tollskog, G. Periodontal Conditions of Adult Regular Dental Care Attendants. *J. Clin. Periodontol*: 20, 714–722. 1993.
8. Malamed, S. F., Gagnon, S., and Leblanc, D. Efficacy of Articaine: A New Amide Local Anesthetic. *JADA*: 2000. 131, 635–642.
9. Choi, H. Private communications. 1999.
10. Park, E., Suh, M., and Lee, C. Color Stability of a Composite Resin. Loma Linda University student project. 2000.
11. Tukey, J. *Exploratory Data Analysis*, Addison-Wesley. 1977.
12. Hogg, R. V., and Craig, A. T. *Introduction to Mathematical Statistics*. Third edition. The Macmillan Company. 1970.
13. Kirk, R. E. *Statistics: An Introduction*. Fourth edition, Harcourt Brace. 1999.

14. Kaocharoen, T., Backer, J., and Nguyen, K. Evaluation of the Strength of a Prefabricated Post on Endodontically Treated Teeth. Loma Linda University student project. 1998.

15. Aranyarachkul, P. Assessment of Human Alveolar Bone Density by Using Volumetric CT Machine. Research protocol. Loma Linda University School of Dentistry. 2001.

16. Brunette, D. M. *Critical Thinking: Understanding and Evaluating Dental Research.* Quintessence Publishing Co., Inc. 1996.

17. Ciuffreda, L., Boylan, R., Scherer, W., Palat, M., and Bacchi, A. An In Vivo Comparison of the Antimicrobial Activities of Four Mouthwashes. *J. of Clinical Dentistry*: 1994. 4, 103–105.

Chapter 4
Probability

4.1 INTRODUCTION

Clinicians and researchers in biomedical and health sciences do far more than simply describe and present their experimental data. They use the data they collect to draw conclusions and make inferences regarding the population of all objects of the kind that they have studied. Inferential statistical methods are enormously powerful techniques that enable us to draw valid conclusions and make accurate predictions of certain characteristics of the population based on the limited number of samples drawn from the population. Proper understanding and correct applications of inferential statistical methods require knowledge of probability. Probability is not only a fundamental tool for inferential statistics but is the foundation for statistical tests, as we shall see in future chapters.

Nothing in life is certain. In everything we do, from patient care to business activities, we gauge the chances of successful outcomes. The following are typical questions that health care professionals have to answer:

1. What is the chance that microleakage will occur when the occlusal surfaces have been sealed with a pit and fissure sealant?
2. What is the chance that the adenocarcinoma cells will recur within 2 years after the malignant tumor has been surgically removed?
3. What is the chance that titanium implants placed in patients who smoke more than 20 cigarettes a day will survive 5 years?
4. Is the probability greater than 90% that the new outbreak of influenza will infect at least 50% of the population in the community within the next 3 months?

Addressing these questions properly requires an adequate knowledge of basic probability. The basic concepts of probability are discussed in the next three sections; those questions are followed by discussions on the conditional probabilities and Bayes theorem. In addition, applications of the conditional probabilities that are also useful in epidemiology are presented.

4.2 SAMPLE SPACE AND EVENTS

Your doctor might inform you that after oral maxillofacial surgery, there is an 80% chance the postoperative pain will dissipate in 2 days. Roughly speaking, **probability** is a numerical assessment of the likelihood of the occurrence of an outcome of a random variable. Probability is a number between 0 and 1, inclusive. It can be expressed in percentages as well as in fractions. The probability *near* 1 indicates that the event is most likely to occur, but it does not necessarily mean it will occur. The probability *near* 0 indicates that the event is not likely to occur, but it does not necessarily mean it will not occur. The probability 1 means that the event involved will occur with certainty. The event that has the probability 1 is called the **sure event**. The probability 0 means that the event involved will not occur. The events with extremely small probabilities of occurrence are referred to as **rare events**. The event with the probability $\frac{1}{2}$ is just as likely to occur as it is not to occur. We will now define a few terms to facilitate our discussions.

Definition 4.2.1. The **sample space** is the set of all possible outcomes of an experiment (or a random variable) and is denoted by Ω (a Greek letter "omega"). The outcomes are sometimes referred to as the sample points.

Definition 4.2.2. Any subset of the sample space is an **event**. Events are denoted by uppercase letters, A, B, C, $\cdots$, or E_1, E_2, E_3, $\cdots$.

Example 4.2.1. A fair coin means the chance of observing a head (H) is just as likely as observing a tail (T). A fair coin is tossed once. The sample space for this experiment consists of H and T, that is, $\Omega = \{H, T\}$, because there are exactly two possible outcomes in an experiment of tossing a coin once.

Example 4.2.2. A fair coin is tossed twice, or two fair coins are tossed once. Then the sample space is given by $\Omega = \{HH, HT, TH, TT\}$. There are four possible outcomes in this experiment. Each outcome is equally likely to occur; therefore, $P\{HH\} = P\{HT\} = P\{TH\} = P\{TT\} = \frac{1}{4}$. We can form a number of events from this sample space. For instance, $A = \{HH, HT, TH\} = \{$at least one H$\}$, $B = \{HT, TH, TT\} = \{$at least one T$\}$, and $C = \{HH, TT\}$. Because the four outcomes are equally likely, and the event A contains 3 outcomes of the sample space, the probability of observing event A is $\frac{3}{4}$. This is denoted by $P(A) = \frac{3}{4}$. Similarly, the probabilities of observing the events B and C are $P(B) = \frac{3}{4}$, and $P(C) = \frac{1}{2}$, respectively.

Example 4.2.3. The Brown family has three children. What is the sample space for the sexes of their three children? Because each of the three children can be either B or G, the sample space consists of 8 outcomes;

$$\Omega = \{BBB, BBG, BGB, BGG, GBB,$$
$$GBG, GGB, GGG\}.$$

Let's assume that the likelihood of a female birth is equal to the likelihood of a male birth; that is, $P(B) = P(G) = \frac{1}{2}$. Then

1. $P(\text{three girls}) = P(GGG) = \frac{1}{8}$.
2. $P(\text{exactly one boy}) = P\{BGG, GBG, GGB\} = \frac{3}{8}$.
3. $P(\text{at least two boys}) = P\{BBB, BBG, BGB, GBB\} = \frac{4}{8} = \frac{1}{2}$.

Example 4.2.4. Suppose we toss a coin n times. Then the sample space, Ω, contains 2^n outcomes. If we tossed a coin five times ($n = 5$), $\Omega = \{2^5 \text{ outcomes}\} = \{32 \text{ outcomes}\}$.

Example 4.2.5. Dr. Brown and Dr. Chen each have 2 patients. At least one of Dr. Brown's patients is male, and Dr. Chen's first patient is male. Assume that the probability of having a male patient is the same as that of having a female patient. (a) What is the probability that both of Dr. Brown's patients are male? (b) What is the probability that both of Dr. Chen's patients are male? Are the two probabilities equal?

Solution. This example can be viewed as a coin tossing experiment where *Male* and *Female* correspond to H and T, with $P(H) = P(T) = \frac{1}{2}$.

(i) Let's first consider all possible outcomes for the sex of Dr. Brown's patients. Dr. Brown has at least one male patient. Therefore, there are three possible outcomes; $\Omega = \{MM, MF, FM\}$. The event $A = \{MM\}$ is the event of our interest. Because $P(\text{Male}) = P(\text{Female})$, the three outcomes are all equally likely. Hence, $P(A) = \frac{1}{3}$.

(ii) All possible outcomes for the sex of Dr. Chen's patients are MM and MF, because her first patient is male; $\Omega = \{MM, MF\}$. These two outcomes are equally likely; thus $P(A) = \frac{1}{2}$, where $A = \{MM\}$. The chance that Dr. Chen has both male patients is greater than the chance that Dr. Brown has both male patients.

The probability of an event can be determined by examining the sample space. Provided that the outcomes are equally likely, the probability of any event A is the number of outcomes in A divided by the total number of outcomes in the sample space;

$$P(A) = \frac{\text{Number of outcomes in } A}{\text{Total number of outcomes in the sample space}}.$$

4.3 BASIC PROPERTIES OF PROBABILITY

To motivate discussions on algebraic operations on events, we will roll a balanced die. If the numbers we will observe from the experiment of rolling a die are equally likely, then the die is said to be balanced. In other words, $P(1) = P(2) = P(3) = P(4) = P(5) = P(6) = 1/6$. The sample space

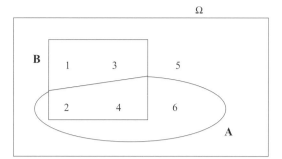

Ω

B 1   3   5

2   4   6

A

Figure 4.3.1   Diagram for event A and event B.

for the die-rolling experiment is $\Omega = \{1, 2, 3, 4, 5, 6\}$. Let A be the event of observing even numbers, that is, $A = \{2, 4, 6\}$, and let B be the event of observing a number less than 5, that is, $B = \{1, 2, 3, 4\}$. The probability of observing the event A is $P(A) = 3/6 = 1/2$, and the probability of observing the event B is $P(B) = 4/6 = 2/3$. What is the probability of observing both event A *and* event B? From Figure 4.3.1, events A and B will be observed if either 2 or 4 turns up. Hence, the probability that both events A and B will occur is, $P(A \text{ and } B) = P\{2, 4\} = 2/6 = 1/3$.

What is the probability that either event A *or* event B will occur? Either event A or event B can be observed if A or B, or both A and B, occur, namely, if any of the faces 1, 2, 3, 4, 6 turns up. These are 5 of the 6 equally likely outcomes. Thus, $P(A \text{ or } B) = P(A \text{ or } B, \text{ or both } A \text{ and } B) = 5/6$. To make the discussions slightly more formal, we need to introduce the following definitions.

Definition 4.3.1.

1. The **union** of the events A and B is the event "A or B, or both A and B," denoted by $A \cup B$ (read, A union B). The probability of A or B, or both A and B, is denoted by $P(A \cup B)$.
2. The **intersection** of the events A and B is the event "both A and B," denoted by $A \cap B$ (read, A intersection B). The probability of A and B is denoted by $P(A \cap B)$.
3. The **complement** of an event A is the event "not A," denoted by A^C or $\overline{A}$. The complementary event, A^C of the event $A = \{2, 4, 6\}$ is $A^C = \{1, 3, 5\}$. The event A consists of even numbers, and its complementary event A^C consists of odd numbers. The complementary event of $B = \{1, 2, 3, 4\}$ is $B^C = \{5, 6\}$.

A complementary event E^C consists of all outcomes outside the event E that lie in the sample space.

4. Two events A and B are said to be **mutually exclusive** if both cannot occur at the same time. Thus, $A = \{2, 4, 6\}$ and $B = \{1, 3, 5\}$ are mutually exclusive.

Example 4.3.1. Suppose the possible drugs prescribed by dentists that may affect smell or taste are ampicillin, benzocaine, codeine, metronidazole, sodium lauryle sulfate toothpaste, and tetracycline. Define events $C = \{$benzocaine, codeine, metronidazole, tetracycline$\}$, $D = \{$ampicillin, codeine, metronidazole, tetracycline$\}$, and $E = \{$ampicillin$\}$.

1. The union of the two events C and D is $C \cup D = \{$ampicillin, benzocaine, codeine, metronidazole, tetracycline$\}$.
2. The intersection of the two events C and D is $C \cap D = \{$codeine, metronidazole, tetracycline$\}$.
3. The complementary events of C and D are: $C^C = \{$ampicillin, sodium lauryle sulfate toothpaste$\}$, and $D^C = \{$benzocaine, sodium lauryle sulfate toothpaste$\}$.
4. The two events C and D are not mutually exclusive, because they have common outcomes: codeine, metronidazole, and tetracycline. They can both occur simultaneously.
5. The events C and E are mutually exclusive.

We now state basic properties of probability.

Properties 4.3.1 (Axioms of Probability) Let A and B be any events defined on the sample space, Ω. Then

1. $P(\Omega) = 1$.
2. $0 \leq P(A) \leq 1$.
3. $P(A) = 1 - P(A^C)$ and $P(A^C) = 1 - P(A)$.
4. If A and B are mutually exclusive, then $P(A \cap B) = 0$.

The first property indicates that the probability of the entire sample space is 1. Any experiment must certainly result in one of the outcomes in the sample space. The third property involving a complementary event is a useful way to calculate the probabilities. It can be used to avoid tedious probability calculations as we shall see in

58

Biostatistics for Oral Healthcare

the later sections. The fourth property implies that if A and B are mutually exclusive, then $P(A \cup B) = P(A) + P(B)$. We note that $A \cup A^C = \Omega$; the union of A and A^C yields the sample space. Clearly, A and A^C are mutually exclusive. The concept of mutually exclusiveness can be extended beyond two events. For example, if no two events among $E_1, E_2, \cdots, E_k$, $(k > 2)$ can occur at the same time, then they are mutually exclusive.

Example 4.3.2. There are 8 differential diagnoses of ulcers of the oral mucosa [1]: (1) aphthous stomatitis, (2) cancer, (3) chancre of syphilis, (4) deep fungal infection, (5) necrotizing sialometaplasia, (6) noma, (7) traumatic ulcer, and (8) tuberculosis. Suppose that only one specific diagnosis of the 8 differential diagnoses is made for a given patient at a time and that the different diagnoses are equally likely to be made. Let events A, B, and C be defined by $A = \{2, 4, 5, 8\}$, $B = \{2\}$, and $C = \{5, 7, 8\}$.

1. The events B and C are mutually exclusive, because they cannot occur simultaneously.
2. $P(B \text{ or } C) = P(B) + P(C) = \frac{1}{8} + \frac{3}{8} = \frac{4}{8} = \frac{1}{2}$.
3. $P(B^C) = 1 - P(B) = 1 - \frac{1}{8} = \frac{7}{8}$, by the third axiom of probability.

Let A be the event that the husband flosses his teeth at least once a day, and B be the event that the wife flosses her teeth at least once daily. If $P(A) = 0.45$, and $P(B) = 0.60$, what can we say about the event $A \cap B$ (A and B), that is, both husband and wife floss their teeth at least once a day? To address this type of situation, we need to introduce the following concept.

Definition 4.3.2. Two events A and B are said to be **statistically independent** or simply **independent** if $P(A \cap B) = P(A) \cdot P(B)$. If the events are not independent, we say they are **dependent**.

In simple terms, if the occurrence or non-occurrence of A does not influence the occurrence or non-occurrence of B, then A and B are statistically independent. If A and B are independent, the probability of the occurrence of both events is obtained by the product of $P(A)$ and $P(B)$. If the event A is independent of the event B, then B is also independent of A.

Example 4.3.3. (i) If the flossing habit of the husband is independent of the flossing habit of the wife, that is, the events A and B are statistically independent, then $P(A \cap B) = P(A)P(B) = (0.45)(0.60) = 0.27$. The chance that both husband and wife floss their teeth at least once a day is 0.27.

(ii) Suppose $P(A) = 0.45$ and $P(B) = 0.60$. If $P(A \cap B) = 0.38$, is the event that the husband flosses his teeth daily statistically independent of the event that the wife flosses her teeth daily? From Definition 4.3.2, if we can show $P(A \cap B) = P(A) \cdot P(B)$, then they are independent events. If $P(A \cap B) \neq P(A) \cdot P(B)$, then the events are not independent. Because $P(A) \cdot P(B) = (0.45) \cdot (0.60) = 0.27 \neq P(A \cap B)$, the events A and B are not independent.

Example 4.3.4. Let X be a random variable describing the probing depths of patients, A be the event that the probing depth is between 2 and 5 mm, and B be the event that the probing depth is between 3 and 7 mm. We can rewrite the events as $A = \{2 \leq X \leq 5\}$ and $B = \{3 \leq X \leq 7\}$. Then $A \cup B = \{2 \leq X \leq 7\}$ and $A \cap B = \{3 \leq X \leq 5\}$. The union of A and B is the event that the patient's probing depth is between 2 and 7 mm, and the intersection of A and B is the event that the patient's probing depth is between 3 and 5 mm. The probability $P(A \cup B)$ would mean the proportion of the patients whose probing depth is between 2 and 7 mm, and $P(A \cap B)$ the proportion of the patients whose probing depth is between 3 and 5 mm.

We now state a useful principle known as the addition rule of probability. We have learned from the axiom of probability that if A and B are mutually exclusive, then $P(A \cup B) = P(A) + P(B)$. A more general case where A and B are not mutually exclusive will be presented.

Addition Rule of Probability:
If A and B are any two events, then $P(A \cup B) = P(A) + P(B) - P(A \cap B)$.

To calculate the probability of the union $P(A \cup B)$, add two probabilities $P(A)$ and $P(B)$ separately, and subtract the probability corresponding to the overlapping area, $A \cap B$ (i.e., A and B), shown in Figure 4.3.2.

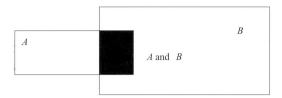

Figure 4.3.2 Overlapping area $A \cap B$.

Example 4.3.5. A dental researcher has been collecting extracted teeth in a jar. The jar contains cuspids, incisors, bicuspids, and molars. Suppose the events are defined by $A = \{$incisor, molar$\}$, $B = \{$cuspid, incisor$\}$, and $C = \{$cuspid, molar$\}$. He estimated the probabilities of A, B, and C by repeatedly drawing a tooth from the jar, one at a time with a replacement: $P(A) = 0.625$, $P(B) = 0.375$, $P(C) = 0.430$, $P(A \cap B) = 0.250$, and $P(A \cap C) = 0.375$. Then by the addition rule of probability

(i) $P(A \cup B) = P(A) + P(B) - P(A \cap B)$
$= 0.625 + 0.375 - 0.250 = 0.750$.
(ii) $P(A \cup C) = P(A) + P(C) - P(A \cap C)$
$= 0.625 + 0.430 - 0.375 = 0.680$.

Example 4.3.6. As part of a thorough dental examination, a patient was required to take a posterior periapical radiograph. Let A be the event Dr. Berry, after reviewing the periapical radiograph, makes the diagnosis that the patient has carious or pathologic lesions (i.e., a positive diagnosis), and B be the event that his associate, Dr. Jarvis, makes a positive diagnosis. If $P(A) = 0.20$, $P(B) = 0.26$, and the chances are 29.0% that either Dr. Berry or Dr. Jarvis makes a positive diagnosis, what is the probability that both dentists make a positive diagnosis?

Solution. From the given information, we have $P(A \cup B) = 0.29$. By applying the addition rule, we obtain $P(A \cap B) = P(A) + P(B) - P(A \cup B) = 0.20 + 0.26 - 0.29 = 0.17$.

There is a 17% chance that both dentists will make a positive diagnosis.

Example 4.3.7. More and more dentists recommend that youngsters who participate in sports activities wear mouthguards to protect their teeth. The chances of suffering an injury to teeth by those who do not wear mouthguards are significantly higher than among those who do. Let E_1 be the event of an injury to teeth when a mouthguard is not used, and E_2 be the event of an injury to teeth when a mouthguard is used. Let $P(E_1) = 0.15$ and $P(E_2) = 0.03$. The Moseley family has two boys, Jack and Tim, who play sports. Jack uses a mouthguard, and Tim doesn't. Suppose the two events E_1 and E_2 are independent. What is the probability that at least one of Mr. Moseley's boys will sustain an injury to his teeth during sports activity?

Solution. The event that at least one of the boys sustains an injury is equivalent to the event that either Jack or Tim sustains an injury. We can express the probability as follows:

P(at least one boy sustains an injury)

$= P$(Jack or Tim sustains an injury)

$= P(E_1 \cup E_2) = P(E_1) + P(E_2) - P(E_1 \cap E_2)$

$= P(E_1) + P(E_2) - P(E_1) \cdot (E_2)$, by independence

$= 0.15 + 0.03 - (0.15) \cdot (0.03) = 0.1755$.

The concepts of statistical independence and mutually exclusiveness can be generalized to the case of $k > 2$.

Definition 4.3.3.

(i) (Multiplication Law of Probability) If E_1, $E_2, \cdots, E_k$ are **mutually independent**, then

$$P(E_1 \cap E_2 \cap \cdot \cap E_k) = P(E_1)P(E_2) \cdots P(E_k).$$

(ii) The events $E_1, E_2, \cdots, E_k$ are **mutually exclusive** if no two events can occur at the same time.

(iii) A set of events $E_1, E_2, \cdots, E_k$ are **mutually exclusive and exhaustive** if no two events can occur at the same time and at least one of the events must occur. Therefore, exactly one of the events must occur.

This first identity is known as the **multiplication law of probability**. If k events are mutually independent, then the probability that k events occur simultaneously is obtained by the product of k individual probabilities. For brevity, the expressions $A \cap B$ and $E_1 \cap E_2 \cap \cdots \cap E_k$ are written as AB and $E_1 E_2 \cdots E_k$. Hereafter, we will write $P(AB)$ instead of $P(A \cap B)$ and $P(E_1 E_2 \cdots E_k)$ instead of $P(E_1 \cap E_2 \cap \cdots \cap E_k)$.

Example 4.3.8. A tooth can be classified into one of the following four categories; $\Omega = \{$healthy, decayed, missing, restored$\}$. Let $E_1 = \{$healthy, missing$\}$, $E_2 = \{$decayed$\}$, $E_3 = \{$restored$\}$, $E_4 = \{$healthy, missing, restored$\}$, $E_5 = \{$healthy$\}$, and $E_6 = \{$missing, restored$\}$.

1. The set of events E_1, E_2, and E_3 is mutually exclusive and exhaustive, because exactly one of the events in the set must occur.
2. However, the set of events E_2, E_3, and E_4 are not mutually exclusive and exhaustive, because E_3 and E_4 can occur at the same time whenever the outcome "restored" is observed.
3. The events E_1, E_2, E_3, and E_6 are not mutually exclusive and exhaustive.
4. The events E_2, E_3, and E_5 are mutually exclusive but not exhaustive.

Example 4.3.9. Suppose in a typical community the fluoride concentration level in the drinking water is 0.7 to 1.1 ppm. A study shows that a patient who resides in such a community has a 21% chance of developing a carious tooth. The study also indicates that the family members are independent of each other in developing carious teeth. Mr. and Mrs. Flossom have twin sons who are about 11 years old. What is the chance that all four members of the Flossom family will develop a carious tooth?

Solution. Let E_1, E_2, E_3, and E_4 denote the events that each of the four members in the Flossom family develop a carious tooth, respectively. Then

P(All four have a carious tooth)
$= P(E_1 E_2 E_3 E_4)$
$= P(E_1)P(E_2)P(E_3)P(E_4)$, by independence
$= (0.21) \cdot (0.21) \cdot (0.21) \cdot (0.21) \simeq 0.0019.$

There is about a 0.2% chance that all four in the family develop a carious tooth.

Frequently, we need to deal with more than two events together. If A is the event that the patient is a heavy smoker and has smoked more than 15 cigarettes since age 22, B the event that he has lived in a fluoridated community, and C is the event that he has the symptoms of a periradicular abscess, then what is the probability that A or B or C occurs? We state the following extension of the addition rule of probability.

Addition Rule of Probability: Let A, B, and C be three events. Then the probability of the occurrence of event A or B or C is given by

$$P(A \text{ or } B \text{ or } C) = P(A \cup B \cup C)$$
$$= P(A) + P(B) + P(C) - P(AB)$$
$$- P(AC) - P(BC) + P(ABC).$$

The event of the occurrence of "A or B or C" is equivalent to the event of the occurrence of "at least one of A, B, and C." The probability is obtained by first adding the three probabilities $P(A)$, $P(B)$, $P(C)$, and subtracting the three probabilities $P(A \cap B)$, $P(A \cap C)$, $P(B \cap C)$, corresponding to the overlapping areas, A and B, A and C, and B and C, and finally, adding the probability $P(A \cap B \cap C)$, corresponding to the overlapping area, A and B and C.

(i) If A, B, and C are mutually exclusive, $P(A \cap B) = 0$, $P(A \cap C) = 0$, $P(B \cap C) = 0$, and $P(A \cap B \cap C) = 0$. Thus, $P(A \cup B \cup C) = P(A) + P(B) + P(C)$.
(ii) If A, B, and C are mutually independent, then

$$P(A \cup B \cup C)$$
$$= P(A) + P(B) + P(C)$$
$$- P(AB) - P(AC) - P(BC) + P(ABC)$$
$$= P(A) + P(B) + P(C) - P(A)P(B)$$
$$- P(A)P(C) - P(B)P(C) + P(A)P(B)P(C).$$

Example 4.3.10. Consider three events A, B, and C:

A = Myocardial infarction patients who have periodontitis and reside in the fluoridated community.
B = Periodontitis patients with osteopetrosis who have myocardial infarction.
C = Osteopetrosis patients residing in the fluoridated community who have periodontitis.

Suppose that $P(A) = 0.12$, $P(B) = 0.06$, $P(C) = 0.09$, $P(AB) = 0.04$, $P(AC) = 0.06$, $P(BC) = 0.03$, and $P(ABC) = 0.02$. The chance that at least one of the three events is observed is

P(at least one of the events A, B, and C happens)
$= P(A \cup B \cup C)$
$= 0.12 + 0.06 + 0.09 - 0.04 - 0.06 - 0.03$
$+ 0.02 = 0.16.$

Example 4.3.11. Let A, B, C be the events that the patient has periodontitis, caries, and needs a root canel treatment. Suppose $P(A) = 0.25$, $P(B) = 0.45$, and $P(C) = 0.60$. (i). Are all the events mutually exclusive? (ii). What is $P(A$ or B or $C)$ if all three are independent?

Solution. (i) $P(A) + P(B) + P(C) = 0.25 + 0.45 + 0.60 = 1.30 > 1.0$. The sum of the three probabilities exceeds 1.0, which implies that there must be at least one pair of events that occur simultaneously. The three events A, B, C are not mutually exclusive.

(ii) $P(A$ or B or $C) = P(A) + P(B) + P(C)$
$\quad - P(A)P(B) - P(A)P(C) - P(B)P(C)$
$\quad + P(A)P(B)P(C)$, by independence
$= 0.25 + 0.45 + 0.60 - (0.25)(0.45)$
$\quad - (0.25)(0.60) - (0.45)(0.60)$
$\quad + (0.25)(0.45)(0.60)$
$= 0.835.$

It may be tempting to think that A and B are mutually exclusive if $P(A) + P(B) < 1.0$. In general, this cannot be true. For example, in the die-rolling experiment let $A = \{2, 5\}$ and $B = \{4, 5\}$. Clearly, $P(A) + P(B) = 2/6 + 2/6 = 4/6 < 1.0$, but A and B are not mutually exclusive.

4.4 INDEPENDENCE AND MUTUALLY EXCLUSIVE EVENTS

One might be tempted to think that if two events A and B are independent, then they are mutually exclusive. This is a common misconception among students. There is no relationship between these two concepts. Two events can be independent but not mutually exclusive, and vice versa. We will present biomedical examples to illustrate that there is no relationship between the two concepts.

Example 4.4.1. The following are examples of two events A and B that are independent, but not mutually exclusive:

1. A = Eruption of mandibular third molar, and B = high caries rate.

2. A = Radiation therapy for head and neck cancer, and B = root caries in a patient age 50 years of age or older.
3. A = Mom has a root fracture, and B = dad has a class II amalgam restoration.
4. A = A patient with the existence of squamous cell carcinoma, and B = a patient with a root fracture.
5. A = Candida infections in the oral cavity, and B = tooth decay.

Example 4.4.2. The following are examples of two events A and B that are not independent, but are mutually exclusive:

1. A = An avulsed tooth that is not replanted, and B = an avulsed tooth that is replanted with subsequent root canal treatment.
2. A = Vital uninflamed coronal pulp is present, and B = gutta-percha is present in the root canal system.
3. A = Tumor in tongue was detected at an advanced age, and B = heavy smoking earlier in life.
4. A = A patient suffers a trauma on a maxillary central incisor, and B = the same patient, 10 years later, having root canal treatment on the same tooth due to pulpal restriction from the trauma.

Example 4.4.3. The following are examples of two events A and B that are independent and mutually exclusive:

1. A = Exfoliation of deciduous dentition, and B = root surface caries in an elderly patient.
2. A = Candidiasis in a newborn child, and B = dental implants in an elderly patient.
3. A = Baby bottle decay at a young age, and B = broken denture at an old age.
4. A = Taking an impression of teeth, and B = filling a cavity.

Example 4.4.4. The following are examples of two events A and B that are not independent and are not mutually exclusive:

1. A = Periradicular lesion, and B = pulpal necrosis.
2. A = Wearing tongue jewelry, and B = fractured lingual cusp of a molar.

3. A = Gross caries in a tooth, and B = acute pulpitis.
4. A = Rampant decay of teeth, and B = xerostomia.
5. A = Formation of heavy plaque, and B = absence of regular toothbrushing.

4.5 CONDITIONAL PROBABILITY

We have discussed how to compute the probability of two or several events occurring at the same time when the events are independent. For example, $P(A$ and B and $C) = P(ABC) = P(A) \cdot P(B) \cdot P(C)$, if events A, B, and C are independent. How can we compute the probability that some events will occur simultaneously if they are not independent (or are dependent)? Let us consider rolling a balanced die. Let A be the event of observing the number 4, and B be the event of observing an even number, that is, $B = \{2, 4, 6\}$. Clearly, $P(A) = \frac{1}{6}$.

However, if a friend rolled a balanced die and told you that an even number was observed, what is the chance that your friend actually observed the number 4? In other words, what is the probability of the occurrence of event A, given that event B occurs? Knowing that an even number has turned up, and that there are only three possible outcomes that are even numbers (4 is one of the three possible even numbers, 2, 4, and 6), you will say the probability of event A, given that event B occurs, is $\frac{1}{3}$.

These two events are related in such a way that the probability of event A depends on the occurrence or non-occurrence of event B. The additional information, provided by event B, improves the probability of event A from $\frac{1}{6}$ to $\frac{1}{3}$. Events A and B are related, because a knowledge of B affects the probability of A. To quantify the probability of simultaneous occurrence of two events when the events are not independent, we introduce the concept of **conditional probability**.

The probabilities we have discussed, $P(A)$, $P(B)$, $P(E_1)$, $P(E_2)$, etc. are sometimes called the unconditional probabilities. Often the conditional probabilities are of greater interest to the health care professionals than unconditional probabilities. Dentists and physicians ask about a patient's lifestyle and individual and family medical histories to ascertain conditional probabilities such as the following:

- If a patient has consumed a fat- and cholesterol-rich diet most of his life, the chances of him developing a myocardial infarction are much greater.
- If a dentist knows that both parents of her patient suffered from osteogenesis imperfecta, she may offer a different treatment plan to the patient, based on the fact that the patient is more likely to develop osteogenesis imperfecta.
- If a patient has a periapical lesion as a consequence of pulpal necrosis and periodontal disease, the dentist will know that the patient might have an odontogenic infection and tooth loss will result with a high likelihood.
- If an individual is known to have been exposed to an influenza-infected environment, his chance of developing influenza is greater than that of individuals who have not been exposed.

Definition 4.5.1. The **conditional probability** of event A, given that event B has occurred, is denoted by $P(A|B)$ and is defined by

$$P(A|B) = \frac{P(A \text{ and } B)}{P(B)} = \frac{P(AB)}{P(B)}.$$

Similarly, the conditional probability of event B, given event A has occurred, is given by

$$P(B|A) = \frac{P(B \text{ and } A)}{P(A)} = \frac{P(BA)}{P(A)} = \frac{P(AB)}{P(A)}.$$

The conditional probabilities, $P(A|B)$ and $P(B|A)$ are not in general equal. They may look alike, but they represent two very different events. They are equal if and only if $P(A) = P(B)$. The vertical line (|) is read "given" or "conditioned on." Keep in mind that $A|B$ here does not mean that A is divided by B. The event B in the conditional probability statement $P(A|B)$ is called the "conditioning event."

Example 4.5.1. Soft-tissue trauma from dentures, oral infections from periodontal disease, and dental caries are known to put the patients at risk of developing osteoradionecrosis. Let A be the event that a patient has oral infections from periodontal disease and dental caries, and B be the event that a patient develops osteoradionecrosis. If $P(A) = 0.08$, $P(B) = 0.06$, and $P(AB) = 0.03$, what is the probability that a patient will develop osteoradionecrosis, given that the patient has oral infection from periodontal disease and dental caries?

Solution. By the definition of the conditional probability,

$$P(B|A) = \frac{P(BA)}{P(A)} = \frac{P(AB)}{P(A)} = \frac{0.03}{0.08}$$
$$= 0.375.$$

Example 4.5.2. Let C be the event that Dr. Tan diagnoses a patient as having acute periodontal disease, and D be the event that Dr. Robinson diagnoses a patient as having acute periodontal disease. If $P(C) = 0.24$, $P(D) = 0.20$, and $P(CD) = 0.16$, what is the chance that Dr. Robinson makes a positive diagnosis, provided that Dr. Tan makes a positive diagnosis?

Solution. The definition of the conditional probability yields

$$P(D|C) = \frac{P(DC)}{P(C)} = \frac{0.16}{0.24} \simeq 0.6667.$$

What is the chance that Dr. Tan makes a positive diagnosis, provided that Dr. Robinson makes a positive diagnosis? Again, using the definition,

$$P(C|D) = \frac{P(CD)}{P(D)} = \frac{0.16}{0.20} = 0.80.$$

Given that one of them has made a positive diagnosis, the chance that the other makes a positive diagnosis is much greater.

In Example 4.5.2, knowledge of conditioning event C improves the probability of event D. If the events A and B are independent, then the following relations hold:

1. If A and B are independent, then A and B^C are independent. To see this, consider the diagram in Figure 4.5.1.

   Events AB and AB^C are mutually exclusive, hence A can be written as the union of these two mutually exclusive events; $A = AB^C \cup AB$. Therefore, $P(A) = P(AB^C) +$

$P(AB)$. Subtracting $P(AB)$ from both sides of this equation, we get

$$P(AB^C) = P(A) - P(AB)$$
$$= P(A) - P(A)P(B),$$
   by independence of A and B.
$$= P(A)[1 - P(B)],$$
   by factoring out the common factor $P(A)$.
$$= P(A)P(B^C),$$
   since $P(B^C) = 1 - P(B)$.

This shows that the independence of A and B implies the independence of A and B^C.

2. $P(A|B) = \dfrac{P(AB)}{P(B)} = \dfrac{P(A)P(B)}{P(B)}$, by independence of A and B
$= P(A)$. [$P(B)$ in the numerator is cancelled against the $P(B)$ in the denominator.]

3. $P(A|B^C) = \dfrac{P(AB^C)}{P(B^C)} = \dfrac{P(A)P(B^C)}{P(B^C)}$
$= P(A)$, by independence of A and B^C

If A and B are independent, then the occurrence or non-occurrence of the conditioning event B does not affect the probability of the occurrence of A. Recall from the previous section, if A and B are independent, then $P(AB) = P(A) \cdot P(B)$. Alternatively, we say that A and B are independent if and only if $P(A|B) = P(A)$. Similarly, A and B are independent if and only if $P(B|A) = P(B)$. In Example 4.5.1, $P(B|A) = 0.375$ and $P(B) = 0.06$. Therefore, A and B are not independent.

Example 4.5.3. Leukoplakia is a white plaque formed on the oral mucous membrane from surface epithelial cells; this condition is suspected to be more prevalent among individuals who chew tobacco. Suppose A is the event that a patient is affected by leukoplakia, and B is the event that a patient chews tobacco. If $P(B) = 0.06$ and $P(AB) = 0.02$, then the probability that the patient is affected by leukoplakia, knowing that he chews tobacco, is

$$P(A|B) = \frac{P(AB)}{P(B)} = \frac{0.02}{0.06} = \frac{1}{3}.$$

If the patient chews tobacco, his chance of being affected by leukoplakia is about 33.3%.

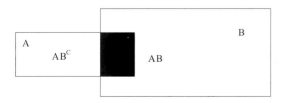

Figure 4.5.1 Events AB and AB^C.

By multiplying $P(A)$ to both sides of the conditional probability equation, we obtain

$$P(A) \cdot P(B|A) = \frac{P(AB)}{P(A)} \cdot P(A).$$

The following formula called the **multiplication law of probability** can be derived.

Multiplication Law of Probability

$$P(AB) = P(A) \cdot P(B|A)$$

or

$$P(AB) = P(B) \cdot P(A|B).$$

As a consequence of the multiplication law of probability, the following relationship holds:

$$P(A) \cdot P(B|A) = P(B) \cdot P(A|B).$$

The application of the multiplication law of probability is described in the next example.

Example 4.5.4. Having a high cholesterol level (say, more than 320 mg per 100 ml of blood) is one of the symptoms that a male patient will likely have a myocardial infarction. Let A be the event of high cholesterol level and B be the event of the male patient developing myocardial infarction. If $P(A) = 0.14$, and $P(B|A) = 0.28$, what is the chance that a male patient, who has a high cholesterol level, will develop a myocardial infarction?

Solution. By the multiplication law, $P(AB) = P(A) \cdot P(B|A) = (0.14)(0.28) = 0.0392$.

Suppose that a conditioning event is the complementary event A^c of event A. Then the conditional probability $P(B|A^c)$ can be stated

$$P(B|A^c) = \frac{P(A^c B)}{P(A^c)}.$$

The same type of the multiplication law as presented above can be derived:

$$P(A^c B) = P(A^c) \cdot P(B|A^c).$$

The unconditional probability $P(B)$ can be expressed in terms of the two multiplication laws we discussed. In Figure 4.5.2, the two mutually exclusive events AB and $A^c B$ are represented by the overlapping and the shaded areas, respectively. Then B is the union of AB and $A^c B$, or

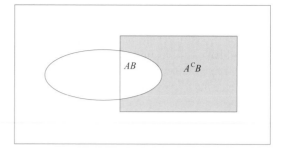

Figure 4.5.2 Events AB and $A^C B$.

$B = AB \cup A^c B$, from which we get

$$P(B) = P(AB) + P(A^C B)$$
$$= P(A) \cdot P(B|A) + P(A^c) \cdot P(B|A^c),$$

by multiplication laws.

Example 4.5.5. Bone resorption visible in radiographs could be strong evidence for periodontal disease. Let A be the event that bone resorption has occurred, and the bone height is below the cementoenamel junction, and let B be the event that the patient has periodontal disease. Suppose the patient data from a large dental clinic indicates that $P(A) = 0.08$, $P(B|A) = 0.90$, and $P(B|A^c) = 0.05$. What is the probability of periodontal disease in the general patient population?

Solution. By the above discussion,

$$P(B) = P(AB) + P(A^C B) = P(A) \cdot P(B|A)$$
$$+ P(A^c) \cdot P(B|A^c)$$
$$= (0.08) \cdot (0.90) + (1.0 - 0.08) \cdot (0.05)$$
$$= 0.118.$$

Example 4.5.6. Suppose A represents the event that the patient is diabetic, and B represents the event that the patient experiences delayed healing after a tooth extraction. If $P(A) = 0.13$, $P(B|A) = 0.74$, and $P(B|A^C) = 0.20$, what is the probability that the patient will experience delayed healing after the extraction?

Similar to Example 4.5.5,

$$P(B) = P(A) \cdot P(B|A) + P(A^c) \cdot P(B|A^c)$$
$$= (0.13) \cdot (0.74) + (0.87) \cdot (0.20)$$
$$= 0.2702.$$

The last two examples illustrate a useful relationship between the unconditional and conditional probabilities. The equation $P(B) = P(A) \cdot P(B|A) + P(A^c) \cdot P(B|A^c)$ can be viewed as the weighted average of the two conditional probabilities. The weights are given by $P(A)$ and $P(A^c)$. The aforementioned result can be extended to the case involving more than two mutually exclusive events. Let $A_1, A_2, \cdots, A_k$ be mutually exclusive and exhaustive events, and B be any given event. We obtain the following total probability law.

Total Probability Law

Let $A_1, A_2, \cdots, A_k$ be mutually exclusive and exhaustive events and B be any given event. Then $P(B) = \sum_{i=1}^{k} P(A_i)P(B|A_i)$. Because $P(A_1) + P(A_2) + \cdots + P(A_k) = 1.0$, $P(B) = \sum_{i=1}^{k} P(A_i)P(B|A_i)$ is the weighted average of k conditional probabilities $P(B|A_i)$. An application of the total probability law is discussed below.

Example 4.5.7. There are three types of early childhood caries (ECC) [2]. Type I ECC is mild to moderate, evidenced by isolated carious lesions involving molars and/or incisors. Type II ECC is moderate to severe, seen as labiolingual caries on maxillary incisors, with or without molar caries and unaffected mandibular incisors. Type III ECC is severe, evidenced by type II including the involvement of lower incisors. Let A_1, A_2, and A_3 be the events representing the three types of ECC and B be the event that a child has bacteremia. Suppose that $P(A_1) = 0.48$, $P(A_2) = 0.30$, and $P(A_3) = 0.22$. If $P(B|A_1) = 0.009$, $P(B|A_2) = 0.01$, and $P(B|A_3) = 0.04$, what is the chance that a child, whether or not he is affected by ECC, has bacteremia?

Solution. First of all, events A_1, A_2, and A_3 are mutually exclusive and exhaustive. By applying the total probability law, we obtain:

$$P(B) = P(A_1)P(B|A_1) + P(A_2)P(B|A_2)$$
$$+ P(A_3)P(B|A_3)$$
$$= (0.48) \cdot (0.009) + (0.30) \cdot (0.01)$$
$$+ (0.22) \cdot (0.04) \simeq 0.016\,1.$$

The chance that a child has bacteremia is 0.0161.

Example 4.5.8. Cancer of the pancreas is rarely curable. It accounts for only 2% of all newly diagnosed cancers in the U.S. each year, but 5% of all cancer deaths. National Cancer Institute data indicates that the highest survival occurs if the tumor is truly localized. Let A be the event that the tumor is localized, and B the event that patients survive at least 5 years. It is known that $P(A) = 0.20$, $P(B|A) = 0.20$, and $P(B|A^c) = 0.0001$. What is the 5-year survival rate of a patient who is recently diagnosed with a pancreatic cancer?

Solution. Because two events A and A^c are mutually exclusive and exhaustive, and $P(A) = 0.20$, we have $P(A^c) = 1 - 0.20 = 0.80$. Using the total probability law, the 5-year survival rate of a patient with a pancreatic cancer can be expressed as

$$P(B) = P(A)P(B|A) + P(A^c)P(B|A^c)$$
$$= (0.20)(0.20) + (0.80)(0.0001)$$
$$= 0.040\,08.$$

4.6 BAYES THEOREM

In the previous section, we pointed out the difference between $P(B|A)$ and $P(A|B)$. We learned from the discussions of the conditional probability that $P(B|A)$ can be found if $P(AB)$ and $P(A)$ are known. What if $P(AB)$ and $P(A)$ are not directly available? Can we still find the conditional probability $P(B|A)$? The theorem formulated by the Reverend Thomas Bayes, known as the Bayes theorem, will address this question. The following are examples of the practical questions that clinicians in dentistry and medicine often ask:

- What is the probability that the patient has the disease, if the test results are positive?
- What is the probability that the patient does not have the disease, if the test results are negative?
- If the patient has periodontal inflammation, what is the chance that he has an acute periodontitis?
- If the patient has no signs of periodontal inflammation, what is the chance that he does not have an acute periodontitis?

Bayes theorem has a wide variety of applications in health sciences [3, 4]. From the multiplication law of probability, we have

$$P(AB) = P(A) \cdot P(B|A) = P(B) \cdot P(A|B).$$

After dividing both sides of $P(A) \cdot P(B|A) = P(B) \cdot P(A|B)$ in the above equation by $P(A)$, we can establish the relationship between $P(B|A)$ and $P(A|B)$:

$$P(B|A) = \frac{P(B) \cdot P(A|B)}{P(A)}.$$

This last equation enables us to compute the conditional probability $P(B|A)$ in terms of the other conditional probability, $P(A|B)$. We may think of A as symptoms and B as the disease.

Example 4.6.1. Whenever the decision has to be made whether to perform an endodontic treatment on a tooth or to extract the tooth, it is important to gain an insight into the probability of success or failure under the given circumstances, such as type of tooth, age of the patient, vital or necrotic pulp, presence or absence of periapical rarefaction, acute or chronic periapical inflammation, etc., especially when the tooth is to be used as an abutment in a complex multitooth restoration [3]. Suppose that A represents the event that the pulp is necrotic, S and F represent success and failure of an endodontic treatment, respectively. If the patient has a necrotic pulp, the chance of failure of the endodontic treatment is 0.16, and if the patient does not have necrotic pulp, the chance of failure is 0.04. Suppose about 10% of patients have necrotic pulp. Among the patients whose endodontic treatment failed, what percent of the patients would have necrotic pulp?

Solution. We can summarize the given information in the example as: $P(A) = P$ (pulp is necrotic) $= 0.10$, $P(F|A) = 0.16$, and $P(F|A^C) = 0.04$. Before we can compute $P(A|F)$, we need to determine $P(F)$. To gain some insights, let us consider the path diagram in Figure 4.6.1.

The event F is observed via the path going through the event A or via the path going through the event A^C. The probabilities of observing these

paths are

$$P(A)P(F|A) = (0.10)(0.16) = 0.016$$

and

$$P(A^C)P(F|A^C) = (0.90)(0.04) = 0.036.$$

Because the two paths are mutually exclusive, we have $P(F) = 0.016 + 0.036 = 0.052$.

From the definition of the conditional probability,

$$P(A|F) = \frac{P(A) \cdot P(F|A)}{P(A)} = \frac{0.016}{0.052} = 0.3077.$$

About 30.8% of the patients had necrotic pulp, given their endodontic treatment failed.

Example 4.6.2. Tooth mobility is important in the development of a prognosis and vital to treatment planning. Mobility is gauged in millimeters by the motion back and forth in a buccal/lingual direction. It is classified into four categories, $E_1 =$ no mobility, $E_2 =$ class I mobility, $E_3 =$ class II mobility, and $E_4 =$ class III mobility. It is estimated that among the general patient population, $P(E_1) = 0.05$, $P(E_2) = 0.40$, $P(E_3) = 0.30$, and $P(E_4) = 0.25$. Let A be the event that the patient brushes and flosses at least once every day. If $P(A|E_1) = 0.86$, $P(A|E_2) = 0.17$, $P(A|E_3) = 0.08$, and $P(A|E_4) = 0.04$, what is the probability that a patient is of class III mobility, knowing that he has been brushing and flossing daily?

Solution. We are interested in the conditional probability $P(E_4|A) = P(AE_4)/P(A)$. Events E_1, E_2, E_3, and E_4 are mutually exclusive and exhaustive, because a tooth can belong to exactly one of the four categories. From the diagram in Figure 4.6.2, we can easily see that event A can be decomposed into four mutually exclusive and exhaustive events,

$$\mapsto A \quad\text{—— } F : P(A)P(F|A) = (0.10)(0.16)$$
$$= 0.016.$$

⊛

$$\mapsto A^C \text{——} F : P(A^C)P(F|A^C) = (0.90)(0.04)$$
$$= 0.036.$$

Figure 4.6.1 Diagram for path probabilities.

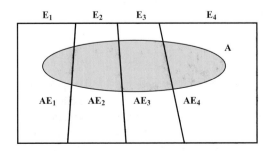

Figure 4.6.2 Diagram of tooth mobility categories and event.

AE_1, AE_2, AE_3, and AE_4 and therefore, the probability $P(A)$ can be written as the sum of $P(AE_1)$, $P(AE_2)$, $P(AE_3)$, and $P(AE_4)$.

$$P(A) = P(AE_1) + P(AE_2) + P(AE_3) + P(AE_4).$$

By applying the multiplication law,

$$P(AE_i) = P(A|E_i)P(E_i), \quad i = 1, 2, 3, \text{ and } 4.$$

$$P(E_4|A) = \frac{P(AE_4)}{P(A)}, \text{ by the definition of}$$
$$\text{conditional probability}$$

$$= \frac{P(A|E_4)P(E_4)}{P(AE_1) + P(AE_2) + P(AE_3) + P(AE_4)}$$

$$= \frac{P(A|E_4)P(E_4)}{P(A|E_1)P(E_1) + P(A|E_2)P(E_2) + P(A|E_3)P(E_3) + P(A|E_4)P(E_4)}$$

$$= \frac{(0.04) \cdot (0.25)}{(0.86) \cdot (0.05) + (0.17) \cdot (0.40) + (0.08) \cdot (0.30) + (0.04) \cdot (0.25)} \simeq 0.069.$$

Example 4.6.2 states that in general, about 25% of teeth are of class III mobility. But if the patient brushes and flosses daily, there is only about 6.9% chance that his teeth are of class III mobility. This new probability information, $P(E_4|A) \simeq 0.069$, can be used to convince patients to brush and floss regularly to maintain good oral health. The concept discussed in Example 4.6.2 can be extended to a case where there are more than three mutually exclusive and exhaustive events. In clinical cases there are often several disease states, for example, stage 1, stage 2, stage 3, and stage 4 carcinoma. Clinicians are interested in predicting the probability of a disease state, given a specific symptom. We state the Bayes theorem.

Bayes Theorem

Let E_1, E_2, $\cdots$, E_k be mutually exclusive and exhaustive events, and A be an event such that $P(A) \neq 0$. Then

$$P(E_i|A) = \frac{P(A|E_i)P(E_i)}{\sum_{j=1}^{k} P(A|E_j)P(E_j)}.$$

As discussed in Example 4.6.2, the expression in the denominator equals $P(A)$. In the clinical case, typically, the event A represents a specific symptom or a set of symptoms, and E_i's represent the disease states, which are mutually exclusive and exhaustive in the sense that at least one disease state must occur, and no two disease states can occur at the same time.

Example 4.6.3. Thoden van Velzen et al. [3] discussed the effect of a complication on the success-failure rate computed for a tooth with a preoperative necrotic pulp and periapical rarefaction. Let A, E_1, E_2, and E_3 represent the events

A = a preoperative necrotic pulp and periapical rarefaction

E_1 = success
E_2 = doubtful
E_3 = failure on the treatment results

The probabilities are given by $P(E_1) = 0.84$, $P(E_2) = 0.07$, and $P(E_3) = 0.09$. These probabilities are sometimes referred to as the *prior probabilities*. Also given are $P(A|E_1) = 0.09$, $P(A|E_2) = 0.09$, and $P(A|E_3) = 0.35$. These are probabilities associated with the event A (a particular symptom), given the occurrence of success, doubtful outcome, and failure, which are mutually exclusive and exhaustive events. These conditional probabilities are sometimes referred to as *likelihoods*. What are the probabilities of observing the events of the treatment results, E_1, E_2, and E_3, given the event A (a preoperative necrotic pulp and periapical rarefaction)?

Solution. By applying Bayes theorem with $k = 3$, we obtain

$$P(E_1|A)$$
$$= \frac{P(A|E_1)P(E_1)}{\sum_{j=1}^{3} P(A|E_j)P(E_j)}$$
$$= \frac{(0.09) \cdot (0.84)}{(0.09)(0.84) + (0.09)(0.07) + (0.35)(0.09)}$$
$$= 0.6667.$$

$P(E_2|A)$

$$= \frac{P(A|E_2)P(E_2)}{\sum_{j=1}^{3} P(A|E_j)P(E_j)}$$

$$= \frac{(0.09)\cdot(0.07)}{(0.09)(0.84) + (0.09)(0.07) + (0.35)(0.09)}$$

$$= 0.0556.$$

$P(E_3|A)$

$$= \frac{P(A|E_3)P(E_3)}{\sum_{j=1}^{3} P(A|E_j)P(E_j)}$$

$$= \frac{(0.35)\cdot(0.09)}{(0.09)(0.84) + (0.09)(0.07) + (0.35)(0.09)}$$

$$= 0.277\,8.$$

Bayes theorem tells us that, given a tooth with a preoperative necrotic pulp and periapical rarefaction, there is about a 66.7% chance that the treatment will be successful, and a 27.8% chance that it will fail.

Example 4.6.4. Suppose a 40-year old male patient has been under stress and smokes a pack of cigarettes a day. During a regular dental examination, white patches on the buccal mucosa were found. The patient is aware of the condition, but no symptoms have surfaced. The dentist was concerned and did the biopsy of the region. The following events are defined.

A = White patches on the buccal mucosa.
B_1 = Lichen planus.
B_2 = Hairy leukoplakia.
B_3 = Focal hyperkeratosis.
B_4 = Follicular keratosis.
B_5 = White spongy nevus.
B_6 = Normal, benign.

Event A represents the symptom, and events $B_1, B_2, \cdots, B_6$ are disease states that are mutually exclusive and exhaustive. If $P(B_1) = 0.24$, $P(B_2) = 0.17$, $P(B_3) = 0.19$, $P(B_4) = 0.11$, and $P(B_5) = 0.17$, suppose $P(A|B_1) = 0.09$, $P(A|B_2) = 0.12$, $P(A|B_3) = 0.15$, $P(A|B_4) = 0.21$, $P(A|B_5) = 0.27$, and $P(A|B_6) = 0.03$. For this 40-year old patient with white patches on buccal mucosa, which one of the six disease states is most likely to occur?

Solution. From the given information and Bayes theorem, we can obtain

$$P(B_6) = 1 - \{P(B_1) + P(B_2) + P(B_3) + P(B_4) + P(B_5)\}$$
$$= 1 - (0.24 + 0.17 + 0.19 + 0.11 + 0.17) = 0.12.$$

$$P(B_1|A) = P(\text{lichen planus} \mid \text{white patches on buccal mucosa}) = \frac{P(A|B_1)P(B_1)}{\sum_{j=1}^{6} P(A|B_j)P(B_j)}$$

$$= \frac{(0.09)(0.24)}{(.09)(.24) + (.12)(.17) + (.15)(.19) + (.21)(.11) + (.27)(.17) + (.03)(.12)} \simeq 0.150\,9.$$

$$P(B_2|A) = P(\text{hairy leukoplakia} \mid \text{white patches on buccal mucosa})$$

$$= \frac{(0.12)\cdot(0.17)}{(.09)(.24) + (.12)(.17) + (.15)(.19) + (.21)(.11) + (.27)(.17) + (.03)(.12)} \simeq 0.142\,6.$$

$$P(B_3|A) = P(\text{focal hyperkeratosis} \mid \text{white patches on buccal mucosa})$$

$$= \frac{(0.15)(0.19)}{(.09)(.24) + (.12)(.17) + (.15)(.19) + (.21)(.11) + (.27)(.17) + (.03)(.12)} \simeq 0.199\,2.$$

$$P(B_4|A) = P(\text{follicular keratosis} \mid \text{white patches on buccal mucosa})$$

$$= \frac{(0.21)(0.11)}{(.09)(.24) + (.12)(.17) + (.15)(.19) + (.21)(.11) + (.27)(.17) + (.03)(.12)} \simeq 0.161\,4.$$

$$P(B_5|A) = P(\text{white spongy nevus} \mid \text{white patches on buccal mucosa})$$

$$= \frac{(0.27)\cdot(0.17)}{(.09)(.24) + (.12)(.17) + (.15)(.19) + (.21)(.11) + (.27)(.17) + (.03)(.12)} \simeq 0.320\,8.$$

$$P(B_6|A) = P(\text{benign} \mid \text{white patches on buccal mucosa})$$

$$= \frac{(0.03)\cdot(0.12)}{(.09)(.24) + (.12)(.17) + (.15)(.19) + (.21)(.11) + (.27)(.17) + (.03)(.12)} \simeq 0.0252.$$

In this example, given the symptom of white patches on buccal mucosa, the disease state of white spongy nevus is most likely to occur with probability 0.3208.

When white patches are found on buccal mucosa (i.e., the event A), the chance of having hairy leukoplakia is about 5.7 times greater (0.1426 vs. 0.0252), and the chance of having white spongy nevus is about 12.7 times greater (0.3208 vs. 0.0252) than the chance that the condition is normal. Although the unconditional probability of B_5 (the event of white spongy nevus) is 0.17, the conditional probability of the disease, given the symptom, is 0.3208. When the symptom is present, the patient is almost twice as likely to have white spongy nevus as he does when the symptom is not present.

4.7 RATES AND PROPORTIONS

This section will examine clinical phenomena in a population, called rates and proportions, which are useful in biomedical and health sciences. In order to assess the study phenomena in a population, we need to quantify them accurately. The events of epidemiologic interest are usually diseases, illnesses, disabilities, or deaths—how they spread, how they infect the population at risk, how to control them—and prediction of the occurrence of a certain type of disease and its impact on the communities. Accurate predictions and clear understanding of diseases and infections will aid in public health policies and in developing preventive measures. We begin the discussion by introducing two of the most fundamental concepts in epidemiology: prevalence and incidence rates. The term *rate* refers to the amount of change taking place in a specified variable with respect to time.

4.7.1 Prevalence and Incidence

Definition 4.7.1. Prevalence rate is the number of people in a defined population who have a specified disease or condition at a fixed point in time divided by the size of the population at that time point. Sometimes this is called **point prevalence rate.** This refers to the probability of currently

having the disease, irrespective of the duration of time the patient has had the disease.

Definition 4.7.2. Incidence rate is the number of new cases (occurrences) of a specified disease, injury, or death during a given time period divided by the size of the population in that specific time interval. This refers to the probability that an individual with no prior disease will develop a new case of the disease over some fixed time period.

It is straightforward to estimate the prevalence rate of a disease, but often it is not a simple matter to determine the denominator for the incidence rate because the population size will change as people move in and out of the communities. It may not always be known how many people were at risk during the study period. It is customary to substitute for the denominator the average of the known population sizes during the specified time period.

Example 4.7.1. A squamous cell carcinoma is a malignant epithelial neoplasm with cells resembling those of the epidermis. It is reported that approximately 50% of squamous cell carcinomas have metastasized at the time of diagnosis. The local chapter of the dental association in the city of Colton contacted dental and medical offices, clinics, and hospitals in the area to collect patient data on squamous cell carcinoma. As of early January there were 128 known cases of squamous cell carcinoma patients who resided in Colton. Between January and June, 43 new cases were reported in the city. The city record shows that as of January, there were 10, 250 people in the city. However, in June there were only 7, 750 residents, because most of the college students left town for the summer. What is the prevalence rate as of January, and what is the incidence rate of squamous cell carcinoma during the period between January and June for the city?

Solution. The prevalence rate as of January is obtained by

Prevalence rate
$$= \frac{\text{The number of known cases as of January}}{\text{The size of the population in the city as of January}}$$
$$= \frac{128}{10, 250} \simeq 0.0125 \text{ (or } 1.25\%).$$

For the incidence rate we need to compute the average population size during the study period from

January to June, that is, $(10, 250 + 7, 750)/2 = 9,000$.

Incidence rate

$$= \frac{\text{The number of new cases in the city between January and June}}{\text{The average size of the population in the city during study period}}$$

$$= \frac{43}{9,000} \simeq 0.0048 \text{ (or approximately, 0.5\%)}.$$

4.7.2 Sensitivity and Specificity

For clinicians in dentistry and medicine, diagnostic tests are important screening tools for determining the presence or absence of a disease or genetic markers, such as the skin test for tuberculosis, the full mouth radiographs for caries detection, and biopsy for malignancy. Other diagnostic tools are home pregnancy test kits, Breathalyzers for police officers, and airport security devices. Diagnostic testing is one of the areas where probability is proven quite useful. In biomedical health sciences, we try to detect the presence or absence of a specified medical condition in human subjects. We have learned in the past that diagnostic tools are not foolproof. They could not always detect the condition when it truly is present, or they falsely indicate the condition in patients when it does not exist at all. The test results fall into one of the four categories.

1. **True positive** ($T+$): The condition is present or the patient has the disease and the diagnostic test detects the condition. The test result is correct and no error has been made.
2. **False negative** ($F-$): The condition is present or the patient has the disease, but the diagnostic test does not detect it. The test result indicates the condition is absent or the patient does not have the disease. The test result is incorrect and an error has been made.
3. **True negative** ($T-$): The condition is absent or the patient does not have the disease, and the diagnostic test indicates that the condition is not present. The test result is correct and no error has been made.
4. **False positive** ($F+$): The condition is absent or the patient does not have the disease, but the diagnostic test indicates that the condition is present. The test result is incorrect and an error has been made.

There are two types of errors: a false positive and a false negative. These can be defined in the context of the conditional probability.

Definition 4.7.3. False positive rate α (Greek letter, alpha) and **false negative rate** β (Greek letter, beta) of a diagnostic test are defined by

$\alpha = P(F+)$
$\quad = P(\text{test result is positive} \mid \text{subject does not have a disease})$
$\quad = P(\text{test result is positive} \mid \text{subject is a true negative}).$

$\beta = P(F-)$
$\quad = P(\text{test result is negative} \mid \text{subject does have a disease})$
$\quad = P(\text{test result is negative} \mid \text{subject is a true positive}).$

False positive and false negative rates describe the probability of obtaining incorrect test results. Two other rates that represent the probability of making correct decisions in diagnostic tests are defined below.

Definition 4.7.4. The **sensitivity rate** of a test is the probability that the test results are positive, given that the patient has the disease:

Sensitivity rate
$\quad = P(\text{test result is positive} \mid \text{subject is a true positive}).$

Definition 4.7.5. The **specificity rate** of a test is the probability that the test results are negative, given that the patient does not have the disease:

Specificity rate
$\quad = P(\text{test result is negative} \mid \text{subject is a true negative}).$

The sensitivity represents the chance that a patient who has the disease is correctly diagnosed

Table 4.7.1. Four categories of diagnostic test results.

	Disease State	
Test Result	Disease	No Disease
Positive (+)	True positive ($T+$)	False positive ($F+$)
Negative (−)	False negative ($F-$)	True negative ($T-$)

as having the disease, and the specificity represents the chance that a patient who does not have the disease is correctly diagnosed as not having the disease. What we have discussed above can be summarized in a simple table (Table 4.7.1).

Example 4.7.2. The hygienists at a university dental clinic screened 220 patients for an acute periodontal disease. Later, a more careful examination was given by periodontists. The results of the periodontal examination indicated that 45 were true positives, 14 false negatives, 26 false positives, and 135 true negatives. Compute the false positive (α), false negative (β), sensitivity and specificity rates.

Solution. The number of patient subjects ($n = 220$) is fixed, but the number of patients with or without a periodontal disease and the number of patients who are tested positive or negative are not fixed. These numbers are in fact random. The results described in the example can be presented in the following table.

	Disease State		
Screening Test by Hygienists	Perio Disease	No Perio Disease	Total Tested
Test positive	45	26	71
Test negative	14	135	149
	59	161	220

By Definition 4.7.3, the false positive rate α is the conditional probability P(test result is positive | subject is a true negative). To compute α, we need to compute P(subject is a true negative) and P(subject is a true negative *and* test result is positive) from the table. The total number of patients with an acute periodontal disease is

$$\text{(true positives)} + \text{(false negatives)} = 45 + 14$$
$$= 59,$$

and the total number of patients without an acute

periodontal disease is

$$\text{(true negatives)} + \text{(false positives)} = 135 + 26$$
$$= 161.$$

It is easy to see that P(subject is a true negative) $= 161/220$, and P(subject is a true negative *and* test result is positive) $= 26/220$. Thus,

$\alpha = P$(test result is positive | subject is a true negative)

$$= \frac{26/220}{161/220} = \frac{26}{161} \simeq 0.1615.$$

A similar argument leads to the calculation of the false negative rate:

$$P\text{(subject is a true positive)} = 59/220,$$

and

$$P\text{(subject is a true positive } and \text{ test result}$$
$$\text{is negative)} = 14/220.$$

Thus,

$\beta = P$(test result is negative | subject is a true positive).

$$= \frac{14/220}{59/220} = \frac{14}{59} \simeq 0.2373.$$

Similarly, the sensitivity and the specificity rates can be estimated from the table as follows.

Sensitivity rate

$= P$(test result is positive | subject is a true positive)

$$= \frac{P\text{(subject is a true positive } and \text{ test result is positive)}}{P\text{(subject is a true positive)}}$$

$$= \frac{45/220}{59/220} = \frac{45}{59} \simeq 0.7627.$$

Specificity rate

$= P$(test result is negative | subject is a true negative)

$$= \frac{P\text{(subject is a true negative } and \text{ test result is negative)}}{P\text{(subject is a true negative)}}$$

$$= \frac{135/220}{161/220} = \frac{135}{161} \simeq 0.8385.$$

Example 4.7.3. *Streptococcus mutans* is a caries-causing organism. Children tend to acquire this organism between the ages of about 1 and 3 years. A new diagnostic technique for detection of *Streptococcus mutans* has been introduced. The manufacturer claims that both sensitivity and specificity rates of the technique are at least 95%. To verify the claim, we have prepared 200 samples with *S. mutans*, and 150 samples without it. The new technique correctly indicated that 191 samples out of 200 contain *S. mutans* and also indicated that 143

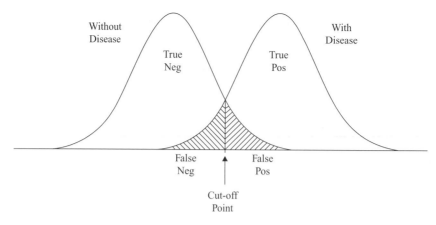

Without   With
Disease   Disease

True   True
Neg   Pos

False   False
Neg   Pos

Cut-off
Point

Figure 4.7.1   Relationship between sensitivity and specificity.

samples of 150 do not contain any *S. mutans*. Does your data support the manufacturer's claims?

Solution.

$$\text{Sensitivity} = \frac{P(\text{subject is a true positive } and \text{ test result is positive})}{P(\text{subject is a true positive})} = \frac{191/350}{200/350} = 0.9550 \ (95.5\%).$$

$$\text{Specificity} = \frac{P(\text{subject is a true negative } and \text{ test result is negative})}{P(\text{subject is a true negative})} = \frac{143/350}{150/350} \simeq 0.9533 \ (95.33\%).$$

Because both sensitivity and specificity rates of the diagnostic technique exceed 95%, the manufacturer's claim is supported and credible.

The most ideal situation, of course, is when both the sensitivity and the specificity rates are 100%, but in practice this is unlikely to happen. No diagnostic techniques are perfect at all times. The relationship between these two rates is depicted in the Figure 4.7.1.

The graph on the right-hand side represents the patients *with* the disease, and the one on the left-hand side represents the patients *without* the disease. The values along the X-axis represent the values of the diagnostic test results, such as blood pressure, hemoglobin, and white blood cell counts. Usually the diagnostic devices have a cut-off point or a threshold value below which the test results are considered negative and above which the test results are considered positive. The vertical line in the middle of the overlapping area in Figure 4.7.1 indicates the cut-off point. Those patients *with* the disease whose diagnostic test value is to the right of the cut-off point are true positives to the left of the cut-off point in the overlapping area are false negatives. These patients do indeed have the disease but the diagnostic test does not so indicate. Those patients *without* the disease, whose diagnostic test value is to the left of the cut-off point, are true negatives and to the right of the cut-off point in the overlapping area are false positives. These patients do not have the disease, but the diagnostic test results erroneously indicate that they do.

By setting the cut-off point at a different location, we can change the sensitivity and specificity rates. If we moved the cut-off point to the right, the number of false negatives would increase, and at the same time, the number of false positives would decrease. Likewise, if we moved the cut-off point to the left, the number of false negatives would decrease, and at the same time, the number of false positives would increase.

In health sciences, what follows the diagnostic test results is an appropriate treatment. The true positives and false positives will be offered an appropriate treatment, whereas the true negatives and false negatives will not. We are faced with a difficult situation in which the false positives, who do not have the disease and therefore do not need the treatment, will be given the treatment. On the other hand, the false negatives, who have the disease and therefore are in need of the treatment, will not be given the treatment. Both situations involve risks to patients.

4.7.3 Relative Risk and Odds Ratio

Clinicians often talk about risk factors; smoking is a risk factor for lung cancer, the positive skin test is a risk factor for tuberculosis, tobacco and alcohol use are the major risk factors for the development of oral cancer, and oral contraceptives and antimalarial agents are risk factors for mucosal pigmentation. A risk factor is neither a necessary nor a sufficient condition for developing the disease. The probability of developing the disease in a group of patients who have the risk factor is likely to be greater than the probability of the disease in a group of patients without the risk factor. **Relative risk** is an important concept that is useful to compare the probabilities of disease in two different groups; one group consists of subjects who have been exposed to the risk factor, and the other consists of subjects who have not been exposed to the risk factor. Two conditional probabilities are involved in the definition of relative risk. Relative risk is defined by the ratio between these two conditional probabilities: the probability of developing the disease, given that a risk factor is present, and the probability of developing the disease, given that a risk factor is not present. The relative risk of D (disease), given that E (exposure) is defined below.

Definition 4.7.6. Let D represent the event of disease and E the event of exposure to a risk factor. Then the complementary event E^C represents the event of non-exposure to a risk factor. The relative risk (RR) is defined by

$$RR = \frac{P(\text{Disease} \mid \text{Exposed to a risk factor})}{P(\text{Disease} \mid \text{Not exposed to a risk factor})}$$
$$= \frac{P(D|E)}{P(D|E^C)}.$$

If D and E are independent, then from the discussions in Section 4.5, the relative risk is

$$RR = \frac{P(D|E)}{P(D|E^C)} = \frac{P(D)}{P(D)} = 1.0.$$

If the events D and E are not independent (or dependent), then the RR will be different from 1.0.

Example 4.7.4. Lung cancer is the number one cause of cancer deaths in both men and women in the United States. Approximately 160, 100 Americans died from lung cancer in 1998. The overwhelming majority of lung cancer, at least 90%, are caused by cigarette smoking [5]. It was estimated that 144, 100 lung cancer deaths per year are caused by smoking. As of 1998 there are about 192.5 million adult Americans, of which 47.2 million are smokers. What is the RR?

Solution. Let D be the event of death due to lung cancer, and let S and S^C be the events representing adult smokers and adult non-smokers, respectively. The conditional probabilities can be expressed

$$P(D|S) = \frac{P(\text{death among smokers})}{P(\text{smokers})}$$
$$= \frac{(144, 100/192, 500, 000)}{(47, 200, 000/192, 500, 000)}$$
$$\simeq 0.0031$$

$$P(D|S^C) = \frac{P(\text{death among non-smokers})}{P(\text{non-smokers})}$$
$$= \frac{(16, 000/192, 500, 000)}{(145, 300, 000/192, 500, 000)}$$
$$\simeq 0.0001.$$

The relative risk is now given by

$$RR = \frac{P(D|S)}{P(D|S^C)} = \frac{0.0031}{0.0001} = 31.$$

The resulting $RR = 31$ means that smokers are 31 times more likely to die from lung cancer than non-smokers. The relative risk is also known as the risk ratio, because it involves the ratio of the risk of a disease in the exposed group to the risk in the unexposed group.

Sensitivity and specificity are interesting and important epidemiologic concepts, but they do not address certain questions that are of great value to clinicians. If a patient is tested positive for a disease, what is the probability that the patient does indeed have the disease? Or if a patient is tested negative, what is the probability that the patient does not have the disease? These questions are related to the concept of the predictive value of diagnostic test results.

Table 4.7.2. The association between risk factor and disease.

| | Disease Status | | |
Risk Factor	Present	Absent	Total
Present	a	b	a + b
Absent	c	d	c + d
Total	a + c	b + d	a + b + c + d

Definition 4.7.7. (i) The **predictive value positive** (PV$^+$) of a diagnostic test is the conditional probability that a subject has the disease, given that the test result is positive, denoted by PV$^+$ = P(disease | test is +).
(ii) The **predictive value negative** (PV$^-$) of a diagnostic test is the conditional probability that a subject does not have the disease, given that the test result is negative, denoted by PV$^-$ = P(no disease | test is −).

Example 4.7.5. Suppose that the probability that a subject has lung cancer, given he is a smoker, is 0.0030, and the probability that a subject has lung cancer, given he is not a smoker, is 0.0001. Then

$$PV^+ = P(\text{disease | test is+})$$
$$= P(\text{lung cancer | smoker}) = 0.0030,$$

and

$$PV^- = P(\text{no disease | test is−})$$
$$= P(\text{no lung cancer | non-smoker})$$
$$= 1 - P(\text{lung cancer | non-smoker})$$
$$= 1 - 0.0001 = 0.9999.$$

Another useful concept of the relative probabilities is that of **odds ratio**. Table 4.7.2 exhibits the association between risk factor and disease. The risk of the disease in the exposed group is $a/(a + b)$, whereas the odds of the disease in the exposed group is a/b.

In sporting events, people often talk about the odds in favor of the home team. Let p be the probability of a success. Then $1 - p$ is the probability of a failure. The odds in favor of the home team's success is given by the proportion $p/(1 - p)$. For example, if $p = 1/2$, then the odds

are $0.5/(1 - 0.5) = 1$. Thus, the home team's win and loss are equally likely. If $p = 0.8$, then the odds are $0.8/(1 - 0.8) = 4$. Namely, the odds are 4 to 1 in favor of the home team's success. So, the home team is 4 times more likely to win than lose. The **odds ratio** is a convenient measure for comparing two different such proportions.

Definition 4.7.8. The **odds ratio** (OR) of two different proportions, p_1 and p_2, are defined by

$$OR = \frac{p_1/(1 - p_1)}{p_2/(1 - p_2)} = \frac{p_1/q_1}{p_2/q_2} = \frac{p_1 q_2}{p_2 q_1}, \text{ by letting}$$
$$q_1 = 1 - p_1 \quad \text{and} \quad q_2 = 1 - p_2.$$

In the context of the association between a risk factor and a disease, the odds ratio represents the odds in favor of a disease for the exposed group divided by the odds in favor of a disease for an unexposed group. That is,

$$OR = \frac{[P(\text{disease | exposed})]/[1 - P(\text{disease | exposed})]}{[P(\text{disease | unexposed})]/[1 - P(\text{disease | unexposed})]}.$$

Using the notation in Table 4.7.2, we can express the odds ratio as

$$OR = \frac{[a/(a + b)]/[b/(a + b)]}{[c/(c + d)]/[d/(c + d)]}$$
$$= \frac{[a/(a + b)] \times [d/(c + d)]}{[c/(c + d)] \times [b/(a + b)]} = \frac{ad}{bc}.$$

Example 4.7.6. It is known that the bacteria associated with acute necrotizing ulcerative gingivitis (ANUG), also known as Vincent's infection or trench mouth, are fusiform bacteria and spirochetes—a fusospirochetal complex. A fusospirochetal complex is a risk factor for ANUG. Suppose that periodontists have collected ANUG data, presented in the table below.

| | ANUG Status | | |
Fusospirochetal Complex	Present	Absent	Total
Present	28	36	64
Absent	6	145	151
Total	34	181	215

Then

$$OR = \frac{ad}{bc} = \frac{(28)(145)}{(36)(6)} = \frac{4,020}{216} \simeq 18.80.$$

The odds in favor of an ANUG for patients with the presence of a fusospirochetal complex is 18.8 times the odds in favor of an ANUG for patients with the absence of a fusospirochetal complex.

Example 4.7.7. The primary factors shown to predispose to implant failure are low bone density (i.e., type IV bone) and smoking [6–9]. Bain reported a prospective study of the early outcomes of 223 implants placed in 78 patients [10]. The patients are divided into two groups: smokers and non-smokers. The failure rate of the implants was observed. An implant removal for any reason or an implant exhibiting more than 50% bone loss was considered a failure. Bain's data are summarized in the following table.

Risk Factor	Results of Implants		Total No. of Implants
	Failure	Success	
Smokers	9	38	47
Non-smokers	10	166	176
Total	19	204	223

Then

$$OR = \frac{ad}{bc} = \frac{(9)(166)}{(38)(10)} = \frac{1,494}{380} \simeq 3.93.$$

The odds in favor of an implant failure for smokers is about 3.93 times the odds in favor of an implant failure for non-smokers.

4.8 EXERCISES

1 How many outcomes are there in an experiment of rolling a die?

2 Write all possible outcomes in an experiment of rolling two dice.

3 Dental patients are classified according to their age: young, middle-aged, and elderly. They also are classified according to their tooth mobility: no mobility, class I, class II, and class III. What is the sample space Ω when you classify the patients according to their age and tooth mobility?

4 Suppose the outcomes in Exercise 3 are equally likely. (a). What is the probability that a middle-aged patient is categorized as having class II mobility? (b). What is the probability that an elderly patient is categorized as having either class II or class III mobility?

5 Suppose that erythema multiforme, lichen planus, pemphigoid, pemphigus vulgaris, and viral disease are all the conditions and diseases that may cause vesiculobullous lesions (blistering) in the human mouth. Assume that only one of the conditions and diseases can develop at a time. The sample space consists of these five conditions and diseases. Let two events be defined by $C = \{$lichen planus, viral disease$\}$ and $D = \{$erythema multiforme, lichen planus, pemphigoid$\}$. Find the events, $C \cup D$, $C \cap D$, C^C and D^C.

6 In the above exercise, let $P(C) = 0.42$, $P(D) = 0.68$, and $P(C \cap D) = 0.26$. What is the chance that you will observe the event C or the event D?

7 Let A be the event that a patient brushes his teeth at least once a day, B be the event that a patient eats carbohydrates, and C be the event that a patient uses a toothpaste that contains fluoride. Suppose $P(A) = 0.76$, $P(B) = 0.15$, $P(C) = 0.47$, $P(A \cup B) = 0.84$, and $P(B \cap C) = 0.12$. Compute the probabilities $P(A \cap B)$ and $P(B \cup C)$.

8 A patient who has gingival bleeding went to an endodontist and later went to a periodontist. Let A and B, respectively, be the events that an endodontist and a periodontist correctly diagnose the patient as having advanced periodontitis. If $P(A) = 0.49$ and $P(B) = 0.57$, what is the probability that both of them correctly diagnose the patient if the two events were statistically independent ?

9 The chance that a father has at least one decayed, missing, filled (DMF) tooth is 0.34, and the chance that a mother has at least one DMF is 0.43. Suppose that the father's having any DMF teeth is statistically independent of the mother's having any DMF teeth. What is the probability that either father or mother has at least one DMF tooth?

10 Suppose that A is the event of a mother having at least one missing tooth and that B is the event of a father having at least one missing tooth. If it is known that $P(A) = 0.10$, $P(B) = 0.20$, and $P(AB) = 0.02$, are the events A and B statistically independent?

11 Flip a pair of fair coins until at least one of them lands on heads. What is the probability that the other coin also has landed on heads?

12 Many factors can influence the condition of the teeth, such as eating habits, toothbrushing, flossing, and fluoridation.

Let

A = the event that a patient brushes her teeth at least twice a day,

B = the event that a patient flosses her teeth at least once a day,

C = the event that a patient lives in a fluoridated community.

Suppose $P(A) = 0.55$, $P(B) = 0.40$, $P(AB) = 0.25$, and $P(C) = 0.75$.

a. Are the events A and B independent?
b. Are the events A, B, and C mutually exclusive?
c. Knowing that a patient brushes her teeth at least twice a day, what is the chance that she flosses her teeth at least once a day?
d. Suppose the chance that a patient whose town drinking water is fluoridated and she flosses her teeth at least once a day is 0.30. Given that a patient flosses her teeth at least once a day, what is the chance that she lives in a fluoridated town?
e. Are the events A and B mutually exclusive?

13 Let A be the event that a canine tooth is carious and B be the event that a canine tooth is fractured. Let $P(A) = 0.25$ and $P(B) = 0.20$. If the probability that a canine tooth is carious, given that it is fractured, is 0.45, what is the chance that a canine tooth is fractured and carious?

14 A jar contains 140 adult molar teeth. The molar teeth are categorized as follows: 30 sound, 20 decayed, 75 restored, and 15 decayed and restored. If you were to select a molar tooth from the jar at random, what are the probabilities of the following events?
a. P(selecting only a decayed tooth).
b. P(selecting any decayed tooth).
c. P(selecting any decayed or any restored tooth).

15 Let A be the event that Dr. Jones diagnoses a patient as having myofacial pain syndrome, and B be the event that Dr. Lam diagnoses a patient as having myofascial pain syndrome. Let $P(A) = 0.15$ and $P(B) = 0.24$. If A and B are statistically independent, what is the $P(A$ or $B)$?

16 Let A^+ be the event of Dr. Chung making a positive diagnosis, and B^+ be the event of Dr. Smith making a positive diagnosis. If at least one of them makes a positive diagnosis, then the patient is referred for further evaluation. Suppose $P(A^+) = 0.24$, $P(B^+) = 0.29$, and $P(A^+B^+) = 0.18$. What is the probability that a patient is referred for further examination?

17 An orthodontics researcher is interested in modeling the distribution of maxillary teeth. He needs to measure the distance from mesial to mesial between two maxillary second bicuspids. This requires all his subjects to have both second bicuspids. Let A be the event that a patient has at least one missing second bicuspid. The age of the subjects is divided into five classes as follows. What is the chance that a patient is 66 or older, given that she has at least one missing second bicuspid?

Age	Population (%)	With a Missing Second Bicuspid (%)
Less than 20	20	5
21–35	15	10
36–50	25	18
51–65	30	23
66 or older	10	45

18 Find an example in dentistry where the Bayes theorem can be applied. Be very specific in defining the events, including the mutually exclusive and exhaustive events.

19 Find an example in dentistry, medicine, and other health care areas to describe the following:
a. Events A and B are independent but not mutually exclusive.
b. Events A and B are independent and mutually exclusive.
c. Events A and B are not independent and not mutually exclusive.
d. Events A and B are not independent but mutually exclusive.

20 A dental clinic is conducting a survey on patients' perception of the quality of the dental care they have received and the competency of the dental professionals they have had at the clinic. They intend to sample 100 patients from the database, which contains a large number of patient records. Ideally, the sample of 100 should represent the entire patient population. The chance that a patient has a private insurance carrier is 0.45, and the chance that a patient is female, is 0.55. What is the probability that a randomly chosen patient from the database is female who has private insurance?

21 Find an example in biological or health sciences that illustrates
a. Two events A and B that are independent but not mutually exclusive.
b. Two events A and B that are not independent but mutually exclusive.
c. Two events A and B that are independent and mutually exclusive.
d. Two events A and B that are not independent and not mutually exclusive.

22 Let E_1 and E_2 be the events that Dr. Anderson and Dr. Lee diagnose a patient as having a mucogingival defect. Suppose $P(E_1) = 0.34$ and $P(E_2) = 0.54$. If $P(E_1 E_2) = 0.25$, what is the chance that at least one of them diagnoses a patient as having a mucogingival defect?

23 Suppose that the probability of a person's having microdontia is 0.05. In a family of four what is the chance that all of them have microdontia if one person's having microdontia is statistically independent of another person's having it?

24 Let E_1 be class I mobility, E_2 be class II mobility, and E_3 be class III mobility, which are mutually exclusive and exhaustive events. It is believed that, among the general patient population, $P(E_1) = 0.40$, $P(E_2) = 0.35$, $P(E_3) = 0.25$. Let A be the event that a patient has been flossing regularly since an early age. Also known are $P(A|E_1) = 0.85$, $P(A|E_2) = 0.10$, $P(A|E_3) = 0.05$. What is the chance that a patient is of class II mobility, knowing that he has been flossing ?

25 A team of dental professionals visited a community in the Southwest. Among the samples of 568 patients they treated, 428 of them had at least two carious teeth. What is the estimated probability that a patient from this area has at most one carious tooth?

26 Suppose that in America, the chance of a person having ECC is about 0.15. There are 7 kids in one neighborhood.What is the chance that all

of them have ECC, if one person's having ECC is independent of another having it?

27 Suppose the chance that an individual is affected by odontodysplasia is 0.08. Mr. and Mrs. Smith have two children. What is the chance that all four of them are affected by odontodysplasia, if an individual being affected by it is statistically independent of another being affected?

28 Let A, B, and C be three events with $P(A) = 0.35$, $P(B) = 0.10$, and $P(C) = 0.25$. If the events are mutually exclusive, what is the probability of observing at least one of the events?

29 It has been observed by the statistics instructors of an elementary statistics course that about 5% of the class earn the letter grade A. Among the students who took a college level calculus course, however, about 85% earn the letter grade A. If 10% of the students in the statistics class took a calculus course, what is the probability that a student took a calculus course and earned an A in the statistics course?

30 It is known that most of the patients brush their teeth at least once daily. Let A be the event that a patient brushes teeth at least once a day, and B be the event that the patient's plaque score is less than 50%. The chance that the patient brushes his teeth at least once a day, given his plaque score is less than 50%, is 0.89. The chance that the patient brushes his teeth at least once daily, given that his plaque score is greater than 50%, is 0.08. If $P(B) = 0.47$, what is the chance that the patient brushes his teeth at least once a day?

31 Let S^+ and S^-, respectively, denote positive and negative symptoms of periodontal inflammation. Let D and D^C, respectively, denote existence and non-existence of an acute periodontal disease. If $P(S^+) = 0.20$, $P(S^-) = 0.80$, $P(D^C S^+) = 0.03$, and $P(DS^-) = 0.016$.
a. What is the probability that a patient does not have an acute periodontal disease, knowing that the patient has positive symptoms of periodontal inflammation?
b. If it is known that the patient showed negative symptoms of periodontal inflammation, what is the probability that the patient has an acute periodontal disease?

32 Furcation defects are classified according to probing, and the treatment of furcations varies, depending on the type and the tooth. The treatment may range from simple management with scaling, root planing, and curettage, to tissue-guided regeneration with bone-grafting material. Let the events be defined

A = Patient's dental health history
B_1 = No furcation involvement
B_2 = Class I furcation
B_3 = Class II furcation
B_4 = Class III furcation.

From past data it is estimated that $P(B_1) = 0.44$, $P(B_2) = 0.28$, $P(B_3) = 0.22$, $P(B_4) = 0.06$, $P(A|B_1) = 0.05$, $P(A|B_2) = 0.14$, $P(A|B_3) = 0.21$, and $P(A|B_4) = 0.26$. Given the patient's dental health history, what is the probability that his tooth will be of class III furcation?

33 Cancer patients undergoing chemotherapy can develop mucositis as part of the side effects of the treatment. Suppose B_1 and B_2 are the events representing the patients who develop mucositis and those who do not, respectively. Let C be the event that the cancer patients are undergoing chemotherapy. $P(B_1) = 0.64$, $P(C|B_1) = 0.76$, and $P(C|B_2) = 0.14$. If we know that a patient has developed mucositis, what is the probability that he is a cancer patient undergoing chemotherapy?

34 Common causes for chronic xerostomia include aging, anticholinergic drugs, autoimmune sialadenitis, neurologic dysfunction, nutritional deficiencies (e.g., vitamin A, vitamin B, and iron), and radiation to the gland. The following is the U.S. population distribution by age (source of data: U.S. Census Bureau, 2000), and the probability of the patients having xerostomia, given the range of their age. What is the chance that the age range of a patient is 60 to 79 years, given that he has xerostomia?

A_1 = 39 or younger, $P(A_1) = 0.568$ $P(B|A_1) = 0.05$
A_2 = 40 − 59 years old, $P(A_2) = 0.268$ $P(B|A_2) = 0.10$
A_3 = 60 − 79 years old, $P(A_3) = 0.131$ $P(B|A_3) = 0.48$
A_4 = 80 or older, $P(A_4) = 0.033$ $P(B|A_4) = 0.89$
B = Patients with xerostomia

35 In January, 2005, 1,825 people were employed by the Riverside County government. It was reported that, at the beginning of the new year

2005, 125 employees were suffering from chronic depression. At the end of the fiscal year in June, 2005, the number of employees suffering from chronic depression increased to 185. Between January and June, 2005, 75 employees left their jobs with the county government for a variety of reasons. Express the incidence rate for the period of January through June, 2005, and the prevalence rate at the end of June, 2005.

36 A team of hygienists and dentists visited a community in South America during spring break. Their visit lasted only a few days. The primary goal they hoped to achieve during their stay was to assess the proportion of children who require root canal treatments. What type of epidemiologic rate is most appropriate for this? Give a short reason why.

37 The results shown in the table below were obtained from a study conducted to evaluate the quality of a pathology laboratory in a major hospital. Eighty-two malignant samples and 181 benign samples of lymph nodes were sent to the laboratory for analysis. Compute the sensitivity and specificity rates.

	True State	
Pathological Result	Malignant	Benign
Positive test result	74	12
Negative test result	8	169
Total	82	181

38 As the uptake of fluoride and other minerals make the tooth surface less acid soluble, enamel becomes more resistant to dental caries throughout the life of the tooth. Suppose that the probability of dental caries among those who live in fluoridated communities is 0.08, and the probability of dental caries among those whose drinking water is not

fluoridated is 0.48. Compute the relative risk, and interpret the result in words.

39 The patients with Addison's disease (hypoadrenocorticism) experience slowly progressive loss of cortisol and aldosterone secretion, usually producing a chronic, steadily worsening fatigue, a loss of appetite, and some weight loss. Hyperpigmentation of the skin or gingiva occurs often enough to raise a strong suspicion of the disease, prompting further evaluation. Suppose there is a 1 in 100 chance that the patient has Addison's disease when he has hyperpigmentation of the gingivae, and a 5 in 10, 000 chance when he does not have hyperpigmentation of the gingivae. What are the predictive value positive and the predictive value negative?

4.9 REFERENCES

1. Sonis, S. T. *Dental Secrets*. Second edition. Hanley & Belfus, Inc. 1999.
2. Wyne, A. H. Nomenclature and Case Definition. *Community Dent. Oral Epidemiol*: 1999, 27, 313–315.
3. Thoden van Velzen, S. K., Duivenvoorden, H. J., and Schuurs, A. H. B. Probabilities of success and failure in endodontic treatment: A Bayesian approach. *Oral Surg*: 1981, 85–90.
4. Jekel, J. F., Elmore, J. G., and Katz, D. L. *Epidemiology, Biostatistics, and Preventive Medicine*. W. B. Saunders Company. 1996.
5. http://ourworld.compuserve.com/homepages/lungcancer.
6. Jaffin, R. A., and Berman, C. L. The excessive loss of Branemark implants in type IV bone: A 5-year analysis. *J. Periodontol*: 1991, 62, 2–4.
7. Bain, C. A., and Moy, P. K. The association between the failure of dental implants and cigarette smoking. *Int. J. Oral Maxillofac. Implants*: 1993, 8, 609–615.
8. De Bruyn, H., and Collaert, B. The effects of smoking on early implant failure. *Clin. Oral Implants Res.*: 1994, 5, 260–264.
9. Jones, J. K., and Triplett, R. G. The relationship of smoking to impaired intraoral wound healing. *J. Oral Maxillofac. Surg.*: 1992, 50, 237–239.
10. Bain, C. A. Smoking and implant failure—Benefits of a smoking cessation protocol. *The Int. J. Oral Maxillofac. Implants*: 1996, 11, 756–759.

Chapter 5

Probability Distributions

5.1 INTRODUCTION

In Chapter 2 we discussed random variables, both discrete and continuous. A discrete random variable assumes a finite or countable number of possible outcomes, such as causes of pulpal death, specialty areas in dentistry and medicine, and types of injuries. A continuous random variable can take on any value within a specified interval or continuum, such as time of healing, root angulation, or amount of anesthetic used. Every random variable has a unique corresponding probability distribution. To draw precise conclusions about a population based on a sample taken from the population, we need to understand the probability distribution corresponding to the population. This chapter will introduce three of the most useful distributions, which have a wide variety of applications in biomedical and health sciences: binomial distribution, Poisson distribution, and normal distribution. For a discrete random variable, the probability distribution gives all possible outcomes and the probabilities associated with the outcomes. These probabilities represent the relative frequency of the occurrence of each outcome in a large number of experiments repeated under identical conditions. The next three sections are devoted to these three probability distributions.

5.2 BINOMIAL DISTRIBUTION

When a fair coin is tossed three times, the sample space consists of eight possible outcomes: TTT, TTH, THT, HTT, HHT, HTH, THH, HHH. Let Y be the random variable (rv) for the number of heads observed, then Y assumes the value 0, 1, 2, 3. Probabilities for the values of the random variable Y can be determined as shown in Table 5.2.1.

Therefore, the probability of observing no heads is $\frac{1}{8}$, one head is $\frac{3}{8}$, two heads is $\frac{3}{8}$, and three heads

is $\frac{1}{8}$. The probability distribution for the number of heads observed from tossing a fair coin three times can be constructed as in Table 5.2.2 below.

There are three different ways to obtain exactly two heads out of three tosses; HHT, HTH, THH. Each outcome is equally likely ($\frac{1}{8}$) because a fair coin is tossed. Hence, $P(Y = 2) = P(HHT) + P(HTH) + P(THH) = \frac{3}{8}$. The two most likely outcomes when a coin is tossed three times are two heads and two tails.

There are many situations in biomedical and health sciences where the investigators are interested in the probability that an event occurs k times out of n trials. For example, we may be interested in (a) the probability of getting 85 responses to 200 questionnaires sent to nurses and dental hygienists to find out about job satisfaction, (b) the probability that 3 out of 18 patients who need an immediate root canal treatment do not have an employer-provided insurance, (c) the probability that at least one member in a family of five has osteogenesis imperfecta, or (d) the probability that 7 out of 25 lymphoma patients undergoing chemoradiation treatment will survive at least 5 years. In each of the cases, the investigators are interested in the probability of obtaining k successes in n trials (or k heads in n coin tosses). Getting k successes in n trials (or k heads in n coin tosses) means k successes *and* $n - k$ failures in n trials (or k heads *and* $n - k$ tails in n coin tosses). Table 5.2.1 reveals that the event of observing two heads is the same as that of observing one tail. Therefore, the probability of observing one tail should be the same as the probability of observing two heads, which is, $\frac{3}{8}$.

A large dental clinic record indicates that 78% of the patients have at least one DMFT, and 22% do not have any decayed, missed, and filled teeth (DMFT) at all. Let X be a random variable that represents the patient's DMFT status. It is convenient to let $X = 0$ if the patient does not have any

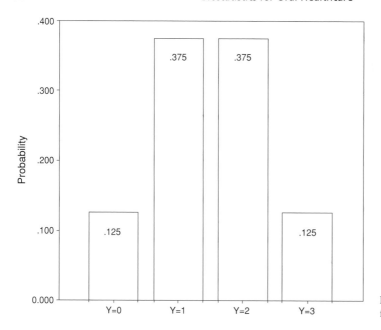

Figure 5.2.1 Probability distribution for the number of heads.

Table 5.2.1. Probabilities for Y = no. of heads.

Number of H's	No heads	One H	Two H's	Three H's
rv	$Y = 0$	$Y = 1$	$Y = 2$	$Y = 3$
Outcome	TTT	TTH THT HTT	HHT HTH THH	HHH
Probability	$\frac{1}{8}$	$\frac{3}{8}$	$\frac{3}{8}$	$\frac{1}{8}$

DMFT, and $X = 1$ if the patient has at least one DMFT. These two outcomes of X are mutually exclusive and exhaustive. Thus, we can express the probabilities associated with the outcomes of X as

$$P(X = 0) = 0.22 = p,$$

and

$$P(X = 1) = 1.0 - p = 1.0 - 0.22 = 0.78$$

For convenience in discussing the binomial distribution, we shall denote the outcome $X = 0$ as "failure" or "tail," and $X = 1$ as "success" or "head." For the validity of our discussions on the binomial distributions, we shall assume

- the number of trials, n, is fixed.
- the n trials are statistically independent.

Table 5.2.2. Probability of the number of heads.

Number of heads, Y	$Y = 0$	$Y = 1$	$Y = 2$	$Y = 3$
Probability, $P(Y = y)$	$\frac{1}{8}$	$\frac{3}{8}$	$\frac{3}{8}$	$\frac{1}{8}$

- the probability of success, p, is constant throughout the trials.

If p and $1 - p$ are the probabilities of obtaining a head and a tail on any given trial (i.e., a coin tossing), the probability of observing 2 heads and 3 tails in 5 tosses in some specific order is $p^2(1 - p)^{5-2} = p^2(1 - p)^3$. Since this probability applies to any outcome of two heads and three tails, we need to count how many of such outcomes there are. In fact, we can write down all possible such outcomes when n is small, as follows:

HHTTT	*TTHTH*
HTHTT	*TTTHH*
HTटHT	*THHTT*
HTTTH	*TTHHT*
THTTH	*TTTHH*

Since there are 10 outcomes that are mutually exclusive, the probability of observing two heads in 5 tosses is $10 \cdot p^2(1 - p)^{5-2}$. To facilitate the discussion, we need to introduce some notation. Given n endodontic patients, $n!$ (read, n factorial) represents the number of distinct ways in which n patients can be ordered. Note that we have n choices for the first position, $(n - 1)$ choices for the second position, $(n - 2)$ choices for the third, and only one choice left for the last position. Hence, the number of ways in which we can order n patients is given by

$$n! = n(n - 1)(n - 2) \cdots (3)(2)(1).$$

For example,

$$5! = 5 \cdot 4 \cdot 3 \cdot 2 \cdot 1 = 120$$
$$4! = 4 \cdot 3 \cdot 2 \cdot 1 = 24$$
$$3! = 3 \cdot 2 \cdot 1 = 6$$
$$2! = 2 \cdot 1 = 2$$
$$1! = 1$$
$$0! = 1, \text{ by convention.}$$

The expression $\binom{n}{k} = \dfrac{n!}{k!(n - k)!}$ describes the number of distinct ways in which k patients can be selected from the total of n patients without regard to order. Read $\binom{n}{k}$ as "n choose k." An experiment where n coins are tossed is statistically equivalent to tossing a coin n times. Let X be a binomial random variable. Using the notation introduced we now can define a binomial probability.

Definition 5.2.1. To define binomial probability, let n be the number of independent trials and p be the probability of success. Then the probability of observing exactly k successes is given by

$$P(X = k) = \binom{n}{k} p^k (1 - p)^{n-k}$$

$$= \frac{n!}{k!(n - k)!} p^k (1 - p)^{n-k}$$

where $k = 0, 1, \cdots, n$

From the definition of $\binom{n}{k}$, it is easy to see

$\binom{n}{k} = \binom{n}{n - k}$. By a simple substitution in the above formula we can establish

$$P(X = k) = \binom{n}{k} p^k (1 - p)^{n-k}$$

$$= \binom{n}{n - k} p^k (1 - p)^{n-k}.$$

The binomial random variable X when the number of trials is n and the probability of success is p is sometimes denoted by $X \sim B(n, p)$ (read $\sim$ as "distributed according to").

Example 5.2.1. Six students always sit in the front row in statistics class. They took the National Board exam at the same time. If the probability of passing the board exam is 0.90, what is the chance that five of the six students passed the exam?

Solution. From the information given in the example, we know that $n = 6$, and $p = P$(passing the exam) $= 0.90$. The probability of our interest is

$$P(X = 5) = \binom{6}{5}(0.90)^5(1.0 - 0.90)^{6-5}$$

$$= \frac{6!}{5!(6 - 5)!}(0.90)^5(0.10)$$

$$= 0.3543.$$

Example 5.2.2. The normal range of the white blood cell (WBC) count for healthy adult is $3,800$ to $10,800$ per cubic millimeter. The white blood cell count of the patients undergoing chemotherapy is expected to drop below the normal range. Suppose that the WBC count of about 45% of the cancer patients fall below $2,000$ per cubic millimeter during treatment. If five lung cancer patients are waiting in Dr. Jackson's office, what is the probability that no more than 40% of them have a WBC count of less than $2,000$ per cubic millimeter?

Solution. The random variable we have here is $X \sim B(5, 0.45)$, where $p = P$(white blood cell count $\leq 2,000$) $= 0.45$. Forty percent of the five patients is equal to two patients, so the probability we need to find is:

$$P(X \leq 2)$$
$$= P(X = 0) + P(X = 1) + P(X = 2)$$
$$= \binom{5}{0}(0.45)^0(0.55)^{5-0} + \binom{5}{1}(0.45)^1(0.55)^{5-1}$$
$$+ \binom{5}{2}(0.45)^2(0.55)^{5-2}$$
$$= \frac{5!}{0!(5 - 0)!}(0.55)^5 + \frac{5!}{1!(5 - 1)!}(0.45)^1(0.55)^4$$
$$+ \frac{5!}{2!(5 - 2)!}(0.45)^2(0.55)^3$$
$$= 0.0503 + 0.2059 + 0.3369 = 0.5931.$$

The probabilities in Example 5.2.2 can be found in the binomial probability table (Table B in the Appendix). The first two columns in the binomial probability table are the number n of trials and the number k of successes observed in the experiment. The top row has the probabilities $p = 0.05$, $0.10, 0.15, \cdots, 0.45$, and 0.50. To find the probability $P(X = 2)$ in the example, go to the row for $n = 5$ and $k = 2$ in Table B. The table value corresponding to $p = 0.45$ is the desired probability, $P(X = 2) = 0.3369$.

The table contains the probabilities for $n = 2, \cdots, 40$ and $p = 0.05, \cdots, 0.45$, and 0.50. What if $p > 0.50$? We can still use Table B to compute the binomial probabilities when $p > 0.50$. Suppose we have a random variable $X \sim B(7, 0.70)$. The probability that $(X = 3)$, that is, the probability of an event of three successes out of seven trials when $p = 0.70$, is

$$P(X = 3) = \binom{7}{3}(0.70)^3(0.30)^{7-3}$$

$$[\text{keep in mind here that } n = 7,$$
$$k = 3, \text{ and } p = 0.70]$$

$$= \binom{7}{7-3}(0.30)^{7-3}(0.70)^3$$

$$= \binom{7}{7-3}(0.30)^{7-3}(0.70)^{7-(7-3)}.$$

In this expression we have $n - k$ and $1 - p$ in place of k and p.

$$= \binom{7}{4}(0.30)^4(0.70)^3 = 0.0972.$$

If $p > 0.50$, then the probability of obtaining k successes in n trials is given by

$$P(X = k) = \binom{n}{k}p^k(1-p)^{n-k}$$

$$= \binom{n}{n-k}(1-p)^{n-k}p^{n-(n-k)}.$$

For $p > 0.50$, $P(X = k)$ is found in Table B by putting $n - k$ in place of k and $1 - p$ in place of p.

Example 5.2.3. As a class project, student dentists were instructed to record probing depth, bleeding index, mobility, furcations, recession and attachment level in their patients' chart. A recent audit of charts indicated that at least one of the six variables is missing from 55% of the charts. Suppose 12 patient charts are randomly selected. What

is the probability that 7 of the charts are missing at least one variable?

Solution. In this problem, $n = 12$, $k = 7$, and $p = 0.55$ so that the probability $P(X = 7)$ is

$$P(X = 7)$$

$$= \binom{12}{7}(0.55)^7(1 - 0.55)^{12-7}$$

$$= \binom{12}{12-7}(1 - 0.55)^{12-7}(0.55)^{12-(12-7)},$$

$$\text{since } p > 0.50,$$

$$= \binom{12}{12-7}(1 - 0.55)^{12-7}(0.55)^{12-(12-7)}$$

$$= \binom{12}{5}(0.45)^5(0.55)^7$$

$$= 0.2225.$$

This is the table value corresponding to $n = 12$, $k = 5$ and $p = 0.45$.

Example 5.2.4. A pontic is an artificial tooth on a fixed partial denture that replaces a lost natural tooth. The design of the pontic is dictated by the boundaries of an edentulous ridge, opposing the occlusal surface, and musculature of tongue, cheeks, and lips. Suppose prosthodontists in a clinic have experienced that 15% of the pontics require some minor adjustments. In other words, the defect rate of the pontic is 15%. Of 10 pontics the dental clinic has prepared for their patients, what is the chance that between 2 and 5 (inclusive) are defects?

Solution. The required probability is given by

$$P(2 \leq X \leq 5) = P(X = 2) + P(X = 3)$$
$$+ P(X = 4) + P(X = 5)$$
$$= 0.2759 + 0.1298 + 0.0401$$
$$+ 0.0085 = 0.4543,$$

from Table B in the Appendix.

Example 5.2.5. An individual who has a type-A influenza (also known as Asian flu) has a 5% chance of infecting a person with whom he comes into close contact and who has had no prior exposure. If the carrier of a type-A influenza comes into close contact with 12 individuals, what is the probability that he will pass the disease on to at least 3 of them?

Solution. Let X be the random variable representing the number of individuals who will be infected by the carrier of the flu virus. Then the possible values X takes on are 0, 1, 2, 3, $\cdots$, 12. The event of interest is "at least 3 of them," which is in boldface in the figure below.

X: 0 1 2 **3 4 5 6 7 8 9 10 11 12**

We can calculate the probability directly from the binomial table with $n = 12$, and $p = 0.05$ by adding 10 terms as in the following expression:

$$P(3 \le X) = P(X = 3) + P(X = 4)$$
$$+ \cdots + P(X = 12).$$

However, the calculation can be simplified if we use the complementary argument discussed in Chapter 4. The event $\{X \le 2\}$ is complementary to the event $\{3 \le X\}$. Therefore, $P(3 \le X)$ can be expressed as

$$P(3 \le X) = 1.0 - P(X \le 2)$$
$$= 1.0 - [P(X = 0) + P(X = 1)$$
$$+ P(X = 2)]$$
$$= 1.0 - (0.5404 + 0.3413 + 0.0988)$$
$$= 0.0195.$$

Example 5.2.6. The principle of guided bone regeneration (GBR) is an established surgical method used in treatment of bone defects, bone augmentation procedures, and implant installment [1]. An unbiased and accurate quantitative evaluation of the amount of regenerated bone in a GBR is critical. Suppose that the past studies with rabbits using stereological methods showed that in 35% of the subjects, the amount of bone regeneration in a 6-month time period was about 23% or greater. A dental researcher has a group of 8 rabbits for an experiment to assess the amount of regenerated bone after placement of degradable membranes covering defects in rabbit calvaria using the principle of GBR. What is the chance that the researcher will observe at least 23% bone regeneration in, at most, 75% of his rabbit samples?

Solution. At least 23% bone regeneration constitutes success. Let X denote the number of rabbits that achieve at least 23% bone regeneration. Thus, $X \sim B(8, 0.35)$. Because 75% of 8 rabbits is 6 rabbits, the probability of "at most 75% of rabbit

samples" can be written as

$$P(X \le 6) = P(X = 0) + P(X = 1)$$
$$+ \cdots + P(X = 6)$$
$$= 1.0 - [P(X = 7) + P(X = 8)],$$

by the complementary event

$$= 1.0 - (0.0034 + 0.0002)$$
$$= 0.9964.$$

Suppose we toss a coin 100 times. If the probability of obtaining a head is $\frac{1}{2}$, $p = P(H) = \frac{1}{2}$. Then we would expect to obtain about 50 heads. If $p = P(H) = \frac{1}{4}$, we would expect to obtain about 25 heads. In statistics, the mean is often referred to as the **expected value**. From this simple observation, it seems reasonable to say that the mean of a binomial distribution is np, that is, the number of trials times the probability of success. We can derive mathematically that the mean is indeed given by np. We state the mean, variance, and standard deviation of a binomial distribution $X \sim B(n, p)$, which will be useful in future discussions.

Mean, $\qquad\qquad \mu = np$

Variance, $\qquad\quad \sigma^2 = np(1 - p) = npq,$

$\qquad\qquad\qquad$ where $q = 1 - p$

Standard deviation, $\sigma = \sqrt{np(1 - p)} = \sqrt{npq}.$

The variance of a binomial distribution becomes smaller and smaller as p approaches 0 or 1. Intuitively, when $p = 0$ there will be no heads observed, and when $p = 1$, every coin toss will result in a head. Therefore, there is no variability. Hence, the variance $np(1 - p) = 0$. The largest variability occurs when $p = \frac{1}{2}$. The variance is maximum when $p = \frac{1}{2}$, as can be seen in Figure 5.2.2.

Example 5.2.7. Health care professionals in medicine and dentistry routinely use latex gloves, which are inexpensive and protect the clinicians from transmission of infection. Regular contact

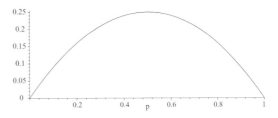

Figure 5.2.2 Plot of p vs. $p(1 - p)$.

with latex-containing products such as rubber gloves can result in an allergy. A survey showed that about 32% of the respondents reported experiencing a latex allergy [2]. In a sample of 125 clinicians, what is the mean and the variance of the number of those who experience a latex allergy?

Solution. With $n = 125$ and $p = 0.32$, substitution in the above formula yields

$$\text{Mean, } \mu = np = 125 \cdot (0.32) = 40$$

and

$$\text{Variance, } \sigma^2 = np(1 - p)$$
$$= 125 \cdot (0.32)(0.68) = 27.2.$$

5.3 POISSON DISTRIBUTION

After the binomial distribution, the Poisson distribution is the second most widely used discrete distribution. The Poisson distribution is useful when n is large and p is small and when the events occur over a period of time, area, volume, or space:

- The number of calls received by the dental assistant for cancellation of an appointment
- The number of cases where oral-dental infections contributed to bacteremia
- The number of false alarms sounded at a nuclear power plant
- The number of neutrophils in a tiny drop of blood sample
- The count of certain bacterial colonies growing on an agar plate
- The number of mistakes in patient charts

The probability of receiving a cancellation call at time t_1 (actually, a small time interval around t_1) is very small. The probability of getting calls at any two time points, t_1 and t_2, are independent. The number of cancellation calls over a day will follow a Poisson distribution. The following assumptions need to be made.

1. The probability of observing one occurrence (one call) is directly proportional to the length of the time interval, Δt.
2. The probability of observing more than one call over this time interval, Δt, is essentially 0.
3. What happens in one interval is independent of what happens in another interval.

Let λ be the average number of occurrences of the event per unit of time (or area or volume) and s be the number of units. Then the **Poisson probability** of observing k occurrences in a period of length s is given by

$$P(X = k) = \frac{(\lambda s)^k e^{-\lambda s}}{k!},$$
$$\text{where } k = 0, 1, 2, 3, \cdots, \text{ and}$$
$$e = 2.7183$$
$$= \frac{\mu^k e^{-\mu}}{k!}, \quad \text{by letting } \mu = \lambda s.$$

Example 5.3.1. Dr. Chung and his partners keep 750 patient charts in their practice. Suppose 1, 125 errors (e.g., typographical errors, sex of a male patient is marked as "F" in the chart, etc.) are randomly scattered among these charts. (i) What is the probability that each patient chart contains exactly 3 errors? (ii) What is the probability that each chart contains at least 3 errors?

Solution (i) Because there are 1, 125 errors randomly distributed in 750 patient charts, each chart has an average of

$$\lambda = \frac{1,125}{750} = 1.5.$$

Since $k = 3$ and $s = 1$ (each patient chart), $\mu = \lambda s = 1.5$. Substituting in the Poisson probability formula given above, we obtain

$$P(X = 3) = \frac{(1.5)^3 e^{-1.5}}{3!} = 0.1255 \text{ (e = 2.7183)}.$$

(ii) $P(\text{chart contains at least 3 errors}) = P(3 \leq X)$

$$= 1.0 - P(X \leq 2), \text{ using the argument of}$$
$$\text{complementary event}$$
$$= 1.0 - [P(X = 0) + P(X = 1) + P(X = 2)]$$
$$= 1.0 - \left[\frac{(1.5)^0 e^{-1.5}}{0!} + \frac{(1.5)^1 e^{-1.5}}{1!} + \frac{(1.5)^2 e^{-1.5}}{2!} \right]$$
$$= 1.0 - (0.2231 + 0.3347 + 0.2510)$$
$$= 0.1912.$$

To facilitate calculation of the Poisson probability, the Poisson probability table is provided in Table C in the Appendix. Table C presents probabilities for $\mu = 0.5, 1.0, 1.5, \cdots, 20.0$, and $k = 0, 1, 2, 3, \cdots, 40$. In the above example, we have computed the probabilities after substituting e with 2.7183. Table C should provide the same values without involving any computations.

Example 5.3.2. The white blood cell count of cancer patients undergoing chemotherapy is closely monitored by the oncologist, who will interrupt the treatment when the patient's WBC count falls below 2,000 per cubic millimeter. Overall, the normal number of leukocytes ranges from 5,000 to 10,000 per cubic millimeter. If the average WBC count for healthy adults is 7,000 per cubic millimeter what is the probability that only 2 white cells are found in a 0.001 mm³ drop of a blood sample taken from a healthy adult individual?

Solution. In this problem, the unit volume is cubic millimeter, the average count per unit is given by $\lambda = 7,000$, $s = 0.001$ mm³, and $k = 2$. We then have $\mu = \lambda s = (7,000)(0.001) = 7$. Thus,

$$P(X = 2) = \frac{\mu^2 e^{-\mu}}{2!} = \frac{(7)^2 e^{-7}}{2!}$$
$$= 0.0223, \quad \text{from Table C.}$$

The chances are about 2.2% that only 2 WBCs are found in a 0.001 mm³ blood sample taken from a healthy adult individual.

Example 5.3.3. Some psychological reports speculate that left-handed people are "smarter" than right-handed people. Suppose that 13% of the population is left-handed. At the American Dental Association meeting, a psychologist was standing at the door to a conference room and asked the dentists if they were left-handed. What is the chance that she will find at least 20 left-handed dentists among the first 100 entering the conference room?

Solution. Let us consider a block of 100 dentists as a unit. Then $\lambda = (0.13)(100) = 13$. Since $s = 1$, $\mu = \lambda s = \lambda$.

P(at least 20 left-handed)

$$= P(20 \le X) = P(X = 20) + P(X = 21)$$
$$+ P(X = 22) + \cdots$$
$$= \frac{(13)^{20} e^{-13}}{20!} + \frac{(13)^{21} e^{-13}}{21!} + \frac{(13)^{22} e^{-13}}{22!} + \cdots$$
$$= 0.0177 + 0.0109 + 0.0065 + 0.0037 + 0.0020$$
$$+ 0.0010 + 0.0005 + 0.0003$$
$$+ 0.0001 + 0.0001 + 0 + \cdots = 0.0428.$$

Example 5.3.4. Emergencies commonly experienced in dental offices involve allergic reactions of the patients to anesthesia, seizures, asthmatic attack, airway obstruction, syncope, laryngospasm, bradycardia, hypoglycemia, and angina pectoris. Suppose a survey showed that on the average a dental office has 3 emergencies in a year. What is the probability that Dr. Baker's dental practice will have 2 emergencies in the next 6 months?

Solution. The time unit in this example is 1 year, and $\lambda = 3$. Because $s = 0.5$ (6 months), $\mu = (3)(0.5) = 1.5$. We seek to find the probability of observing 2 emergencies in 6 months:

$$P(X = 2) = \frac{\mu^2 e^{-\mu}}{2!} = \frac{(1.5)^2 e^{-1.5}}{2!} = 0.2510.$$

There is a 25.1% chance that Dr. Baker's office will have 2 emergencies in six months.

For a Poisson distribution with parameter μ, the mean and variance are both equal to μ, and the standard deviation is $\sqrt{\mu}$. This fact gives us a preliminary indication that if we have a discrete data set where the mean and variance are approximately equal, then the data set is likely to have come from a Poisson distribution.

5.4 POISSON APPROXIMATION TO BINOMIAL DISTRIBUTION

We learned in Section 5.2 that the binomial distribution with parameters n and p has the mean $\mu = np$ and variance $\sigma^2 = np(1 - p)$. Consider the case where n is large and p is small. When p is small (close to 0), $(1 - p)$ is close to 1.0. If $(1 - p)$ is approximately equal to 1.0, then the variance $np(1 - p)$ is approximately np. This implies that the mean and variance are both equal to np (approximately). This simple observation suggests that the Poisson distribution can be used to approximate the binomial distribution. We will state the following useful rule: *The binomial distribution, $B(n, p)$, where n is large and p is small can be approximated by a Poisson distribution with parameter $\mu = np$.*

As we have seen before, the binomial distribution involves $\binom{n}{k}$ and $(1 - p)^{n-k}$. For a large value of n, it could be time consuming to calculate the probabilities. In comparison it would be much simpler to compute the Poisson probability $\mu^k e^{-\mu}/k!$.

Example 5.4.1. The incidence of cleft lip with or without cleft palate is known to be 1 in 700 to 1, 000 births in the United States. Suppose the incidence rate is 1 in 1, 000. If the number of births per year in a large metropolitan area is about 18, 500, what are the chances that there will be 20 new births with cleft lip over a 1-year period in the area?

Solution. The exact binomial probability is obtained by letting $n = 18, 500$ and $p = 0.001$. That is,

$$P(X=20)= \binom{18,500}{20}(0.001)^{20}(0.999)^{18,500-20}.$$

Even with a calculator in hand this is not a simple task. Using the Poisson approximation with $\mu = \lambda s = \dfrac{1}{1000}(18,500) = 18.5$, we can obtain:

$$P(X = 20) = \frac{(18.5)^{20}e^{-18.5}}{20!} = 0.0837,$$

either by direct calculation or from Table C.

For an adequate approximation one is advised to use the Poisson approximation if $n \geq 100$ and $p \leq 0.01$.

5.5 NORMAL DISTRIBUTION

Continuous random variables arise when quantities are measured on a continuous span. Some examples may include a remission period of a patient who is undergoing a cancer treatment, the amount of blood lost during a surgery, the survival time of a gold crown, the bone height of a patient who needs a titanium implant, mercury concentration in amalgam, the amount of carbon monoxide in the air, or the shear strength of a composite material. In these situations, we usually round off our measurements to the nearest whole unit or to a few decimals, regardless of how precise and accurate the measuring instrument might be and how capable the technicians are. Of all the continuous probability distributions, the normal distribution is the most popular and widely used in statistics. The

normal distribution is tremendously important in the analysis of every aspect of experimental data in biomedical and health sciences, engineering, and social sciences.

Many continuous random variables, such as weight and blood pressure, have distributions that are bell-shaped. A histogram for systolic blood pressure data representing 100 randomly selected college students is presented in Figure 5.5.1(a). As we increase the sample size, we may obtain the histograms in Figure 5.5.1(b) and 5.5.1(c), which look approximately like a graph of the normal density function in (d). The normal density function is *informally* referred to as the normal distribution or normal curve. However, the normal density and normal distribution are not the same. As there are many different binomial distributions, $B(n, p)$, with different parameters n and p, there are many different normal distributions. Each normal distribution has a density function of the form

$$f(x) = \frac{1}{\sqrt{2\pi}\sigma}e^{-\frac{1}{2\sigma^2}(x-\mu)^2}$$

where μ is the mean and σ is the standard deviation of the normal distribution (σ^2 is the variance of the normal distribution). The mean and standard deviation, (μ, σ) uniquely determine a particular normal distribution. We will not use this mathematical equation at all in this book. Instead, we will work with the standard normal probability table (Table D in the Appendix).

5.5.1 Properties of Normal Distribution

The graph of the normal distribution is a symmetric, bell-shaped curve centered at its mean, μ. Figure 5.5.2 shows that for the normal distribution, its mean, median, and mode are equal and located at the center of the distribution. The normal distribution curve is unimodal. The area bounded by the normal curve and the horizontal axis is 1.0. The normal probabilities can be found by corresponding areas under the curve. The height of the normal distribution is given by $\dfrac{1}{\sqrt{2\pi}\sigma}$. When $\sigma = 1$, the height of the curve is $\dfrac{1}{\sqrt{2\pi}} = 0.39894$. The larger the values of σ, the larger the dispersion and, therefore, the flatter the normal distribution will be as shown in Figure 5.5.3.

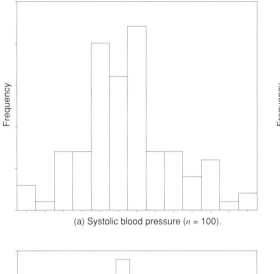

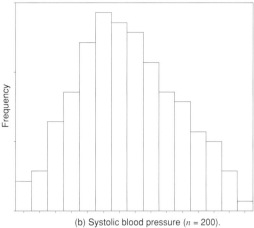

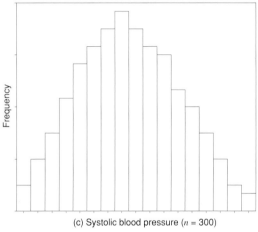

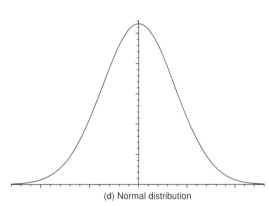

(a) Systolic blood pressure ($n = 100$).

(b) Systolic blood pressure ($n = 200$).

(c) Systolic blood pressure ($n = 300$)

(d) Normal distribution

Figure 5.5.1   Histograms for systolic blood pressure data.

The area under the normal curve that lies

- within $\mu \pm \sigma$ (within one SD of the mean) is approximately 0.683 (68.3%),
- within $\mu \pm 2\sigma$ (within two SD of the mean) is about 0.955 (95.5%), and
- within $\mu \pm 3\sigma$ (within three SD of the mean) is about 0.997 (99.7%).

The bell-shaped curve extends indefinitely in both directions. The curve comes closer and closer to the horizontal axis without ever touching it, regardless of how far we go in either direction away from the mean. The area under the curve beyond 4 standard deviations from the mean is negligibly small; thus, from a practical standpoint, we may rarely have to extend the tails of the normal

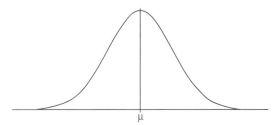

Figure 5.5.2   The normal distribution is centered at its mean.

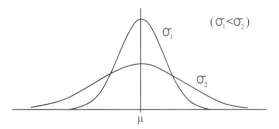

Figure 5.5.3   The standard deviation determines the shape.

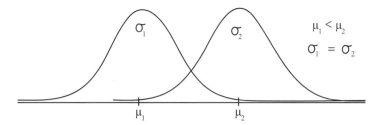

Figure 5.5.4 Two normal distributions with unequal means and equal standard deviation.

distribution more than 4 or 5 standard deviations away from its mean.

As mentioned, a normal distribution is uniquely determined by two parameters, μ and σ. This means that there can be only one normal distribution with a given mean and a given standard deviation. In Figure 5.5.3, the two curves have equal means but unequal standard deviations. The flatter normal distribution has a larger SD. Two normal distributions with unequal means but equal standard deviations are displayed in Figure 5.5.4. The one on the right has a larger mean μ than the one on the left ($\mu_1 < \mu_2$). Similarly, two normal curves with unequal means and unequal standard deviations are shown in Figure 5.5.5 ($\mu_1 < \mu_2$ and $\sigma_1 < \sigma_2$).

The properties regarding the area under the curve discussed apply only to a unimodal, symmetric distribution such as normal distributions. If the data is not unimodal and symmetric, the following **Chebychev's inequality** can be used to specify the proportion of the spread in terms of the standard deviation. Chebychev's inequality applies no matter what the shape of the distribution.

Chebychev's Inequality

The proportion of the values from a data set that will fall within k standard deviations of its mean is *at least* $1 - \left(\dfrac{1}{k^2}\right)$, where $k \geq 1$.

For example, if $k = 1.5$, then $1 - \left(\dfrac{1}{1.5^2}\right) = 0.5556$. This implies that *at least* 55.56% of the data will fall within 1.5 standard deviations of its mean. For $k = 2$, $1 - \left(\dfrac{1}{2^2}\right) = 0.75$. Thus, *at least* 75% of the data will fall within 2 standard deviations of its mean. For $k = 3$, $1 - \left(\dfrac{1}{3^2}\right) = 0.8889$. Hence, *at least* 88.89% of the data will fall within 3 standard deviations of its mean. Chebychev's inequality provides a conservative proportion of the measurements that fall within $k \cdot SD \pm$ mean, regardless of the shape of the distribution.

5.5.2 Standard Normal Distribution

A random variable X that has the normal distribution with the mean μ and the variance σ^2 is denoted by $X \sim N(\mu, \sigma^2)$. Hence, $X \sim N(0, 1)$ indicates that a random variable X has mean $= 0$ and variance $= 1$. A normal distribution with a mean $\mu = 0$ and a variance $\sigma^2 = 1$ (that is, a standard deviation $\sigma = 1$) is referred to as the **standard normal distribution**. It is neither feasible nor necessary to provide normal probability tables for all possible values of μ and σ^2. The standard normal probability table can be used for all cases, because normally distributed random variables can

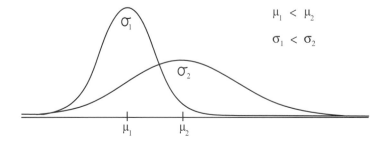

Figure 5.5.5 Two normal distributions with unequal means and standard deviation.

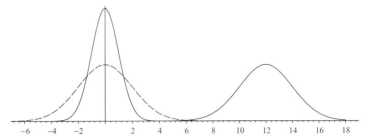

Figure 5.5.6 Transformation of X to the standard normal curve.

be transformed into the standard normal distribution by

$$Z = \frac{X - \mu}{\sigma}$$

This formula will make the conversion from $X \sim N(\mu, \sigma^2)$ to $Z \sim N(0, 1)$. The transformed X values are referred to as Z **scores** or Z **values**. The Z score represents the number of standard deviations that a particular value of X is away from the mean μ. The transformation has a physical meaning. The normal curve on the right-hand side in Figure 5.5.6 has mean $\mu = 12$ and variance $\sigma^2 = 4$. The numerator of the above formula $X - \mu$ has the same effect as pulling the curve to the left until the center of the curve (i.e., $\mu = 12$) comes to the point zero (i.e., $\mu = 0$). After this process is done, the normal curve is located where the dotted normal curve is in the figure. The center of the dotted normal curve is at zero. The dotted normal distribution has mean $\mu = 0$ and variance $\sigma^2 = 4$. The denominator σ in the formula, that is, dividing $X - \mu$ by σ, has the same effect as squeezing the dotted curve so that the curve is pushed up until it completely coincides with the graph of the standard normal distribution. In case of a normal distribution with the mean $\mu = 0$ and the variance $\sigma^2 < 1$, say, $X \sim N(0, 0.5)$ shown in Figure 5.5.7, dividing $X - \mu$ by σ has the same effect as flattening the curve until it coincides with the standard normal curve.

Example 5.5.1. Suppose the amount of time the dental hygienists spend with their patients for prophylaxis is normally distributed with a mean of 50 min. and a standard deviation (SD) of 6 min. Letting X be the random variable representing the amount of time, we can write $X \sim N(50, 36)$. We can easily transform X to Z scores. The table below presents the selected values of X and their corresponding Z scores.

X Values (in min.)	Z Scores
42	$\dfrac{X - 50}{6} = \dfrac{42 - 50}{6} = -1.33$
50	$\dfrac{X - 50}{6} = \dfrac{50 - 50}{6} = 0$
55	$\dfrac{X - 50}{6} = \dfrac{55 - 50}{6} = 0.83$
68	$\dfrac{X - 50}{6} = \dfrac{68 - 50}{6} = 3.0$

5.5.3 Using Normal Probability Table

In this section we will discuss how to use Table D in the Appendix to compute the necessary normal probabilities. The first column of Table D lists the digits in the ones and tenths places of non-negative values (represented hereafter as z) from 0.0 to 3.9. In the first row across the top of the table are the

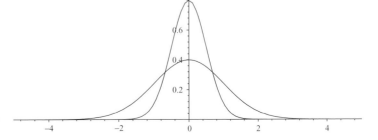

Figure 5.5.7 Two normal curves with mean zero but unequal variance.

digits in the one-hundredth place (second digit below the decimal). The table values represent the probabilities corresponding to the entire area under the standard normal curve to the left of a given *z* score.

Example 5.5.2. Find the probability $P(Z \leq 1.65)$.

Solution. The probability $P(Z \leq 1.65)$ corresponds to the area under the standard normal curve to the left of the score $z = 1.65$.

z	.00	.01	.02	.03	.04	**.05**	.06	.07	.08	.09
0.0						·				
0.1						·				
0.2						·				
·						·				
·						·				
1.5						↓				
1.6	·	·	·	·	→	**.9505**				
1.7										
1.8										

We need to look up *z* score 1.65 in Table D. Go to 1.6 in the first column and .05 in the top row. The table entry value 0.9505 where 1.6 and .05 meet is the probability, that is, $P(Z \leq 1.65) = 0.9505$.

From Figure 5.5.8 we can see that the area under the curve to the left of zero is the same as the area under the curve to the right of zero; that is, $P(Z \leq 0) = P(Z \geq 0) = 0.5$. Indeed Table D gives $P(Z \leq 0) = 0.5$.

By the symmetric property of the standard normal distribution, $P(Z \leq -z) = P(Z \geq z)$. The probabilities for $-z$ are not provided in Table D, but we will learn to find such probabilities using the symmetric property. The probability $P(Z \leq -z)$ refers to the left tail and the probability $P(Z \geq z)$

refers to the right tail of the standard normal distribution. Keep in mind that $P(Z = z) = 0$ because the area under the curve at $Z = z$ is zero. Consequently,

$$P(Z \leq z) = P(Z < z) + P(Z = z)$$
$$= P(Z < z) + 0 = P(Z < z).$$

Example 5.5.3. (i) Find $P(Z \leq 1.96)$. In Figure 5.5.8 place a tick mark at $z = 1.96$. The corresponding probability is the entire area under the curve to the left of 1.96. In Table D, find the first two digits 1.9 in the first column headed *Z*. Follow that row over to the column labeled by the third digit, 0.06, to find the desired probability of 0.9750.

(ii) Find $P(Z \leq -2.43)$. This probability is not included in the table, but notice that from the symmetric property of the normal distribution $P(Z \leq -2.43) = P(Z \geq 2.43)$. Thus, this problem is equivalent to finding $P(Z \geq 2.43)$, which is the area to the right of $z = 2.43$, that is, the right tail of the standard normal distribution. Recall that the entire area under the normal curve is 1.0. Therefore, we can express

$$P(Z \geq 2.43) = 1 - P(Z < 2.43)$$
$$= 1 - P(Z \leq 2.43), \text{ since } Z \text{ is a}$$
$$\text{continuous random variable.}$$
$$= 1 - 0.9925 = 0.0075.$$

Hence, $P(Z \leq -2.43) = 0.0075$.

(iii) Find $P(Z \geq -1.28)$. In Figure 5.5.8, place a tick mark at $z = -1.28$. The probability is the same as the area to the right of $z = -1.28$. The area to the right of $z = -1.28$ is equal to $1 -$ [the area to the left of -1.28]. Using the probabilistic expression, we can write $P(Z \geq -1.28) = 1 - P(Z \leq -1.28)$. We need to compute $P(Z \leq -1.28)$ in a similar manner as in (ii) above. That is, $P(Z \leq -1.28) = 1 - P(Z \leq 1.28) = 1 - 0.8997. = 0.1003$. The desired probability then is

$$P(Z \geq -1.28) = 1 - P(Z \leq -1.28)$$
$$= 1 - [1 - P(Z \leq 1.28)]$$
$$= 1 - 0.1003 = 0.8997.$$

(iv) Find $P(1.27 \leq Z \leq 3.15)$. This probability corresponds to the area under the standard normal curve between $z = 1.27$ and $z = 3.15$. Geometrically, this area is [the area to the left of 3.15] − [the

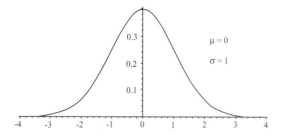

Figure 5.5.8   Standard normal curve.

area to the left of 1.27]. Hence, we can rewrite $P(1.27 \leq Z \leq 3.15)$ as

$$P(1.27 \leq Z \leq 3.15)$$
$$= P(Z \leq 3.15) - P(Z \leq 1.27)$$
$$= 0.9992 - 0.8980 = 0.1012.$$

In Example 5.5.3 we have demonstrated how to find a variety of different standard normal probabilities using Table D. We will continue to discuss a few more examples dealing with the normal probability distributions.

Example 5.5.4. Ascorbic acid is one of the principal ingredients contained in vitamin C tablets. It is found in fresh fruits and vegetables, such as citrus fruits, tomatoes, and cabbage. A deficiency of ascorbic acid is known to lead to scurvy; the pathologic signs of scurvy, confined mainly to the connective tissues, include hemorrhages, loosening of teeth, gingivitis, and poor wound healing. Suppose the amount of ascorbic acid contained in vitamin C tablets is normally distributed with the mean of 450 mg and the SD of 15 mg. What proportion of the vitamin C tablets would contain ascorbic acid between 425 mg and 475 mg?

Solution. Let X be the random variable for the amount of ascorbic acid. The desired proportion of the vitamin C tablets can be expressed as $P(425 \leq X \leq 475)$. First, we need to transform X to the standard normal. Because $\mu = 450$ and $\sigma = 15$,

$$P(425 \leq X \leq 475)$$
$$= P\left[\frac{425 - 450}{15} \leq \frac{X - \mu}{\sigma} \leq \frac{475 - 450}{15}\right]$$
$$= P(-1.67 \leq Z \leq 1.67)$$
$$= P(Z \leq 1.67) - P(Z \leq -1.67)$$
$$= 0.9525 - 0.0475 = 0.9050.$$

Therefore, 90.5% of the tablets would contain ascorbic acid between 425 mg and 475 mg.

Example 5.5.5. Suppose that the bite force in 5- to 10-year-old healthy children was measured and found to be normally distributed with the mean $\mu = 80.8$ lbs and the SD $\sigma = 14.4$ lbs [3]. What is the probability that a healthy 8-year-old male patient who regularly brushes his teeth twice a day would have the bite force of at least 70 lbs?

Solution. Letting Y be the random variable denoting the bite force, we can write the probability as

$$P(70 \leq Y) = P\left[\frac{70 - 80.8}{14.4} \leq \frac{Y - \mu}{\sigma}\right]$$
$$= P(-0.75 \leq Z)$$
$$= 1 - P(Z \leq -0.75)$$
$$= 1.0 - P(Z \geq 0.75).$$

One should be able to draw the standard normal curve and graphically indicate the areas corresponding to the probabilities to understand the equalities in the above expressions.

$$P(Z \geq 0.75) = 1.0 - P(Z \leq 0.75)$$
$$= 1.0 - 0.7734 = 0.2266.$$

By substitution, $P(70 \leq Y) = 1.0 - P(Z \geq 0.75) = 1.0 - 0.2266 = 0.7734$.

The probability is 0.7734 that the patient has the bite force of at least 70 lbs.

In the above example, some of the intermediary steps could have been avoided by noticing that the area under the standard normal curve to the right of -0.75 is equal to the area to the left of 0.75 by the symmetric property, which implies $P(-0.75 \leq Z) = P(Z \leq 0.75)$.

Example 5.5.6. Pocket depth, usually expressed in millimeters, is the measurement of the distance between the gingival crest and the base of the pocket. If the probability distribution of the pocket depths of smokers is normal with the mean $\mu = 3.5$ mm and the variance $\sigma^2 = 0.64$, what is the chance that a randomly chosen smoker has a pocket depth no more than 5.0 mm?

Solution. Suppose we let Y be the random variable representing the pocket depth. Then the problem can be written as $P(Y \leq 5.0)$. By transformation,

$$P(Y \leq 5.0) = P\left[\frac{Y - \mu}{\sigma} \leq \frac{5.0 - 3.5}{0.8}\right]$$
$$= P(Z \leq 1.875)$$

Note that $z = 1.875$ is the midpoint between 1.87 and 1.88. From Table D, $P(Z \leq 1.87) = 0.9693$ and $P(Z \leq 1.88) = 0.9700$. We will approximate the probability $P(Z \leq 1.875)$ by the midpoint between 0.9693 and 0.9700, that is, the average of the two probabilities. This approximation technique is called the linear interpolation.

$$P(Z \leq 1.875) = \frac{0.9693 + 0.9700}{2} = 0.9697.$$

A randomly chosen smoker has a 96.97% chance that his pocket depth will not exceed 5.0 mm.

Example 5.5.7. Karjalainen et al. [4] investigated the relationship between the occurrence of caries and diabetes in children and adolescents with insulin-dependent diabetes mellitus. One of the variables they observed was salivary pH in the subjects with decayed and/or filled teeth. The average salivary pH was 7.4 and the SD was 0.3. Suppose the probability distribution of the salivary pH level is approximately normal. Dr. Chung has filled two mandibular molar teeth in a 12-year-old patient who is an insulin-dependent diabetic. What is the probability that the salivary pH level of Dr. Chung's patient is no less than 7.0 but no more than 7.5?

Solution. The desired probability can be expressed as

$$P(7.0 \leq X \leq 7.5)$$
$$= P \left[\frac{7.0 - 7.4}{0.3} \leq \frac{X - \mu}{\sigma} \leq \frac{7.5 - 7.4}{0.3} \right]$$
$$= P(-1.33 \leq X \leq 0.33)$$
$$= P(X \leq 0.33) - P(X \leq -1.33)$$
$$= 0.6293 - (1.0 - 0.9082) = 0.5375.$$

5.5.4 Further Applications of Normal Probability

In the preceding section we have studied several examples for finding appropriate probabilities using the standard normal probability table. In this section, we will discuss examples that illustrate applications combining both binomial and normal distributions.

Example 5.5.8. Dentists who treat patients with insulin-dependent diabetes mellitus (IDDM) should be concerned about hypoglycemia before undertaking any outpatient treatment. The IDDM patients are likely to experience greater bone resorption, and, therefore, the survival time of an implant placed in the IDDM patients may be considerably shorter. Suppose a retrospective study shows that the survival times of titanium implants

for these patients are approximately normally distributed with the average survival time of 34 months and the variance of 28. What is the chance that 2 of 6 patients with IDDM will have their implants function beyond 40 months?

Solution. First, we should compute the probability of an implant surviving beyond 40 months, that is, $P(40 \leq Y)$. Let p be the probability of success. Then, because $\mu = 34$ and $\sigma = \sqrt{28} = 5.3$, we have

$$p = P(40 \leq Y) = P \left[\frac{40 - 34}{5.3} \leq \frac{Y - \mu}{\sigma} \right],$$
$$\text{since } Y \sim N(34, 28)$$
$$= P(1.13 \leq Z) = 1.0 - P(Z \leq 1.13) = 0.1292.$$

Let X be the binomial random variable with parameters $n = 6$ and $p = 0.1292$. The chance that 2 of 6 patients have their implants function at least 40 months is given by

$$P(X = 2) = \binom{6}{2} p^2 (1 - p)^{6-2}$$
$$= \frac{6!}{2!(6-2)!} \times (0.1292)^2 (0.8708)^4$$
$$= (15) \cdot (0.0167) \cdot (0.5750)$$
$$= 0.1440.$$

Example 5.5.9. Veneered stainless steel (VSS) crowns are one of the treatment options to restore severely carious anterior teeth. Although these VSS crowns are esthetically pleasing, the veneers can fracture. A study was conducted to determine the fracture resistance of these veneers by placing the crowns in the Instron universal testing machine and loading them to failure. The peak loads at failure were approximately normal with the mean $\mu = 68.49$ kg and the standard deviation $\sigma = 18.07$ [5]. Dr. Hernandez prepared 4 VSS crowns for his patients. What is the probability that none of the veneers will fracture at the load strength of 70 kg?

Solution. That none of the veneers will fracture at the load strength of 70 kg means that, for all 4 veneers, fracture will occur at the load strength higher than 70 kg. First, we need to calculate the probability that fracture occurs at the load strength higher than 70 kg;

$$p = P(70 < Y) = P\left[\frac{70 - 68.49}{18.07} \leq \frac{Y - \mu}{\sigma}\right]$$

$$= P(0.08 < Z)$$

$$= 1.0 - P(Z \leq 0.08) = 0.4681.$$

P(none of the veneers will fracture at the load strength of 70 kg)

$= P$ (all 4 veneers will fracture at the load strength higher than 70 kg)

$$= \binom{4}{4} p^4 (1-p)^{4-4}$$

$$= \frac{4!}{4!(4-4)!}(0.4681)^4(0.5319)^0 = 0.0480.$$

The desired probability that none of the veneers will fracture at the load strength of 70 kg is 0.0480.

Example 5.5.10. Provisional restorations play a critical role in the success of restorative treatment. The provisional restoration must maintain its surface integrity throughout the restorative process. A study was performed to evaluate the microhardness of a contemporary prosthodontic provisional material (bis-acryl resin composites). Knoop hardness was measured for the samples with a microhardness tester. Knoop hardness is a means of measuring surface hardness by resistance to the penetration of an indenting tool made of diamond [6]. Suppose the Knoop hardness for this provisional material is normally distributed with $\mu = 17.20$ and $\sigma^2 = 4.41$, that is, $Y \sim N(17.20, 4.41)$. What is the probability that at least 2 of the 5 provisional restorations have Knoop hardness between 15 and 20?

Solution. We need to compute the binomial probability of "success."

$$p = P(15 \leq Y \leq 20)$$

$$= P\left[\frac{15 - 17.2}{2.1} \leq \frac{Y - \mu}{\sigma} \leq \frac{20 - 17.2}{2.1}\right]$$

$= P(-1.05 \leq Z \leq 1.33)$, this probability corresponds to the area under the standard normal curve between $Z = -1.05$ and $Z = 1.33$.

$$= P(Z \leq 1.33) - P(Z \leq -1.05)$$

$$= P(Z \leq 1.33) - [1.0 - P(Z \leq 1.05)]$$

$$= 0.9082 - (1.0 - 0.8531) = 0.7613.$$

Let X be the binomial random variable with parameters $n = 5$ and $p = 0.7613$, $X \sim B(5, 0.7613)$. The probability P(at least 2 of the 5 provisional restorations have Knoop hardness between 15 and 20) $= P(2 \leq X)$.

$$P(2 \leq X) = 1.0 - [P(X = 0) + P(X = 1)]$$

$$= 1.0 - \left[\binom{5}{0}(0.7613)^0(0.2387)^5\right.$$

$$\left. + \binom{5}{1}(0.7613)^1(0.2387)^4\right]$$

$$= 0.9868.$$

5.5.5 Finding the $(1-\alpha)$ 100th Percentiles

In the previous sections, we have learned how to transform a normal variable to the standard normal variable and how to calculate the probabilities using the normal probability table provided in the Appendix. To make the transformation, we used the simple formula $Z = (X - \mu)/\sigma$. Conversely, given the above transformation, we can obtain X in terms of a Z score by a simple algebraic manipulation: $X = \mu + Z \cdot \sigma$.

Consider the following problem. A speedy ambulance response time can save many lives in critical situations. Public officials in the city of Riverside have been monitoring the ambulance response times within the city limits. Suppose the distribution of the response time is approximately normal with the mean of 10 minutes and the standard deviation of 2.5 minutes. The city mayor wishes to know what the response time is for the 95% of the 911 emergency calls. In other words, the mayor wants to know the 95th percentile of the ambulance response time. We can use the normal probability table (Table D) to solve the problem. First, let $Z_{1-\alpha}$ denote the $(1 - \alpha)100^{th}$ percentile point of the standard normal distribution. If $\alpha = 0.05$, the $Z_{1-\alpha} = Z_{1-0.05} = Z_{0.95}$ denotes the 95th percentile on the standard normal distribution. We can find the 95th percentile, $Z_{0.95}$, by following the steps described below.

Step 1. In Table D, look for the probability 0.95. Although 0.95 does not appear in the table, note that it is the midpoint between 0.9495 and 0.9505. The z scores corresponding to 0.9495 and 0.9505 are 1.64 and 1.65, respectively.

Table 5.5.1. Standard normal probability table.

z	.00	.01	.02	.03	**.04**	**.05**	.06	.07	.08	.09
0.0					.	.				
0.1					.	.				
0.2					.	.				
.					.	.				
.					.	.				
1.5					↓	↓				
1.6	.	.	.	$\longrightarrow$	.9495	.9505				
1.7										

Step 2. By an approximation technique known as linear interpolation, take the midpoint between 1.64 and 1.65, that is, 1.645 as the corresponding z score to the probability 0.95, so that $Z_{0.95} = 1.645$.

We can use $Z_{0.95} = 1.645$ to answer the mayor's question. In the identity $X = \mu + Z \cdot \sigma$, we make substitutions for $\mu = 10$, $\sigma = 2.5$, and $Z_{0.95} = 1.645$; $X = \mu + Z \cdot \sigma = 10 + (1.645)(2.5) = 14.113$. Therefore, the emergency vehicles can respond to 95% of the calls within 14.113 minutes (see Table 5.5.1).

Definition 5.5.2. The $(1 - \alpha)100^{\text{th}}$ percentile, $Z_{1-\alpha}$ is sometimes referred to as the upper α^{th} percentile, and the αth percentile, Z_α is sometimes referred to as the lower α^{th} percentile. For example, the 95th percentile point, $Z_{0.95}$ is referred to as the upper 5th percentile, and the 5th percentile, $Z_{0.05}$ is referred to as the lower 5th percentile.

Example 5.5.11. A carving skill test is given to all aspiring dental students to evaluate their ability to shape and form restorations with instruments. Suppose the carving skill scores are normally distributed with $\mu = 78$ and $\sigma = 7.5$. If it is known that the applicants to dental schools score in the top 10%, what is the minimum carving skill test score of the successful applicants?

Solution. Because the top 10% score corresponds to the 90th percentile point, first we need to find $Z_{0.90}$. This is equivalent to finding the z value that yields 0.10 of the area under the standard normal curve to the right of the z value. From Table D we get $Z_{0.90} = 1.28$ (approximately). One can obtain $Z_{0.90} = 1.282$ by the use of the linear interpolation technique. Substitution in the equation

$X = \mu + Z \cdot \sigma$ gives

$$X = \mu + Z \cdot \sigma = 78 + (1.28)(7.5) = 87.6.$$

Thus, a minimum carving skill score of 87.6 is needed for dental school admissions.

Example 5.5.12. For an optimal orthodontic bonding system, the bond strength must be high enough to prevent failure and the damage to the enamel involved in achieving the bond must be minimized. It should also be possible to remove the orthodontic brackets in such a way that minimal damage is caused to the teeth. The etching technique that uses phosphoric acid results in good bond strength, but some enamel loss occurs. A profilometer was used to determine the surface enamel loss (μm). If the amount of the surface loss is normally distributed with the mean of 6.4 and the standard deviation of 1.5 [7], find the lower and upper 2.5th percentiles.

Solution. The area to the right of the upper 2.5th percentile and the area to the left of the lower 2.5th percentile under the standard normal curve are both equal to 0.025. As illustrated in Figure 5.5.9, the probability corresponding to the area between the lower and upper 2.5th percentiles is 0.95. The 95% of the standard normal population falls between the lower and upper 2.5th percentiles. The upper 2.5th percentile is the same as the 97.5th percentile, $Z_{0.975}$. The lower 2.5th percentile is given by $Z_{0.025} = -Z_{0.975}$ by the symmetric property. From Table D the z score corresponding to the probability 0.975 is 1.96. Hence, the upper 2.5th percentile $Z_{0.975} = 1.96$ and the lower 2.5th percentile $Z_{0.025} = -1.96$. Substituting these percentiles in the formula $X = \mu + Z \cdot \sigma$, we get

The lower 2.5th percentile:

$$X = \mu + Z_{0.025} \cdot \sigma = 6.4 + (-1.96)(1.5) = 3.46.$$

The upper 2.5th percentile:

$$X = \mu + Z_{0.975} \cdot \sigma = 6.4 + (1.96)(1.5) = 9.34.$$

5.5.6 Normal Approximation to the Binomial Distribution

Binomial distribution was introduced earlier in this chapter to evaluate the probability of k successes

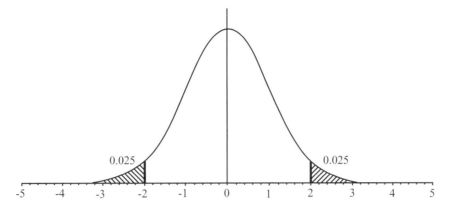

Figure 5.5.9 Lower and upper 2.5th percentiles.

in n independent trials. Recall that a binomial distribution possesses the following characteristics:

1. There is a fixed number of trials.
2. The trials are independent.

central limit theorem, which is presented in Chapter 6.) To illustrate the normal approximation, let's consider $p = 0.35$, and $n = 5$, 10, and 15. From Table B in the Appendix, we obtain the values in the following table.

$n = 5, \; p = 0.35$		$n = 10, \; p = 0.35$		$n = 15, \; p = 0.35$			
k	$P(X = k)$	k	$P(X = k)$	k	$P(X = k)$	k	$P(X = k)$
0	0.1160	0	0.0135	0	0.0016	8	0.0710
1	0.3124	1	0.0725	1	0.0126	9	0.0298
2	0.3364	2	0.1757	2	0.0476	10	0.0096
3	0.1812	3	0.2522	3	0.1110	11	0.0024
4	0.0488	4	0.2377	4	0.1793	12	0.0004
5	0.0053	5	0.1536	5	0.2123	13	0.0001
		6	0.0689	6	0.1906	14	0.0000
		7	0.0212	7	0.1319	15	0.0000
		8	0.0043				
		9	0.0005				
		10	0.0000				

3. Each trial can result in exactly two possible outcomes.
4. The probability p of a success must remain the same from trial to trial.

The calculation of the binomial probability when n is large becomes tedious and time consuming. For a binomial distribution, $X \sim B(n, p)$, if p is close to 0.5, then the shape of the binomial distribution looks similar to the normal distribution, as n increases. The larger n gets and the closer p is to 0.5, the more similar the shape of the binomial distribution is to the normal distribution. Intuitively, this suggests that we can use the normal distribution to approximate the binomial distribution. (Theoretical justification is based on the

Figure 5.5.10 shows three binomial mass functions with $n = 5$, 10, 15, and $p = 0.35$. There is empirical evidence that as n increases, the shape of the binomial mass functions become closer to the normal distribution. Because the mean and variance of a binomial distribution are np and $np(1 - p)$, or npq, it seems quite natural to use $N(np, npq)$, the normal distribution with the mean np and the variance npq, as an approximation. When n is relatively small and p is close to 0 or 1, the normal approximate is not accurate. Even for large n, the binomial distribution when p is close to 0 or 1 will be either positively or negatively skewed. The normal approximation to the binomial distribution is recommended when $npq \geq 5$. Notice that if $npq \geq 5$,

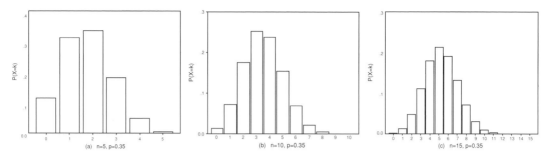

Figure 5.5.10 Binomial mass functions.

then $np \geq 5$ because q is smaller than or equal to 1.0. Suppose $n = 10$ and $p = 0.42$. Because $npq = (10)(0.42)(0.58) = 2.436 < 5.0$, the normal approximation should not be used in this case. We will restate the theorem next.

Normal Approximation to the Binomial Distribution

Let X be a binomial random variable with parameters n and p. Then for large n, X is approximately normal with mean np and variance npq.

Suppose we want to compute the probability $P(a \leq X \leq b)$, where $X \sim B(n, p)$. It appears reasonable to approximate the probability by the area under the normal curve between a and b. It turns out that a better approximation to this probability is given by the area under the normal curve between $a - \frac{1}{2}$ and $b + \frac{1}{2}$. We note that $P(X = 0)$ and $P(X = n)$ are better approximated by the areas to the left of $n + \frac{1}{2}$ and to the right of $n - \frac{1}{2}$, respectively, under the normal curve. In summary,

1. $P(a \leq X \leq b)$

$$\simeq P\left[\frac{(a-0.5)-np}{\sqrt{npq}} \leq \frac{X-np}{\sqrt{npq}} \leq \frac{(b+0.5)-np}{\sqrt{npq}} \right]$$

$$= P\left[\frac{(a-0.5)-np}{\sqrt{npq}} \leq Z \leq \frac{(b+0.5)-np}{\sqrt{npq}} \right]$$

2. $P(X = 0)$

$$\simeq P\left[\frac{X-np}{\sqrt{npq}} \leq \frac{0.5-np}{\sqrt{npq}} \right] = P\left[Z \leq \frac{0.5-np}{\sqrt{npq}} \right]$$

3. $P(X = n)$

$$\simeq P\left[\frac{(n-0.5)-np}{\sqrt{npq}} \leq \frac{X-np}{\sqrt{npq}} \right]$$

$$= P\left[\frac{(n-0.5)-np}{\sqrt{npq}} \leq Z \right]$$

4. $P(X = a)$

$$\simeq P\left[\frac{(a-0.5)-np}{\sqrt{npq}} \leq \frac{X-np}{\sqrt{npq}} \leq \frac{(a+0.5)-np}{\sqrt{npq}} \right]$$

$$\text{for } 0 < a < n$$

$$= P\left[\frac{(a-0.5)-np}{\sqrt{npq}} \leq Z \leq \frac{(a+0.5)-np}{\sqrt{npq}} \right]$$

Example 5.5.13. Suppose that the chance of orthodontic treatment lasting more than 30 months is about 0.20. Dr. Elderidge receives, on average, 160 new patients a year. What is the probability that between 30 and 50 of these patients will require the treatment longer than 30 months?

Solution. Because $npq = 160 \cdot (0.20)(0.80) = 25.6 > 5.0$, we may use the normal approximation to compute the probability $P(30 \leq X \leq 50)$. Now the mean and variance of the binomial random variable X are $np = 32.0$ and $npq = 160 \cdot (0.20)(0.80) = 25.6$. Using the formula

$$P(30 \leq X \leq 50)$$

$$\simeq P\left[\frac{(30-0.5)-32}{\sqrt{25.6}} \leq Z \leq \frac{(50+0.5)-32}{\sqrt{25.6}} \right]$$

$$= P\left[\frac{-2.5}{5.0596} \leq Z \leq \frac{18.5}{5.0596} \right]$$

$$= P(-0.49 \leq Z \leq 3.66)$$

$$= P(Z \leq 3.66) - P(Z \leq -0.49)$$

$$= 0.9999 - 0.3121 = 0.6878.$$

Example 5.5.14. Physical abuse of a child is defined as a non-accidental injury or trauma to the body of a child. Hospital data over a 5-year period indicated that 49% of abused children exhibited facial and intraoral trauma [8]. Parkview Community Hospital ER had 28 child maltreatment cases in one week. What is the probability that exactly one-half of those children exhibited facial and intraoral trauma?

Solution. Let $p = P$(abused child exhibit facial and intraoral trauma) $= 0.49$. Then $np = 28(0.49) = 13.72$, and $npq = 28(0.49)(0.51) = 6.9972 > 5.0$. Thus, using the normal approximation to the binomial distribution, we have

$$P(X = 14)$$
$$\simeq P\left[\frac{(14 - 0.5) - 13.72}{\sqrt{6.9972}} \leq \frac{X - np}{\sqrt{npq}}\right.$$
$$\left.\leq \frac{(14 + 0.5) - 13.72}{\sqrt{6.9972}}\right]$$
$$= P(-0.08 \leq Z \leq 0.29)$$
$$= P(Z \leq 0.29) - P(Z \leq -0.08)$$
$$= 0.1460.$$

The normal distribution is the most frequently used theoretical model in statistics. It can serve as a model for many phenomena in biomedical, epidemiologic, and health sciences that are approximately normally distributed. It provides an excellent approximation to the binomial distribution (and to other distributions) when n is sufficiently large. When n is large, it is too laborious to calculate the exact binomial probabilities. One of its most important applications is as a model for the sampling distribution of statistics based on a large number of observations. The sampling distribution will be discussed in Chapter 6.

5.6 EXERCISES

1 Suppose that the chances of a patient's being equally female or male are 50%. Sixteen patients have an appointment with Dr. Johnson. The outcome that is most likely to happen is that Dr. Johnson will examine
a. 16 female patients
b. 16 male patients
c. 9 female and 17 male patients
d. 17 female and 9 male patients
e. 8 female and 8 male patients.

2 Compute the following.

a. $\binom{12}{4}$ b. $\binom{12}{0}$ c. $\binom{12}{12}$ d. $6!$

3 Discuss why $\binom{n}{k}$ and $\binom{n}{n-k}$ are equal.

4 Most patients trust that the dental and medical instruments used in their treatment are sterilized and free from any bacteria. They may also trust that the same instruments will not be used on the next patients before they are resterilized. The Public Health Department took a random sample of 126 dental and medical practices and found that 12% of them have infection control problems. Let X be the number of practices with infection control problems.
a. Explain why X is a binomial random variable
b. What are n and p?

5 The chance that a gold crown functions 10 years or longer is about 0.20. Dr. Shin placed 6 gold crowns last week. What is the probability that 3 of the 6 crowns will still function 10 years from now?

6 The data collected on *Streptococcus sanguis* by a group of hygiene students indicate that it can be found in about 20% of the healthy individuals' oral cavities. Dr. Danton typically treats 15 patients a day. What is the probability that he will find *S. sanguis* in the oral cavity of at least 3 of his next 10 patients?

7 Dental patients are classified into three categories based on their oral hygiene status; poor, fair, and good. Let P(poor hygiene) $= 0.32$, P(fair hygiene) $= 0.43$, and P(good hygiene) $= 0.25$. Poor oral hygiene can cause serious periodontitis. Of 12 patients arriving at a dental clinic, what is the chance that between 5 and 8 (inclusive) patients have poor oral hygiene?

8 An exposure incident defined by OSHA (Occupational Safety and Health Administration) is an occurrence that puts clinicians at risk of a biomedical or chemical contact on the job, such as eye, skin, mucous membrane, or parenteral contact with blood or other potentially infectious fluids. It is required that all exposure incidents be reported to OSHA. Suppose that only 75% of the exposure incidents are reported and 25% are ignored. What is the chance that Arrowhead Dental Clinic reported only 9 of the 15 exposure incidents last year?

9 The average number of patients diagnosed with pancreatic cancer is about 6.5 per 100, 000 individuals per year. If the number of patients diagnosed with pancreatic cancer follows the Poisson distribution, what is the probability that during a given year

a. exactly 10 patients with pancreatic cancer live in a community with approximately 100, 000 people?
b. there are at least three cases in the community?
c. there are two or fewer cases in the community?

10 Suppose in a water sample taken from a dental water line on average there are five organisms.

a. What is the probability that the next sample contains four organisms?
b. What is the probability that at least three organisms will be found in the next sample?
c. What is the probability that no more than two organisms will be found?

11 Loma Linda Community Hospital receives 3.5 ER patients per hour on average between 11:00 pm and 7:00 am. What is the chance that the hospital would get 30 ER patients during this period?

12 To evaluate the Poisson approximation, compare the Poisson approximation to the exact binomial probabilities for $n = 100$, $p = 0.01$, and $k = 0, 1, 2, 3, 4, 5, 6, 7$, and 8.

13 About 4% of the dental and medical bills are uncollectable for various reasons. Dr. Johnson and his partners have about 1, 000 outstanding patient bills. What is the chance that 45 of those bills are uncollectable?

14 A survey on quality care indicates that one of the major factors affecting patient satisfaction is the waiting time before they are examined by the health care professionals. Suppose the distribution of patient waiting time is not known. What percent of the patients would have to wait $\pm 1.5\sigma$ of the average waiting time?

15 Suppose a random variable X describes the pocket depth, and it is found to be approximately normally distributed with the mean of 3.2 mm and the standard deviation of 1.5 mm. A 66-year-old male patient has a pocket depth of 5.7 mm. What is the standardized normal score of his pocket depth?

16 According to a study, the actual amount of anesthetic contained in the bottle labeled 5 cc. is normally distributed with the mean of 5.4 cc. and the SD of 1.8 cc. Let X be the amount of anesthetic. Then $X \sim N(5.4, 3.24)$.

a. Transform the random variable X to a standard normal.
b. Find $P(-2.04 \le Z \le 1.97)$.
c. Find $P(-2.12 \le Z \le -0.59)$.
d. What is the probability that a given bottle contains more than 7.0 cc.?
e. What proportion of the anesthetic bottles labeled 5 cc. contain more than 8.0 cc.?

17 The historical data indicate that the scores of the National Board Exam Part I taken during the second year in dental school are normally distributed with the mean score of 77.8 and the variance of 19.4. In order to pass the exam one must score at least 75. Compute the percent of students who passed this year's exam.

18 Find the following percentiles using Table D (standard normal probabilities) in the Appendix.
a. 10th   b. 75th   c. 85th   d. 97.5th

19 Educational outcomes assessment of the predoctoral dental curriculum has long been a concern of educators and dental practitioners. The curricular guidelines were developed by the American Association of Dental Schools to prescribe course contents and to ensure that dental schools provide sufficient instruction to prepare competent future dental clinicians. To evaluate the success of these efforts, an outcomes assessment test consisting of a didactic test and a test of clinical diagnostic skills was given to a group of 4th year dental students. Suppose the scores are normally distributed with the mean of 66.3 and the variance of 64.6. Find 25th, 50th, 90th, 95th and 99th percentiles of the test results.

20 Root resorption is an undesirable side effect of orthodontic treatment. Acar et al. [9] investigated the effects on root resorption of continuous force application by means of elastics. Elastics were worn 24 hours per day for 9 weeks. At the end of the 9th week, the teeth were extracted. The samples were then appropriately prepared and the resorbed root area was calculated as a percentage of the total root area seen in each composite. Suppose that these percentages are approximately normal with the mean of 11% and the standard deviation of 2.6%. What are the lower and upper 5th percentiles?

21 The length of time endodontists spend with their patients at each visit is known to be normally distributed with the mean $\mu = 20$ min and the standard deviation $\sigma = 5$ min. Suppose an endodontist starts treating a patient at 11:45 am. What is the probability that he will complete the treatment by 12:15 pm?

22 Dr. Johnny is an orthodontist. In the above exercise, what is the chance that Dr. Johnny spends either less than 15 min or more than 25 min with a randomly chosen patient?

23 The National Board Exam Part II scores are normally distributed. If the mean score is 78 and the variance is 28, what proportion of the students have scored between 75 and 85?

24 If the annual household dental and medical expenditure in the State of California is approximately normal with $\mu = \$11,450$ and $\sigma = \$2,750$. What is the probability that a randomly chosen household in California spends between $10,000 and $13,000 a year?

25 The salivary flow rate of adult patients is known to be normally distributed with the mean of 1.2 ml/min and SD of 0.3 ml/min. If nine patients were selected at random and their salivary flow rate was measured, what is the chance that exactly three of them have the flow rate less than 1.0 ml/min?

26 Composite bonding agent is used by many dental practitioners as the surface treatment for denture teeth. The shear bond strength of composite to acrylic resin denture teeth was measured in megapascals. Suppose the probability distribution of the shear bond strength is normal with $\mu = 7.33$ and $\sigma = 1.52$. Dr. Danbury prepared 45 central incisors and canines of acrylic resin denture teeth in the last 6 months. How many of them would have a shear bond strength greater than 6.5 MPa?

27 Many dental and medical students carry a large amount of educational loans while in school. A survey shows, however, that surprisingly about 16% of the students have less than $20,000 in loans. Out of 150 dental and medical students who were randomly sampled, what is the chance that between 25 and 35 students have less than $20,000 in loans?

28 Separation of instruments while performing root canals is something that has plagued all practitioners. A study [10] shows that with rotary nickel-titanium instruments at 333.33 rpm file distortion

and/or separation is four times as likely to occur than at 166.67 rpm. Suppose that the probability of file distortion or separation at 333.33 rpm is 0.15. Out of 80 files, what is the probability that at least 50 will not be damaged at this rate?

29 In Exercise 28, what is the chance that between 25 and 50 files will not be distorted or separated?

30 Microleakage can occur at the abutment-implant interface in osseointegrated implants and may cause malodor and inflammation of peri-implant tissues. Using colored tracing probes driven by a 2-atm pressure system, the interface microleakage of certain implants was determined spectrophotometrically [11]. Suppose microleakage at the abutment-implant interface occurs at the rate of 18 per 100 when closing torque is about 15 N.cm. Dr. Camp and his associates placed 60 implants so far this year. What is the chance that no more that 10 of the implants would have microleakage at the abutment-implant interface?

31 Dr. Camp has two hygienists working in his practice. For the purpose of scheduling patient appointments, it is important to know something about the distribution of time it takes for the hygienists to complete prophylaxis. Suppose he has learned from a hygiene journal that the distribution of time the hygienists spend in patient contact is normal with $\mu = 58$ min and $\sigma^2 = 50$. One of his hygienists has 12 patients to treat. What is the probability that she will be able to complete prophylaxis in 50 min for at least 9 of her patients?

32 The volume of the cranial cavity, denoted by a random variable Y, is a great concern to orthodontists. Suppose that Y is normally distributed with the mean of $1,500$ cc and standard deviation of 200 cc.
a. What is the probability that the volume of the cranial cavity of a 14-year-old male patient is less than 1,400?
b. Dr. Jung has 14 patients sitting in 14 chairs in his practice. Find the probability that between 5 and 8 patients have cranial cavity volume of at most 1,400 cc.
c. Find the 95th percentile of the distribution of Y.

33 It is known that about 95% of bacteria-causing odontogenic infections respond to penicillin and that about 6% of the population is allergic to penicillin. Suppose 850 patients have been given a dose of penicillin VK, 500 mg every 6 hours for a week. Find the probability that no more than 30 of these patients would have an allergic reaction.

34 The percentage of mercury concentration in an amalgam restoration is known to range from 25% to 65%. Suppose the chance that mercury concentration in amalgam exceeding the 50% level is 0.28. Of 26 amalgam samples Dr. Lang has prepared, what is the probability that at least 7 of them have mercury concentration higher than 50%?

35 Bacteria and their by-products are known to cause periapical inflammation. Thus, endodontic treatment is focused on preventing microorganisms from entering the root canal system or eliminating them if already present. The tightness of root canal fillings is essential to prevent bacteria from invading the periapex. The estimated rate of leakage in roots coronally sealed with a certain type of temporary filling over 30 days is 35%. Arrowhead Dental Clinic treated 25 endodontic patients with this temporary filling. What is the probability that the temporary filling experienced leakage in no more than 5 patients?

5.7 REFERENCES

1. Buser, D., Bragger, U., Lang, N. P., and Nyman, S. Regeneration and enlargement of jaw bone using guided tissue regeneration. *Clinical Oral Implants Research*. 1990. 1: 22–32.
2. Hemsley, C., and Jones, L. Occupational hazards of latex and powdered gloves in the dental profession. Student project. Loma Linda University School of Dentistry. 2001.
3. Bakke, M., Holm, B., Jensen, B. L., Michler, L., and Moller, E. Unilateral, isometric bite force in 8 68-year-old women and men related to occlusal factors. *Scand J Dent Res*. 1990: 98, 149–58.
4. Karjalainen, K. M., Knuuttila, M. L. E., and Käär, M. L. Relationship between caries and level of metabolic balance in children and adolescents with insulin-dependent diabetes mellitus. *Caries Research*. 1997: 31, 13–18.
5. Hoffer, J. Evaluation of three bonding agents in the repair of fractured veneered stainless stain crowns. MA thesis, Loma Linda University. 2001.
6. Zwemer, T. J. *Mosby's Dental Dictionary*. Mosby, Inc. 1998.
7. van Waveren Hogervosrst, W. L., Feilzer, A. J., and Pralh-Andersen, B. The air-abrasion technique versus the conventional acid-etching technique: A quantification of surface enamel loss and a comparison of shear bond strength. *Am J. Orthod Dentofacial Orthop*. 2000: 117, 20–26.
8. Jessee, S. A. Physical manifestations of child abuse to the head, face and mouth: A hospital survey. *J. of Dentistry for Children*. 1995: 245–249.
9. Acar, A., Canyürek, Ü., Kocaaga, M., and Erverdi, N. Continuous vs. discontinuous force application and root resorption. *The Angle Orthodontist*. 1999: 69, 159–163.
10. Gabel, W.P., Hoen, M. Steiman, H. R., Pink, F., and Dietz, R. Effect of rotational speed on nickel-titanium file distortion. *J. of Endodontics*. 1999: 25, 752–785.
11. Gross, M., Abramovich, I., and Weiss, E. I. Microleakage at the abutment-implant interface of osseointegrated implants: A comparative study. *J. Oral Maxillofac. Implants*. 1999: 14, 94–100.

Chapter 6

Sampling Distributions

6.1 INTRODUCTION

In Chapter 5 we introduced theoretical probability distributions—binomial, Poisson, and normal—where the population mean and variance are assumed to be known. However, in most practical situations these parameters are not known. In these cases the unknown parameters must be estimated from the data in order to describe the distributions and to estimate the associated probabilities for certain events. One of the most basic concepts of statistical inference is the **sampling distribution** of the sample mean ($\overline{X}$), which we introduced in Chapter 3. This chapter focuses on the sampling distribution of the sample mean; in later chapters we shall consider the sampling distributions of other statistics.

To illustrate the concept of a sampling distribution, let's consider a population of 5 maxillary molar and premolar teeth contained in a jar. Each tooth is marked with a number: 1, 2, 3, 4, or 5. We will draw a sample of 3 teeth from the jar without replacement. The population mean of the numbers marked on the 5 teeth is

$$\mu = \frac{1+2+3+4+5}{5} = 3.0.$$

Now let's draw a random sample of 3 teeth. There are $\binom{5}{3} = 10$ possible samples:

$(1, 2, 3)$, $(1, 2, 4)$, $(1, 2, 5)$, $(1, 3, 4)$, $(1, 3, 5)$, $(1, 4, 5)$, $(2, 3, 4)$, $(2, 3, 5)$, $(2, 4, 5)$, $(3, 4, 5)$.

The sample mean of each sample is 2.0, 2.33, 2.67, 2.67, 3.0, 3.33, 3.0, 3.33, 3.67, and 4.0. Each sample is equally likely, so each sample has the probability $\frac{1}{10}$. Thus, we have the sample means with the equal probability of $\frac{1}{10}$ as summarized in Table 6.1.1.

6.2 SAMPLING DISTRIBUTION OF THE MEAN

Suppose that the investigators are interested in the hemoglobin level of patients with the unknown population mean μ. The sample mean $\overline{X}$ is called an estimator of the parameter μ. Let's select two different samples of size n taken from the same population. The sample means for these two samples are likely to be different unless all the patients in the population have precisely the same level of hemoglobin. Now, consider the set of all possible samples of size n that can be selected from the population. As we can imagine, the values of $\overline{X}$ in all these samples will likely be different due to inherent uncertainty involved with different samples. It is very important that the samples represent accurately the population from which they are drawn. Any sample that does not represent the population properly will lead to biased conclusions.

Suppose we wish to draw a conclusion about the hemoglobin level of patients based on a sample of size n. If all of the n patients included in the sample are undergoing chemotherapy, the sample mean, which is the estimate of the population mean of patients' hemoglobin level, is likely to be too low, since the chemotherapy tends to decrease the hemoglobin level in cancer patients. Let the sample mean of the first sample of size n be $\overline{X}_1$, the sample mean of the second sample of size n be $\overline{X}_2$, $\cdots$, and the sample mean of the nth sample of the same size n be $\overline{X}_n$. At this point it is very helpful to consider these sample means as representative of all possible samples of size n that could have been drawn from the population. In other words, think of $\overline{X}$ as a random variable with possible outcomes $\overline{x}_1, \overline{x}_2, \cdots, \overline{x}_n$, and so on. If each sample mean in this case is treated as a unique observed value, the probability distribution of $\overline{X}$ is known as a **sampling distribution** of sample means of size n.

Table 6.1.1. Sampling distribution of the mean of three teeth numbers.

Sample Mean, $\overline{X}$	Probability, $P(\overline{X} = x)$
2.0	$\frac{1}{10}$
2.33	$\frac{1}{10}$
2.67	$\frac{2}{10}$
3.0	$\frac{2}{10}$
3.33	$\frac{2}{10}$
3.67	$\frac{1}{10}$
4.0	$\frac{1}{10}$

Definition 6.2.1. The **sampling distribution** of $\overline{X}$ is the distribution of values of $\overline{X}$ over the sample space consisting of all possible samples of size n.

Sampling distributions play an important role in statistical inference because they describe the sample to sample variability of statistics computed from random samples taken under a variety of different situations. Sampling distributions will be used extensively in future chapters, especially when the hypothesis testing is discussed. Consider now a large number of random samples of size n. If we compute the average of these sample means $\overline{X}$, we see that this average is approximately equal to the population mean μ. In fact, the mean of the sample means drawn from a population with mean μ is precisely the same as μ. This remark will become clearer as we discuss examples later. *The mean (expected value) of the sample means $\overline{X}$ is equal to the population mean μ.* This statement holds true for any population regardless of its underlying distribution function. In statistics, this estimator $\overline{X}$ is called an **unbiased estimator** of the unknown population mean μ. There are other unbiased estimators available, such as the **sample median** and the **average of the maximum and the minimum** of the observed values. There are advantages to working with $\overline{X}$. When the population is normally distributed, $\overline{X}$ is known to have the smallest variance among all unbiased estimators.

6.2.1 Standard Error of the Sample Mean

As we saw in Section 6.1, the sample mean of the first sample was 2.0, and the sample mean of the

second sample was 2.33, and so on. In general, the values of the sample means $\overline{X}$ of the same size n, drawn repeatedly from a population with the mean μ and variance σ^2, vary from one sample to the next. It is intuitively clear that a larger sample would likely yield more accurate estimates than a smaller sample. Therefore, we prefer to estimate the parameters μ and σ^2 from larger samples than from smaller samples. Bear in mind that in practice we do not repeatedly select samples of size n from a given population. Statistical inferences are made based on a single sample of size n. This practice is justified by the properties of the sampling distribution of the sample mean. We would expect that the averages of the random samples would be clustered together around the population mean, and the variability of $\overline{X}$'s is smaller than the variability of individual observations. That is, there is less variability among the sample means than there is among the individual observations.

Figure 6.2.1 below shows four random samples of size $n = 5$ drawn from a given population with the mean μ and variance σ^2. The individual observed values are marked by "$\star$" and the sample mean of each sample is marked by "$\downarrow$" on the line, and denoted by $\overline{X}_1$, $\overline{X}_2$, $\overline{X}_3$, and $\overline{X}_4$ below the line. When all the observed values and the sample means are projected and superimposed on the same horizontal line at the bottom of the figure, it is easy to see that the range of $\overline{X}$'s is much smaller than the range of the individual observations. How much smaller is the variability of the sample means than the variability of the individual observations? Using the properties of linear combination of random variables, we can show the following. If you are not interested in the details of the following derivation, you may skip it.

$$\text{Var}(\overline{X}) = \text{Var}\left(\frac{1}{n}\sum_{i=1}^{n} X_i\right) = \left(\frac{1}{n^2}\right)\text{Var}\left(\sum_{i=1}^{n} X_i\right)$$

$$= \left(\frac{1}{n^2}\right)\sum_{i=1}^{n}\text{Var}(X_i) = \left(\frac{1}{n^2}\right)\cdot n \cdot \sigma^2$$

$$= \frac{\sigma^2}{n}, \text{ since } \text{Var}(X_i) = \sigma^2 \text{ for}$$

$$i = 1, 2, \cdots, n.$$

Thus, the variance and the standard deviation of the sample mean $\overline{X}$ is given by $\frac{\sigma^2}{n}$ and $\sigma/\sqrt{n}$. Namely, the variance of the sample mean is smaller

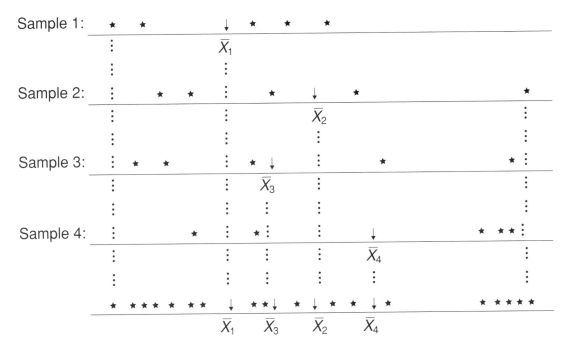

Figure 6.2.1 Variability of $\overline{X}$'s is smaller than the variability of individual observations.

than the variance of the individual observations by the factor of the sample size n, and the standard deviation of the sample mean is smaller than the SD of the individual observations by the factor of $\sqrt{n}$.

Definition 6.2.2. Let $X_1, X_2, \cdots, X_n$ be a random sample taken from a population with the mean μ and variance σ^2. The set of sample means $\overline{X}$'s of the random samples of size n drawn from this population has variance given by $\dfrac{\sigma^2}{n}$ and the SD $\sigma/\sqrt{n}$. The SD $\sigma/\sqrt{n}$ is referred to as the **standard error of the sample mean** or the **standard error (SE)**.

1. The variance of the sample mean $\overline{X}$ is denoted by $\text{Var}(\overline{X})$ or $\sigma^2(\overline{X})$.
2. The standard error is denoted by $SE(\overline{X})$, $\sigma(\overline{X})$, or some denote it by $\sigma_{\overline{X}}$.

It is important to understand that the SE $\sigma/\sqrt{n}$ is *not* the standard deviation of an individual observation X_i, but of the sample mean $\overline{X}$. As the sample size n increases, the denominator of $\sigma/\sqrt{n}$ increases and, consequently, the SE decreases. When a given population is normal with parameters μ and σ^2, the sampling distribution of $\overline{X}$ is also normal.

Let $X_1, X_2, \cdots, X_n$ be a random sample from a normal distribution with the mean μ and the variance σ^2. Then the sample mean $\overline{X}$ has a normal distribution with the mean μ, the variance $\dfrac{\sigma^2}{n}$, and the standard error $\sigma/\sqrt{n}$. That is, $\overline{X} \sim N\left(\mu, \dfrac{\sigma^2}{n}\right)$.

Example 6.2.1. Sunlight is a major etiological factor for malignant melanoma. The prognosis is dependent primarily on the depth of the tumor: the thicker the lesion, the poorer the prognosis. Suppose that for patients who are diagnosed with malignant melanoma in the sunbelt region, the distribution of the depth of the melanoma tumor is normal with $\mu = 2.3$ mm and $\sigma^2 = 0.8$. If 9 melanoma patients were randomly selected in this region, what is the SE of the sample mean of the depth of their tumor?

Solution. Since $\sigma = \sqrt{0.8} = 0.8944$ and $n = 9$, the SE is given by

$$\frac{\sigma}{\sqrt{n}} = \frac{0.8944}{\sqrt{9}} = 0.298\,1.$$

Note that the SE $\sigma/\sqrt{n} = 0.2981$ is much smaller than the SD $\sigma = 0.8944$. If the sample size were larger, say $n = 16$, the SE would be $\sigma/\sqrt{n} = 0.8944/\sqrt{16} = 0.223\,6$. In Example 6.2.1, the distribution of $\overline{X}$ is normal because the underlying distribution of the depth of the tumor is normal.

Example 6.2.2. Greenbaum and Zachrisson [1] investigated post-orthodontic patients to determine the effect of palatal expansion therapy on the periodontal supporting structures, located at the buccal aspects on the maxillary first permanent molars. The patients were treated with a rapid maxillary expansion technique using a tissue-bone, fixed, split acrylic appliance. Their study showed that the average increase in maxillary first molar width was 4.6 mm with the standard deviation of 1.6 mm. Suppose these parameters represent the mean and variance of the increase in maxillary first molar width for the population of orthodontic patients who underwent a rapid maxillary expansion (RME) treatment. Find the standard error of the sample mean for a random sample of 5 patients who underwent RME treatment.

Solution. The population SD is $\sigma = 1.6$, and the sample size $n = 5$. Hence, the SE is

$$\frac{\sigma}{\sqrt{n}} = \frac{1.6}{\sqrt{5}} = 0.715\,5.$$

In this example the underlying distribution of the magnitude of the increase in maxillary first molar width is not specified. Whether the underlying distribution is known or not, the SE of the sample mean $\overline{X}$ is obtained by dividing σ by $\sqrt{n}$.

We have stated that if the underlying distribution is normal, then the sampling distribution of $\overline{X}$ is also normal with mean $= \mu$ and SE $= \sigma/\sqrt{n}$. Similar to what we did in Section 5.5.2, a transformation can be made to convert $\overline{X}$ to a standard normal, that is, $\dfrac{\overline{X} - \mu}{\sigma/\sqrt{n}}$ has a standard normal distribution with $\mu = 0$ and $\sigma^2 = 1$.

Let $X_1, X_2, \cdots, X_n$ be normally distributed with mean μ and variance σ^2. Then

$$Z = \frac{\overline{X} - \mu}{\sigma/\sqrt{n}} \sim N(0, 1).$$

Example 6.2.3. Dr. Provine and his colleagues used calcium sulfate grafts in conjunction with a

sinus lift procedure in sinus augmentation for endosseous implants. The calcium sulfate was placed around the endosseous implants after the implants had been installed. Two months later, implant integration in the newly formed bone was measured in percent (%), which is normally distributed with mean μ and variance σ^2. Let's assume that μ and σ^2 are known to be 84.5 and 36, respectively. Suppose there are 18 patients who have received this procedure. (i) What is the sampling distribution of $\overline{X}$? (ii) What is the chance of obtaining an average implant integration percent higher than 82.8% from a random sample of $n = 7$?

Solution. (i) The expected value of the sample mean is 84.5%, as given in the problem. The variance is $\dfrac{\sigma^2}{n} = \dfrac{36}{18} = 2.0$, and since the underlying distribution is normal, $\overline{X}$ has a normal distribution $\overline{X} \sim N(\mu, \dfrac{\sigma^2}{n}) = N(84.5, 2.0)$.

(ii) We need to find the probability that the sample mean is greater than 82.8. From the given information in the problem, we have $\sigma = 6.0$ and $n = 7$. Therefore, the standard error is $\sigma/\sqrt{n} = 6/\sqrt{7} = 2.27$, and the desired probability is

$$P(\overline{X} \geq 82.8) = P\left(\frac{\overline{X} - \mu}{\sigma/\sqrt{n}} \geq \frac{82.8 - 84.5}{2.27}\right)$$
$$= P(Z \geq -0.75) = 0.7734.$$

6.2.2 Central Limit Theorem

If the underlying distribution is normal, then the distribution of the sample mean is also normal, with mean μ and variance $\dfrac{\sigma^2}{n}$. The question is, what is the sampling distribution of the sample mean when the underlying distribution of the population from which the random sample is selected is *not* normal? The answer to this question is provided by the central limit theorem.

Central Limit Theorem

Let $X_1, X_2, \cdots, X_n$ be a random sample from a distribution with the mean μ and variance σ^2. Then for a sufficiently large sample n, the sampling distribution of $\overline{X}$ is approximately normal;

$$\overline{X} \overset{\circ}{\sim} N\left(\mu, \frac{\sigma^2}{n}\right)$$

Many distribution functions we encounter in practice are not normal. This remarkable theorem enables us to perform a variety of statistical inferences based on the approximate normality of the sample mean, even though the distribution of individual observations is not normal. The larger the sample size, the more accurate is the normal approximation. We present several examples where the central limit theorem is applied to compute the probabilities.

Example 6.2.4. Suppose a group of 64 dental patients gave the investigators informed consent to participate in a study designed to test a new anticaries vaccine. If the mean and variance of the level of fluorocal salivarius found in the saliva of these patients after the vaccine was given are 11.2 mg and 12.9, what is the probability that their sample mean is between 11.0 and 12.0 mg?

Solution. Since the underlying distribution is not known, but the sample size $n = 64$ is sufficiently large, we can use the central limit theorem (CLT) to find the probability by the normal approximation. The standard error is $\sigma/\sqrt{n} = \sqrt{12.9}/\sqrt{64} = 0.45$. Thus, we can express

$P(11.0 \leq \overline{X} \leq 12.0)$

$\overset{\circ}{\sim} P\left(\dfrac{11.0 - 11.2}{0.45} \leq \dfrac{\overline{X} - \mu}{\sigma/\sqrt{n}} \leq \dfrac{12.0 - 11.2}{0.45}\right)$

$= P(-0.44 \leq Z \leq 1.78)$

$= P(Z \leq 1.78) - P(Z \leq -0.44)$

$= 0.9625 - 0.3300 = 0.632\,5.$

Example 6.2.5. CD4$^+$ T lymphocytes play a central role in regulating the cell-mediated immune response to infection. The human immunodeficiency virus (HIV), which causes AIDS, attacks CD4$^+$ cells. Uninfected individuals have on the average about 1, 100 cells per milliliter of blood. Suppose the standard deviation of the CD4$^+$ cell count for an uninfected subject is around 260. Out of a random sample of 125 uninfected individuals, find the 95th percentile of the sample mean of the CD4$^+$ cell count of these individuals.

Solution. Since the distribution of the cell count is unknown, we will use the CLT to find the 95th

percentile of the sample mean. From the given information, the standard error is computed $\sigma/\sqrt{n} = 23.\,26$. We need to find the value $\overline{x}$ such that the equation $P(\overline{X} \leq \overline{x}) = 0.95$ holds. That is,

$$P(\overline{X} \leq \overline{x}) \overset{\circ}{\sim} P\left(\frac{\overline{X} - \mu}{\sigma/\sqrt{n}} \leq \frac{\overline{x} - 1100}{23.26}\right)$$

$$= P\left(Z \leq \frac{\overline{x} - 1100}{23.26}\right)$$

$$= P(Z \leq Z_{0.95}) = 0.95.$$

Therefore, we have $Z_{0.95} = \dfrac{\overline{x} - 1100}{23.26}$ and we know from Table D and Section 5.5.5 that $Z_{0.95} = 1.645$. By substituting $Z_{0.95}$ with 1.645 in the equation $Z_{0.95} = \dfrac{\overline{x} - 1100}{23.26}$, we obtain a linear equation $\dfrac{\overline{x} - 1100}{23.26} = 1.645$. We now have to solve the equation for $\overline{x}$: $\overline{x} - 1100 = (23.26) \cdot (1.645) = 38.\,263$. Adding 1, 100 to both sides of the above equation, we get $\overline{x} = 1,138.263$. So, the 95th percentile of the sample mean of the CD4$^+$ cell count of these 125 individuals is *approximately* 1, 138.263.

Example 6.2.6. Find the lower and upper limits that encompass 95% of the means of the samples of size 125 drawn from the population described in the above example. Since 2.5% of the area under the standard normal curve lies above 1.96, and the same amount 2.5% lies below -1.96 (see Section 5.5.5), and $\mu = 1, 100$ and $\sigma/\sqrt{n} = 23.\,26$,

$P(\overline{x}_1 \leq \overline{X} \leq \overline{x}_2)$

$= P\left(\dfrac{\overline{x}_1 - 1100}{23.26} \leq \dfrac{\overline{X} - \mu}{\sigma/\sqrt{n}} \leq \dfrac{\overline{x}_2 - 1100}{23.26}\right)$

$\overset{\circ}{\sim} P\left(\dfrac{\overline{x}_1 - 1100}{23.26} \leq Z \leq \dfrac{\overline{x}_2 - 1100}{23.26}\right)$

$= P(Z_{0.025} \leq Z \leq Z_{0.975})$

$= P(-1.96 \leq Z \leq 1.96).$

From the above relationship, we get two linear equations

$$\frac{\overline{x}_1 - 1100}{23.26} = -1.96 \quad \text{and} \quad \frac{\overline{x}_2 - 1100}{23.26} = 1.96.$$

By solving the equations for $\overline{x}_1$ and $\overline{x}_2$, we obtain

$$\overline{x}_1 = (23.26) \cdot (-1.96) + 1, 100 = 1, 054.41$$

and

$$\overline{x}_2 = (23.26) \cdot (1.96) + 1, 100 = 1, 145.59.$$

This indicates that approximately 95% of the means of the samples of the size of 125 individuals fall between 1,054.41 and 1,145.59 CD4+ cell counts.

6.3 STUDENT *t* DISTRIBUTION

It should be familiar by now that the distribution of the sample mean $\overline{X}$ is normally distributed with mean μ and variance $\dfrac{\sigma^2}{n}$ when the random samples are drawn from a normal population that has mean μ and variance σ^2. The value of σ^2 is assumed to be known. In practice the value of σ^2 is rarely known. In fact, if μ is not known, σ^2 is likely to be unknown. That is, the value of σ is not likely to be known. When σ is not known, it must be estimated from data. We discussed in Chapter 3 that the sample SD

$$S = \sqrt{\frac{\sum_{i=1}^{n}(X_i - \overline{X})^2}{n-1}}$$

is an estimator of σ. If we replaced σ with its estimator S in the expression $\dfrac{\overline{X} - \mu}{\sigma/\sqrt{n}}$, would it still have the standard normal distribution? If not, what would be the distribution of the statistic $\dfrac{\overline{X} - \mu}{S/\sqrt{n}}$? It is well known that this statistic has the **Student *t* distribution** or *t* distribution with $(n-1)$ degrees of freedom. We will let *t* denote the statistic,

$$t = \frac{\overline{X} - \mu}{S/\sqrt{n}}.$$

The shape of the *t* distribution looks very similar to the standard normal distribution, except that it has longer tails and is associated with a special feature called the degrees of freedom. In Figure 6.3.1 the standard normal curve and the *t* distribution are displayed. The one with longer left and right tails is *t* distribution with $(n-1)$ degrees of freedom.

The general characteristics of the *t* distributions include the following.

1. The *t* random variable is continuous.
2. The graph of the density of the *t* random variable is symmetric and bell-shaped.
3. The mean, median, and mode are equal to 0 and located at the center of distribution.
4. Each *t* distribution is identified by a parameter δ (a Greek letter delta), called degrees of freedom.
5. The degree of freedom is always a positive integer.
6. The parameter is a shape parameter in the sense that as δ increases, the variance of the *t* distribution decreases. The variance σ^2 of the *t* distribution is larger than 1.0. Hence, the *t* distribution is more dispersed than the standard normal distribution.
7. As degrees of freedom increase, the *t* distribution approaches the standard normal distribution.

The degrees of freedom are the number of values that are free to vary after a sample statistic has been calculated. For example, if the average of 3 values is 5, then 2 of the 3 values are free to vary. But once 2 values have been chosen, the third value must be a specific value so that the sum of the 3 values is 15, because $15/3 = 5$. In this case, the degree of freedom is $3 - 1 = 2$. Some may get the idea that the degrees of freedom are always one less than the sample size $(n-1)$. In many situations it is true that the degrees of freedom $\delta = n - 1$, but in other situations it is not. However, the degrees of freedom are all expressed in

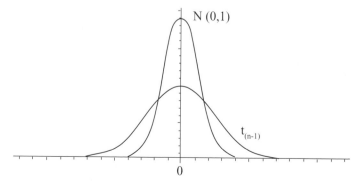

Figure 6.3.1 Standard normal and *t* distributions.

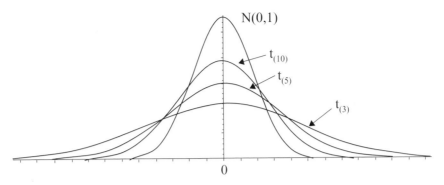

Figure 6.3.2 Standard normal and t distributions with different degrees of freedom.

terms of the sample size (i.e., $\delta = n - 1$) and thus, increasing the sample size is the same as increasing the degrees of freedom. There are four bell-shaped curves in Figure 6.3.2. The tallest curve in the middle with the shortest tails and the smallest variance is the standard normal, and the other three curves with longer tails represent the t distributions. The

first column of Table E. As we move from left to right across the row, stop at the entry that has 2.57, or approximately 2.57. In this example, we have an entry that contains 2.5706, as indicated in the table. The corresponding percentile to 2.5706 is 0.975 in the top row. Hence, $P(t_{(5)} \le 2.57)$ is approximately 0.975.

df (δ)	0.55	0.60	0.65	0.70	0.75	0.80	0.85	0.90	0.95	**0.975**	0.98	0.985	$\cdots$
1										.			
2										.			
3										.			
4										$\downarrow$			
5	.	.	.	.	.	.	.	.	$\longrightarrow$	**2.5706**	.		
6													

t distribution with the longest tails is associated with the smallest degrees of freedom (or smallest sample size). We can see in Figure 6.3.2 that as the degrees of freedom increases, the t distribution becomes closer and closer to the standard normal.

The percentiles of the t distribution are provided in Table E in the Appendix. The values in the first column of Table E are the degrees of freedom ranging from 1 to ∞ (read ∞ as "infinity"). The symbol ∞ represents the degrees of freedom greater than 120. In the first row across the top of Table E are the percentiles. The table entry values are percentiles that correspond to the degrees of freedom. The probability that the t random variable with the degrees of freedom δ having the values less than (or equal to) t is denoted by $P(t_{(\delta)} \le t)$.

Example 6.3.1. Find the probability $P(t_{(5)} \le 2.57)$.

Solution. This is a t random variable with the degrees of freedom (df), $\delta = 5$. To find the probability, go to the degrees of freedom $\delta = 5$ in the

Similar to the standard normal distribution, this probability $P(t_{(5)} \le 2.57) = 0.975$ indicates that the entire area to the left of $t = 2.57$ under the t distribution with the degrees of freedom 5 is 0.975. The area to the right of $t = 2.57$ is then 0.025. To see how closely the t distribution approaches the standard normal distribution as the degrees of freedom increase, let us consider the following table. Table 6.3.1 $t_{(0.975)}$ denotes the 97.5[th] percentile. With the specific degrees of freedom we will use $t_{(\delta, 0.975)}$ to denote the 97.5[th] percentile of the t distribution associated with δ degrees of freedom. The table illustrates that the t distribution rapidly approaches the standard normal distribution as the degrees of freedom become larger.

Example 6.3.2. Find the probability $P(t_{(19)} \le -0.86)$.

Solution. This is the t distribution with the degrees of freedom 19. Table E does not include any negative entry values, but the symmetric property of the t distribution will allow us to find the desired

Table 6.3.1. Comparison between t and Z distributions.

Degrees of Freedom	$t_{(0.975)}$	$Z_{(0.975)}$
$\delta = \quad 5$	2.5706	1.96
10	2.2281	1.96
20	2.0860	1.96
40	2.0211	1.96
60	2.0003	1.96
80	1.9901	1.96
100	1.9840	1.96
120	1.9799	1.96
∞	1.96	1.96

probability, just as it does in the standard normal distribution. The probability $P(\mathbf{t}_{(19)} \leq -0.86)$ is equal to the area to the left of $t = -0.86$ under the t distribution with $\delta = 19$, which is precisely the same as the area to the right of $t = 0.86$ by the symmetric property. Therefore, it can be expressed

$$P(\mathbf{t}_{(19)} \leq -0.86) = P(\mathbf{t}_{(19)} \geq 0.86), \text{ by symmetry}$$
$$= 1.0 - P(\mathbf{t}_{(19)} \leq 0.86)$$
$$= 1.0 - 0.8 = 0.20.$$

It is quite straightforward to find the percentiles of the t distribution for a given δ from Table E. For example, $t_{(14, 0.75)} = 0.6924$, $t_{(24, 0.90)} = 1.3178$, $t_{(24, 0.95)} = 1.7109$, and $t_{(30, 0.975)} = 2.0423$.

Example 6.3.3. Find $t_{(35, 0.95)}$.

Solution. Table E does not show the degrees of freedom $\delta = 35$. However, it provides the 95th percentiles for the degrees of freedom $\delta = 30$ and $\delta = 40$. We can use the method of linear interpolation as described below.

df	0.90	0.95	0.975
29	.	.	.
30	.	1.6973	.
35	$\longrightarrow$		
40	.	1.6839	.
50	.	.	.

The 95th percentiles corresponding to the degrees of freedom $\delta = 30$ and $\delta = 40$ are provided by the table; $t_{(30, 0.95)} = 1.6973$ and $t_{(40, 0.95)} = 1.6839$. Since $\delta = 35$ is the midpoint between 30 and 40, by the method of linear interpolation the 95th percentile corresponding to the degrees of freedom $\delta = 35$ will be the midpoint between $t_{(30, 0.95)}$ and

$t_{(40, 0.95)}$. Thus,

$$t_{(35, 0.95)} = \frac{(1.6973 + 1.6839)}{2} = 1.690\,6.$$

Example 6.3.4. Let X be a random variable describing the angle between subnasale (SN) plane and mandibular plane in orthodontics. Suppose X is normally distributed. A study was performed to evaluate the long-term stability of deep overbite correction in Class II Division 2 malocclusion and to search for predictor variables of post-retention overbites [3]. After treatment, cephalograms of 29 patients were analyzed, and the angle between the SN plane and mandibular plane for each patient was measured. If you were to take a random sample of 29 patients repeatedly after treatment, what is the sampling distribution of the statistic

$$t = \frac{\overline{X} - \mu}{S/\sqrt{n}}?$$

Solution. Since σ is not known, the standard error $\sigma/\sqrt{n}$ of $\overline{X}$ is to be estimated by $S/\sqrt{n}$. The statistic $t = \dfrac{\overline{X} - \mu}{S/\sqrt{n}}$ has the t distribution with the degrees of freedom $\delta = n - 1 = 29 - 1 = 28$.

One of the key assumptions of the t distribution is that the underlying population distribution is normal. Under this assumption the sampling distribution of $\overline{X}$ is normal for any sample size n, and by a statistical property the numerator and denominator of the statistic $t = \dfrac{\overline{X} - \mu}{S/\sqrt{n}}$ are statistically independent. What if the population distribution of X is not normal? It is known that when n is sufficiently large and the distribution of X is unimodal and symmetric, we still have an adequate approximation. We will elaborate on this later when we introduce the t test. The t distribution will be used often throughout the next several chapters when confidence intervals and hypothesis testing are introduced.

6.4 EXERCISES

1 Let the random variable X be normally distributed with $\mu = 136.2$ and $\sigma^2 = 86.4$. Find the variance and the standard error of $\overline{X}$ when the sample size $n = 20$.

2 The dental fees for a root canal treatment vary from one office to another. According to a survey conducted by an insurance company, the distribution of the fees is normal with the mean of $1,100 and the SD of $50. To compare the fees in Riverside County to the nation as a whole, we took a sample of eight dental offices in the county. What is the sampling distribution of the average cost of a root canal treatment in Riverside County?

3 Suppose the salivary flow rate of adult patients is known to be normally distributed with the mean of 6.2 ml/min and the SD of 2.2 ml/min. If nine dental and medical students were selected at random, what is the SE of their average salivary flow rate?

4 Suppose that the survival time of the patients who underwent a surgical procedure to remove a brain tumor is normally distributed with the mean of 82 months and the SD of 18 months. Eight brain tumor patients were surgically treated at the Riverside Community Hospital last month. What is the chance that the average survival time of these patients will exceed 90 months?

5 In exercise 3 above, what is the probability that the sample mean of salivary flow rate is between 5.0 and 7.3 ml/min?

6 Advanced lymphoma is one of the deadliest cancers. The distribution of survival time in months to death of a patient after the illness is diagnosed is not known, but the mean and SD are given as 17.8 months and 6.5 months, respectively. Thirty-two patients have just been diagnosed with an advanced case of lymphoma. What is the probability that their average survival time is at least 15 months?

7 Investigators have found it difficult to simultaneously and reliably evaluate bite force in the intercuspal position with the area and location of occlusal contacts. Hidaka et al. [2] reports that occlusal contact area at maximum voluntary clenching level has the mean of 30.2 mm^2 and the SD of 10.7 mm^2. If the area of occlusal contact of 38 randomly selected adult patients is to be measured, what is the chance that the sample mean of their occlusal contact area is greater than 33.0 mm^2?

8 Cholesterol is a lipid common to all animals. In most cases, the cholesterol levels in the human body range from about 135 to 250 mg per 100 ml of blood. If the mean cholesterol level is 190 and the SD is 17.5, find the lower and upper limits that enclose 95% of the mean of a sample of size 25 drawn from the population. Assume that the cholesterol levels are normally distributed.

9 In Exercise 8, find the lower and upper limits that enclose 95% of the means of samples of size 35 drawn from the population, instead of 25. Compare the limits obtained to those in Exercise 8.

10 Find the probabilities:
a. $P(\mathbf{t}_{(7)} \leq 0.40)$,
b. $P(\mathbf{t}_{(10)} \leq -1.37)$,
c. $P(\mathbf{t}_{(5)} \geq -0.73)$,
d. $P(0.68 \leq \mathbf{t}_{(24)} \leq 2.17)$,
e. $P(-0.88 \leq \mathbf{t}_{(9)} \leq -0.26)$.

11 Find the appropriate percentiles:
a. $t_{(5,0.75)}$,
b. $t_{(7,0.90)}$,
c. $t_{(13,0.95)}$,
d. $t_{(25,0.975)}$,
e. $t_{(45,0.95)}$,
f. $t_{(9,0.995)}$.

12 Suppose a random variable Y has t distribution associated with the degrees of freedom 17. Determine the percentage of the approximate area under the t distribution:

a. to the left of 1.069,
b. to the right of 2.110,
c. between -0.863 and 1.333,
d. between -0.689 and -0.257.

6.5 REFERENCES

1. Greenbaum, K. R., and Zachrisson, B. U. The effect of palatal expansion therapy on the periodontal supporting tissues. *Am. J. Orthod.* 1982: 81, 12–21.
2. Hidaka, O., Iwasaki, M., Saito, M. and Morimoto, T. Influence of clenching intensity on bite force balance, occlusal contact area, and average bite pressure. *J. Dent. Res.* 1999: 78, 1336–1344.
3. Kim, T., and Little, R. M. Postretention assessment of deep overbite correction in Class II Division 2 malocclusion. *The Angle Orthodontist*. 1999: 69, 175–186.

Chapter 7

Confidence Intervals and Sample Size

7.1 INTRODUCTION

A statistic used to approximate an unknown population parameter is called an estimator for the parameter. For example, the sample mean $\overline{X}$ and sample variance S^2 are estimators for the population mean μ and population variance σ^2. There are two different estimation methods. One method is **point estimation**. A statistic $\overline{X}$ is called a point estimator for μ because a particular set of sample data is used to calculate $\overline{X}$ and yields a single value or point on the real number scale. The value that $\overline{X}$ yields for a particular data is called an estimate and is denoted by $\overline{x}$ (a bar over the lowercase x). Likewise, a statistic S is a point estimator for σ. Many scientific papers present the sample mean, along with the sample SD S, and the sample size n. We learned in previous chapters that two different samples are likely to result in different sample means due to an inherent variability in the samples. This inherent variability is not reflected in the sample mean. Therefore, it is difficult to know how close the estimate $\overline{x}$ is to the true mean μ. For large samples, most of the observed values are expected to fall very close to μ. But the fact is, there will always be some difference between $\overline{x}$ and μ. It would be helpful to know how close the estimate is to the unknown true population parameter and to answer the question, How confident are we of the accuracy of the estimate?

The other method of estimation that reflects sample-to-sample variability is called an **interval estimation**. An **interval estimator** provides an interval that is a range of values based on a sample. We hope that the interval provided will contain the population parameter being estimated. This interval, referred to as **confidence interval**, is a random variable whose endpoints L and U are statistics involving $\overline{X}$. An interval estimator is often preferred because it enables us to get an idea of not only the value of the parameter, but the accuracy of the estimate. A confidence interval for μ is an interval (L, U), which contains the true mean with some prespecified degree of certainty. L is called the **lower confidence limit** and U the **upper confidence limit** (or **lower limit** and **upper limit**). For example, a 95% confidence interval is an interval (L, U) such that $P(L \leq \mu \leq U) = 0.95$. The probability associated with a confidence interval is the measure of our confidence that the mean μ is between L and U. This probability is called a **confidence coefficient** or **confidence level**. The degree of confidence desired is determined and controlled by the researcher. Scientific investigators often present 95% confidence intervals for the parameters of their interest in the reports. A correct interpretation of a 95% confidence interval for μ is that when it is used in repeated sampling from the same population, 95% of the intervals that result will contain the unknown true population mean μ, and 5% will fail to contain μ. This is illustrated in Figure 7.1.1. It should be noted that a 95% confidence interval (L, U) (1) does *not* imply 95% of the population values lie within the interval, and (2) does *not* imply μ is a random variable that assumes a value within the interval.

In this chapter we will discuss how to construct confidence intervals for mean μ when σ is known, for mean μ when σ is *not* known, for proportion p, for variance σ^2, and standard deviation σ.

7.2 CONFIDENCE INTERVALS FOR THE MEAN μ AND SAMPLE SIZE n WHEN σ IS KNOWN

Chapter 6 discussed the theoretical properties of a distribution of sample means. We will now use these properties in making statistical inferences. Suppose X is a random variable that has mean μ and SD σ. The statistic $Z = \dfrac{\overline{X} - \mu}{\sigma/\sqrt{n}}$ has a standard

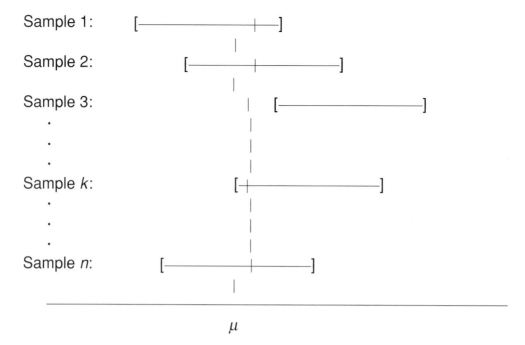

Figure 7.1.1 95% of the confidence intervals are expected to contain μ.

normal distribution if X is normally distributed. If it is not normally distributed, then by the central limit theorem, it has an approximately standard normal distribution, provided that the sample size n is sufficiently large ($n \geq 30$). For a standard normal variable Z, the probability is $0.95 = 1 - 0.05$ that it lies between $Z_{0.05/2} = Z_{0.025} = -1.96$ and $Z_{1-(0.05/2)} = Z_{0.975} = +1.96$. That is, $P(-1.96 \leq Z \leq 1.96) = 0.95$. By substituting $\dfrac{\overline{X} - \mu}{\sigma/\sqrt{n}}$ for Z, we have $P(-1.96 \leq \dfrac{\overline{X} - \mu}{\sigma/\sqrt{n}} \leq 1.96) = 0.95$. We can multiply all three terms of the inequality inside the parentheses by the factor $\dfrac{\sigma}{\sqrt{n}}$ without altering the probability, and thus we obtain the expression $P\left(-1.96 \cdot \dfrac{\sigma}{\sqrt{n}} \leq \overline{X} - \mu \leq 1.96 \cdot \dfrac{\sigma}{\sqrt{n}}\right) = 0.95$.

Subtracting $\overline{X}$ from each term in the inequality yields

$$P\left(-\overline{X} - 1.96 \cdot \dfrac{\sigma}{\sqrt{n}} \leq -\mu \leq -\overline{X} + 1.96 \cdot \dfrac{\sigma}{\sqrt{n}}\right) = 0.95$$

and multiplying by -1, which reverses the direction of the inequality and the signs of the terms,

gives

$$P\left(\overline{X} - 1.96 \cdot \dfrac{\sigma}{\sqrt{n}} \leq \mu \leq \overline{X} + 1.96 \cdot \dfrac{\sigma}{\sqrt{n}}\right) = 0.95.$$

The above probability statement says the chances are 95% that the parameter μ is contained in a random interval

$$\left(\overline{X} - 1.96 \cdot \dfrac{\sigma}{\sqrt{n}}, \overline{X} + 1.96 \cdot \dfrac{\sigma}{\sqrt{n}}\right).$$

This interval is called a 95% confidence interval. The endpoints of the confidence interval, $L = \overline{X} - 1.96 \cdot \dfrac{\sigma}{\sqrt{n}}$ and $U = \overline{X} + 1.96 \cdot \dfrac{\sigma}{\sqrt{n}}$ are called the **lower** and **upper confidence limits**. We are 95% confident that this interval will contain mean μ. We should keep in mind that $\overline{X}$ is a random variable, and therefore, the interval

$$\left(\overline{X} - 1.96 \cdot \dfrac{\sigma}{\sqrt{n}}, \overline{X} + 1.96 \cdot \dfrac{\sigma}{\sqrt{n}}\right)$$

is random and has a 95% chance that it contains the unknown parameter μ. The parameter μ is a fixed constant that happens to be unknown. Once the confidence interval has been determined, either μ lies within the confidence limits or it does not (i.e., μ lies outside the confidence limits). In general, a

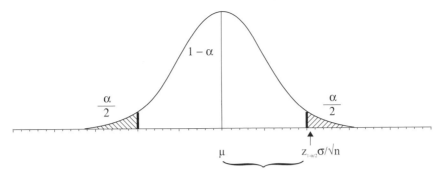

Figure 7.2.1 Distribution of the sample mean.

$(1 - \alpha)100\%$ confidence interval when σ is known is given by

$$\left(\overline{X} - Z_{1-\alpha/2} \cdot \frac{\sigma}{\sqrt{n}}, \overline{X} + Z_{1-\alpha/2} \cdot \frac{\sigma}{\sqrt{n}} \right)$$

For a 95% confidence interval, $\alpha = 0.05$, $(1 - \alpha)100\% = 0.95\%$ and $Z_{1-\alpha/2} = Z_{0.975} = 1.96$. Sometimes, the above confidence interval is expressed as

$$\overline{X} \pm Z_{1-\alpha/2} \cdot \frac{\sigma}{\sqrt{n}}.$$

The term $Z_{1-\alpha/2} \cdot \dfrac{\sigma}{\sqrt{n}}$ is referred to as the *maximum error of estimate*. As we can see in Figure 7.2.1 the probability is $1 - \alpha$ that the mean of a large random sample from an infinite population will differ from the population mean by at most $Z_{1-\alpha/2} \cdot \dfrac{\sigma}{\sqrt{n}}$. For a given value of α, say $\alpha = 0.05$, 95% of the sample means will fall within this error limit on either side of the population mean μ. Let E denote the maximum error of estimate.

Example 7.2.1. Suppose X is a random variable representing the amount of organic sulfur contained in 500 mg methyl sulfonyl methane (MSM) tablets. Organic sulfur plays an important role in the maintenance of joint cartilage. The formula for MSM requires that each tablet should contain 85 mg of organic sulfur. To assess how well the requirement is being followed, 24 MSM tablets were randomly selected. Analytical results show that on the average the tablets contain about 80.5 mg of organic sulfur. If, based on experience, the amount of organic sulfur found in MSM tablets is normally distributed with $\sigma = 14.2$ mg, construct a 95% confidence interval for mean μ.

Solution. Since $\sigma = 14.2$ and $n = 24$, the standard error is

$$\frac{\sigma}{\sqrt{n}} = \frac{14.2}{\sqrt{24}} = 2.898\,6.$$

We also have $\overline{X} = 80.5$ and $Z_{1-\alpha/2} = Z_{0.975} = 1.96$. By substitution in the above formula, the 95% confidence interval is

$$\left(\overline{X} - Z_{1-\alpha/2} \cdot \frac{\sigma}{\sqrt{n}}, \overline{X} + Z_{1-\alpha/2} \cdot \frac{\sigma}{\sqrt{n}} \right)$$

$$= (80.5 - (1.96)(2.8986), 80.5 + (1.96)(2.8986))$$

$$= (74.8187, 86.1813) \simeq (74.82, 86.18).$$

$$L = 74.82 \qquad U = 86.18$$
$$\downarrow \qquad\qquad \downarrow$$

70	75	80	85	90

Before a random sample of $n = 24$ is drawn, we can say that there is a 95% chance that the population mean μ lies between 74.82 and 86.18, approximately.

Example 7.2.2. Pumice prophylaxis has long been accepted as a prerequisite for achieving enamel etching during orthodontic bonding procedures. Lindauer et al. [1] conducted a study to determine whether pumice prophylaxis, performed before acid etching, enhances the bond strength and retention rate of orthodontic brackets. A laboratory test was performed in which brackets were bonded to $n = 13$ extracted premolars after surface preparation protocols, and the shear bond strengths were calculated and recorded in megapascals (1×10^6 N/m^2). Suppose the distribution of the shear bond strength is known to be normal with a specified $\sigma = 4.6$. If the average bond strength of the 13 premolar samples is 9.6 MPa, construct a 99% confidence interval for μ.

Solution. It is easy to see that $\alpha = 0.01$ from $(1 - \alpha)100\% = 99\%$. From Table D, $Z_{1-\alpha/2} = Z_{0.995} = 2.58$ (using the method of linear interpolation). The standard error is $\dfrac{\sigma}{\sqrt{n}} = \dfrac{4.6}{\sqrt{13}} = 1.2758$. Hence, a 99% confidence interval is obtained by

$$\left(\bar{X} - Z_{1-\alpha/2} \cdot \frac{\sigma}{\sqrt{n}}, \bar{X} + Z_{1-\alpha/2} \cdot \frac{\sigma}{\sqrt{n}}\right)$$

$$= (9.6 - (2.58)(1.2758), 9.6 + (2.58)(1.2758))$$

$$= (6.3084, 12.8916).$$

There is a 99% chance that the population mean μ lies between 6.3 MPa and 12.9 MPa, approximately.

Example 7.2.3. The recent introduction of new bonding agents has led some dentists to suggest that certain endodontically treated posterior teeth could be restored with a bonded restoration instead of a full-coverage crown or onlay. Steele and Johnson [2] performed the fracture-resistance test of endodontically treated premolars restored with 4-META bonding agent (MOD prep, root canal treatment, composite resin plus bonding agent). They used 56 mature maxillary premolars extracted for periodontal reasons, which were free of caries, previous restorations, and preexisting fractures. These teeth were subjected to compressive fracture tests, and the average fracture strength was 47.2 kg. Suppose that the SD σ of the fracture strength from their previous experience is about 9.3 kg. Construct a 90% confidence interval for the population mean fracture strength.

Solution. Since the confidence level is 90%, we know $\alpha = 0.10$. In order to construct a 90% confidence interval, first we need to find the SE and $Z_{1-\alpha/2}$. From the discussions in Chapter 6 we have $Z_{0.95} = 1.645$, and $\dfrac{\sigma}{\sqrt{n}} = \dfrac{9.3}{\sqrt{56}} = 1.2428$. By substitution,

$$\left(\bar{X} - Z_{1-\alpha/2} \cdot \frac{\sigma}{\sqrt{n}}, \bar{X} + Z_{1-\alpha/2} \cdot \frac{\sigma}{\sqrt{n}}\right)$$

$$= (45.1556, 49.2444).$$

Table 7.2.1. Confidence intervals for the mean fracture strength.

Confidence Coefficient	Confidence Interval
90%	(45.16, 49.24)
95%	(44.76, 49.64)
99%	(43.99, 50.41)

In practice 90%, 95%, and 99% are the most commonly used confidence coefficients, and therefore, it is useful to keep in mind that $Z_{0.95} = 1.645$, $Z_{0.975} = 1.96$, and $Z_{0.995} = 2.58$. In Example 7.2.3, what if we required a different level of confidence? Table 7.2.1 presents confidence intervals for the mean fracture strength under three different confidence coefficients.

The table shows that for a given n and σ, the confidence interval becomes wider (narrower) as the confidence coefficient increases (decreases). Similarly, given a sample size n and the confidence coefficient, the larger the variance, the wider the confidence interval, and given the variance σ^2 and the confidence coefficient, the larger the sample size, the narrower the confidence interval. The factors that influence the confidence intervals are

- Sample size n
- Variance σ^2
- Confidence coefficient

We now present some applications of the concept of maximum error of estimate.

Example 7.2.4. Gangas et al. [3] studied 29 female patients with high low-density lipoprotein (LDL) cholesterol during 6 months of therapy with pravastatin. At the end of the study period the average LDL cholesterol level X of these women was 130.3 mg/dL. If the random variable X has a normal distribution with $\sigma = 6.1$, what can they assert with probability 0.95 about the maximum error of their estimate?

Solution. Substituting $Z_{0.975} = 1.96$, $\sigma = 6.1$, and $n = 29$ in the definition of maximum error of estimate,

$$E = Z_{1-\alpha/2} \cdot \frac{\sigma}{\sqrt{n}} = 1.96 \cdot \frac{6.1}{\sqrt{29}} = 2.2202.$$

With probability 0.95 they can assert that the error will be at most 2.2202.

We can use the formula $E = Z_{1-\alpha/2} \cdot \dfrac{\sigma}{\sqrt{n}}$ to determine the sample size necessary to achieve a desired degree of precision. Suppose we want to use the sample mean of a large random sample to estimate the population mean and to be able to assert with probability $1 - \alpha$ that the error of the estimate will not exceed some prespecified level E. This can be done by solving the equation $E = Z_{1-\alpha/2} \cdot \dfrac{\sigma}{\sqrt{n}}$ for n.

$$n = \left(\frac{Z_{1-\alpha/2} \cdot \sigma}{E} \right)^2$$

Example 7.2.5. Dental fluorosis occurs as a result of excessive fluoride intake during tooth development. Some children may receive a substantial intake from soft drinks. Suppose we want to use the sample mean of a random sample to estimate the population mean of the fluoride level in soft drinks and to be able to assert with probability 0.99 that our error will be no more than 0.15 ppm. If it is reasonable to assume that the distribution of the fluoride level is normal and the SD $\sigma = 0.32$ ppm, how large a sample will we need?

Solution. We can obtain the necessary sample n by substitution in the above formula, $Z_{0.995} = 2.58$, $\sigma = 0.32$, and $E = 0.15$.

$$n = \left(\frac{Z_{1-\alpha/2} \cdot \sigma}{E} \right)^2 = \left(\frac{2.58 \cdot 0.32}{0.15} \right)^2 = 30.294.$$

We need to round up to the nearest integer $n = 31$. Rounding off to $n = 30$ will not meet the requirement. Thus, a random sample of size $n = 31$ (31 soft drink samples) is required.

As we can see, the formula $n = \left(\dfrac{Z_{1-\alpha/2} \cdot \sigma}{E} \right)^2$ cannot be used unless we know the value of the population SD σ. In practice, we begin with a relatively small sample and then use the sample SD S as an estimate of σ to determine if more data is needed. As with the confidence intervals there are three factors that influence the determination of sample size: $Z_{1-\alpha/2}$, variance σ^2, and maximum error E. Table 7.2.2 presents the comparison of sample size. It shows how the sample size requirement changes as $Z_{1-\alpha/2}$ σ^2 and E vary.

When a random variable of our interest is normally distributed and σ is known, the standard

Table 7.2.2. Comparison of sample size.

$Z_{1-\alpha/2}$	E	σ^2	n
$Z_{0.95} = 1.645$	0.5	4	44
		8	87
	1.5	4	5
		8	10
$Z_{0.975} = 1.96$	0.5	4	62
		8	123
	1.5	4	7
		8	14

normal distribution can be used to construct confidence intervals regardless of the sample size. When the sample size is large enough ($n \geq 30$), the distribution of the sample means will be approximately normal (by central limit theorem) even if the underlying distribution deviates from normality. If $n \geq 30$, then S can be substituted for σ in the formula, and the standard normal distribution can be used to find confidence intervals for the population means.

7.3 CONFIDENCE INTERVALS FOR THE MEAN μ AND SAMPLE SIZE n WHEN σ IS NOT KNOWN

It was assumed in our discussions of the confidence interval $\overline{X} \pm Z_{1-\alpha/2} \cdot \sigma / \sqrt{n}$ that the SD σ is known. From a practical standpoint this assumption is unrealistic. In most scientific investigations, the studies are being conducted for the first time. Thus, there is no way to know either the mean or the variance of the population of our interest prior to the study. As discussed in Chapter 3, unknown population parameters must be estimated from the available data. In this section, we will consider realistic situations of making statistical inferences on the mean μ when the population variance σ^2 is not known. Since the value of σ is not known, it must be estimated. In fact, when σ in the statistic $Z = \dfrac{\overline{X} - \mu}{\sigma/\sqrt{n}}$ is replaced by its estimate S, we get $t = \dfrac{\overline{X} - \mu}{S/\sqrt{n}}$, which has the t distribution with the degrees of freedom $\delta = n - 1$. Detailed discussions on t distributions were presented in Section 6.3. It is now easy to determine a $(1 - \alpha)100\%$ confidence interval for μ when σ is not known.

All the algebraic arguments given in the previous section will hold true, except that $Z_{1-\alpha/2}$ and σ are replaced by $t_{(\delta,1-\alpha/2)}$ and S. We state a general formula for a confidence interval for μ with an unknown σ.

Let $X_1, X_2, \cdots, X_n$ be a random sample of size n from a normal distribution with mean μ and variance σ^2. Then a $(1-\alpha)100\%$ confidence interval for μ is given by

$$\left(\overline{X} - t_{(n-1,1-\alpha/2)} \cdot \frac{S}{\sqrt{n}}, \overline{X} + t_{(n-1,1-\alpha/2)} \cdot \frac{S}{\sqrt{n}}\right)$$

or

$$\overline{X} \pm t_{(n-1,1-\alpha/2)} \cdot \frac{S}{\sqrt{n}}.$$

Example 7.3.1. Glass ionomer cement (GI) is one of several new classes of adhesive luting agents recently introduced as an alternative to zinc phosphate cement. GI has been shown to reduce microleakage, increase retention, and improve physical properties, compared with zinc phosphate cements [4]. Different factors might influence the hydraulic response and therefore the film thickness of different classes of adhesive luting agents. Let X be a random variable representing the film thickness of GI. White et al. [5] measured the film thickness (micrometers) of GI with a load of 5 kg applied vertically to the plates. The sample mean and sample SD of 10 samples are $\overline{X} = 19.9$ and $S = 1.3$. If X is normally distributed, find a 95% confidence interval for μ.

Solution. The degree of freedom is $n - 1 = 10 - 1 = 9$; the sample SE is $S/\sqrt{n} = 1.3/\sqrt{10} = 0.4111$; and from Table E in the Appendix we get $t_{(n-1,1-\alpha/2)} = t_{(9,0.975)} = 2.2622$. By substituting in the formula, a 95% confidence interval for μ is given by

$$\left(\overline{X} - t_{(n-1,1-\alpha/2)} \frac{S}{\sqrt{n}}, \overline{X} + t_{(n-1,1-\alpha/2)} \frac{S}{\sqrt{n}}\right)$$
$$= (19.9 - (2.2622)(0.4111), 19.9$$
$$+ (2.2622)(0.4111))$$
$$= (18.97, 20.83).$$

Example 7.3.2. Posterior crossbite is one of the most frequently observed malocclusions of the deciduous and mixed dentition periods. The prevalence of this malocclusion is regarded to be 8–12% [6, 7]. To evaluate specific dental and skeletal changes during the treatment of posterior crossbite using expansion plates, investigators selected 13 children with posterior crossbite in the mixed dentition between the ages of 8 and 11. The subjects were treated with the use of expansion plates for about a year. Let Y represent post-treatment maxillary intermolar width, which is one of the variables of their interest. Assume that Y is approximately normally distributed. Erdinc et al. [8] reported that the sample mean and sample SD of the post-treatment maxillary intermolar width of the 13 patients are 46.8 mm and 2.3 mm, respectively. Construct a 90% confidence interval for μ.

Solution. Since it is given that Y is approximately normally distributed, $n = 13$, $\overline{Y} = 46.8$, and $S = 2.3$, we can use the formula discussed above. From Table E we can obtain $t_{(n-1,1-\alpha/2)} = t_{(13-1,0.95)} = 1.7823$, and $S/\sqrt{n} = 2.3/\sqrt{13} = 0.6379$. By making appropriate substitutions, we get

$$\left(\overline{Y} - t_{(n-1,1-\alpha/2)} \cdot \frac{S}{\sqrt{n}}, \overline{Y} + t_{(n-1,1-\alpha/2)} \cdot \frac{S}{\sqrt{n}}\right)$$
$$= (45.6631, 47.9369).$$

We have seen that some students have difficulty in deciding whether to use $Z_{(1-\alpha/2)}$ or $t_{(n-1,1-\alpha/2)}$ when constructing confidence intervals for the mean μ. When the variable is normally distributed and σ^2 (or σ) is known, $Z_{(1-\alpha/2)}$ values are to be used regardless of the sample size n. When $n \geq 30$ and σ is not known, the estimate S can be used with a $Z_{(1-\alpha/2)}$ value. When $n < 30$ and σ is not known, the estimate S can be used with a $t_{(n-1,1-\alpha/2)}$ value as long as the variable is approximately normal. Bear in mind that the key assumption here is that the underlying distribution is normal. The validity of the assumption can be checked roughly by constructing a stem-and-leaf plot or a histogram. This approach, based on the t distribution, works well if the observations exhibit an approximately bell-shaped curve. This is true for discrete observations as well. However, if observations are far from being normal, statistical procedures based on the t distribution should not be used. In such cases, appropriate non-parametric methods should be employed. Non-parametric techniques are presented in Chapter 14.

The method presented in Section 7.2 to determine the maximum error we risk with

$(1 - \alpha)100\%$ confidence when estimating the population mean with a sample mean can be readily adapted to the cases discussed in this section when σ is not known. Simply substitute S for σ, and $t_{(n-1,1-\alpha/2)}$ for $Z_{(1-\alpha/2)}$ in the formula.

Definition 7.3.1. The maximum error of extimate is defined by $E = t_{(n-1,1-\alpha/2)} \cdot \dfrac{S}{\sqrt{n}}$

Example 7.3.3. It is well known in dentistry that dental anxiety is one of the leading factors in avoiding dental treatments. To quantify the level of anxiety among dental-phobic patients, a researcher selected 15 patients at random and measured their pulse rates while the patients were sitting in the dental chair. She compared these rates to their normal pulse rates in their home environment and recorded the differences. If the average of the 15 observations is $\overline{X} = 28.7$ beats per min with the SD $S = 5.3$, with probability 99%, what can the researcher say about the maximum error if she wants to use $\overline{X}$ to estimate μ?

Solution. Substituting $n = 15$, $\dfrac{S}{\sqrt{n}} = \dfrac{5.3}{\sqrt{15}} = 1.3685$ and $t_{(14,0.995)} = 2.9768$ in the above formula,

$$E = t_{(n-1,1-\alpha/2)} \cdot \frac{S}{\sqrt{n}} = (2.9768)(1.3685)$$

$$= 4.0738.$$

If she uses $\overline{X} = 28.7$ to estimate the true unknown mean increase in pulse rate of her patients, she can say with probability 99% that the error will not exceed 4.07 beats per minute.

7.4 CONFIDENCE INTERVALS FOR THE BINOMIAL PARAMETER p

We have dealt with the binomial parameter p when the binomial probability was discussed in Section 5.2, where a counting principle was introduced. Data are obtained by counting rather than measuring. For example,

1. the number of smokers among health science professionals' patients.
2. the number of hygienists who prefer ultrasonic scalers for routine prophylaxis and periodontal instrumentation over hand-held scalers.

3. the number of endodontic patients who experience severe pain and/or swelling following root canal treatment.
4. the number of patients whose mortality rates returned to the level of that for the general population after undergoing bone marrow transplantation.

In these examples, we typically collect data to estimate the population proportion p by a sample proportion $\frac{X}{n}$, where X is the number of times that an event of our interest, such as a patient who smokes, has occurred in n independent trials. If a study shows that in a random sample of 185 hygienists, 152 prefer ultrasonic scalers, then $\frac{X}{n} = \frac{152}{185} \simeq 0.82$. We can use this value as a point estimate of the true unknown proportion of hygienists who prefer ultrasonic scalers. Throughout the discussion in this section we will assume that the conditions of the binomial distribution are satisfied. That is, we have n independent trials, and for each trial the probability p of success has the same constant value. The proportion p is the parameter we want to estimate. We introduce the following notation for our discussion: Let p be the true population proportion, and $\hat{p}$ (read "p" hat) be the sample proportion given by

$$\hat{p} = \frac{X}{n} \quad \text{and} \quad \hat{q} = 1 - \hat{p} = 1 - \frac{X}{n} = \frac{n - X}{n}.$$

Example 7.4.1. In a recent survey of 68 endodontic patients who underwent root canal treatment, 27 have experienced severe pain and/or swelling following the treatment. Find $\hat{p}$ and $\hat{q}$.

Solution. Since $n = 68$ and $X = 27$, $\hat{p} = \dfrac{X}{n} = \dfrac{27}{68} = 0.3971$ (or 39.71%), and $\hat{q} = 1 - \dfrac{X}{n} = \dfrac{n - X}{n} = \dfrac{68 - 27}{68} = 0.6029$ (or 60.29%).

We can also obtain $\hat{q}$ by using the relation $\hat{q} = 1 - \hat{p} = 1 - 0.3971 = 0.6029$.

We know from Section 5.5.6 that the binomial distribution can be approximated by a normal distribution with mean np and variance npq when both are greater than 5. Recall that this approximation requires that n must be sufficiently large. In fact, for large values of n, the statistic

$$Z = \frac{X - np}{\sqrt{np(1-p)}} = \frac{X - np}{\sqrt{npq}}$$

has *approximately* the standard normal distribution, $N(0, 1)$. As discussed in Section 7.2,

$$P(-Z_{1-\alpha/2} \le Z \le Z_{1-\alpha/2}) = 1 - \alpha.$$

Replacing Z by $\frac{X - np}{\sqrt{npq}}$, we have

$$P\left(-Z_{1-\alpha/2} \le \frac{X - np}{\sqrt{npq}} \le Z_{1-\alpha/2}\right)$$

$$= P(-Z_{1-\alpha/2}\sqrt{npq} \le X - np \le Z_{1-\alpha/2}\sqrt{npq}),$$

subtracting X from each term, we get

$$= P(-X - Z_{1-\alpha/2}\sqrt{npq} \le -np$$
$$\le -X + Z_{1-\alpha/2}\sqrt{npq}),$$

dividing each term by $-n$ yields

$$= P\left(\frac{X}{n} - Z_{1-\alpha/2} \cdot \sqrt{\frac{pq}{n}} \le p\right.$$

$$\left.\le \frac{X}{n} + Z_{1-\alpha/2} \cdot \sqrt{\frac{pq}{n}}\right) = 1 - \alpha.$$

Note that $\sqrt{\frac{pq}{n}}$ is the SE of a proportion, that is, the SD of the sampling distribution of a sample proportion $\frac{X}{n}$. By replacing p by its estimate $\hat{p} = \frac{X}{n}$, we derive the following $100(1-\alpha)\%$ large sample confidence interval for p. We refer to it as a large sample confidence interval because a sufficiently large sample size n is required for the normal approximation.

A $100(1-\alpha)\%$ **large sample confidence interval for a proportion** p is given by;

$$\left(\hat{p} - Z_{1-\alpha/2} \cdot \sqrt{\frac{\hat{p}\hat{q}}{n}}, \hat{p} + Z_{1-\alpha/2} \cdot \sqrt{\frac{\hat{p}\hat{q}}{n}}\right),$$

where $\hat{q} = 1 - \hat{p}$.

Example 7.4.2. A retrospective study was conducted on the durability and life span of restorations in primary molars of pediatric patients treated at a dental school clinic. The histories of crowned primary molars were followed for up to 9 years

and their durability assessed in terms of crown replacements and length of service, using appropriate definitions for failure and success. Of 331 crowns studied, 291 were successful either to tooth exfoliation or to the end of the study [9]. Construct a 95% confidence interval for the true proportion p of successful crowns.

Solution. Since $n = 331$ and $X = 291$, the sample proportion is $\hat{p} = \frac{X}{n} = \frac{291}{331} = 0.879$. We note that npq is greater than 5. Substituting $Z_{1-\alpha/2} = Z_{0.975} = 1.96$ in the formula, we obtain

$$\left(\hat{p} - Z_{1-\alpha/2} \cdot \sqrt{\frac{\hat{p}\hat{q}}{n}}, \hat{p} + Z_{1-\alpha/2} \cdot \sqrt{\frac{\hat{p}\hat{q}}{n}}\right)$$

$$= (0.879 - 1.96\sqrt{\frac{(0.879)(0.121)}{331}}, 0.879$$

$$+ 1.96\sqrt{\frac{(0.879)(0.121)}{331}}) = (0.844, 0.914).$$

A 95% confidence interval for p is given by $(0.844, 0.914)$. Bear in mind this interval either contains the parameter it is intended to estimate or it does not. We actually do not know which is the case, but we can be 95% confident that the proportion of success is between 84.4% and 91.4%.

Example 7.4.3. Coronal leakage should be taken into account as a potential etiological factor in the failure of root canal treatment. An endodontist has performed an experiment to evaluate the effectiveness of the pigmented glass ionomer cement he uses as an intraorifice barrier to prevent coronal microleakage. He sampled 135 extracted human teeth with a single canal. The teeth were instrumented, obturated, and placed in a glass vial filled with red broth. Three weeks later he examined his samples for microleakage and found 9 had leakage. Find a 99% confidence interval for the true proportion of coronal microleakage.

Solution. The sample size is $n = 135$ and the number of leakage is $X = 9$, so the sample proportion is $\hat{p} = \frac{X}{n} = \frac{9}{135} = 0.0667$. Since $Z_{1-\alpha/2} = Z_{0.995} = 2.58$ and the sample size is large enough, by substitution

$$\left(\hat{p} - Z_{1-\alpha/2} \cdot \sqrt{\frac{\hat{p}\hat{q}}{n}}, \hat{p} + Z_{1-\alpha/2} \cdot \sqrt{\frac{\hat{p}\hat{q}}{n}} \right)$$

$$= \left(0.067 - 2.58\sqrt{\frac{(0.067)(0.933)}{135}}, \right.$$

$$\left. 0.067 + 2.58\sqrt{\frac{(0.067)(0.933)}{135}} \right)$$

$$= (0.011, 0.123).$$

Similar to our discussions in Section 7.2, the maximum error of estimate is $E = Z_{1-\alpha/2} \cdot \sqrt{\frac{pq}{n}}$. From this equation we can determine the minimum sample size required for a confidence interval for p by solving the above equation for n. Thus, the minimum sample size required for $100(1 - \alpha)\%$ confidence interval for p is:

$$n = pq \left(\frac{Z_{1-\alpha/2}}{E} \right)^2.$$

If necessary, round up to obtain a whole number for n.

Of course, p is not known in the formula. We cannot use the formula unless we have some ideas about the possible values of p. If some approximate value of p is known, that value can be used. Otherwise, we should use $p = 0.5$. We saw in Section 5.2 that pq achieves its maximum when $p = 0.5$. With $p = 0.5$, the sample size n will be larger than necessary. In this case, we can say that the probability is at least $1 - \alpha$ that our error will not exceed E.

Example 7.4.4. Hormone replacement therapy (HRT) is used by an increasing number of women to relieve menopausal problems. A protective effect against bone loss and cardiovascular disease has been demonstrated. One study [10] reported that estrogen replacement therapy prolonged survival in women when coronary artery disease was present. However, concern has been raised about an increased incidence of breast cancer after HRT use, especially after more than 10 years of use [11]. A clinical study is designed to estimate the proportion of women who develop breast cancer after having been on HRT at least 10 years. If the

research team wants to assert with the probability of at least 0.95 that its error will not exceed 0.015, how large a sample should they take (a) if it is known from the past studies that the true proportion lies between 0.01 and 0.05; and (b) if they have no idea what the true proportion might be?

Solution. (i) Since p is known to be in the interval between 0.01 and 0.05, we take $p = 0.05$. Substituting $p = 0.05$, $Z_{1-\alpha/2} = 1.96$, and $E = 0.015$ in the formula for n, we obtain

$$n = pq \left(\frac{Z_{1-\alpha/2}}{E} \right)^2 = (0.05) \cdot (0.95) \cdot \left(\frac{1.96}{0.015} \right)^2$$

$$= 811.0044.$$

Rounding up to the nearest integer, we get the required sample size $n = 812$ subjects.

(ii) By substitution with $p = 0.5$, $Z_{1-\alpha/2} = 1.96$, and $E = 0.015$, we have

$$n = (0.5) \cdot (0.5) \cdot \left(\frac{1.96}{0.015} \right)^2 = 4268.4.$$

Rounding up to the nearest integer, we obtain the required sample size $n = 4,269$ subjects.

7.5 CONFIDENCE INTERVALS FOR THE VARIANCES AND STANDARD DEVIATIONS

In previous sections we have illustrated how to construct confidence intervals for means and proportions. This section is devoted to discussing how to find confidence intervals for variances and SDs. We studied in Chapter 3 that location parameters, such as mean, median, and mode, are not enough to adequately describe data. Variances and SDs were introduced to represent the dispersion of data. In drug manufacturing, keeping variability as small as possible is the key step to providing the "right" dosage level for the patients. To discuss confidence intervals for σ^2 we need to introduce another probability distribution function, called the χ^2 distribution. Read χ^2 as "chi-square" (χ is a Greek letter). Like the t distribution, the **chi-square distribution** is associated with the degree of freedom. The shape of the chi-square distribution is determined by the degree of freedom associated with it. It is a well-known fact in statistics that the χ^2 distribution is obtained from the values of $(n - 1)S^2/\sigma^2$, where the random samples are

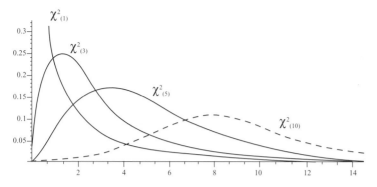

Figure 7.5.1 χ^2 densities for different degrees of freedom.

taken from an underlying population that is normally distributed with the variance σ^2. Some characteristics of the χ^2 distribution are as follows.

1. Like the t distribution, the χ^2 distribution is a family of distributions whose shapes depend on the associated degrees of freedom.
2. The degrees of freedom δ is equal to $n-1$.
3. Unlike the normal and t distributions, the χ^2 distribution takes on non-negative values between 0 and ∞ (infinity).
4. Unlike the normal and t distributions, the χ^2 distribution is positively skewed for small values of δ (small degrees of freedom). As δ increases, the distribution becomes less and less skewed. In fact, for sufficiently large degrees of freedom δ, the χ^2 distribution approaches a normal distribution with mean $\mu = \delta$ and variance $\sigma^2 = 2\delta$. Whether δ is small or large, the mean and the variance of the χ^2 distribution are given by δ and 2δ, respectively. In other words, the mean μ of the χ^2 distribution is the same as the degrees of freedom, and the variance σ^2 is twice the degrees of freedom.

Figure 7.5.1 shows the χ^2 distribution with four different values for degrees of freedom δ; $\delta = 1$, 3, 5, and 10. As we can see in the figure, the shape of the χ^2 distribution appears less and less skewed as the degrees of freedom increase.

Table F in the Appendix gives the percentile values for the χ^2 distribution for $p = 0.005, 0.01, 0.025, 0.05, 0.10, 0.90, 0.95, 0.975, 0.99,$ and 0.995. The first column of the table shows the degrees of freedom δ. The degrees of freedom in Table F ranges from $\delta = 1$ to $\delta = 100$. The entire area under each χ^2 distribution is equal to 1.0. As in the t distribution, $(1-\alpha)100^{\text{th}}$ percentile of the χ^2 distribution with the degrees of freedom δ is denoted by $\chi^2_{(\delta,1-\alpha)}$.

Let X be a random variable that has the χ^2 distribution with the degrees of freedom δ. Then $P(X \leq \chi^2) = 1 - \alpha$. After replacing X by $\chi^2_{(\delta)}$ to indicate that X is distributed according to the χ^2 distribution with the degrees of freedom δ, we may write $P(\chi^2_{(\delta)} \leq \chi^2_{(\delta,1-\alpha)}) = 1 - \alpha$.

The probability $P(\chi^2 \leq \chi^2_{(\delta,1-\alpha)})$ corresponds to the area to the left of the point $\chi^2_{(\delta,1-\alpha)}$

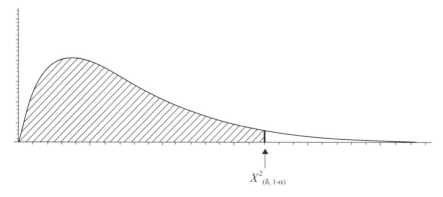

Figure 7.5.2 $P(X^2 \leq X^2_{(\delta,1-a)})$ corresponds to the area to the left of the point $X^2_{(\delta,1-a)}$ under the curve.

surrounded by the χ^2 curve and the x-axis shown in Figure 7.5.2.

Example 7.5.1. Find the appropriate percentile points for the following.

(i) $P(\chi^2_{(6)} \le \chi^2) = 0.90$,

(ii) $P(\chi^2_{(24)} \le \chi^2) = 0.95$, and

(iii) $P(\chi^2_{(15)} \le \chi^2) = 0.975$.

Solution. Using Table F in the Appendix, we can find the values $\chi^2_{(\delta, 1-\alpha)}$.

(i) $\chi^2_{(6, 0.90)} = 10.645$,

(ii) $\chi^2_{(24, 0.95)} = 36.415$, and

(iii) $\chi^2_{(15, 0.05)} = 4.601$.

For the χ^2 distribution with the degrees of freedom $\delta = 6$, 90% of the population lies below 10.645, or the area encompassed by the χ^2 curve, and the X-axis and the vertical line drawn at 10.645 is 0.90.

Example 7.5.2. Find the following probabilities.

(i) $P(\chi^2_{(7)} \le 2.83)$,

(ii) $P(\chi^2_{(20)} \le 37.57)$, and

(iii) $P(\chi^2_{(35)} \le 53.16)$.

Solution. The first two probabilities are readily available from Table F. The table does not contain the degrees of freedom $\delta = 35$ but it includes $\delta = 30$ and 40. Since $\delta = 35$ is the midpoint between 30 and 40, we will apply the linear interpolation method to approximate the probability. In the table, 53.16 is between 46.979 for $\delta = 30$ and 59.342 for $\delta = 40$ under $P = 0.975$. In fact, 53.16 is the midpoint between 46.979 and 59.342. Thus, $P(\chi^2_{(35)} \le 53.16) = 0.975$.

df (δ)	.	0.950	0.975	0.990	.
.		.	.	.	.
30	.	43.773	46.979	50.892	.
35	$\rightarrow$	$\rightarrow$	**53.16**		.
40	.	55.758	59.342	63.691	.
.		.	.	.	.

　Recall that if the variable X is normally distributed, then the statistic $\chi^2 = \frac{(n-1)S^2}{\sigma^2}$ has the χ^2 distribution with the degrees of freedom $(n-1)$, where S^2 is the sample variance. Similar to t distribution, $\chi^2_{(n-1, \alpha/2)}$ and $\chi^2_{(n-1, 1-\alpha/2)}$ denote

the $(\alpha/2)100^{\text{th}}$ and $(1-\alpha/2)100^{\text{th}}$ percentiles of the χ^2 distribution with the degrees of freedom $(n-1)$. Therefore, a $(1-\alpha)100\%$ confidence interval for σ^2 is given by $\frac{(n-1)S^2}{\chi^2_{(n-1, 1-\alpha/2)}} \le$

$\sigma^2 \le \frac{(n-1)S^2}{\chi^2_{(n-1, \alpha/2)}}$, and a $(1-\alpha)100\%$ confidence

interval for σ is given by $\sqrt{\frac{(n-1)S^2}{\chi^2_{(n-1, 1-\alpha/2)}}} \le \sigma \le$

$\sqrt{\frac{(n-1)S^2}{\chi^2_{(n-1, \alpha/2)}}}$.

Example 7.5.3. Let X be the random variable denoting the mucogingival distance, which is normally distributed. To estimate the mean and variance of the mucogingival distance for adult patients, a periodontist took a random sample of 24 patients and measured the distance X in millimeters. She has obtained $S^2 = 4.74$. Find a 95% confidence interval for the variance.

Solution. Since $(1-\alpha)100\% = 95\%$, $\alpha = 0.05$. The sample size $n = 24$ means the degree of freedom is $n - 1 = 23$. We now find the percentiles from Table F; $\chi^2_{(n-1, \alpha/2)} = \chi^2_{(23, 0.025)} = 11.689$ and $\chi^2_{(n-1, 1-\alpha/2)} = \chi^2_{(23, 0.975)} = 38.076$. By substitution in the formula, we get

$$\frac{(23)(4.74)}{38.076} \le \sigma^2 \le \frac{(23)(4.74)}{11.689}.$$

Calculations lead to $2.86 \le \sigma^2 \le 9.33$.

Thus, a 95% confidence interval for σ^2 is $(2.86, 9.33)$. A 95% confidence interval for the standard deviation σ is obtained by taking the square root $(\sqrt{2.86}, \sqrt{9.33}) = (1.69, 3.05)$.

Example 7.5.4. Dilution of 5.25% sodium hypochlorite before its use as an endodontic irrigant has been recommended. To evaluate the effect of dilution on the solvent action of sodium hypochlorite, 9 necrotic tissue specimens were exposed to 5.25% sodium hypochlorite and the percent X of tissue weight change was measured. Suppose X is normally distributed and the sample of 9 specimens yielded the sample SD of 14.26% [12]. Construct a 90% confidence interval for σ.

Solution. Since $S = 14.26$, $S^2 = 203.35$. The degree of freedom is given by $n = 9 - 1 = 8$. From

Table F we get $\chi^2_{(n-1,\alpha/2)} = \chi^2_{(8,0.05)} = 2.733$, and $\chi^2_{(n-1,1-\alpha/2)} = \chi^2_{(8,0.95)} = 15.507$. Substitution in the formula yields

$$\sqrt{\frac{(8)(203.35)}{15.507}} \leq \sigma \leq \sqrt{\frac{(8)(203.35)}{2.733}}.$$

Thus, a 90% confidence interval for σ is given by (10.24, 24.40).

7.6 EXERCISES

1 Changes in dental arch dimensions that occur as a result of growth and treatment are of interest to orthodontists and must be carefully considered when planning treatment. To study the changes in arch length, thirty-three 13-year old males have been recruited, and their arch length measurements were made. The sample mean of the 33 measurements was 77.9 mm. Let Y be the random variable for maxillary arch length. Suppose Y has a normal distribution with the SD $\sigma = 4.1$ mm. Find a 90% confidence interval for the population mean arch length of 13-year-old males.

2 To study whether or not there are any differences in changes between females and males, the investigators took twenty-nine 13-year-old females and measured their arch length. The sample mean of the 29 arch length measurements was 74.7 mm. Suppose that the arch length has a normal distribution with the SD $\sigma = 3.2$ mm. Find a 95% confidence interval for the population mean arch length of 13-year-old females.

3 Fifteen fully developed maxillary anterior teeth were artificially stained with human hemoglobin to evaluate objectively in vitro the effectiveness of bleaching. The bleaching agents were applied twice over a 1-week period, and the changes in tooth shade were analyzed using a sphere spectrophotometer, which measures the color "white." Let X be a random variable describing the amount of changes in "white" color. The average change of the 15 samples was 7.24. Suppose X has a normal distribution and our past experience indicates that the SD is known to be 1.73. Construct a 99% confidence interval for the mean μ.

4 In Exercise 3, suppose the investigators took 25 fully developed maxillary anterior teeth instead of

15. Discuss how this would affect the 99% confidence intervals for μ.

5 In Example 7.2.5, discuss why rounding off to $n = 30$ will not meet the requirement.

6 It is reasonable to assume that the level of triglycerides (milligrams per decaliter) is normally distributed. A previous study indicates that the variance σ^2 among male subjects is 86.4. We want to use the sample mean of a random sample to estimate the population mean of the triglyceride level and want to be able to assert with probability 0.85 that our error will be no more than (at most) 2.75 mg/dL. How large a sample will we need?

7 Eight dentists work in a large clinic. Let X be a random variable for the amount of time they spent in patient contact. Suppose the SD of X is 8.5 min. What can we say with probability 95% about the maximum error of estimate of the mean μ of their patient contact time? Assume X is normally distributed.

8 Cardiologists want to estimate the average duration of chest pain experienced by AMI (acute myocardial infarction) patients. Suppose that the duration is normally distributed with variance $\sigma^2 = 424$. Chest pain data were collected from 24 AMI patients who have been admitted to a coronary care unit. With what probability can you assert that the maximum error of estimate will be no greater than 10 min?

9 Public Health Department officials are concerned about the oral hygiene of inner city children. Twenty schoolchildren were randomly selected to assess the overall oral hygiene conditions. Dental examination of these children showed that the average pocket depth is 6.2 mm with the SD of 2.4 mm. Suppose that the distribution of children's pocket depth is approximately normal. With probability 95%, what is the maximum error the officials make when they use 6.2 mm to estimate the true average pocket depth of inner city children?

10 If the officials in Exercise 9 want to reduce the maximum error by 50%, how many more children should they select? Assume that the sample mean and the sample SD will stay the same.

11 Suppose in Example 7.3.2 the investigators collected the following post-treatment mandibular intercanine width of 10 subjects from the group of

13 patients. Find a 99% confidence interval for the population mean μ.

Subject	Mandibular Intercanine Width
1	26.5
2	24.6
3	26.4
4	27.3
5	26.0
6	25.8
7	27.0
8	24.8
9	25.2
10	24.1

12 A university clinic offers a flu vaccine each year. The flu vaccine does not protect individuals from being infected by the flu virus. It only reduces the probability of infection. Of 375 individuals who were given a flu vaccine, 64 had the flu during the last flu season. Construct a 90% confidence interval for the proportion of the people who will not get the flu after receiving a flu shot.

13 The heat produced by dental implant osteotomy preparation at different speeds and the effects of heat production on the prognosis of implant treatment are controversial [13]. To study the relationship between drill speed at 30,000 rpm and heat production, rabbits will be used. Heat production will be measured in vivo during osteotomy preparation in the rabbit tibia. Temperature will be recorded while an osteotomy is being drilled 1 mm from the thermocouple receptor site. Distilled water is to be used as coolant in conjunction with drilling. The goal is to estimate the proportion of the heat measurements that exceed 33.0° C. If you want to assert with the probability of at least 0.90 that its error will not exceed 0.025, how large a sample will you need?

14 The breakage of the esthetically desirable ceramic bracket has been considered a major clinical problem because it prolongs the orthodontic treatment and leads to compromises in its final outcome. Broken ceramic brackets are uncomfortable to the patients and difficult to remove. Internal causes for ceramic breakage are porosity and cracks, the presence of localized stresses and scratches, an inadequate heat treatment, and an improper design and material [14]. To improve the quality of the ceramic brackets, the manufacturer has designed an impact resistance test. A focus of the test is to estimate the proportion of brackets that survive the impact test. Suppose the manufacturer wishes to claim, with the probability of at least 0.99, that its error is no greater than 0.03. How large a sample will it need?

15 The prevalence of hypodontia in children with clefts, both inside and outside the cleft region, is being studied. It is known that hypodontia prevalence rate is 0.77 from the past studies. How large a sample would you need if you want to assert with the probability of at least 0.95 that the maximum error of your estimate of the prevalence rate is less than 0.02?

16 Quality of patient care includes a quiet environment in the hospital ward area. To assess their quality patient care, Loma Linda Community Hospital administrators collected noise level data at 23 randomly selected time points during January in the ward area. Suppose the noise level is normally distributed. Their data yielded the sample mean of 52.5 decibels and the sample SD of 5.2 decibels. The administrators would like to know a 99% confidence interval for the true mean noise level in the hospital.

17 Tooth size ratios represent a valid diagnostic tool that allows for an educated prediction of treatment outcomes and may also limit the necessity for diagnostic setups for complex cases. A proper relationship of the total mesiodistal width of the maxillary dentition to the mesiodistal width of the mandibular dentition will favor an optimal post-treatment occlusion [15]. Suppose the maxillary-to-mandibular tooth size relationship is observed, and the ratio is known to be normally distributed. A sample of 31 patients is selected, and the sample variance of the ratio of these 31 patients is 2.72. Construct a 85% confidence interval for the standard deviation σ.

18 Homocysteine is a by-product of protein processing, which is known to be one of the serious artery clogging villains. Patients can lower homocysteine levels by taking vitamins, such as folic acid, vitamins B-6 and B-12. Doctors took 29 patients and measured their daily intake of folic acid, which is assumed to be normally distributed. From the measurements they obtained, the sample SD

$S = 34$ micrograms. Find a 90% confidence interval for the population variance σ^2.

19 Silicon nitride is a high-performance ceramic characterized by high wear resistance, good fatigue life, and fracture toughness. Its elastic modulus in the porous state is similar to that of bone. These properties are indicative of its potential as a material for orthopedic prostheses [16]. Suppose investigators studied its fracture toughness in megapascals using 41 samples. The investigators are interested in estimating the standard deviation of fracture toughness X. Suppose X is normally distributed and $S^2 = 784$. Find a 95% confidence interval for σ.

20 The parathyroid hormone regulates calcium levels in blood. Blood calcium levels increase when the production of parathyroid hormone increases. This high blood calcium level can lead to kidney stones, making a person urinate large volumes, and be constantly thirsty. It also leaches calcium from bones, weakening them and making them vulnerable to fractures. A high calcium level can dull a person's thinking. If the level is quite high, it can eventually put a person into a coma. An endocrinologist estimated the SD of the blood calcium level to be 0.25 mg/dL based on 12 patients he examined last week. Find a 99% confidence interval for σ assuming the distribution of the blood calcium level is normal.

7.7 REFERENCES

1. Lindauer, S. J., et al. Effect of pumice prophylaxis on the bond strength of orthodontic brackets. *Am. J. Orthod. and Dentofacial Orthopedics*: 1997, 111, 599–605.
2. Steele, A., and Johnson, B. R. In vitro fracture strength of endodontically treatred premolars. *J. of Endodontics*, 1999: 25, 6–9.
3. Gangas, G., et al. Gender difference in blood thrombogenicity in hyperlipidemic patients and response to pravastatin. *Am. J. of Cardiology*, 1999, 84, 639–643.
4. Tjan, A. J., and Li, T. Dentition and fit of crowns cemented with an adhesive resin. (abstract) *J. Dent Res*. 1990, 69, 123.
5. White, S. N., et al. Effect of seating force on film thickness of new adhesive luting agents. *J. Prosthet. Dent*. 1992: 68, 476–481.
6. Kutin, G., and Hawes, R. R. Posterior crossbite in the deciduous and mixed dentition. *Am. J. Orthod*. 1969, 56, 491–504.
7. Hanson, M. I., Barnard, L. W., and Case, J. L. Tongue thrust preschool children. Part II: Dental occlusal patterns. *Am. J. Orthod*. 1970, 57, 15–22.
8. Erdinc, A. E., Turkoz, U., and Erbay, E. A comparison of different treatment techniques for posterior crossbite in the mixed dentition. *Am. J. Dentofacial Orthop*. 1999, 116, 287–300.
9. Messer, L. B., and Levering, N. J. The durability of primary molar restorations: II. Observations and predictions of success of stainless steel crowns. *Pediatric Dentistry*; 1988, 10, 81–85.
10. Sullivan, J. M., et al. Estrogen replacement and coronary artery disease: Effects on survival in postmenopausal women. *Arch. Intern. Med*: 1990, 150, 2557–2562.
11. Grodstein, F., et al. Postmenopausal hormone therapy and mortality. *N. Engl. J. Med*: 1997, 336, 1769–1775.
12. Iyer, S., Weiss, C., and Mehta, A. Effects of drill speed on heat production and the rate and quality of bone formation in dental implant osteotomies. Part I: Relationship between drill speed and heat production. *Int. J. Prosthodont*: 1997,10, 411–414.
13. Matasa, C. G. Impact resistance of ceramic brackets according to ophthalmic lenses standards. *Am. J. Orthod. Dentofacial Orthop*: 1999, 115, 158–165.
14. Hand, R. E., et al. Analysis of the effect of dilution on the necrotic tissue dissolution property of sodium hypochlorite. *J. of Endod*: 1978, 4, 60–64.
15. Santoro, M., et al. Mesiodistal crown dimensions and tooth size discrepancy of the preeminent of Dominican Americans. *Angle Orthodontist*: 2000, 70, 303–307.
16. Lin, S., Shi, S., LeGeros, R. Z., and LeGeros, J. P. Three-dimensional finite element analyses of four designs of a high-strength silicon nitride implant. *Implant Dent*: 2000, 9, 53–60.

Chapter 8

Hypothesis Testing: One-Sample Case

8.1 INTRODUCTION

Statistical inference is a process of drawing conclusions regarding a population based on the limited information from a sample taken from the population of our interest. There are different statistical approaches to making decisions about the population. One that has received much attention is **hypothesis testing**, which has a wide range of applications in biomedical and health sciences, as well as other disciplines. Statistical hypothesis testing can be applied to address conjectures such as the following:

- Wearing a mouthguard is an effective way to prevent trauma to teeth during sports activities.
- The prevalence of decayed, missing, filled teeth (DMFT) in children with cleft lip/palate is higher than in those without cleft lip/palate.
- Alcohol consumption, like smoking, might be related to periodontal diseases.
- Patients treated with nifedipine tend to have gingival enlargement.
- A 5-year survival rate of oral and pharyngeal cancer is higher for white patients than for black patients.
- Bleach is much more effective than a dish washing soap in eliminating microorganisms such as salmonella, pseudomonas, staphylococcus, and candida.
- Apolipoprotein E E4 allele is strongly associated with late-onset familial Alzheimer's disease.

In hypothesis testing, the researchers must clearly define the population under investigation, state the hypotheses to be tested, specify the significance level (this will be defined later), select a sample from the population, collect data, select a test statistic, perform the calculations required for the statistical test, draw a conclusion, and, finally, develop appropriate interpretations of the conclusion.

Scientific investigations involve learning from data. Researchers state hypotheses on the basis of the statistical evidence contained in the sample data. The hypothesis is either *rejected*, meaning the evidence from the sample indicates enough to say with a certain degree of confidence that the hypothesis is false, or *accepted*, meaning there is not enough evidence to reject the hypothesis. Suppose we want to show that a new cholesterol-reducing drug is more effective than the current one. We hypothesize that they are equally effective. Since we hypothesize that there is no difference in medical effectiveness between the two drugs, this type of hypothesis is called the **null hypothesis** and is denoted by H_0. The hypothesis that we accept when the null hypothesis is rejected is called the **alternative hypothesis**, denoted by H_1.

In our system of criminal justice, the accused is presumed innocent until proven guilty "beyond reasonable doubt." The null hypothesis we make in court proceedings is the presumption of innocence. The alternative hypothesis is "the defendant is guilty." In the U.S. justice system, the burden of proof lies with the prosecution to convince the jury that the defendant is guilty. The two hypotheses must be formulated together so that we know when to reject the null hypothesis. For example, the investigators are testing the null hypothesis H_0 that the average birth weight of full-term babies born in the U.S. is $\mu \leq 7.5$ lbs versus the alternative hypothesis H_1 that $\mu > 7.5$ lbs. They would reject H_0 only if the sample mean is much greater than 7.5 lbs. The hypothesis being proposed by the scientific investigators is the alternative hypothesis. Thus the alternative hypothesis is sometimes referred to as the *research hypothesis*.

8.2 CONCEPTS OF HYPOTHESIS TESTING

To illustrate some of the underlying concepts of testing a statistical hypothesis, suppose a claim was made by emergency room staff that the average waiting time for emergency room patients is about 30 minutes. The hospital administration considers reorganizing the emergency room staff. They want to test the null hypothesis that the average waiting time is 30 minutes versus the alternative hypothesis that the average waiting time is not 30 minutes, that is, either longer or shorter than 30 minutes. We can state the hypotheses as follows:

$$H_0 : \mu = 30 \quad \text{vs.} \quad H_1 : \mu \neq 30.$$

A member of the ER staff is assigned to observe 25 patients at random, carefully recording their arrival time and the time they are attended by the medical staff. Suppose the hospital administration has decided to accept the claim if the mean waiting time of the random sample of 25 patients is between 27 and 33 minutes. Otherwise, H_0 will be rejected. This is a criterion for making a decision whether to accept or reject the ER staff's claim. As we discussed in detail in Chapter 6, the sample mean is a random variable. Since the decision is made based on a sample, the value of the sample mean of 25 patients may be greater than 33 minutes or less than 27 minutes, even though the true mean of the waiting time is between 27 and 33 minutes. This situation will lead them to make a wrong decision, because according to their criterion they will reject the claim that is true. Therefore, it seems reasonable to evaluate the chances of making a wrong decision, given a decision criterion. Let's assume that the waiting time is normally distributed and the SD σ of the waiting time is known to be 6.75.

The chance that the sample mean of the waiting time is shorter than 27 or longer than 33, given that the true mean is 30, is $P(\overline{X} \leq 27) + P(\overline{X} \geq 33)$. We can calculate these probabilities

$$P(\overline{X} \leq 27) = P\left(Z \leq \frac{27 - 30}{6.75/\sqrt{25}}\right)$$
$$= P(Z \leq -2.22) = 0.0132,$$

and

$$P(\overline{X} \geq 33) = P\left(Z \geq \frac{33 - 30}{6.75/\sqrt{25}}\right)$$
$$= P(Z \geq 2.22) = 0.0132.$$

So $P(\overline{X} \leq 27) + P(\overline{X} \geq 33) = 0.0132 + 0.0132 = 0.0264$.

The probability of observing a sample mean that is less than 27 or greater than 33 is given by the combined area under the normal curve to the left of $\overline{x} = 27$ and to the right of $\overline{x} = 33$ shown in Figure 8.2.1. That is, the chance that they reject H_0 purely due to chance, even though the null hypothesis is true, is 0.0264. This probability is small enough to be considered as an acceptable risk. If, however, the probability were 0.0784 instead of 0.0264, the hospital administrators will have to decide if they are willing to take the risk in light of the consequences of an error.

We now consider the other possibility, that is, accepting H_0 (or failing to reject H_0) when the null hypothesis is false. Suppose the true mean waiting time is 34 minutes. The chance that the sample mean of 25 patients is between 27 and 33 minutes is

$$P(27 \leq \overline{X} \leq 33)$$
$$= P\left(\frac{27 - 34}{6.75/\sqrt{25}} \leq Z \leq \frac{33 - 34}{6.75/\sqrt{25}}\right)$$
$$= 0.2296,$$

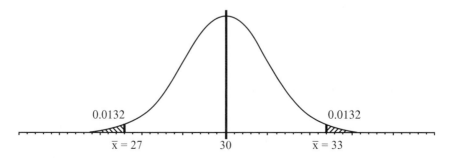

Figure 8.2.1 Normal distribution with $\mu = 30$.

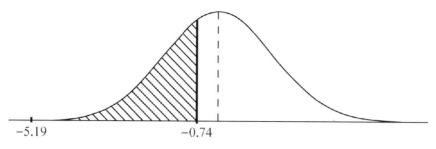

Figure 8.2.2   The shaded area corresponds to $P(-5.19 \leq Z \leq -0.74)$.

which is the same as the entire area between $z = -5.19$ and $z = -0.74$ under the standard normal curve in Figure 8.2.2. But this area is approximately the same as the entire area to the left of $z = -0.74$ under the normal curve. Why?

The above probability 0.2296 is the probability of erroneously accepting H_0 when the true mean waiting time is indeed $\mu = 34$ minutes. The example we described is typical of statistical hypotheses tests, which is summarized in the table below.

	H_0 Is True	H_0 Is False
Accept H_0	Correct decision	Incorrect decision
Reject H_0	Incorrect decision	Correct decision

What we have discussed is analogous to a jury trial in a court of law. The defendant who is on trial is either innocent or guilty in the same way that the null hypothesis is either true or false. Relevant evidence (data) is presented during the trial. The jury finds the defendant either innocent or guilty after the deliberation. If the jury finds the defendant not guilty when he truly is innocent, the right verdict is delivered. On the other hand, if the jury finds him innocent when he truly is guilty, the wrong verdict is delivered. As the above table indicates, two types of incorrect decisions can be made: rejecting H_0 when it is true, and accepting H_0 when it is false. We define two types of errors in hypothesis testing.

Definition 8.2.1. We say a **type I error** is committed if the null hypothesis is rejected when it is true, and a **type II error** is committed if the null hypothesis is accepted when it is false.

Notation 8.2.1. The probability of committing a type I error is denoted by the Greek letter α (alpha), and the probability of committing a type II error is

denoted by the Greek letter β (beta). That is, $P(\text{a type I error}) = \alpha$ and $P(\text{a type II error}) = \beta$.

We will present a few examples to illustrate how the hypotheses can be stated.

Example 8.2.1. A new drug is being developed by a pharmaceutical company for the treatment of lung cancer. The company will release the drug only if a clinical trial indicates that it is effective on a majority of lung cancer patients. The company's scientists are confident that the drug is effective, but they wish to make the claim based on the statistical evidence. Let p be the proportion of lung cancer patients for whom the drug is effective. How would you state the hypotheses?

Solution. The company wishes to prove the drug is effective in a majority of lung cancer patients, which means the proportion $p > 0.5$. Thus, the null and alternative hypotheses can be stated as

$$H_0 : p \leq 0.5 \quad \text{vs.} \quad H_1 : p > 0.5.$$

Example 8.2.2. Due to dental anxiety experienced by the patients, their pulse rate tends to increase while the patients are sitting in the dental chair. Suppose the average pulse rate of the dental patients during the treatment is 105 beats per minute. Research is being conducted to test what effect soothing music might have on the patients: increased pulse rate, decreased pulse rate, or no changes at all. State the null and alternative hypotheses.

Solution. Letting μ be the average pulse rate of the patients while sitting in the dental chair, we state H_0: $\mu = 105$ vs. H_1: $\mu \neq 105$. The null hypothesis specifies that there is no change in the mean pulse rate. The alternative hypothesis states that the mean pulse rate is different from 105, either lower or higher than 105 beats/min.

Example 8.2.3. Both dental and medical societies have an obligation to become aware of the methods of bacterial spread. In recent years, the dental profession has increased measures to prevent potential vehicles of transmission for clinicians and patients. Bacterial contamination can occur every day. For instance, airborne bacteria are produced during dental procedures in the oral cavity. It has been generally known that in the immediate site of operation, a cavitron produces no more than 75, 000 bacterial counts per cubic foot, much less than a high-speed handpiece. But recently, dental researchers have begun to suspect that the level of bacterial contamination produced by a cavitron might be higher, and they wish to confirm their suspicion. State the appropriate hypotheses.

Solution. Let μ denote the average amount of aerosols produced by a cavitron during dental procedures. Since the investigators speculate that μ is at least 75, 000, we state the hypotheses as:

$$H_0 : \mu \leq 75, 000 \quad \text{vs.} \quad H_1 : \mu > 75, 000.$$

If the null hypothesis in Example 8.2.3 is rejected when it is true, then a type I error is committed. The sample data indicated that a cavitron produced more bacteria-ridden aerosols by chance (i.e., more than 75, 000), even though it really doesn't. In this case, a cavitron might not necessarily produce bacteria-ridden aerosols more than 75, 000, but the investigators wrongly concluded that it does. Therefore, they have committed a type I error. On the other hand, a cavitron might produce aerosols much less than 75, 000 by chance, even if it really doesn't, thereby leading the investigators to accept the null hypothesis, that is false. In this case, they have committed a type II error.

We emphasize that the investigator's decision to reject or accept the null hypothesis in some sense does not prove much. The only definitive way to prove anything statistically is to observe the entire population, which is not easy to accomplish. The decision to accept or reject the null hypothesis is made on the basis of a random sample and thus of a probabilistic concept as discussed in Chapter 6. When there is a large difference between the observed mean from the sample (say, the sample mean is 118 in Example 8.2.2) and the hypothesized mean ($\mu = 105$ in Example 8.2.2), the null hypothesis is probably false. We would not expect the mean $\overline{X}$ of a single random sample to be exactly equal to the hypothesized value 105, even if the true mean is $\mu = 105$. Some discrepancy is expected between $\overline{X}$ and 105 due to chance. But if the discrepancy is large, we would be inclined to believe that H_0 is false and that it should be rejected. Therefore, we conclude that the population mean μ could not be 105 beats/min. In this situation, statisticians say that a test result is **statistically significant**. If the sample mean $\overline{X}$ is close to 105, that is, if the statistical evidence is not strong enough to doubt the validity of the null hypothesis, we accept H_0. Instead of saying "accept H_0," some authors prefer to say "not enough evidence to reject H_0." There is a good reason for this. The true population mean could be some value other than 105, but the random sample we have selected did not contain enough evidence to prove it. The key question in hypothesis testing is how large a difference do we need to observe in order to reject the null hypothesis? As we explained in the above discussion, when H_0 is rejected, we take a risk of rejecting a null hypothesis that is true. It is customary in statistics that we reject H_0 if the probability is less than or equal to 0.05 of observing a discrepancy between $\overline{X}$ and 105 at least as large as the one you just observed. Such a probability is called the significance level. We state the following definitions.

Definition 8.2.2. The **significance level** is the maximum probability of committing a type I error and is denoted by α.

Definition 8.2.3. The **power** of a hypothesis test is defined as

$$1 - \beta = 1 - P(\text{a type II error}).$$

Definition 8.2.4. The **test statistic** is a statistic based on which the hypothesis is to be tested. For example, the sample mean $\overline{X}$ is a test statistic for testing the hypothesis in Example 8.2.3.

The ideal case, of course, is when both P(type I error) $= \alpha$ and P(type II error) $= \beta$ are equal to 0. However, this is unrealistic to expect unless the sample size is increased without a bound ($n = \infty$). The best we can do in the hypothesis-testing procedure is to limit the probability of committing a type I error and try to minimize the probability of committing a type II error. The significance level sets the limit on the risk of making a type I error. Statisticians usually specify $\alpha = 0.05$. But the investigators can be flexible with the selection of the significance level α, depending upon circumstances. In many medical and pharmaceutical studies α is typically specified by a value lower than 0.05, for example, 0.01.

Once again, this situation is analogous to a court trial. At the end of a trial, the judge issues a statement to the members of the jury to the effect that if they must find the defendant guilty, find him guilty "beyond reasonable doubt." The American judicial system recognizes the fact that there is a risk of wrongly convicting an innocent man by the jury, that is, committing a type I error. To protect against potentially devastating consequences, the judge is setting a limit on the probability of committing a type I error. This limit is specified by "beyond reasonable doubt," which is equivalent to the significance level in hypothesis testing. The jury must now try to minimize the chance of finding the defendant "not guilty" when he truly is guilty. After specifying the significance level, an appropriate **critical value** or critical values must be selected using the probability tables provided in the Appendix.

Definition 8.2.5. The critical value(s) defines the **rejection region**, which is the range of values of a test statistic for which there is a significant difference, and therefore the null hypothesis should be rejected. The **acceptance region** is the range of values of a test statistic for which the null hypothesis is accepted.

Definition 8.2.6. When the rejection region is on either the right-hand side or the left-hand side of the mean, the test is called a **one-tailed test**. When the rejection region is on both sides of the mean, the test is called a **two-tailed test**.

The critical value can be on either the right-hand side or left-hand side of the mean for a one-tailed test. It depends on the inequality sign of the alternative hypothesis. In Example 8.2.3, the critical value is on the right-hand side. If the direction of the inequality was reversed in the statement of the alternative hypothesis (i.e., $H_1: \mu < 75{,}000$), then the critical value will be on the left-hand side of the mean. For a two-tailed test the critical values are on both sides of the mean. Example 8.2.2 is a two-tailed test for which the rejection region is on both sides. The procedures for testing statistical hypotheses can be summarized as follows:

Step 1. State the hypotheses to be tested.
Step 2. Specify the significance level α.
Step 3. Choose a test statistic and perform the required calculations for the statistical test.
Step 4. Find the critical value and define the rejection region.
Step 5. Decide to accept or reject H_0.
Step 6. Draw conclusions and make interpretations.

8.3 ONE-TAILED Z TEST OF THE MEAN OF A NORMAL DISTRIBUTION WHEN σ^2 IS KNOWN

We will explain how to obtain the critical value using the example of the average birth weight of full-term babies discussed in the previous section. We shall assume the distribution of the birth weight is normal with a known variance $\sigma^2 = 1.74$. The standard deviation (SD) is $\sigma = \sqrt{1.74} = 1.32$. In that example, the null and alternative hypotheses are stated as

$$H_0 : \mu \leq 7.5 \text{ lbs.} \quad \text{vs.} \quad H_1 : \mu > 7.5 \text{ lbs.}$$

Suppose that the investigators selected the significance level $\alpha = 0.05$. Since this is a one-tailed test with the critical value lying on the right side, we need to look for a z value such that 5% of the area falls to the right and 95% to the left of the z value. It can be shown that the best test in this type of situation is a test based on the sample mean $\overline{X}$. If $\overline{X}$ is sufficiently larger than 7.5 lbs, we reject H_0. Otherwise, we accept H_0. If the true mean birth weight of full-term babies is less than 7.5 lbs, then most likely the values of $\overline{X}$ will tend to be less than 7.5. If H_1 is true, then the values of $\overline{X}$ will tend to be much larger than 7.5. How large should $\overline{X}$ be for H_0 to be rejected? Let c denote the critical value. Then, H_0 will be rejected if $c \leq \overline{X}$. Given the significance level $\alpha = 0.05$, we can find the critical value c from the relation $P(\text{a type I error}) = \alpha$.

$$P \text{ (a type I error)} = P(c \leq \overline{X})$$
$$= P\left(\frac{c - 7.5}{\sigma/\sqrt{n}} \leq Z\right) = 0.05.$$

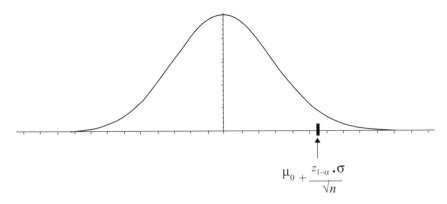

$$\mu_0 + \frac{z_{1-\alpha} \cdot \sigma}{\sqrt{n}}$$

Figure 8.3.1 The critical value for a one-tailed test.

This indicates that $\dfrac{c - 7.5}{\sigma/\sqrt{n}}$ corresponds to the upper 5th percentile or 95th percentile on the standard normal distribution. Using the notation from Chapter 5, we have

$$\frac{c - 7.5}{\sigma/\sqrt{n}} = z_{1-\alpha}.$$

Since $\alpha = 0.05$, $z_{1-\alpha} = z_{0.95}$. Thus we get $\dfrac{c - 7.5}{\sigma/\sqrt{n}} = z_{0.95}$. Solving the equation for c by multiplying both sides of the equation by $\sigma/\sqrt{n}$ and adding 7.5, we obtain the critical value $c = 7.5 + z_{1-\alpha}\sigma/\sqrt{n}$.

Instead of 7.5 lbs in the statement of the hypotheses, we will use μ_0 to indicate an unspecified but known birth weight. Replacing 7.5 with μ_0, we can state the hypotheses as

$$H_0 : \mu \leq \mu_0 \quad \text{vs.} \quad H_1 : \mu > \mu_0.$$

The critical value c is then given by $c = \mu_0 + z_{1-\alpha}\sigma/\sqrt{n}$. This critical value is indicated in Figure 8.3.1 for the significance level α.

The best procedure to test the above hypotheses H_0: $\mu \leq \mu_0$ vs. H_1: $\mu > \mu_0$ is based on a sample mean $\overline{X}$. Suppose that the investigators observed the birth weight of 16 full-term babies born at a local hospital and that the mean weight was 8.2 lbs. Letting $\alpha = 0.05$, we obtain the critical value

$$c = \mu_0 + \frac{z_{1-\alpha} \cdot \sigma}{\sqrt{n}} = 7.5 + \frac{(1.645) \cdot (1.32)}{\sqrt{16}}$$

$$= 8.0429.$$

Since $\overline{X} = 8.2$ is greater than $c = 8.0429$, we reject the null hypothesis H_0 and conclude that

the average birth weight of full-term babies is statistically significantly higher than 7.5 lbs at the significance level $\alpha = 0.05$. If $\overline{X}$ had been less than $c = 8.0429$, we would have accepted H_0. The hypothesis-testing procedure we have just demonstrated can be summarized as follows:

- Hypotheses: H_0: $\mu \leq \mu_0$ vs. H_1: $\mu > \mu_0$
- Significance level: α
- Test statistic: $\overline{X}$ or $Z = \dfrac{\overline{X} - \mu_0}{\sigma/\sqrt{n}}$
- Critical value: $c = \mu_0 + z_{1-\alpha}\sigma/\sqrt{n}$
- Reject H_0 if $\overline{X} > \mu_0 + \dfrac{z_{1-\alpha} \cdot \sigma}{\sqrt{n}}$, or accept H_0 if $\overline{X} \leq \mu_0 + \dfrac{z_{1-\alpha} \cdot \sigma}{\sqrt{n}}$.

The acceptance and rejection regions for testing the birth weight hypotheses are shown in Figure 8.3.2.

The rejection region defined by $\overline{X} > \mu_0 + z_{1-\alpha}\sigma/\sqrt{n}$ can be rewritten by subtracting μ_0 from both sides of the inequality sign and dividing both sides by $\dfrac{\sigma}{\sqrt{n}}$,

$$\frac{\overline{X} - \mu_0}{\sigma/\sqrt{n}} > z_{1-\alpha}.$$

Therefore, we can express the test criteria in terms of the standardized values, $Z = \dfrac{\overline{X} - \mu_0}{\sigma/\sqrt{n}}$. Given the hypotheses H_0: $\mu \leq \mu_0$ vs. H_1: $\mu > \mu_0$, we reject H_0 if $Z = \dfrac{\overline{X} - \mu_0}{\sigma/\sqrt{n}} > z_{1-\alpha}$, or accept H_0 if

$$Z = \frac{\overline{X} - \mu_0}{\sigma/\sqrt{n}} \leq z_{1-\alpha}.$$

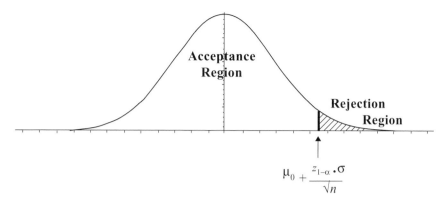

Figure 8.3.2 Acceptance and rejection regions for $H_0: \mu \le \mu_0$ vs. $H_1: \mu > \mu_0$.

Assuming $\alpha = 0.05$, the null hypothesis H_0 is rejected if $Z = \dfrac{\overline{X} - \mu_0}{\sigma/\sqrt{n}} > 1.645$, or accepted if $Z = \dfrac{\overline{X} - \mu_0}{\sigma/\sqrt{n}} \le 1.645$. Under the null hypothesis H_0, the test statistic $Z = \dfrac{\overline{X} - \mu_0}{\sigma/\sqrt{n}}$ has the standard normal distribution $N(0, 1)$. This type of hypothesis test, based on the test statistic Z, is referred to as the **one-sample Z test**. Suppose in the statement of the above hypotheses that we have discussed, the inequalities were reversed, that is, $H_0: \mu \ge \mu_0$ vs. $H_1: \mu < \mu_0$. The critical value will be on the left-hand side of the mean and is given by $c = \mu_0 + \dfrac{z_\alpha \cdot \sigma}{\sqrt{n}}$. For the significance level $\alpha = 0.05$, $z_\alpha = z_{0.05} = -1.645$, SD $\sigma = 1.32$ and $n = 16$,

$$c = 7.5 + \frac{(-1.645)(1.32)}{\sqrt{16}} = 6.9572$$

Thus, the null hypothesis is rejected if $\overline{X} < 6.9572$, or accepted if $\overline{X} > 6.9572$. Similarly, we may express the test criteria as follows: Given the hypotheses

$$H_0: \mu \ge \mu_0 \text{ vs. } H_1: \mu < \mu_0,$$
$$\text{reject } H_0 \text{ if } \overline{X} < \mu_0 + z_\alpha \cdot \sigma/\sqrt{n},$$
$$\text{or accept } H_0 \text{ if } \overline{X} \ge \mu_0 + z_\alpha \cdot \sigma/\sqrt{n}.$$

Equivalently, reject H_0 if $Z = \dfrac{\overline{X} - \mu_0}{\sigma/\sqrt{n}} < z_\alpha$, or accept H_0 if $Z = \dfrac{\overline{X} - \mu_0}{\sigma/\sqrt{n}} \ge z_\alpha$.

The rejection and acceptance regions of the test are shown in Figure 8.3.3.

Example 8.3.1. For many years, conscious sedation has been a popular pharmacological approach in the management of young uncooperative children who need invasive dental and medical procedures. The waiting time Y after drug admin-

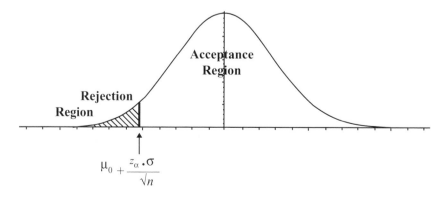

Figure 8.3.3 Acceptance and rejection regions for $H_0: \mu \ge \mu_0$ vs. $H_1: \mu < \mu_0$.

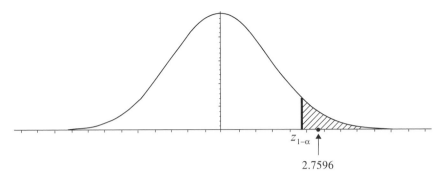

Figure 8.3.4 Rejection and acceptance regions for the test in Example 8.3.1.

istration for sedation is believed to be normally distributed. For the children who are at least 36 months old, the average waiting time is about 55 minutes. Some pediatric clinicians claim that they have waited longer and were determined to prove it. They observed 22 sedation appointments and recorded the waiting time for each appointment. The sample mean of these 22 observations is 61 minutes. Suppose the variance of the waiting time Y is 104. State the hypotheses and perform an appropriate test at the significance level $\alpha = 0.05$.

Solution. Since the clinicians claim that the waiting time is longer than 55 min., we can state the hypotheses $H_0: \mu \leq 55$ vs. $H_1: \mu > 55$. We now calculate the test statistic with $\sigma = \sqrt{104} = 10.1980$ and $n = 22$.

$$Z = \frac{\overline{X} - \mu_0}{\sigma/\sqrt{n}} = \frac{61 - 55}{10.1980/\sqrt{22}} = 2.7596.$$

Since $z_{1-\alpha} = 1.645$ and $z = 2.7596 > z_{1-\alpha}$, we reject H_0 and conclude that the average waiting time is statistically significantly longer than 55 minutes at the significance level $\alpha = 0.05$. The rejection and acceptance regions are shown in Figure 8.3.4.

Example 8.3.2. The risk of mandibular canal penetration during endosteal implant placement is a concern for both the implant surgeon and the patient. At the time of surgery, intrusion in the mandibular canal results in an increase in hemorrhage, impairs visibility, and increases the potential of fibrous tissue formation at the contact of the implant. To protect the patients during the placement of posterior mandibular endosteal implants, the zone of safety is defined as an area within the

bone safe to place implants, without fear of impingement on the mandibular neurovascular bundle [1]. Suppose the zone of safety is a random variable X that is normally distributed with the known variance $\sigma^2 = 3.49$. It is generally known that the average zone of safety for the implant patient is 9.64 mm². Dr. Laurent suspects from her clinical experience that patients in their 60s, 70s, or older have the zone of safety substantially smaller than 9.64 mm². To confirm her suspicion, she has measured the zone for 8 patients in their 60s, and 10 patients in their 70s based on their panoramic radiographs. The sample mean of the 18 observations was $\overline{X} = 8.48$ mm². (a) State the appropriate hypotheses; and (b) test her suspicion at the significance level $\alpha = 0.05$.

Solution. (i) Let μ denote the average zone of safety for the older patients. The hypotheses can be stated $H_0: \mu \geq 9.64$ vs. $H_1: \mu < 9.64$.
(ii) We compute the test statistics by substituting $\sigma = 1.87$ and $n = 18$

$$Z = \frac{\overline{X} - \mu_0}{\sigma/\sqrt{n}} = \frac{8.48 - 9.64}{1.87/\sqrt{18}} = -2.64.$$

Since $z_\alpha = z_{0.05} = -1.645$ and $-2.64 < z_{0.05} = -1.645$, we reject H_0 at the significance level $\alpha = 0.05$. So the average zone of safety for the older patients is statistically significantly smaller than that for the general implant patients. The rejection and acceptance regions of the test are illustrated in Figure 8.3.5.

Example 8.3.3. Imperfect spacing between the primary incisors and malalignment of the permanent incisors may suggest the need for orthodontic intervention. Without sufficient data, decisions to treat are based on individual judgment rather

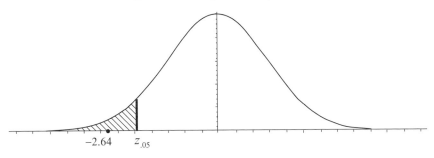

Figure 8.3.5 Rejection and acceptance regions for the test in Example 8.3.2.

than clinical evidence. A study was undertaken to determine whether slipped contact arrangement (distal-lingual surface of mandibular permanent lateral incisors overlapping the facial surface of the primary canines at the end of incisor transition) should be considered when children undergo early orthodontic treatment for teeth crowding [2]. Suppose 37 children presenting with slipped contact arrangement were studied. The space deficiency, denoted by Y, between primary canines for ideally aligned permanent incisors was measured. The sample mean $\overline{Y}$ of the space deficiency is 3.24 mm, with $\sigma = 1.82$ mm. Is the sample mean of 3.24 mm statistically significantly wider than the "standard" value of 3.00 mm? Test the hypotheses at the significance level $\alpha = 0.05$.

Solution. The hypotheses we wish to test can be stated as H_0: $\mu \leq 3.0$ vs. H_1: $\mu > 3.0$. We note that the distribution of the space deficiency Y is not known. But, since the sample size $n = 37$ is large enough, the central limit theorem (see Section 6.22) can be applied. The standard error is obtained by $\alpha/\sqrt{n} = 1.82/\sqrt{37} = 0.299\,2$. Thus, the test statistic

$$Z = \frac{\overline{Y} - \mu_0}{\sigma/\sqrt{n}} \overset{\circ}{\sim} N(0, 1) \text{ by the central limit theorem}$$

$$= \frac{3.24 - 3.0}{1.82/\sqrt{37}} = 0.8021 < z_{1-\alpha} = 1.645.$$

The calculated z value is in the acceptance region. Therefore, we accept the null hypothesis. No statistically significant difference from the "standard" value has been detected at $\alpha = 0.05$.

In the above examples, we have specified the significance level $\alpha = 0.05$ because this value is commonly used in most areas of scientific investigations. Readers should keep in mind that

hypothesis tests can be performed at different significance levels, for instance $\alpha = 0.10$, 0.05, 0.01, as pointed out in the previous section. The choice of the α level depends on the seriousness of the consequence of the type I error. The more serious the consequence, the smaller the α level should be. You may have encountered many research reports containing a **p value** (a **probability value**). We will state the definition of a p value, and will discuss that a significance test can be performed by obtaining the p value for the test.

Definition 8.3.1. The **p value** of a test is the probability that the test statistic assumes a value as extreme as, or more extreme than, that observed, given that the null hypothesis is true.

Recall our discussions on the conditional probability in Chapter 4. We see that the p value is really the conditional probability of observing "extreme" data, given the null hypothesis: $P(D \mid H_0)$. This conditional probability $P(D \mid H_0)$ is different from the conditional probability $P(H_0 \mid D)$, as we learned in Chapter 4. A small value of $P(D \mid H_0)$ does not imply a small value of $P(H_0 \mid D)$. The p values can be obtained by using a statistical software package or the probability tables provided in the Appendix. It is customary for scientific articles to report the test statistic that was employed, the value of the test statistic, and the p value. Suppose an article in the *Journal of American Dental Association* reports a p value of 0.0212 for a statistical hypothesis test based on the test statistic $Z = \dfrac{\overline{X} - \mu_0}{\sigma/\sqrt{n}} = 2.03$. Then the probability of observing $Z = \dfrac{\overline{X} - \mu_0}{\sigma/\sqrt{n}}$ greater than or equal to 2.03 is 0.0212 if the null hypothesis were true. Intuitively, if the p value were very small, then the

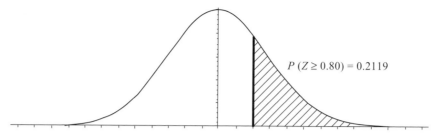

Figure 8.3.6 The p value $P(Z \geq 0.80)$.

chances that the null hypothesis is true might be small. This will lead us to reject the null hypothesis at the significance level $\alpha = 0.05$, but not at $\alpha = 0.01$. We will show how to find a p value for the Z test.

Example 8.3.4. The observed value of the test statistic in Example 8.3.3 is $z = 0.8021$, which is not included in Table D in the Appendix, since the standard normal probability table is limited. We will have to round it off to the nearest hundredth so that we have $z = 0.80$. By the definition, the p value is the probability that the test statistic Z is greater than this observed value 0.80 ("more extreme than that observed" means greater than 0.80), that is,

$$p = P(0.80 \leq Z) = 1 - 0.7881 = 0.2119.$$

Since the p value of the Z test is 0.2119, which is much larger than the significance level $\alpha = 0.05$, we accept the null hypothesis. The p value is shown in Figure 8.3.6.

Example 8.3.5. Periodontists have claimed that the average pocket depth of smokers is 7.5 mm, which is much deeper than that for non-smokers. Based on his own experiences with periodontal patients he has treated, Dr. Pang is suspicious of this claim. In fact, he hypothesized that the pocket depth of smokers is deeper than that for non-smokers but less than 7.5 mm. The sample mean of his 14 patients who are smokers is 6.25 mm. Let's assume that the distribution of the pocket depth for smokers is normal, with the known standard deviation of 2.15 mm. State the hypotheses and perform the test using the p value.

Solution. The hypotheses that Dr. Pang needs to test can be stated as: $H_0: \mu = 7.5$ vs. $H_1: \mu < 7.5$. The standard error is obtained by $\dfrac{\sigma}{\sqrt{n}} = \dfrac{2.15}{\sqrt{14}} =$

0.5746. Thus, the test statistic is

$$Z = \frac{\overline{X} - \mu_0}{\sigma / \sqrt{n}} = \frac{6.25 - 7.5}{0.5746} = -2.175.$$

The p value is the probability of observing the values less than $z = -2.175$, because those values to the left of -2.175 are more extreme than the z value that was obtained. We can express

$$p = P(Z \leq -2.175) = P(2.175 \leq Z),$$

by symmetry

$$= 1 - P(Z \leq 2.175) = 0.0148.$$

Since the p value 0.0148 is smaller than $\alpha = 0.05$, we reject H_0 at the significance level $\alpha = 0.05$ and conclude that the average pocket depth of smokers is significantly shallower than the 7.5 mm previously claimed by the periodontists. The p value of the test is shown in Figure 8.3.7.

We have performed statistical testing hypotheses using the p value. As we saw in the examples discussed, the importance of the p value is that it tells us exactly how significant the test results are on the basis of the observed data. Students and researchers in biomedical and health sciences frequently ask how small the p value has to be for the results to be considered statistically significant. Here are some crude guidelines many investigators use.

- If $p \geq 0.05$, then the results are not statistically significant.
- If $0.01 \leq p < 0.05$, then the results are significant.
- If $0.001 \leq p < 0.01$, then the results are highly significant.
- If $p < 0.001$, then the results are very highly significant.

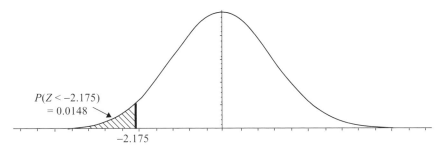

Figure 8.3.7 The p value $P(Z \leq -2.175)$.

Remember that the p value represents the probability, that is, the chance that the investigators mistakenly find the results significant due to an error. In a jury trial, the p value represents the probability that, based on the evidence, the jury wrongly finds the defendant guilty when he is really innocent.

Keep in mind that, depending upon particular situations, these guidelines may not be entirely adequate. A pharmaceutical company that is about to introduce a new drug may not consider the results statistically significant unless the p value is less than 0.01. In the first three examples, we took the critical value approach to establish whether or not the results from the hypothesis tests are statistically significant. In the last two examples, the p value approach was taken. We can take either one of the two approaches, though the p value approach is more precise because it yields an exact value, and it is more popular among the practitioners.

8.4 TWO-TAILED Z TEST OF THE MEAN OF A NORMAL DISTRIBUTION WHEN σ^2 IS KNOWN

In Section 8.3, the alternative hypothesis was stated in a specific direction ($H_1 : \mu > 3.0$ or H_1: $\mu < 7.5$) relative to the null hypothesis, assuming that we have prior knowledge regarding the direction. However, in many situations this knowledge may not be available. If the null hypothesis is false, we would have no idea if the alternative mean is smaller or larger than the null mean.

To explain a two-tailed test, let's consider complete denture prosthodontics. Although the prevalence rate of edentulous conditions has been decreasing, the great number of edentulous patients warrants the continuing efforts of basic and clinical research on removable partial dentures. Residual ridge resorption is an inevitable consequence of tooth loss and denture wearing. Suppose the amount of residual ridge resorption in women in their 60s and 70s who wear dentures is approximately normally distributed with mean 2.0 mm and SD 0.36 mm. It is not known whether residual ridge resorption in men in the same age range who wear dentures is more or less than that in women. We assume that the amount of residual ridge resorption in men is also approximately normally distributed with unknown mean and SD 0.36 mm. We wish to test the hypotheses H_0: $\mu = 2.0$ vs. H_1: $\mu \neq 2.0$. Suppose 12 male patients in their 60s and 70s who wear dentures were examined and the mean residual ridge resorption was found to be 1.8 mm. What can we conclude from the test? This is an example of a two-tailed test, since the alternative mean can be either less or more than the null mean of 2.0 mm. A reasonable decision rule for the two-tailed test is to reject H_0 if the test statistic is either too small or too large. That is, $Z \leq c_1$ or $Z \geq c_2$. As in the one-tailed test, these values will be determined by a type I error. Since

$$\begin{aligned} \alpha &= P(\text{type I error}) \\ &= P(\text{reject } H_0 \text{ when } H_0 \text{ is true}) \\ &= P(\text{reject } H_0 | H_0 \text{ is true}). \end{aligned}$$

We can see that c_1 and c_2 should be determined such that the following relationship is satisfied.

$$\begin{aligned} P(\text{reject } H_0 | H_0 \text{ is true}) \\ &= P(Z \leq c_1 \text{ or } Z \geq c_2 | H_0 \text{ is true}) \\ &= P(Z \leq c_1 | H_0 \text{ is true}) + P(Z \geq c_2 | H_0 \text{ is true}) \\ &= \alpha. \end{aligned}$$

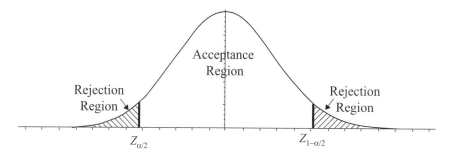

Figure 8.4.1   Rejection regions of a two-tailed test.

Assigning the type I error evenly to $P(Z \leq c_1 | H_0$ is true) and $P(Z \geq c_2 | H_0$ is true), we have

$$P(Z \leq c_1 | H_0 \text{ is true}) = P(Z \geq c_2 | H_0 \text{ is true})$$
$$= \alpha/2.$$

Since $Z \sim N(0, 1)$, it follows that $c_1 = z_{\alpha/2}$ and $c_2 = z_{1-\alpha/2}$. For $\alpha = 0.05$, we obtain $c_1 = z_{\alpha/2} = z_{0.025} = -1.96$ and $c_2 = z_{1-\alpha/2} = z_{0.975} = 1.96$. This indicates the rejection regions are to the left of $c_1 = z_{\alpha/2}$ and to the right of $c_2 = z_{1-\alpha/2}$, which are left and right tails of the standard normal distribution shown in Figure 8.4.1.

We summarize the two-tailed test for the mean of a normal distribution with known variance where the best test is based on

$$Z = \frac{\overline{X} - \mu_0}{\sigma/\sqrt{n}}.$$

Given the hypotheses $H_0: \mu = \mu_0$ vs. $H_1: \mu \neq \mu_0$ at the significance level α,

we reject H_0 if $\overline{X} < \mu_0 + z_{\alpha/2} \cdot \dfrac{\sigma}{\sqrt{n}}$,   or

$$\overline{X} > \mu_0 + z_{1-\alpha/2} \cdot \frac{\sigma}{\sqrt{n}}, \quad \text{and}$$

we accept H_0 if $\mu_0 + z_{\alpha/2} \cdot \dfrac{\sigma}{\sqrt{n}} \leq \overline{X}$

$$\leq \mu_0 + z_{1-\alpha/2} \cdot \frac{\sigma}{\sqrt{n}}$$

Equivalently, we reject H_0 if $Z = \dfrac{\overline{X} - \mu_0}{\sigma/\sqrt{n}} < z_{\alpha/2}$,

or $Z = \dfrac{\overline{X} - \mu_0}{\sigma/\sqrt{n}} > z_{1-\alpha/2}$,   and

we accept H_0 if $z_{\alpha/2} \leq \dfrac{\overline{X} - \mu_0}{\sigma/\sqrt{n}} \leq z_{1-\alpha/2}$.

Example 8.4.1. Dental injury is a traumatic event related to many factors, including dentofacial morphology. Dr. Bailey examined pretreatment lateral cephalograms from his patient files and learned that external gap (distance between labrale superior and labrale inferior) is approximately normally distributed with mean 19.0 mm and SD 5.1 mm [3]. She wishes to determine whether or not the patients who had injured their maxillary incisors before orthodontic treatment would have a shorter or longer external gap. She has collected lateral cephalograms of 64 patients who had experienced the trauma and calculated the mean external gap of 20.7 mm. Suppose the distribution of the external gap is normal with SD $\sigma = 5.1$ mm. State the hypothesis and perform a statistical test at the significance level $\alpha = 0.05$.

Solution. Dr. Bailey is not certain whether the average external gap μ of injured patients is shorter or longer than that of uninjured patients. Thus, we can state a two-tailed test hypothesis, $H_0: \mu = 19.0$ vs. $H_1: \mu \neq 19.0$. We now compute the test value

$$Z = \frac{\overline{X} - \mu_0}{\sigma/\sqrt{n}} = \frac{20.7 - 19.0}{5.1/\sqrt{64}} = 2.67.$$

The observed test statistic $z = 2.67 > z_{0.975} = 1.96$. Hence, we reject the null hypothesis at the significance level $\alpha = 0.05$ and conclude that the mean external gap of trauma patients is statistically significantly longer than the mean of uninjured patients.

As noted in the previous section, we can also use the p value method to perform the test. If the observed test statistic $z \leq 0$, the p value is twice the area under the standard normal curve to the left of z, the left tail area. If the observed test statistic $z > 0$, the p value is twice the area under the standard normal curve to the right of z, the right tail area. The area under the standard normal curve

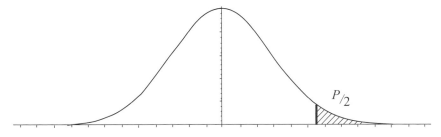

Figure 8.4.2 The *p* value for a two-tailed test.

should be multiplied by 2, because in a two-tailed test, extreme values are measured by the absolute value of the test statistic. These areas are illustrated in Figure 8.4.2 and Figure 8.4.3.

The *p* value for a two-tailed test is given by

$$
p = \begin{cases} 2 \cdot P\left(\dfrac{\overline{X} - \mu_0}{\sigma/\sqrt{n}} < z \right) \\[2mm] \qquad = 2 \cdot P(Z < z) \text{ if } z \le 0 \\[3mm] 2 \cdot \left[1 - P\left(\dfrac{\overline{X} - \mu_0}{\sigma/\sqrt{n}} < z \right) \right] \\[2mm] \qquad = 2 \cdot [1 - P(Z < z)] \text{ if } z > 0. \end{cases}
$$

Example 8.4.2. Compute the *p* value of the test in Example 8.4.1.

Solution. Since $Z = 2.67$, the *p* value is twice the area under the standard normal curve to the right of $z = 2.67$. That is, $p = 2 \cdot P(Z > 2.67) = 2 \cdot [1 - P(Z \le 2.67)] = 2(0.0038) = 0.0076$. Hence, the result is highly significant with the *p* value of 0.0076. This *p* value is illustrated in Figure 8.4.4.

Example 8.4.3. Homocysteine is a by-product of protein processing. It is as much an artery-clogging villain as cholesterol is in contributing to heart attacks and strokes. A study was conducted to investigate if there exists any difference in homocysteine levels between adult males living in the Southwest and those in the Midwest. Suppose past medical data indicated that the level of homocysteine of those living in the Southwest is normally distributed with mean 14 mg/dL and SD 3.26 mg/dL. Assume that the distribution of the homocysteine levels of midwestern counterparts is also normal, with the same known standard deviation, $\sigma = 2.26$ mg/dL. Investigators randomly selected 15 individuals from the Midwest, and their homocysteine levels were measured. If the sample mean of the 15 observations was $\overline{X} = 13$ mg/dL, what conclusions can be drawn from this evidence?

Solution. It is clear that the we need to have a two-tailed alternative hypothesis;

$$H_0 : \mu = 14.0 \quad \text{vs.} \quad H_1 : \mu \ne 14.0.$$

From the given information we compute the test value

$$Z = \frac{\overline{X} - \mu_0}{\sigma/\sqrt{n}} = \frac{13.0 - 14.0}{3.26/\sqrt{15}} = -1.19.$$

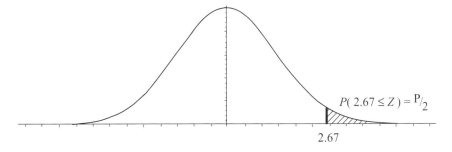

2.67

Figure 8.4.3 The *p* value for a two-tailed test.

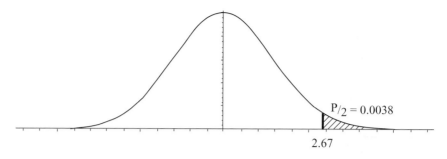

Figure 8.4.4   The *p* value for a two-tailed test in Example 8.4.2.

Since $z = -1.19 < 0$, the *p* value is obtained by

$$p = 2 \cdot P(Z < -1.19)$$
$$= 2 \cdot [1 - P(Z \geq 1.19)]$$
$$= 0.2340 > \alpha = 0.05.$$

The test result is not significant, and therefore we accept the null hypothesis. There is no significant difference in mean homocysteine level between those living in the Southwest and those in the Midwest with the *p* value of 0.2340.

Example 8.4.4. Porcelain-fused-to-metal (PFM) crowns are produced with a variety of marginal designs to achieve the best fit and appearance. The metal butt margin and the porcelain butt margin are known to be the more popular designs. Suppose 32 subjects who required 51 PFM crowns with potential supragingival facial margins were selected from patients who were treated with the porcelain butt design at a large dental school clinic. The measurements in microns (μm) of the marginal opening were made after cementation. Suppose that the distribution of the margins of the metal butt crowns after cementation are approximately normal with mean 48 μm and SD 13.6 μm. The sample mean of the marginal opening of the 51 PFM crown porcelain butt design measured with an SEM (scanning electron microscope) on replicas derived from elastomeric impressions is 44 μm. Assume that these marginal openings are normally distributed with the same known SD $\sigma = 13.6$ μm. Is the mean marginal opening for the porcelain butt margin significantly different from that of the metal butt margin?

Solution. We have a two-tailed alternative hypothesis; H_0: $\mu = 48$ vs. H_1: $\mu \neq 48$. From the given

information we compute the test value with $n = 51$, $\overline{X} = 44$, $\mu_0 = 48$, and $\sigma = 13.6$.

$$Z = \frac{\overline{X} - \mu_0}{\sigma/\sqrt{n}} = \frac{44 - 48}{13.6/\sqrt{51}} = -2.10.$$

Since $z = -2.10 < 0$, the *p* value is obtained by $p = 2 \cdot P(Z < -2.10) = 0.0358 < \alpha = 0.05$. The result is significant, and thus we reject the null hypothesis H_0. The porcelain butt margin has a statistically significantly lower average marginal opening with the *p* value 0.0358.

Would the conclusions be different if we had a one-tailed alternative hypothesis? Let's state a one-tailed alternative hypothesis as H_0: $\mu = 48$ vs. H_1: $\mu < 48$. From the previous discussions we know that the rejection region is in the left-hand tail of the standard normal distribution. In fact, the *p* value is given by $p = P(Z < -2.10) = 0.0179$. We would, of course, reject the null hypothesis. Suppose the investigators stated a one-tailed alternative hypothesis as H_0: $\mu = 48$ vs. H_1: $\mu > 48$. The *p* value is obtained by $p = 1 - P(Z < -2.10) = 0.9821$. Thus we accept the null hypothesis if we use a one-tailed test and the sample mean is on the opposite side of the null mean from the alternative hypothesis. In the above example, the sample mean $\overline{X} = 44$ is less than the null mean $\mu = 48$, which is on the opposite side from H_1. In general, a two-tailed test has an advantage because we do not need prior knowledge as to which side of the null hypothesis is the alternative hypothesis. Because the two-tailed tests are more widely used in biomedical and health sciences literature, we will focus more on the two-tailed cases in our future discussions.

8.5 *t* TEST OF THE MEAN OF A NORMAL DISTRIBUTION

In all of our discussions in the previous two sections, we assumed knowledge of the variance of the underlying distribution. However, in most cases the information on the variance is not available. Therefore, it is more realistic to assume that the variance of the underlying distribution is not known. How can we then conduct the hypothesis testing? We learned in Section 6.3 that if X_1, $X_2, \cdots, X_n$ are a random sample from a normal distribution $N(\mu, \sigma^2)$ and the variance σ^2 is estimated by the sample variance S^2, then the random variable

$$t = \frac{\overline{X} - \mu_0}{S/\sqrt{n}}$$

follows a *t* distribution with the degrees of freedom $(n - 1)$. It makes very good sense to base the significance test on a *t* statistic. The unknown population SD σ in a *Z* test statistic is replaced by the sample SD S. The critical values c_1 and c_2 are determined in the same way as the *Z* tests. That is, under the null hypothesis

$$P(t < t_{n-1,\alpha/2}) = P(t > t_{n-1,1-\alpha/2}) = \frac{\alpha}{2}.$$

Hence, $c_1 = t_{n-1,\alpha/2} = -t_{n-1,1-\alpha/2}$, by the symmetric property of a *t* distribution, and

$$c_2 = t_{n-1,1-\alpha/2}.$$

In the following we summarize a *t* test when σ^2 is not known.

Given the hypothesis H_0: $\mu = \mu_0$ vs.

$H_1 : \mu \neq \mu_0$ at the significance level α,

we reject H_0 if $\overline{X} < \mu_0 + t_{n-1,\alpha/2} \cdot \dfrac{S}{\sqrt{n}}$, or

$$\overline{X} > \mu_0 + t_{n-1,1-\alpha/2} \cdot \frac{S}{\sqrt{n}}, \text{ and}$$

we accept H_0 if $\mu_0 + t_{n-1,\alpha/2} \cdot \dfrac{S}{\sqrt{n}} \leq \overline{X}$

$$\leq \mu_0 + t_{n-1,1-\alpha/2} \cdot \frac{S}{\sqrt{n}}.$$

Equivalently, we reject H_0 if

$$t = \frac{\overline{X} - \mu_0}{S/\sqrt{n}} < t_{n-1,\alpha/2}, \text{ or}$$

$$t = \frac{\overline{X} - \mu_0}{S/\sqrt{n}} > t_{n-1,1-\alpha/2}, \text{ and}$$

we accept H_0 if

$$t_{n-1,\alpha/2} \leq \frac{\overline{X} - \mu_0}{S/\sqrt{n}} \leq t_{n-1,1-\alpha/2}.$$

The rejection and acceptance regions of a *t* test are illustrated in Figure 8.5.1.

The *p* value for a one-sample two-tailed *t* test for a mean of normal distribution can be computed as described below:

If $t = \dfrac{\overline{X} - \mu_0}{S/\sqrt{n}} < 0$, then

$p = 2 \cdot P(t_{n-1} < t) = 2 \cdot$ [area to the left of t under a *t* distribution with $df = n - 1$].

If $t = \dfrac{\overline{X} - \mu_0}{S/\sqrt{n}} \geq 0$, then

$p = 2 \cdot P(t_{n-1} \geq t) = 2 \cdot$ [area to the right of t under a *t* distribution with $df = n - 1$].

Example 8.5.1. Although obstructive sleep apnea (OSA) patients tend to be obese, a significant

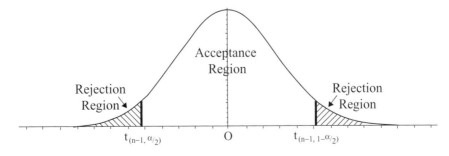

Figure 8.5.1 Rejection and acceptance regions of a two-tailed *t* test.

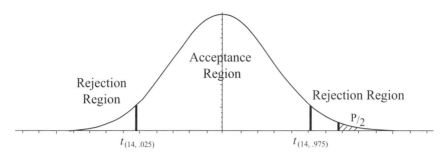

Figure 8.5.2   Rejection regions and the *p* value of a two-tailed *t* test.

number of them are not. A recent study suggested that fat deposition around the neck may be a factor associated with OSA in non-obese patients [4]. Suppose that apnea hypopnea index (AHI), an index used to quantify the degree of obstructive sleep apnea, is normally distributed and that the average AHI for non-obese patients, whose body mass index is less than 25, is 7.65. It has been Dr. Johnston's experience that AHI for obese patients (say, BMI > 35) is not much different from that of the non-obese. To validate his assertion Dr. Johnston took a sample of 15 obese patients and measured their AHI. The mean ($\overline{X}$) and variance (S^2) of his measurements are 9.77 and 11.14, respectively. State the hypotheses and perform a test at the significance level $\alpha = 0.05$.

Solution. Dr. Johnston's hypotheses can be stated as $H_0: \mu = 7.65$ vs. $H_1: \mu \neq 7.65$. Since the population variance σ^2 is not known, but the sample variance S^2 is calculated from the data, we need to perform a two-tailed *t* test with $\overline{X} = 9.77$, $S = \sqrt{11.14} = 3.3377$, and $n = 15$. The test statistic is

$$t = \frac{\overline{X} - \mu_0}{S/\sqrt{n}} = \frac{9.77 - 7.65}{3.3377/\sqrt{15}}$$
$$= 2.4600 > t_{n-1,1-\alpha/2} = t_{14,0.975} = 2.145.$$

Hence, we reject the null hypothesis and conclude that the mean AHI of the obese patients is statistically significantly higher than that of the non-obese at the significance level of $\alpha = 0.05$. The *p* value is obtained by

$$p = 2 \cdot P(t \leq t_{n-1})$$
$$= 2 \cdot P(2.460 \leq t_{(14)}) < 2 \cdot P(2.415 \leq t_{(14)})$$
$$= 2(0.015) = 0.030.$$

The *p* value is less than the specified significance level $\alpha = 0.05$. This is an example of a two-tailed

t test. The rejection regions and the *p* value are illustrated in Figure 8.5.2.

Example 8.5.2. Coronary heart disease is the leading cause of morbidity and mortality throughout the world. Emingil et al. [5] investigated the possible association between periodontal health and coronary heart disease in patients with acute myocardial infarction (AMI) and chronic coronary heart disease (CCHD). Based on the physical examination done prior to admission into a clinical trial, it was determined that the average level of triglycerides for the patients with AMI is 196.49 mg/dl. Suppose the investigators claimed that the triglyceride level for the patients with the CCHD should be lower than that for the patients in the AMI group. To confirm their claim, the investigators randomly selected 27 patients with CCHD and observed their triglyceride levels. The data yielded $\overline{X} = 155.23$ mg/dl and $S = 88.04$ mg/dl. Assume that the triglyceride levels are normally distributed. How would you state the hypotheses for the investigators, and what could you conclude?

Solution. Since the investigators claim that the triglyceride levels for the patients with CCHD should be lower than 196.49 mg/dl, we state the hypotheses as $H_0: \mu = 196.49$ vs. $H_1: \mu < 196.49$. As in Section 8.4, we need to perform a one-tailed *t* test with $\overline{X} = 155.23$, $S = 88.04$, and $n = 27$. The test statistic is

$$t = \frac{\overline{X} - \mu_0}{S/\sqrt{n}} = \frac{155.23 - 196.49}{88.04/\sqrt{27}}$$
$$= -2.4352 < t_{n-1,\alpha} = t_{26,0.05}$$
$$= -1.7056.$$

Hence, we reject the null hypothesis at the significance level $\alpha = 0.05$ and conclude that the mean

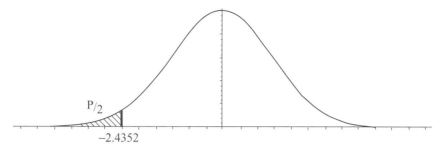

Figure 8.5.3 The *p* value of the one-tailed *t* test in Example 8.5.2.

triglyceride level for the patients with CCHD is statistically significantly lower than that for the patients with AMI. The *p* value is obtained by

$$p = P(t_{n-1} \leq t)$$
$$= P(t_{26} \leq -2.4352) < P(t_{26} \leq -2.2958)$$
$$= 0.015, \text{ from the } t \text{ table.}$$

The *p* value is less than the specified significance level $\alpha = 0.05$. The result is significant with the *p* value less than 0.015. The *p* value is illustrated in Figure 8.5.3.

When the sample size *n* is larger than 30 and the population SD σ is not known, we can use the *Z* test, because by the central limit theorem the distribution of the test statistic $\dfrac{\overline{X} - \mu_0}{S/\sqrt{n}}$ follows approximately standard normal, $N(0, 1)$. As discussed in the previous chapters, the larger the sample size *n*, the better the normal approximation is. When $n \leq 30$ and σ are not known, the *t* test must be used.

In the preceding sections, we explained the concept of the probability of obtaining an observed difference purely due to chance alone. If the probability is sufficiently small, we conclude that such difference is unlikely to have occurred by chance. We stated in Example 8.5.2 that "the mean triglycerides level for the patients with CCHD is significantly lower than that for the patients with AMI." The difference between 155.23 mg/dl and 196.49 mg/dl is **statistically significant** because the probability of the observed difference $(196.49 - 155.23 = 41.26)$ arising by chance is sufficiently small, less than 0.015. The two test statistics we have used, *Z* test and *t* test, depend on three elements:

1. The observed difference between means, $\overline{X} - \mu_0$

2. The standard deviation σ of the underlying distribution, in the case of the *Z* test, and sample standard deviation *S*, in case of the *t* test

3. The sample size, *n*.

How would the sample size affect the magnitude of the observed mean difference to achieve the *p* value < 0.05 so that the results are significant? In Example 8.4.4, the average porcelain butt margin of 44 μm was significantly lower than 48 μm with the *p* value 0.0358. The observed mean difference was $\overline{X} - \mu_0 = 4$ μm and the sample size was $n = 51$. Table 8.5.1 illustrates the relationship between the sample size and the observed mean difference necessary to achieve statistical significance.

For the sample size $n = 1,000$, the observed mean difference of 0.84 μm is statistically significant. However, from the standpoint of a clinician, the magnitude of the difference 0.84 μm in marginal opening may mean absolutely nothing. In other words, the observed mean difference of 0.84 μm may *not* be **clinically significant**. Readers should keep in mind that *what is statistically significant is not necessarily clinically significant, and vice versa*. See an excellent article by Hujoel et al. [6]. Readers should realize from Table 8.5.1 that any observed difference can eventually become statistically significant if we can

Table 8.5.1. Relationship between the sample size and mean difference.

n	$\overline{X}$ (in μm)	μ_0	$|\overline{X} - \mu_0|$	*p*
50	44.23	48	3.77	0.05
100	45.33	48	2.67	0.05
500	46.81	48	1.19	0.05
1,000	47.16	48	0.84	0.05
2,000	47.41	48	0.59	0.05
5,000	47.62	48	0.38	0.05

afford to keep increasing the sample size. This is one of the few unpleasant aspects of a testing hypothesis procedure.

8.6 THE POWER OF A TEST AND SAMPLE SIZE

We have explained the appropriate hypothesis tests based on the sample mean $\overline{X}$, assuming that the underlying distribution is normal. Of course, we could have selected a test statistic that is based on the sample median, instead of the sample mean. However, the best test is the one that is built on the sample mean; the best in the sense of the power of a test. The **power** of a hypothesis test, denoted by $1 - \beta$, was defined earlier in this chapter as

$$1 - \beta = 1 - P(\text{a type II error})$$
$$= P(\text{Reject the null hypothesis} \\ \text{when it is false})$$
$$= P(\text{Reject } H_0 | H_0 \text{ is false}).$$

The power of a test is the conditional probability of rejecting H_0, given that H_0 is false. For the hypotheses $H_0: \mu = \mu_0$ vs. $H_1: \mu < \mu_0$, we reject H_0 if $\overline{X} < \mu_0 + z_\alpha \dfrac{\sigma}{\sqrt{n}}$ and accept H_0 if $\overline{X} \geq \mu_0 + z_\alpha \dfrac{\sigma}{\sqrt{n}}$. Thus, the power of the test is given by

$$1 - \beta = P(\text{Reject } H_0 | H_0 \text{ is false})$$
$$= P\left(\overline{X} < \mu_0 + z_\alpha \frac{\sigma}{\sqrt{n}} | \mu < \mu_0 \right).$$

The above power $1 - \beta$ assumes different values at different values of μ under H_1. Specifically, at $\mu = \mu_1 < \mu_0$, the sample mean $\overline{X}$ has a normal distribution $N\left(\mu_1, \dfrac{\sigma^2}{n} \right)$. For example, at $\mu = \mu_1 < \mu_0$, the power of the test is

$$P\left(\frac{\overline{X} - \mu_1}{\sigma/\sqrt{n}} < \frac{(\mu_0 + z_\alpha \cdot \sigma/\sqrt{n}) - \mu_1}{\sigma/\sqrt{n}} \right)$$
$$= P\left(Z < \frac{(\mu_0 + z_\alpha \cdot \sigma/\sqrt{n}) - \mu_1}{\sigma/\sqrt{n}} \right)$$
$$= P\left(Z < z_\alpha + \frac{\mu_0 - \mu_1}{\sigma/\sqrt{n}} \right).$$

The rejection region and the power of test are shown in Figure 8.6.1.

The area to the left of the point $\mu_0 + Z_\alpha \cdot \sigma/\sqrt{n}$ under H_1 under the normal curve corresponds to the power, and the area to the left of the same point $\mu_0 + Z_\alpha \cdot \sigma/\sqrt{n}$ under H_0 under the normal curve corresponds to the type I error α (the significance level). The power is an important property of a test that tells us how likely it is the test can detect a significant difference, given that the alternative hypothesis is true. When the power is low, the chances are small that the test will detect a significant difference even if there exists a real difference. Often a small sample size results in a low power to detect a statistically as well as a clinically significant difference. After presenting examples to show how to calculate the power of a test, we shall discuss the relationship between the power of a test and the sample size.

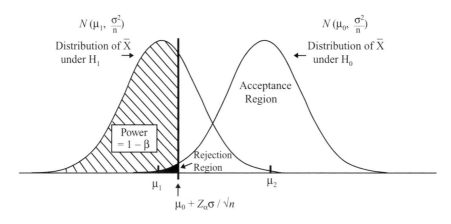

Figure 8.6.1 Rejection region and power of the one-sample test.

Example 8.6.1. Calculate the power of the test used for testing the hypothesis in Example 8.3.5 at the alternative mean $\mu_1 = 4.0, 4.5, 5.0, 5.5, 6.0, 6.5$, and 7.0 mm when $\alpha = 0.05$.

Solution. Substituting $n = 14$, $\sigma = 2.15$, $z_\alpha = -1.645$, and $\mu_0 = 7.5$ in the formula, we get at $\mu_1 = 4.0$,

$$P\left(Z < z_\alpha + \frac{\mu_0 - \mu_1}{\sigma/\sqrt{n}}\right)$$

$$= P\left(Z < -1.645 + \frac{7.5 - 4.0}{2.15/\sqrt{14}}\right)$$

$$= P(Z < 4.45) = 1.0;$$

at $\mu_1 = 4.5$, $P\left(Z < z_\alpha + \frac{\mu_0 - \mu_1}{\sigma/\sqrt{n}}\right)$

$$= P\left(Z < -1.645 + \frac{7.5 - 4.5}{2.15/\sqrt{14}}\right)$$

$$= P(Z < 3.58) = 1.0;$$

at $\mu_1 = 5.0$, $P\left(Z < z_\alpha + \frac{\mu_0 - \mu_1}{\sigma/\sqrt{n}}\right)$

$$= P\left(Z < -1.645 + \frac{7.5 - 5.0}{2.15/\sqrt{14}}\right)$$

$$= P(Z < 2.71) = 0.9966;$$

Continuing the calculations using the standard normal probability table at the other alternative mean μ_1, we obtain the power of the test presented in Table 8.6.1.

We note that as the alternative mean increases, that is, as μ_1 gets closer to μ_0, the power of the test decreases. This is to be expected since the closer μ_1 and μ_0 are, the smaller the observed mean difference. Therefore, it would be more "difficult" for the test to detect a significant difference. For the power of a test for H_0: $\mu = \mu_0$ vs. H_1: $\mu > \mu_0$ the

null hypothesis is rejected if

$$\frac{\overline{X} - \mu_0}{\sigma/\sqrt{n}} > z_{1-\alpha}.$$

By multiplying both sides by $\sigma/\sqrt{n}$ and adding μ_0 to both sides, we get $\overline{X} > \mu_0 + z_{1-\alpha}\sigma/\sqrt{n}$. So the power of the test for H_0: $\mu = \mu_0$ vs. H_1: $\mu > \mu_0$ is given by

$$\text{power} = 1 - \beta$$
$$= P(\overline{X} > \mu_0 + z_{1-\alpha} \cdot \sigma/\sqrt{n} \mid H_0 \text{ is false}).$$

At a specific value of the alternative mean $\mu = \mu_1$, power

$$= P(\overline{X} > \mu_0 + z_{1-\alpha} \cdot \sigma/\sqrt{n} | \mu = \mu_1)$$

$$= P\left(\frac{\overline{X} - \mu_1}{\sigma/\sqrt{n}} > \frac{(\mu_0 + z_{1-\alpha} \cdot \sigma/\sqrt{n}) - \mu_1}{\sigma/\sqrt{n}}\right)$$

$$= P\left(Z > z_{1-\alpha} + \frac{\mu_0 - \mu_1}{\sigma/\sqrt{n}}\right), \text{ where } \mu_1 > \mu_0.$$

For a one-tailed Z test for H_0: $\mu = \mu_0$ vs. H_1: $\mu < \mu_0$, the power of the test is

$$1 - \beta = P\left(Z < z_\alpha + \frac{\mu_0 - \mu_1}{\sigma/\sqrt{n}}\right), \quad \mu_1 < \mu_0.$$

For a one-tailed Z test for H_0: $\mu = \mu_0$ vs. H_1: $\mu > \mu_0$, the power of the test is

$$1 - \beta = P\left(Z > z_{1-\alpha} + \frac{\mu_0 - \mu_1}{\sigma/\sqrt{n}}\right), \quad \mu_1 > \mu_0.$$

It is clear from the above formulas that the power of a test depends on the following factors: α, σ, n, and $|\mu_0 - \mu_1|$, that is, the magnitude of the difference between μ_0 and μ_1.

1. If the significance level α is small, then z_α is small. Hence, the power decreases.
2. If the alternative mean, which is moving away from the null mean, that is, $|\mu_0 - \mu_1|$ is larger, then the power increases.
3. If the SD σ of individual measurements increases, then the power decreases.
4. If the sample size increases, then the power increases.

The power of a two-tailed test is obtained in a similar way to a one-tailed test. For example, consider hypotheses H_0: $\mu = \mu_0$ vs. H_1: $\mu \neq \mu_0$. The null hypothesis is rejected if

$$\overline{X} < \mu_0 + z_{\alpha/2} \cdot \frac{\sigma}{\sqrt{n}}, \text{ or } \overline{X} > \mu_0 + z_{1-\alpha/2} \cdot \frac{\sigma}{\sqrt{n}}.$$

Table 8.6.1. Power of the test in Example 8.3.5.

μ_1 (alternative mean)	$1 - \beta$ (power of the test)
4.0	1.0
4.5	1.0
5.0	0.9966
5.5	0.9671
6.0	0.8352
6.5	0.5359
7.0	0.2206

The power of the test at a specific alternative mean $\mu = \mu_1$ is given by

$$1 - \beta = P(\overline{X} < \mu_0 + z_{\alpha/2} \cdot \sigma/\sqrt{n} \mid \mu = \mu_1)$$
$$+ P(\overline{X} > \mu_0 + z_{1-\alpha} \cdot \sigma/\sqrt{n} \mid \mu = \mu_1)$$
$$= P\left(Z < z_{\alpha/2} + \frac{\mu_0 - \mu_1}{\sigma/\sqrt{n}} \right)$$
$$+ P\left(Z > z_{1-\alpha/2} + \frac{\mu_0 - \mu_1}{\sigma/\sqrt{n}} \right).$$

The power of a two-tailed test for H_0: $\mu = \mu_0$ vs. H_1: $\mu \neq \mu_0$ is given by

$$1 - \beta = P\left(Z < z_{\alpha/2} + \frac{\mu_0 - \mu_1}{\sigma/\sqrt{n}} \right)$$
$$+ P\left(Z > z_{1-\alpha/2} + \frac{\mu_0 - \mu_1}{\sigma/\sqrt{n}} \right).$$

Example 8.6.2. Calculate the power of the test used for testing the hypothesis in Example 8.4.4 at the alternative mean $\mu_1 = 40, 42, 43, 44, 45, 46, 47, 48, 49, 50, 51, 52, 53, 54,$ and 55 μm when $\alpha = 0.05$.

Solution. Substituting $n = 51$, $\sigma = 13.6$, $z_{\alpha/2} = -1.96$, $z_{1-\alpha/2} = 1.96$, and $\mu_0 = 48$ in the above formula, we obtain the following.

At $\mu_1 = 40$,

$$P\left(Z < z_{\alpha/2} + \frac{\mu_0 - \mu_1}{\sigma/\sqrt{n}} \right)$$
$$+ P\left(Z > z_{1-\alpha/2} + \frac{\mu_0 - \mu_1}{\sigma/\sqrt{n}} \right)$$
$$= P\left(Z < -1.96 + \frac{48 - 40}{13.6/\sqrt{51}} \right)$$
$$+ P\left(Z > 1.96 + \frac{48 - 40}{13.6/\sqrt{51}} \right)$$
$$= P(Z < 2.24) + P(Z > 6.16)$$
$$= 0.9875 + 0 = 0.9875.$$

At $\mu_1 = 42$,

$$P\left(Z < z_{\alpha/2} + \frac{\mu_0 - \mu_1}{\sigma/\sqrt{n}} \right)$$
$$+ P\left(Z > z_{1-\alpha/2} + \frac{\mu_0 - \mu_1}{\sigma/\sqrt{n}} \right)$$

Table 8.6.2. Power of the test in Example 8.6.2.

μ_1	$1 - \beta$	μ_1	$1 - \beta$
40	0.9875	49	0.0757
41	0.9573	50	0.1814
42	0.8830	51	0.3520
43	0.7471	52	0.5557
44	0.5557	53	0.7471
45	0.3520	54	0.8830
46	0.1814	55	0.9573
47	0.0757	56	0.9875
48	0.05		

$$= P\left(Z < -1.96 + \frac{48 - 42}{13.6/\sqrt{51}} \right)$$
$$+ P\left(Z > 1.96 + \frac{48 - 42}{13.6/\sqrt{51}} \right)$$
$$= P(Z < 1.19) + P(Z > 5.11)$$
$$= 0.8830 + 0 = 0.8830.$$

Continuing the similar calculations at another alternative mean μ_1, we obtain the power of the test presented in Table 8.6.2.

The power of the test increases as the alternative mean μ_1 moves away from the null mean μ_0 in either direction. In other words, as the observed mean difference increases, so does the power of the test. We have described the power in terms of the Z test, but the power of the t test is precisely the same except we replace z_α (or $z_{\alpha/2}$) and $z_{1-\alpha}$ ($z_{1-\alpha/2}$) by $t_{n-1,\alpha}$ (or $t_{n-1,\alpha/2}$) and $t_{n-1,1-\alpha}$ ($t_{n-1,1-\alpha/2}$), and σ by S in the formulas presented above.

Investigators often ask statisticians "what is an appropriate sample size for my experiment?" An answer to this question depends on several factors, such as SD σ, the significance level α, the power $1 - \beta$, and the difference to be detected. In practice, typical values for the power are 80%, 85%, 90%, 95%, 97.5%, and 99%. Suppose the difference between the null mean and the alternative mean is $|\mu_0 - \mu_1|$, and SD σ is known. What sample size do we need for the test to be able to detect the specified difference with probability $1 - \beta$ when the test is conducted at the significance level α? The following formulas for the sample size can be derived from the expression for the power of the test. Suppose that the observations are normally distributed with mean μ and known variance σ^2. Let α be the significance level of the test. The sample size, required to detect a significant difference with probability $1 - \beta$, is given by the following formulas.

For a one-tailed test: $n = \dfrac{\sigma^2(z_{1-\alpha} + z_{1-\beta})^2}{(\mu_0 - \mu_1)^2}.$

For a two-tailed test: $n = \dfrac{\sigma^2(z_{1-\alpha/2} + z_{1-\beta})^2}{(\mu_0 - \mu_1)^2}.$

Example 8.6.3. A titanium implant method is being tested for previously infected bones. Suppose the effectiveness of the titanium implant is determined by the amount of bone growth 1 year after the implant is placed. The average bone growth for the patients with no history of previous infection is about 3.2 mm. Dr. Simmon believes from her clinical experience that the bone growth of the patients with a history of previous infection is slower than those with no such medical history. In order to confirm her belief, Dr. Simmon wishes to test her hypotheses at the significance level $\alpha = 0.05$. In fact, she wants to detect a significant difference of 0.9 mm with probability 0.90. Assume that the amount of bone growth is normally distributed with variance $\sigma^2 = 2.68$. How many patients with a history of previous bone infection does she need for her research?

Solution. From the description of Dr. Simmon's research project, she should have a one-tailed alternative hypothesis stated as $H_0: \mu = 3.2$ vs. $H_1: \mu < 3.2$. We are given $\sigma^2 = 2.68$, $z_{1-\alpha} = z_{0.95} = 1.645$, $z_{1-\beta} = z_{0.90} = 1.282$, and $(\mu_0 - \mu_1)^2 = (0.9)^2 = 0.81$. By substituting in the first formula, we get the required sample size

$$n = \frac{\sigma^2(z_{1-\alpha} + z_{1-\beta})^2}{(\mu_0 - \mu_1)^2}$$

$$= \frac{(2.68)(1.645 + 1.282)^2}{0.81} = 28.346.$$

To achieve the 90% power of detecting a significant difference of 0.9 mm she needs 29 patients for her study.

If we rounded off $n = 28.346$ to the nearest whole number, we would have $n = 28$. With $n = 28$ we will achieve the power slightly less than 90%. Therefore, we should always round up to the next integer and get $n = 29$. The sample size $n = 29$ will yield the power slightly higher than 90%.

Example 8.6.4. Let X be the random variable representing the mesiodistal width of a tooth taken as the distance between contact points on the proximal surfaces. Dental investigators use a Digimatic caliper to measure the width, accurate to 0.01 mm. A study suggested that X is normally distributed with mean μ and SD σ, which is known to be 0.30. The study also suggested that the mean of the mesiodistal width of left lateral incisors for the noncleft patients is approximately 6.00 mm. The investigators suspect that the width of left lateral incisors for the cleft patients ought to be different from that of the noncleft. If they wish to test at the significance level $\alpha = 0.05$ and have a 95% power of detecting a minimum difference $|\mu_0 - \mu_1| = 0.25$ mm, what would be the required sample size?

Solution. We have a two-tailed alternative hypothesis stated as $H_0: \mu = 6.00$ vs. $H_1: \mu \neq 6.00$. From the given information we know $\sigma^2 = (0.30)^2 = 0.09$, $z_{1-\alpha/2} = z_{0.975} = 1.96$, $z_{1-\beta} = z_{0.95} = 1.645$, and $(\mu_0 - \mu_1)^2 = (0.25)^2 = 0.0625$. By substituting in the second formula, we obtain the required sample size

$$n = \frac{\sigma^2(z_{1-\alpha/2} + z_{1-\beta})^2}{(\mu_0 - \mu_1)^2}$$

$$= \frac{(0.09)(1.96 + 1.645)^2}{0.0625} = 18.714.$$

To achieve the 95% power of detecting a significant difference of 0.25 mm they need 19 teeth samples for the study.

These two examples indicate that a required sample size depends on several factors:

- The sample size decreases (increases) as the difference between null mean and alternative mean, $|\mu_0 - \mu_1|$ increases (decreases).
- The sample size increases as the smaller significance level α is chosen.
- The sample size increases as the power $1 - \beta$ increases.
- The sample size increases as the variance σ^2 increases.

To see the effect of the variance, let's increase the SD in Example 8.6.4 from $\sigma = 0.30$ to $\sigma = 0.60$, leaving all other factors intact. Then the required sample size is

$$n = \frac{\sigma^2 (z_{1-\alpha/2} + z_{1-\beta})^2}{(\mu_0 - \mu_1)^2}$$

$$= \frac{(0.36)(1.96 + 1.645)^2}{0.0625} = 74.857.$$

When the SD σ is increased to 0.6, we need to increase the sample size from $n = 19$ to $n = 75$. Theoretically, a twofold increase in σ results in a fourfold increase in the required sample size. The suggested level of the power $1 - \beta$ is typically 80% or higher. In most of the scientific experiments the investigators would like to have the power around 85%–95%. The key questions we should keep in mind when we determine the sample size are: How can we estimate σ^2, and what is an appropriate value to specify μ_1? Usually, at the beginning of an experiment, values for σ^2 and μ_1 are not available. The researchers will have to decide what a scientifically and clinically reasonable difference $|\mu_0 - \mu_1|$ is. In the absence of any data, the variance σ^2 has to be estimated from previous similar studies or prior knowledge of similar experiments. A small-scale pilot study is most valuable in acquiring knowledge to estimate σ^2 and μ_1. It must be stressed that the sample size obtained using the above formulas is crude rather than precise.

8.7 ONE-SAMPLE TEST FOR A BINOMIAL PROPORTION

In this section we will describe a one-sample test for a binomial proportion. Many clinical and experimental results in biomedical and health sciences are expressed in proportions or fractions, for example, the proportion of patients with myocardial infarction who develop heart failure, the proportion of patients who become infected after an oral surgery, the proportion of patients whose implant failure occurs within 1 year, and the proportion of patients who exhibit symptoms of hypocalcemia. We will explain the significance test for such proportions based on the sample proportion $\widehat{p}$, which was defined in Section 7.4. We will assume that the conditions for the normal approximation to the binomial distribution are met. We explained in Section 7.4 that the proportion $\widehat{p}$ is

approximately normally distributed:

$$\widehat{p} \ \overset{\circ}{\sim} \ N\left(p_0, \frac{p_0 q_0}{n}\right), \quad \text{where } q_0 = 1 - p_0.$$

A transformation yields, $Z = \dfrac{\widehat{p} - p_0}{\sqrt{p_0 q_0 / n}} \overset{\circ}{\sim} N(0, 1)$.

A Medical Expenditure Panel Survey was conducted in 1996 to determine the distribution of diagnostic and preventive, surgical, and other dental visit types received by U.S. children, aged 0 to 18 years. The survey results showed that about 39.3% of children had a diagnostic or preventive visit, 4.1% had a surgical visit, and 16.2% had a visit for restorative/other services [7]. The authors report profound disparities in the level of dental services obtained by children, especially among minority and poor youth. Their findings suggest that Medicaid fails to assure comprehensive dental services for eligible children. Improvements in oral health care for minority and poor children are necessary if national health objectives for 2010 are to be met successfully [7]. Suppose we wish to find out if the proportion of the U.S. adults, aged 19 or older, who have a diagnostic or preventive visit is different from that of the youth group, 0 to 18 years of age. For this purpose we took a random sample of 70 adults and found out that 25 of them (about 35.7%) had a diagnostic or preventive visit. How does this 35.7% compare to 39.3% for the youth group? Here we have $p_0 = 0.393$ (39.3% for the youth group). Appropriate hypotheses we need to test are H_0: $p = 0.393$ vs. H_1: $p \neq 0.393$.

Since $np_0 q_0 = 70(0.393)(0.607) = 16.7 > 5.0$, the normal approximation to the binomial distribution is valid. The expected value and variance of $\widehat{p}$ under the null hypothesis H_0 are p_0 and $\dfrac{p_0 q_0}{n}$. The test statistic Z is given by $Z = \dfrac{\widehat{p} - p_0}{\sqrt{p_0 q_0 / n}} \overset{\circ}{\sim} N(0, 1)$. It is clear that a one-sample test for a binomial proportion is performed precisely the same as a one-sample Z test for the normal mean we studied in Section 8.4.

One-Sample Test for a Binomial Proportion

To test hypotheses H_0: $p = p_0$ vs. H_1: $p \neq p_0$, we use the test statistic

$$Z = \frac{\widehat{p} - p_0}{\sqrt{p_0 q_0 / n}} \ \overset{\circ}{\sim} \ N(0, 1).$$

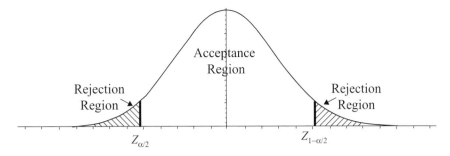

Figure 8.7.1 The rejection and acceptance regions for the binomial proportion.

We reject H_0 if $Z < z_{\alpha/2}$ or $Z > z_{1-\alpha/2}$, and accept H_0 if $z_{\alpha/2} < Z < z_{1-\alpha/2}$.

The rejection and acceptance regions are shown in Figure 8.7.1 above.

In the Medical Expenditure Panel Survey example we have $p_0 = 0.393$, $q_0 = 0.607$, $n = 70$, and $\hat{p} = 0.357$. The value of the test statistic is

$$Z = \frac{\hat{p} - p_0}{\sqrt{p_0 q_0/n}} = \frac{0.357 - 0.393}{\sqrt{(0.393)(0.607)/70}} = -0.67.$$

Since $z_{\alpha/2} = -1.96 < Z < z_{1-\alpha/2} = 1.96$, the null hypothesis is accepted at the significance level $\alpha = 0.05$. We therefore conclude that there is no statistically significant difference in the proportion of patients in those two groups who had a diagnostic or preventive visit.

The p value of the test is calculated in much the same manner as with the two-tailed tests. The calculation of the p value depends on whether the sample proportion $\hat{p} \leq p_0$ or $\hat{p} > p_0$. If $\hat{p} \leq p_0$, then the p value is 2 times the area to the left of z under the standard normal curve. If $\hat{p} > p_0$, then the p value is 2 times the area to the right of z under the standard normal curve. Another way to describe the p value is that if the z value is negative, then the p value is 2 times the area to the left of z under the standard normal curve. If the z value is positive, then the p value is 2 times the area to the right of z.

Computation of the p Value for Testing a Binomial Proportion

Let the test statistic be given by $Z = \dfrac{\hat{p} - p_0}{\sqrt{p_0 q_0/n}}$.

If $\hat{p} \leq p_0$, then p value $= 2 \cdot P(Z \leq z)$.
If $\hat{p} \geq p_0$, then p value $= 2 \cdot P(Z \geq z)$.

The p value of the above example is

$$p \text{ value} = 2 \cdot P(Z \leq -0.67)$$
$$= 2 \cdot [1 - P(Z \leq 0.67)]$$
$$= 0.5028 > 0.05.$$

Example 8.7.1. Hypersensitivity of the teeth is a pathologic condition in which the teeth are sensitive to thermal, chemical, and physical stimuli. The patients with dentin hypersensitivity experience pain from hot/cold and sweet/sour solutions and foods. The pain may be experienced when hot/cold air touches the teeth. It varies in degrees from mild to excruciating. Dentin hypersensitivity occurs due to exposure of dentinal tubules as a result of attrition, abrasion, erosion, fracture, or chipping of the tooth, or a faulty restoration [8]. Suppose that a past study showed that 5% potassium nitrate solution reduced dentin hypersensitivity in 48% of the cases. To compare the effectiveness of a 40% formalin solution with that of 5% potassium nitrate solution, the investigators took a sample of 81 patients who suffer from dentin hypersensitivity. Of these 81 patients, 49 of them expressed that 40% formalin solution did significantly reduce the pain. What could you conclude about the effectiveness of the two desensitizing agents?

Solution. Since no prior knowledge is available regarding the effectiveness of 40% formalin solution relative to 5% potassium nitrate solution, we wish to test the hypotheses H_0: $p = 0.48$ vs. H_1: $p \neq 0.48$. It is given that $p_0 = 0.48$, $q_0 = 1 - 0.48 = 0.52$, $n = 81$, $\hat{p} = 49/81 = 0.60$. The normal approximation is valid because $np_0 q_0 = 81(0.48)(0.52) = 20.22 > 5.0$. We compute the test statistic

$$Z = \frac{\hat{p} - p_0}{\sqrt{p_0 q_0/n}} = \frac{0.60 - 0.48}{\sqrt{(0.48)(0.52)/81}} = 2.16.$$

Let's now compute the p value of the test.

$$p \text{ value} = 2 \cdot P(Z > 2.16)$$
$$= 2 \cdot (1 - 0.9846) = 0.0308 < 0.05.$$

Since $Z > z_{1-\alpha/2} = 1.96$, the null hypothesis is rejected at $\alpha = 0.05$. We conclude that the 40% formalin solution is statistically significantly more effective in reducing the level of pain in dentin-hypersensitive patients than the 5% potassium nitrate solution with the p value of 0.0308.

Example 8.7.2. In the game of basketball, the free throw is an important aspect of the game. A couple of free throws at the last minute can decide the outcome of a game. Using his or her legs properly at the free throw line is a critical technique to develop. Men's basketball coach, Mr. Jackson, knows that as the game progresses, the players' legs get tired, and consequently, their free throw percentage drops. He compared the free throw percentages of the first half and the second half of the games his team has played over the last few seasons, and learned that the free throw percentages (FT%) in the second half is significantly lower. The tired legs definitely affect their FT%. In fact, his team's statistic shows that the FT% of the second half is a disappointing 57%, compared to 79% in the first half. He thinks that the women's basketball team experiences a similar drop in FT% in the second half. However, he has no idea if their percentage will be as low as his team's 57%. Mr. Jackson obtained the FT% data of 105 women's basketball games in the last 4 seasons, and found out their average second-half FT% is 68%. What would you say to Mr. Jackson, based on his data?

Solution. Mr. Jackson's hypotheses can be stated as H_0: $p = 0.57$ vs. H_1: $p \neq 0.57$. Since $np_0 q_0 = 105(0.57)(0.43) = 25.736 > 5.0$, the normal approximation can be applied. Substituting $p_0 = 0.57$, $q_0 = 1 - 0.57 = 0.43$, $n = 105$, and the sample proportion $\widehat{p} = 0.68$ in the test statistic, we obtain

$$Z = \frac{\widehat{p} - p_0}{\sqrt{p_0 q_0 / n}} = \frac{0.68 - 0.57}{\sqrt{(0.57)(0.43)/105}} = 2.28.$$

Let's now compute the p value of the test.

$$p \text{ value} = 2 \cdot P(Z > 2.28) = 0.0226 < 0.05.$$

Since $Z > z_{1-\alpha/2} = 1.96$, the null hypothesis is rejected at the significance level $\alpha = 0.05$. The women's free throw percentage in the second half is statistically significantly better than that of the men's team. The p value of the test is 0.0226.

Because the test is based on the normal approximation, the p values obtained in the above examples are approximate. For a small sample case where the normal approximation to the binomial distribution is not valid, we can use an exact binomial method to perform the test. Interested readers are referred to Fisher and Van Belle [9].

Example 8.7.3. The primary factors known to predispose one to implant failure are low bone density (type IV bone, [10]) and smoking. Suppose that a study with a group of implant patients who are moderate to heavy smokers revealed that about 13% have type IV bone. Dr. Samuelson, who is an implantologist, wanted to investigate how the prevalence rate of low bone density among the smokers will compare to the prevalence rate of type IV bone for the non-smokers. His examination of 74 implant patients indicated that only 7 patients had type IV bone. Do the two groups have a significantly different prevalence rate? Test the hypothesis using the p value method.

Solution. One can perform the hypothesis test by mimicking the examples we discussed in this section. Technical details are left to the readers as an exercise problem.

8.8 ONE-SAMPLE χ^2 TEST FOR THE VARIANCE OF A NORMAL DISTRIBUTION

So far in this chapter our discussions have been focused on testing the hypotheses for the mean of a normal distribution. In this section, we introduce a hypothesis testing procedure for the variance of a normal distribution. Let $X_1, X_2, \cdots, X_n$ be a random sample from a normal population $N(\mu, \sigma^2)$. Suppose we wish to test the hypotheses H_0 : $\sigma^2 = \sigma_0^2$ vs. H_1 : $\sigma^2 \neq \sigma_0^2$. We shall describe how to perform this type of test.

The number of adults seeking orthodontic treatment is increasing. It has been estimated up to 40% of all orthodontic patients are adults. Adult

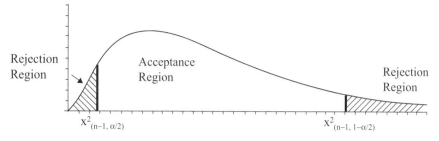

Figure 8.8.1 Rejection and acceptance regions of the χ^2 test.

patients present a challenge to orthodontists because they have high aesthetic demands and often have dental conditions that may complicate treatment, such as tooth wear, poorly contoured restorations, and periodontal disease. In some adults, a black triangular space may appear between the maxillary central incisors and the cervical gingival margin after orthodontic treatment. This open gingival embrasure may appear unaesthetic [11]. The area of gingival embrasure is assumed to be normally distributed. Suppose a past study showed that the variance of the area of normal gingival embrasure is $\sigma^2 = 3.08$. Would the variance of the area of open gingival embrasure among adult patients be significantly different? We can state the hypotheses as $H_0 : \sigma^2 = 3.08$ vs. $H_1 : \sigma^2 \neq 3.08$. Investigators took a sample of 23 patients with an open gingival embrasure. From the measurements of the area, they have calculated the sample variance $S^2 = 4.31$. Under the null hypothesis H_0, the test statistic is

$$\chi^2 = \frac{(n-1)S^2}{\sigma^2} \sim \chi^2_{(n-1)}, \quad \text{that is,}$$

a χ^2 with $(n-1)$ degrees of freedom.

The critical values are determined by $P\left(\chi^2 < \chi^2_{(n-1,\alpha/2)}\right) = \frac{\alpha}{2} = P\left(\chi^2 > \chi^2_{(n-1,1-\alpha/2)}\right)$.

So the critical values are $c_1 = \chi^2_{(n-1,\alpha/2)}$ and $c_2 = \chi^2_{(n-1,1-\alpha/2)}$, which define the rejection and acceptance regions. Figure 8.8.1 illustrates these regions for the distribution of $\chi^2 = \frac{(n-1)S^2}{\sigma_0^2}$ under H_0.

To complete the test for the example, let's compute the test statistic with $n - 1 = 23 - 1 = 22$, $\sigma_0^2 = 3.08$, and $S^2 = 4.31$;

$$\chi^2 = \frac{(n-1)S^2}{\sigma_0^2} = \frac{(23-1)(4.31)}{3.08} = 30.786.$$

From Table F (the χ^2 probability table) in the Appendix we obtain

$$c_1 = \chi^2_{(22,0.025)} = 10.98 \quad \text{and}$$
$$c_2 = \chi^2_{(22,0.975)} = 36.78.$$

Since the computed test statistic $\chi^2 = 30.786$ is between $\chi^2_{(22,0.025)} = 10.98$ and $\chi^2_{(22,0.975)} = 36.78$, we accept H_0 at the significance level $\alpha = 0.05$ and conclude that the variance of the area of an open gingival embrasure is not statistically significantly different from the variance of the area of a normal gingival embrasure. This χ^2 test procedure can be summarized as follows.

One-Sample χ^2 Test for the Variance of a Normal Distribution

Given the hypotheses

$H_0 : \sigma^2 = \sigma_0^2$ vs. $H_1 : \sigma^2 \neq \sigma_0^2$, and the test statistic

$$\chi^2 = \frac{(n-1)S^2}{\sigma_0^2},$$

reject H_0 if $\chi^2 < \chi^2_{(n-1,\alpha/2)}$ or $\chi^2 > \chi^2_{(n-1,1-\alpha/2)}$, and accept if $\chi^2_{(n-1,\alpha/2)} < \chi^2 < \chi^2_{(n-1,1-\alpha/2)}$.

Example 8.8.1. Periodontal probing is done routinely during a dental examination and has become an important diagnostic tool to determine the presence and severity of periodontal disease. Clinicians have used a handheld probe that is non-pressure controlled with visual measurement recording, and, therefore, the degree of accuracy may not be high as well as the precision level of the instrument may be low. Historical data indicates that the variance of the pocket depth by a handheld probe is 2.8. Recently, a medical equipment company has introduced a pressure-controlled

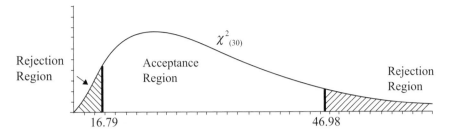

Figure 8.8.2 Rejection and acceptance regions of the χ^2 test in Example 8.8.1.

computerized probe. It is not certain whether or not this computerized probe would necessarily have a higher level of precision than the traditional handheld probe. The clinic director decided to undertake a study to evaluate the variability of the new instrument. He will purchase the computerized probe for his clinic only if the study proves its superiority. A clinician took 31 pocket depth measurements and reported the sample variance $S^2 = 2.2$. We may assume that the pocket depth is normally distributed. Would you recommend that the clinic director purchase the new equipment? Use the significance level $\alpha = 0.05$.

Solution. The hypotheses we need to test can be stated as $H_0 : \sigma^2 = 2.8$ vs. $H_1 : \sigma^2 \neq 2.8$. Substituting $n - 1 = 31 - 1 = 30$, $S^2 = 2.2$, and $\sigma_0^2 = 2.8$, we obtain the test statistic

$$\chi^2 = \frac{(n-1)S^2}{\sigma_0^2} = \frac{(30)(2.2)}{2.8} = 23.571.$$

From Table F in the Appendix we can easily find the critical values,

$$\chi^2_{(n-1,\alpha/2)} = \chi^2_{(30,0.025)} = 16.79 \text{ and}$$

$$\chi^2_{(n-1,1-\alpha/2)} = \chi^2_{(30,0.975)} = 46.98.$$

We see that the computed χ^2 test statistic value is between the critical values;

$$\chi^2_{(n-1,\alpha/2)} = 16.79 < 23.571 < \chi^2_{(n-1,1-\alpha/2)}$$
$$= 46.98.$$

Thus, we accept the null hypothesis and conclude that the computerized probe is not statistically significantly more precise than the handheld probe at the significance level $\alpha = 0.05$. The formula for the p value of a one-sample χ^2 test of a normal distribution is given below. The rejection and acceptance regions of the test are illustrated in Figure 8.8.2.

The p Value of a One-Sample χ^2 Test

Given the hypotheses

$$H_0 : \sigma^2 = \sigma_0^2 \text{ vs. } H_1 : \sigma^2 \neq \sigma_0^2, \text{ and the test}$$

statistic $\chi^2 = \dfrac{(n-1)S^2}{\sigma_0^2}$.

If $S^2 \leq \sigma_0^2$, then the p value $= 2 \cdot P(\chi^2_{(n-1)} \leq \chi^2)$.
If $S^2 > \sigma_0^2$, then the p value $= 2 \cdot P(\chi^2_{(n-1)} > \chi^2)$.

So the p value of the test in Example 8.8.1 is given by

p value
$$= 2 \cdot P\left(\chi^2_{(n-1)} \leq \chi^2\right), \text{ since } S^2 = 2.2 \leq \sigma_0^2 = 2.8$$
$$= 2 \cdot P\left(\chi^2_{(30)} \leq 23.571\right) > 2 \cdot P\left(\chi^2_{(30)} \leq 20.599\right)$$
$$= 2(0.100) = 0.200.$$

The p value is a little larger than 0.200. Figure 8.8.3 illustrates the p value.

Example 8.8.2. Recently, the researchers in dental and medical sciences have shown considerable interest in putative relationships between oral and systemic diseases. Kowolik et al. [12] hypothesized that dental plaque accumulation in healthy subjects would elicit a systemic inflammatory response. During the experiment, their healthy subjects were refrained from all oral hygiene practices for 3 weeks, thus permitting the accumulation of bacterial plaque. One variable that they observed was the total neutrophil counts. Suppose their previous similar experiment with a group of young subjects, aged 21 to 30, showed that the mean and standard deviation of their neutrophil counts ($x 10^9/l$) were 2.61 and 0.27, respectively. Suppose investigators wondered how the variability of the neutrophil counts would compare if the experimental group also included patients in their 30s to 60s. To find out, they took a random sample of

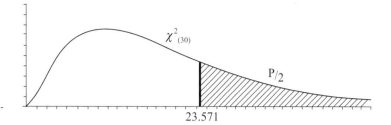

Figure 8.8.3 The *p* value test in Example 8.8.1.

26 patients. A similar experiment yielded the sample standard deviation 0.37 for the total neutrophil counts of these 26 patients. Is there a significant difference in the variance between the two groups?

Solution. The hypotheses will be stated as before, $H_0 : \sigma^2 = (0.27)^2$ vs. $H_1 : \sigma^2 \neq (0.27)^2$. Using the test statistic given in this section and by substitution, we have

$$\chi^2 = \frac{(n-1)S^2}{\sigma_0^2} = \frac{25(0.37)^2}{(0.27)^2} = 46.948.$$

The critical values can be found from the χ^2 probability table (Table F in the Appendix);

$$\chi_{(n-1,\alpha/2)}^2 = \chi_{(25,0.025)}^2 = 13.12 \text{ and}$$
$$\chi_{(n-1,1-\alpha/2)}^2 = \chi_{(25,0.975)}^2 = 40.65.$$

Since the computed test statistic $\chi^2 = 46.948 > \chi_{(25,0.975)}^2 = 40.65$, we reject the null hypothesis at the significance level $\alpha = 0.05$. The *p* value is

p value
$$= 2 \cdot P\left(\chi_{(n-1)}^2 > \chi^2\right),$$
$$\text{since } S^2 = (0.37)^2 > \sigma_0^2 = (0.27)^2$$
$$= 2 \cdot P\left(\chi_{(30)}^2 > 46.948\right)$$
$$< 2 \cdot P\left(\chi_{(30)}^2 > 46.928\right)$$
$$= 2(0.0050) = 0.0100.$$

The variability of the total neutrophil counts for the group with a wider age range is statistically significantly greater with the *p* value slightly less than 0.0100. The difference in the variance between the two groups is highly significant.

8.9 EXERCISES

1 Medical investigators found that about 20% of the population age 65 or older are given medications that are rarely appropriate for people their age. At least part of the problem is the way doctors are trained; pediatrics is mandatory in all U.S. medical schools, but geriatric care tends to get glossed over [13]. Suppose that, motivated by this finding and the rapidly growing population of senior citizens, some medical schools have revamped their curricula to include training in geriatric care. These medical schools like to believe that their new curricula should have reduced the percentage of inappropriate prescriptions by their graduates.
a. State the null and alternative hypotheses.
b. Discuss in the context of the above problem what happens if a type I error is committed.

2 School teachers who are concerned with oral hygiene habits of children claimed that on the average, children spend about 30 seconds brushing their teeth. To test this claim, investigators take a random sample of 50 children, ages 5 to 7. All are healthy, free of developmental delays, and capable of properly applying dentifrice to a toothbrush. The time spent brushing is to be carefully observed for the study.
a. State the null and alternative hypothesis.
b. Discuss in the context of the above problem how a type II error can be committed and what a type II error means.

3 In women, lung cancer has surpassed breast cancer as the leading cause of cancer death. Cigarette smoking causes 85% of lung cancers in American men, and passive smoking also increases the risk of lung cancer, causing 25% of the lung cancers seen in non-smokers. Chromosomal defects are also associated with lung cancer. Suppose it has been known that after successful chemoradiation treatments the average remission period of lung cancer patients is 7.5 years. The researchers have developed a new treatment and hope to demonstrate clinically that it is much more effective in extending the remission period beyond 7.5 years.

a. How should the researchers formulate the hypotheses?
b. State the consequences of committing a type I and a type II error.

23.2	24.5	22.1	22.4	23.6	21.4
22.0	24.0	24.8	25.6	23.2	22.8

4 Vitamin E is a popular and powerful antioxidant, which is effective in preventing the oxidation of polyunsaturated fatty acids. A study showed that the addition of 100 IU or more of vitamin E per day resulted in a reduction by 40% of the risk of heart disease [14]. Public health officials vaguely speculated that adult Americans consume approximately 20 IU per day on the average. To confirm this figure, investigators selected 35 subjects at random and carefully monitored their vitamin E intake. The sample mean $\overline{X}$ of the 35 individuals was 25 IU. Suppose the amount of vitamin E intake by adult Americans has a normal distribution with the standard deviation $\sigma = 5.2$ IU. Has the public health department significantly underestimated the average intake of vitamin E? Use the significance level $\alpha = 0.05$.

5 Base metal alloys have been used with varying degrees of success for metal-ceramic restorations. One shortcoming of these alloys is the technique sensitivity associated with the soldered joints. The strength X of a certain nickel-base alloy is assumed to be normally distributed, $X \sim N(\mu, 6889)$. Sixteen alloy samples were tested for the flexure stress measured in megapascals. If the mean flexure stress of these 16 samples is 703 MPa, is this significantly lower than 750 MPa, which is claimed by the manufacturer? Test the hypotheses at the significance level $\alpha = 0.05$.

6 Brown rice is being sold in a bag labeled 25 kg. Mr. Chang, who owns a grocery store, buys the brown rice from California rice growers. He weighed a few bags and found all were under the labeled value. This led him to believe that the average weight of the 25-kg rice bag is actually less than 25 kg. To ensure that his customers are getting what they pay for, he has selected at random 12 bags from the last week's shipment. The following lists the weight of his samples. You may assume that the weights are normally distributed with $\sigma^2 = 4.2$.
a. State the appropriate hypotheses.
b. Perform the test by using the p value.
c. Draw a conclusion for Mr. Chang.

7 Perform a hypothesis test H_0: $\mu = 2.0$ vs. H_1: $\mu \neq 2.0$ described at the beginning of Section 8.4 at the significance level $\alpha = 0.05$.

8 Studies on antimicrobial action and induction of tissue repair by intracanal medications have shown calcium hydroxide to be an effective therapeutic agent. The manufacturer's brochure suggested that the mean inhibition zone against *S. aureus* is about 6.0 mm in diameter. The scientists suspect that calcium hydroxide is far more effective than what is believed by the manufacturer and that the inhibition zone has to be substantially greater than 6.0 mm. The agar diffusion test, with 15 samples, yielded the mean inhibition zone of 7.1 mm. Suppose the zone of inhibition is normally distributed with the SD $\sigma = 2.23$ mm. What conclusion can be drawn? (Use $\alpha = 0.05$.)

9 An experiment was conducted to investigate the effect of physical exercise on the reduction of the weight of individuals who have the body mass index (BMI) of 30 or higher. The researchers put 28 study subjects on an exercise regimen while controlling their diet during the investigation. A similar study, done in the past, showed that there is on the average a decrease of 3.2 in body mass index. Since the new study is at least a week longer than the previous studies, they expect to see a slightly larger drop in BMI. At the end of the study they obtained the mean decrease of 3.8 in BMI. The amount of reduction in BMI is known to be normally distributed with the SD of 1.52. What can you conclude? What is the p value? (Use $\alpha = 0.05$.)

10 Root-end preparations made with diamond-coated ultrasonic tips (DUST) are being evaluated with respect to extracanal cracks that originate on the root surface and extend into the dentin. For the study, 20 incisors were instrumented and obturated. The investigators hypothesized that preparations made with DUST would be different from preparations made with conventional ultrasonic tips (CUST). Past data indicate that the distribution of extracanal cracks for CUST is approximately normal with mean 2.87 mm. Dye penetration was measured after immersion of the incisor samples in Pelikan ink for 5 days. Suppose the average crack size for DUST, based on these 20 samples, is 2.60 mm. If we assume that the standard deviation of the size of the cracks is $\sigma = 1.08$ mm, state the appropriate hypotheses and perform the hypothesis test using the p value method.

11 Patients want their implants to function at least 10 years and fully expect their dentists to guarantee any damages to implants within 10 years to be corrected at no cost to them. To assess if this expectation is realistic or not, Dr. Quinn decided to collect retrospective data from the patient charts. He had randomly selected 27 charts of the patients who have had titanium implants placed by him and his associates. His data showed that the average survival time of implants is 11.26 years. Suppose that the distribution of implant survival time is normal with a known SD $\sigma = 2.13$ years. Based on this evidence, would you advise Dr. Quinn that it is reasonably safe for him to give his patients a 10-year guarantee on the titanium implants?

12 The salivary flow rate of adult patients is normally distributed with mean 1.2 ml/min and SD 0.3 ml/min. Nine dental patients were chosen at random from a group of habitual gum chewers. Suppose the average salivary flow rate of these patients is 1.6 ml/min. Do gum chewers have a significantly higher rate of salivary flow? State the hypotheses and test at the significance level $\alpha = 0.05$.

13 Dental researchers have collected data on bonding strength Y of an experimental dental material they have developed. Suppose that the null mean bonding strength of the control product is 150 lbs/mm^2. Assume that the random variable Y has a normal distribution with an unknown variance σ^2. On the basis of 20 observations of the experimental material, they obtained the sample mean of 154 lbs/mm^2 and the SD $S = 4.52$. The researchers stated their hypotheses as $H_0: \mu = 150$ vs. $H_1: \mu \neq 150$. Perform a test using the p value method.

14 Xtra-Seal and Belton are sealants widely used by practicing dentists. The lifetime distribution of the sealants is approximately normal. Suppose a study suggested that the average lifetime of Xtra-Seal is 75.6 months. To compare the lifetime of Belton to that of Xtra-Seal, Dr. Jung selected 25 patient charts of those who were treated with Belton and found out that the sample mean of these 25 observations was 77.4 months and the sample SD was 9.75 months. What can you conclude from the evidence? Explain, based on the p value of the test.

15 Calculate the power of the test used for testing the hypotheses in Excercise 11 at the alternative mean $\mu_1 = 5.5, 6.0, 6.5, 7.0$, and 7.5 years. What can you say about the behavior of the power as μ_1 becomes closer to the null mean?

16 Calculate the power of the test used for testing the hypotheses in Exercise 12 at several selected values of the alternative mean, and discuss the behavior of the power as the observed mean difference $|\mu_1 - \mu_0|$ changes.

17 Calculate the power of the test used for testing the hypotheses in Exercise 13 at $\mu_1 = 130, 135, 140, 145, 150, 155, 160, 165$ and 170 lbs/mm^2.

18 Which one of the following statements best describes the difference between statistically significant and clinically significant?

a. I typically treat 26 patients a day but it was hectic yesterday treating 35 patients. This turned out to be a blessing in disguise because my office manager was taking a patient satisfaction survey for me and she was able to collect more data.

b. When I perform statistical hypothesis testing, I let my significance level $\alpha = 0.05$, but when I get involved with a clinical test, I let my significance level $\alpha = 0.10$.

c. My partner in the clinic collected a large amount of data on osseous integration from his patients over the years. He is still collecting data because he believes that the data he currently has is not clinically significant enough. However, my statistical analysis of the current data indicates that the results are statistically significant.

d. A study suggested that in their 80s about 25% of the patients had at least one carious tooth. However, a recent study conducted last year indicated that about 24.5% of the patients had at least one carious tooth. This difference is statistically significant, based on 2,106 patients. Public health officials are happy about the statistically significant reduction in the rate. I did well in my statistics course when I was in dental school; I always tried my best to understand the statistical concepts rather than regurgitate the formulas. The results may be statistically significant but clinically inconsequential.

e. As a statistically savvy physician, I understand the concept of variability perfectly well. About 35% of my patients, who are 65 years of age or older, need to be medicated for hypertension. My estimation of standard deviation of the proportion of hypertensive patients from year to year is 8%. This is a clinically significant number, compared to any other doctor I know. But this may not be statistically significant because I specified the significance level $\alpha = 0.005$, instead of $\alpha = 0.05$ when I did the comparison study with other physicians.

19 Poor oral hygiene is a serious cause of periodontal disease. Clinicians have realized that smokers are much more likely to have poor oral hygiene, and, therefore, their periodontal pocket depth (PPD) is deeper than that for the general patient population. Let a random variable Y denote the PPD. Assume that Y is normally distributed with mean μ and known variance $\sigma^2 = 2.44$, and that the mean PPD of the general population is 4.0 mm. Suppose investigators want to detect a minimum difference $|\mu_0 - \mu_1| = 1.2$ mm with probability 0.90. If a hypothesis test is to be performed at the significance level $\alpha = 0.05$, what is the required sample size?

20 Agents with carbamide peroxide (CP) in various concentrations are widely prescribed for at-home tooth whitening. It is not clear if the more concentrated gels will whiten teeth to a greater extent. Dental researchers plan to conduct a double-blind study of human subjects to evaluate whether a 15% CP tooth-whitening system is more effective than a 10% CP system [15]. Suppose that the values of the Vita Lumin shade guide is normally distributed and that the variance σ^2 of teeth shade for the patients who use CP at various concentrations is known to be 4.56. A pilot study with 20 human subjects suggests that in the 15% CP system the mean teeth shade, measured by Vita Lumin, is 4.19.

a. State the appropriate hypotheses.

b. Suppose the test is conducted at the significance level $\alpha = 0.05$. If the researchers wish to detect a difference $|\mu_0 - \mu_1| = 1.75$ with probability of 0.95, what sample size would you recommend?

21 Suppose a survey with practicing MDs showed about 43% have a solo practice and the remainder 57% have a partnership, association, are employed with HMO or government, etc. Upon reading this survey report, a dental researcher was curious about the proportion of DDSs who have a solo practice. She has randomly selected 450 dentists listed in the ADA directory and mailed a similar survey questionnaire to these DDSs. By the end of the month she had received 118 responses. The sample proportion of a solo practice based on these responses was $\widehat{p} = 0.38$. Is the proportion of a solo practice among DDSs different from that among physicians? Use the significance level $\alpha = 0.05$. (a) State the hypotheses. (b) Test the hypothesis at the significance level $\alpha = 0.05$.

22 Interpret the result of the hypothesis test described in Example 8.7.2.

23 Dental injury is a traumatic event with many causative factors. Dentofacial morphology is thought to be a major factor. Other factors related to dental injury include behavior, environment, and accident-proneness [16]. Suppose a study was conducted with orthodontic patients with injured incisors. Their cephalograms were visually examined by orthodontists, and 62% of the cases have been correctly identified as having injured incisors. A question was, based on their cephalograms, would they be able to correctly identify the patients with non-injured incisors as having no injured incisors? To pursue this question the investigators prepared 90 cephalograms of patients with non-injured incisors and found out that 56% of them were correctly identified as having non-injured incisors. Is there a significant difference in correct identification between injured and non-injured incisors? State the hypotheses and perform an appropriate test at the significance level $\alpha = 0.05$.

24 The materials involved in orthodontic bonding have changed constantly since the acid etch technique permitted adhesion of acrylic filling materials to enamel surfaces. A study suggested that the mean and SD of bonding strength of a widely used material are 6.95 MPa and 3.04 MPa. The variation of this popular material is unacceptably large. Orthodontists are considering a competing material and hope that it will have a lower variance. However, since it is brand new, no one knows if its variability in bonding strength is smaller or larger. To evaluate the quality of the new material, investigators conducted an experiment with 24 samples in their biomaterials research lab and the sample SD of 2.43 MPa was obtained from the data. What can you conclude? Use the p value method.

8.10 REFERENCES

1. Misch, C. E., and Crawford, E. A. Predictable mandibular nerve location – A clinical zone of safety. *Int. J. Oral Implant.* 1990, 7, 37–40.
2. Hartmann, C. R., Hanson, P. R., and Pincsak, J. J. Mandibular intercanine width increase without intervention in children with slipped contacts. *Pediatr Dent.* 2001, 23, 469–475.
3. Ben-Bassat, Y., Brin, I., and Brezniak, N. Can maxillary incisor trauma be predicted from cephalometric measurements? *Am. J. Orthod. Dentofacial Orthop*: 2001, 120, 186–189.
4. Pae, E., and Ferguson, K. A. Cephalometric characteristics of nonobese patients with severe OSA. *Angle Orthod*: 1999, 69: 408–412.
5. Emingil, G., et al. Association between periodontal disease and acute myocardial infarction. *J. Periondontol.*: 2000, 71, 1882–1886.
6. Hujoel, P. P., Armitage, G. C., and Garcia, R. I. A perspective on clinical significance. *J Periodontol*: 2000, 71, 1515–1518.
7. Marcek, M., Edelstein, B. L., and Manski, R. J. An analysis of dental visits in U.S. children, by category of service and sociodemographic factors. *Am. Acad. of Pediatric Dent*: 2000, 23, 383–389.
8. Kishore, A., Mehrotra, K. K., and Saimbi, C. S. Effectiveness of desensitizing agents. *J. of Endodontics*: 2002, 28, 34–35.
9. Fisher, L. D., and Van Belle, G. *Biostatistics: A Methodology for the Health Sciences.* John Wiley & Sons, Inc. 1993.
10. Jaffin, R. A., and Berman, C. L. The excessive loss of Bränemark implants in type IV bone: A 5 year analysis. *J. Periodontol*: 1991, 62, 2–4.
11. Kurth, J. R., and Kokich, V. G. Open gingival embrasures after orthodontic treatment in adults: Prevalence and etiology. *Am. J. Orthod. Dentofacial. Orthop*: 2001, 120, 116–123.
12. Kowolik, M. J., et al. Systemic neutrophil response resulting from dental plaque accumulation. *J. Periodontol*: 2001, 72, 146–151.
13. Gupta, S. Not for the elderly. *Time*, December 24, 2001.
14. Stampfer M., Hennekens C., Manson J, et al. Vitamin E consumption and the risk of coronary disease in women. *N Eng J Med*: 1993, 328, 1444–1449.
15. Kihn, P. E., et al. A clinical evaluation of 10 percent vs. 15 percent carbamide peroxide tooth-whitening agents. *JADA*: 2000, 131, 85–91.
16. Ben-Bassat, Y., Brin, I., and Brezniak, N. Can maxillary incisor trauma be predicted from cephalometric measurements? *Am J Orthod Dentofacial Orthop*: 2001, 120, 186–189.

Chapter 9

Hypothesis Testing: Two-Sample Case

9.1 INTRODUCTION

All of the statistical test procedures we studied in Chapter 8 were one-sample problems. In this chapter we will discuss hypothesis testing of two-sample cases. In most of the practical situations in biomedical health sciences, it is much more common to compare the means of two independent populations. One random sample is drawn from the first population and one from the second in such a way that these two random samples are statistically independent of each other. Typically, two groups receive different treatments, or two groups are compared under two different conditions—one is referred to as an experimental group (or treatment group) and the other a control group. Here are some examples to illustrate two-sample problems that arise in the real world applications.

1. A study was conducted to evaluate the efficacy of desensitizing agents for the treatment of dentin hypersensitivity in which one group was treated with distilled water and the other group with 40% formalin solution.
2. A study was conducted to determine whether an expectant mother's alcohol consumption has any effect on the bone mineral content of her newborn baby.
3. Is there any difference in percent carbon monoxide in the air between downtown L.A. and San Bernardino, California?
4. An investigation was performed to compare the shear bond strength of composite to metal with two commercially available chemical bonding systems: a silicoating system and a nitrogenous heterocycle-acrylonitrile system.
5. Is the sealability of preventive resin restorations prepared conventionally better than those prepared with air-abrasion in the presence of acid etching?

All these examples involve a comparison between two populations. Most questions in scientific research are concerned with the detection of a significant mean difference between two groups. This chapter is devoted to comparing two populations with respect to their means, proportions and variances.

9.2 TWO-SAMPLE Z TEST FOR COMPARING TWO MEANS

Consider two independent normal populations with unknown means μ_1 and μ_2. We assume that the variances of the populations, σ_1^2 and σ_2^2, are known. The variances are not necessarily equal. Suppose random samples of size n_1 and n_2 are taken from the respective populations. Then it is well-known that the sampling distribution of the difference between the sample means is normal. That is, the sampling distribution of $\overline{X}_1 - \overline{X}_2$ is normal. Even if the underlying distributions are not normal, the sampling distribution of $\overline{X}_1 - \overline{X}_2$ is approximately normal for sufficiently large n_1 and n_2. It can be shown that the expected value (mean) and variance of $\overline{X}_1 - \overline{X}_2$ are

$$\mu_1 - \mu_2 \quad \text{and} \quad \frac{\sigma_1^2}{n_1} + \frac{\sigma_2^2}{n_2}.$$

Thus, the **standard error** (SE) of $\overline{X}_1 - \overline{X}_2$ is $\sqrt{\frac{\sigma_1^2}{n_1} + \frac{\sigma_2^2}{n_2}}$. In summary, if two random samples of size n_1 and n_2 are taken from two independent normal populations with unknown means μ_1 and μ_2 and known variances σ_1^2 and σ_2^2, then the sampling distribution of $\overline{X}_1 - \overline{X}_2$ is given by

$$\overline{X}_1 - \overline{X}_2 \sim N\left(\mu_1 - \mu_2, \frac{\sigma_1^2}{n_1} + \frac{\sigma_2^2}{n_2}\right)$$

or

$$\frac{(\overline{X}_1 - \overline{X}_2) - (\mu_1 - \mu_2)}{\sqrt{\frac{\sigma_1^2}{n_1} + \frac{\sigma_2^2}{n_2}}} \sim N(0, 1).$$

If the variances are equal, that is, $\sigma^2 = \sigma_1^2 = \sigma_2^2$, then the variance of $\overline{X}_1 - \overline{X}_2$ is $\sigma^2 \left(\frac{1}{n_1} + \frac{1}{n_2} \right)$. The above expressions can be rewritten as

$$\overline{X}_1 - \overline{X}_2 \sim N \left(\mu_1 - \mu_2, \sigma^2 \left(\frac{1}{n_1} + \frac{1}{n_2} \right) \right)$$

or

$$\frac{(\overline{X}_1 - \overline{X}_2) - (\mu_1 - \mu_2)}{\sigma \sqrt{\frac{1}{n_1} + \frac{1}{n_2}}} \sim N(0, 1).$$

Suppose investigators wish to compare the clinical shear bond strength of the two most widely used orthodontic adhesives; Orthobond (Vivident) and Unibond (Orthobite). For this study, $n_1 = 15$ Orthobond and $n_2 = 12$ Unibond samples were prepared and their strength was tested using an Instron machine. From the measurements of the shear bond strength, they have estimated $\overline{X}_1 = 9.28$ kg and $\overline{X}_2 = 8.13$ kg. Assume that the shear bond strength is normally distributed with known variances $\sigma_1^2 = 4.75$ and $\sigma_2^2 = 4.37$. The investigators' goal is to test the hypotheses:

$$H_0 : \mu_1 = \mu_2 \text{ vs. } H_1 : \mu_1 \neq \mu_2.$$

By subtracting μ_2 from both sides of the null and alternative hypothesis, we have an equivalent hypothesis H_0: $\mu_1 - \mu_2 = 0$ vs. H_1: $\mu_1 - \mu_2 \neq 0$. In light of the statements of the hypothesis, it appears reasonable to form a test statistic based on $\overline{X}_1 - \overline{X}_2$. In fact, we can use

$$\frac{(\overline{X}_1 - \overline{X}_2) - (\mu_1 - \mu_2)}{\sqrt{\frac{\sigma_1^2}{n_1} + \frac{\sigma_2^2}{n_2}}}$$

as a basis for the above hypothesis test. Because this test statistic has the standard normal distribution, testing the hypothesis proceeds precisely the same as the one-sample Z test. Let's compute the value of the test statistic by substituting the appropriate values under the null hypothesis (that is, H_0: $\mu_1 - \mu_2 = 0$):

$$Z = \frac{(\overline{X}_1 - \overline{X}_2) - (\mu_1 - \mu_2)}{\sqrt{\frac{\sigma_1^2}{n_1} + \frac{\sigma_2^2}{n_2}}}$$

$$= \frac{(9.28 - 8.13) - 0}{\sqrt{\frac{4.75}{15} + \frac{4.37}{12}}} = 1.39.$$

At the significance level $\alpha = 0.05$, the critical values are $z = -1.96$ and $z = 1.96$, as we saw in Chapter 8. Therefore, the null hypothesis is accepted. We can also compute the p value.

$$p \text{ value} = 2 \cdot P(Z > 1.39) = 0.1646 > 0.05.$$

Thus, we accept H_0 and conclude that there is no statistically significant difference in the mean shear bond strength between the two orthodontic adhesives. The rejection and acceptance regions of this two-sample Z test is depicted in Figure 9.2.1.

Two-Sample Z Test

Suppose we want to test the hypothesis H_0: $\mu_1 = \mu_2$ vs. H_1: $\mu_1 \neq \mu_2$ at the significance level $\alpha = 0.05$ for two independent normal populations with known variances σ_1^2 and σ_2^2. Under H_0: $\mu_1 = \mu_2$, compute the test statistic

$$Z = \frac{(\overline{X}_1 - \overline{X}_2)}{\sqrt{\frac{\sigma_1^2}{n_1} + \frac{\sigma_2^2}{n_2}}}$$

Reject H_0 if $Z < -Z_{1-\alpha/2} = Z_{\alpha/2}$ or $Z > Z_{1-\alpha/2}$ and accept H_0 if $-Z_{1-\alpha/2} \leq Z \leq Z_{1-\alpha/2}$.

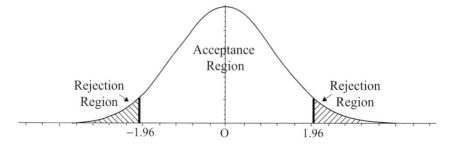

Figure 9.2.1 Rejection and acceptance regions of two-sample Z test.

9.3 TWO-SAMPLE t TEST FOR COMPARING TWO MEANS WITH EQUAL VARIANCES

In general, σ_1^2 and σ_2^2 are not known. Therefore, they must be estimated from the data. From the two samples we select, the sample variances are obtained by S_1^2 and S_2^2, respectively. We assume in this section that the variances are unknown but equal $\sigma^2 = \sigma_1^2 = \sigma_2^2$. The sample variances, S_1^2 and S_2^2, will be used to estimate the population variance σ^2. The best estimate of σ^2 is given by the pooled estimate from two independent samples:

$$S_p^2 = \frac{(n_1 - 1)S_1^2 + (n_2 - 1)S_2^2}{n_1 + n_2 - 2}.$$

Note that S_p^2 is a weighted average of S_1^2 and S_2^2, where the weights are defined by the number of degrees of freedom in each sample. The weights $w_1 = \dfrac{n_1 - 1}{n_1 + n_2 - 2}$ and $w_2 = \dfrac{n_2 - 1}{n_1 + n_2 - 2}$ are assigned to S_1^2 and S_2^2, respectively. The pooled estimate of the variance S_p^2 has $n_1 + n_2 - 2$ degrees of freedom, $n_1 - 1$ from the first sample and $n_2 - 1$ from the second sample. Greater weight is given to the sample variance of the larger sample. If $n_1 = n_2$, then the pooled estimate S_p^2 is the simple arithmetic average of S_1^2 and S_2^2. As we have done in the one-sample case, we will replace σ by the pooled sample SD, S_p in the formula in the previous section and get

$$t = \frac{(\overline{X}_1 - \overline{X}_2) - (\mu_1 - \mu_2)}{S_p\sqrt{\dfrac{1}{n_1} + \dfrac{1}{n_2}}}.$$

Under the null hypothesis H_0: $\mu_1 - \mu_2 = 0$, we have $t = \dfrac{(\overline{X}_1 - \overline{X}_2)}{S_p\sqrt{\dfrac{1}{n_1} + \dfrac{1}{n_2}}} \sim t_{(n_1+n_2-2)}.$

The above statistic has a t distribution with $n_1 + n_2 - 2$ degrees of freedom. A two-sample t test for independent samples when the variances are unknown but equal can be summarized as follows.

Two-Sample t Test with Equal Variances

Suppose we want to test the hypothesis H_0: $\mu_1 = \mu_2$ vs. H_1: $\mu_1 \neq \mu_2$ at the significance level $\alpha = 0.05$ for two independent normal populations with unknown but equal variances. Compute the test statistic

$$t = \frac{(\overline{X}_1 - \overline{X}_2)}{S_p\sqrt{\dfrac{1}{n_1} + \dfrac{1}{n_2}}}, \quad \text{where } S_p \text{ is the sample SD}$$

given by $\sqrt{\dfrac{(n_1 - 1)S_1^2 + (n_2 - 1)S_2^2}{n_1 + n_2 - 2}},$

Reject H_0 if $t < -t_{(n_1+n_2-2,1-\alpha/2)} = t_{(n_1+n_2-2,\alpha/2)}$ or $t > t_{(n_1+n_2-2,1-\alpha/2)}$, and accept H_0 if $-t_{(n_1+n_2-2,1-\alpha/2)} \leq t \leq t_{(n_1+n_2-2,1-\alpha/2)}$.

The p value of the two-sample t test can be calculated the same as the one-sample case:

If $t = \dfrac{(\overline{X}_1 - \overline{X}_2)}{S_p\sqrt{\dfrac{1}{n_1} + \dfrac{1}{n_2}}} \leq 0,$

$$p = 2 \cdot P(t_{(n_1+n_2-2)} < t)$$
$$= 2 \cdot (\text{area to the left of } t \text{ under } t_{(n_1+n_2-2)} \text{ distribution}).$$

If $t = \dfrac{(\overline{X}_1 - \overline{X}_2)}{S_p\sqrt{\dfrac{1}{n_1} + \dfrac{1}{n_2}}} > 0,$

$$p = 2 \cdot P(t_{(n_1+n_2-2)} \geq t)$$
$$= 2 \cdot (\text{area to the right of } t \text{ under } t_{(n_1+n_2-2)} \text{ distribution}).$$

These p values are shown in Figure 9.3.1 and Figure 9.3.2.

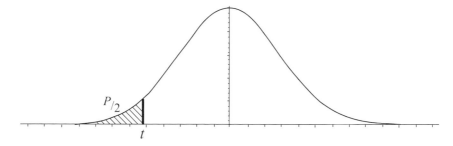

Figure 9.3.1 *P* value when $t \leq 0$.

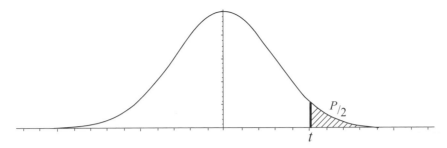

Figure 9.3.2 *P* value when $t \geq 0$.

We present a couple of examples to illustrate a two-sample t test.

Example 9.3.1. Localized gingival recessions are among the indications for mucogingival surgery. They may require treatment because of functional considerations or because of their esthetic implications. Caffesse and Guinard [1] studied 26 localized gingival recessions: 14 of them treated with a lateral sliding flap procedure and 12 treated with a coronally repositioned flap procedure. Six months after the treatment with the respective procedure, the change in mucogingival line was measured. Suppose that the change in mucogingival line is normally distributed and that both procedures have the same population variances. From the measurements the investigators computed the following sample means and sample variances, $\overline{X}_1 = 4.50$ mm, $\overline{X}_2 = 4.33$ mm, $S_1^2 = 1.27$, and $S_2^2 = 1.07$. The investigators wish to test if there is any difference in mean changes between the two procedures. Perform the test at the significance level $\alpha = 0.05$.

Solution. The hypothesis can be stated as follows: H_0: $\mu_1 = \mu_2$ vs. H_1: $\mu_1 \neq \mu_2$. Two independent samples were drawn, one with $n_1 = 14$ and the other with $n_2 = 12$. Since $S_1^2 = 1.27$ and $S_2^2 = 1.07$, we can obtain the pooled estimate of the variance σ^2,

$$S_p^2 = \frac{(n_1 - 1)S_1^2 + (n_2 - 1)S_2^2}{n_1 + n_2 - 2}$$

$$= \frac{(14-1)(1.27)+(12-1)(1.07)}{14 + 12 - 2} = 1.1783.$$

So the SE of $\overline{X}_1 - \overline{X}_2$ is given by

$$S_p\sqrt{\frac{1}{n_1} + \frac{1}{n_2}} = \sqrt{1.1783} \cdot \sqrt{\frac{1}{14} + \frac{1}{12}} = 0.4270.$$

We now compute the t statistics value by substitution,

$$t = \frac{(\overline{X}_1 - \overline{X}_2)}{S_p\sqrt{\dfrac{1}{n_1} + \dfrac{1}{n_2}}} = \frac{4.50 - 4.33}{0.4270} = 0.3981.$$

The critical values are $t_{(24,0.975)} = 2.064$ and $t_{(24,0.025)} = -t_{(24,0.975)} = -2.064$. Because $t = 0.3981$ falls in the acceptance region, $-2.064 < t = 0.3981 < 2.064$, we accept the null hypothesis and conclude that there is no statistically significant difference in mean changes in mucogingival line on the recipients 6 months after the treatment between a lateral sliding flap and a coronally repositioned flap procedure at the significance level $\alpha = 0.05$. We can reach the same conclusion using the p value method.

$$p = 2 \cdot P(0.3981 \leq t_{(24)}) > 2 \cdot P(0.531 \leq t_{(24)}),$$

from the t table in the Appendix

$$= 2(0.30) = 0.60.$$

The p value is slightly larger than 0.60, which is much greater than $\alpha = 0.05$.

Example 9.3.2. The success of endodontic therapy depends on the method and quality of instrumentation, irrigation, disinfection, and the tridimensional obturation of the root canal system. Vertical condensation of warm gutta-percha and lateral condensation with a standardized cone are the techniques widely used for the obturation of the root canal system. These techniques are evaluated in the presence of a smear layer. Twenty-four well-preserved extracted human central incisors with straight roots were selected to evaluate the smear layer influence on the apical seal of the obturation techniques. The root canals of 12 teeth samples ($n_1 = 12$) were obturated with the first technique and 12 ($n_2 = 12$) with the second technique. To compare the effectiveness of the two techniques, apical leakage was assessed by measuring the linear penetration of methylene blue dye with a stereomicroscope [2]. Suppose that the linear penetration is normally distributed and that the variances of penetration for these obturation techniques are the same. The sample means and the sample variances are calculated from the data: $\overline{X}_1 = 5.2$ mm, $\overline{X}_2 = 4.1$ mm, $S_1^2 = 1.96$, and $S_2^2 = 1.0$. Perform a hypothesis test to detect a significant difference in mean between the obturation techniques at the significance level $\alpha = 0.05$.

Solution. The hypotheses we want to test can be stated as $H_0: \mu_1 = \mu_2$ vs. $H_1: \mu_1 \neq \mu_2$. If the sample sizes for the two independent samples are $n_1 = 12$ and $n_2 = 12$, and $S_1^2 = 1.96$ and $S_2^2 = 1.0$, we obtain the pooled estimate of the variance σ^2.

$$S_p^2 = \frac{(n_1 - 1)S_1^2 + (n_2 - 1)S_2^2}{n_1 + n_2 - 2}$$
$$= \frac{(12 - 1)(1.96) + (12 - 1)(1.0)}{12 + 12 - 2} = 1.48.$$

We now compute the value of the t statistic by substitution,

$$t = \frac{(\overline{X}_1 - \overline{X}_2)}{S_p\sqrt{\frac{1}{n_1} + \frac{1}{n_2}}} = \frac{5.2 - 4.1}{1.2166\sqrt{\frac{1}{12} + \frac{1}{12}}}$$
$$= 2.2147$$

The critical values are $t_{(22, 0.975)} = 2.074$ and $t_{(22, 0.025)} = -t_{(22, 0.975)} = -2.074$. Because $t = 2.2147$ falls in the rejection region, $t_{(22, 0.975)} < 2.2147$, we reject the null hypothesis and conclude that there is a statistically significant mean difference. In fact, the lateral condensation with a standardized cone in the presence of a smear layer is significantly more effective in preventing apical leakage than vertical condensation of warm gutta-percha. The p value is obtained by $p = 2 \cdot P(2.2147 < t_{(22)}) < 2 \cdot P(2.183 < t_{(22)}) = 0.04$.

9.4 TWO-SAMPLE t TEST FOR COMPARING TWO MEANS WITH UNEQUAL VARIANCES

In the previous section we discussed a two-sample t test for comparing means of two independent normal populations when the variances are not known but assumed to be equal. In this section we discuss the situations in which the variances are unknown and unequal. One sample of size n_1 is drawn from a normal population $N(\mu_1, \sigma_1^2)$ and another sample of size n_2 is drawn from a normal population $N(\mu_2, \sigma_2^2)$. We wish to test the hypothesis $H_0: \mu_1 = \mu_2$ vs. $H_1: \mu_1 \neq \mu_2$. Instead of using the pooled estimate S_p^2 of the variance, we replace σ_1^2 and σ_2^2 in the formula in Section 9.2 by their estimates S_1^2 and S_2^2 and obtain the test statistic

$$t = \frac{(\overline{X}_1 - \overline{X}_2)}{\sqrt{\frac{S_1^2}{n_1} + \frac{S_2^2}{n_2}}}.$$

Unlike the case with equal variances, the above statistics $t = \dfrac{(\overline{X}_1 - \overline{X}_2)}{\sqrt{S_1^2/n_1 + S_2^2/n_2}}$ when $\sigma_1^2 \neq \sigma_2^2$ has an approximately t distribution with the degrees of freedom δ^* [3]. The quantity δ^* is approximated by

$$\delta = \frac{(S_1^2/n_1 + S_2^2/n_2)^2}{(S_1^2/n_1)^2/(n_1 - 1) + (S_2^2/n_2)^2/(n_2 - 1)}.$$

The δ is known as Satherthwaite approximation. The approximate degrees of freedom δ may not be an integer, in which case, round it down to the nearest integer δ^*. Satherthwaite showed that

$$t = \frac{(\overline{X}_1 - \overline{X}_2)}{\sqrt{S_1^2/n_1 + S_2^2/n_2}} \text{ is approximately } t_{(\delta^*)}.$$

We round the degrees of freedom δ down to the nearest integer, rather than up, to take a conservative approach. This means it is slightly less likely to reject the null hypothesis.

Two-Sample t Test for Comparing Two Normal Means with Unequal Variances

1. For testing the hypothesis $H_0: \mu_1 = \mu_2$ vs. $H_1: \mu_1 \neq \mu_2$, we compute the statistic

$$t = \frac{(\overline{X}_1 - \overline{X}_2)}{\sqrt{S_1^2/n_1 + S_2^2/n_2}}$$

2. Obtain the approximate degrees of freedom δ,

$$\delta = \frac{(S_1^2/n_1 + S_2^2/n_2)^2}{(S_1^2/n_1)^2/(n_1 - 1) + (S_2^2/n_2)^2/(n_2 - 1)}.$$

3. Round δ down to the nearest integer, δ^*.
4. Reject H_0 if $t < t_{(\delta^*, \alpha/2)}$ or $t > t_{(\delta^*, 1-\alpha/2)}$, and accept H_0 if $t_{(\delta^*, \alpha/2)} \leq t \leq t_{(\delta^*, 1-\alpha/2)}$.

The p value is calculated in the same manner as before except the approximated degrees of freedom δ^* must be used. If the value of the test statistic

$$t = \frac{(\overline{X}_1 - \overline{X}_2)}{\sqrt{S_1^2/n_1 + S_2^2/n_2}} \leq 0, \text{ then}$$

$$p = 2 \cdot P(t_{(\delta^*)} < t)$$
$$= 2 \cdot (\text{area to the left of } t \text{ under the}$$
$$t \text{ distribution with the degrees of}$$
$$\text{freedom } \delta^*).$$

If the value of the test statistic

$$t = \frac{(\overline{X}_1 - \overline{X}_2)}{\sqrt{S_1^2/n_1 + S_2^2/n_2}} > 0, \text{ then}$$

$$p = 2 \cdot P(t_{(\delta^*)} > t)$$
$$= 2 \cdot (\text{area to the right of } t \text{ under the } t$$
$$\text{distribution with the degrees of}$$
$$\text{freedom } \delta^*).$$

Example 9.4.1. Investigators selected 34 subjects to study the permanent dentition in deciduous anterior crossbites. Based on the radiographs, the subjects were divided into two groups. One group comprised 17 subjects whose anterior crossbite self-corrected during the transitional state (Group A). The other group was composed of 17 subjects whose anterior crossbite persisted during the transitional dentition (Group B) [4]. Lateral cephalometric radiographs were traced to measure posterior facial height in millimeters. Suppose that the distribution of posterior facial height for both groups is normal with unequal variances. What would you conclude from the data about the mean of the posterior facial height of the two groups? The investigators summarized their research data in the table below.

	Group A	Group B
Sample size	$n_1 = 17$	$n_2 = 17$
Sample mean	$\overline{X}_1 = 46.9$	$\overline{X}_2 = 48.7$
Sample variance	$S_1^2 = 4.25$	$S_2^2 = 2.94$

Solution. The hypothesis we wish to test can be stated as $H_0: \mu_1 = \mu_2$ vs. $H_1: \mu_1 \neq \mu_2$. Following the steps described, we compute the test statistic

$$t = \frac{(\overline{X}_1 - \overline{X}_2)}{\sqrt{S_1^2/n_1 + S_2^2/n_2}}$$
$$= \frac{(46.9 - 48.7)}{\sqrt{4.25/17 + 2.94/17}} = -2.7678.$$

To approximate the degrees of freedom, we compute

$$\delta = \frac{(S_1^2/n_1 + S_2^2/n_2)^2}{(S_1^2/n_1)^2/(n_1 - 1) + (S_2^2/n_2)^2/(n_2 - 1)}$$
$$= \frac{(4.25/17 + 2.94/17)^2}{(4.25/17)^2/(17 - 1) + (2.94/17)^2/(17 - 1)}$$
$$= 30.972.$$

By rounding it down to the nearest integer, we get $\delta^* = 30$. Since $t_{(\delta^*, 1-\alpha/2)} = t_{(30, 0.975)} = 2.042$, and $t_{(\delta^*, \alpha/2)} = t_{(30, 0.025)} = -2.042$, and $t = -3.0753 < t_{(30, 0.025)} = -2.042$, we reject the null hypothesis. Group B has a statistically significantly larger mean posterior facial height at the significance level $\alpha = 5\%$. The p value is given by

$$p = 2 \cdot P(t_{(\delta^*)} < t) = 2 \cdot P(t_{(\delta^*)} < -2.7678)$$
$$< 2 \cdot P(t_{(30)} < -2.581) = 0.015.$$

The p value is less than 0.015.

Example 9.4.2. Rheumatoid arthritis (RA) is associated with an increased mortality rate for cardiovascular disease. This may relate to insulin resistance and dyslipidemia, which were both reported to correlate with the acute phase response in RA [5]. A study was conducted to compare the metabolic variables between a control group and an experimental group. The control group was composed of 81 subjects who are free of RA, and the experimental group composed of 83 subjects who suffer from inflammatory arthritis. One of the metabolic variables under investigation was insulin level (μ microunits per milliliter), which is assumed to be normally distributed. Insulin levels were measured for each subject in the study, and their sample mean and sample variances are $\overline{X}_1 = 5.2, \overline{X}_2 = 8.2$ mm, $S_1^2 = 5.29$ and $S_2^2 = 22.09$. Assume that the population variances σ_1^2 and σ_2^2 for the two groups are not equal. Do the two groups have significantly different mean insulin levels?

Solution. By simple substitution we get the values of test statistic and the approximate degrees of freedom,

$$t = \frac{(\overline{X}_1 - \overline{X}_2)}{\sqrt{S_1^2/n_1 + S_2^2/n_2}} = \frac{(5.2 - 8.2)}{\sqrt{5.29/81 + 22.09/83}}$$

$$= -5.2109$$

and

$$\delta^* = \frac{(S_1^2/n_1 + S_2^2/n_2)^2}{(S_1^2/n_1)^2/(n_1 - 1) + (S_2^2/n_2)^2/(n_2 - 1)}$$

$$= \frac{(5.29/81 + 22.09/83)^2}{(5.29/81)^2/(81-1) + (22.09/83)^2/(83-1)}$$

$$= 119.79.$$

By rounding it down to the nearest integer, we get $\delta^* = 119$. The degrees of freedom 119 is not found in the t table. We will take $\delta^* = 120$, which is the closest value in Table E in the Appendix. Since $t_{(\delta^*,1-\alpha/2)} = t_{(120,0.975)} = 1.980$, and $t_{(\delta^*,\alpha/2)} = t_{(120,0.025)} = -1.980$, and the calculated $t = -5.2109 < t_{(120,0.025)} = -1.980$, we reject the null hypothesis. Therefore, we conclude that the patients with inflammatory arthritis have a statistically significantly higher mean insulin level at the significance level $\alpha = 5\%$. The p value can be obtained by

$$p = 2 \cdot P(t_{(\delta^*)} < t) = 2 \cdot P(t_{(120)} < -5.2109)$$
$$< 2 \cdot P(t_{(120)} < -3.373) = 0.001.$$

The p value is less than 0.001. So the difference in mean insulin levels between the control and experimental groups is highly significant.

The examples of two-sample hypothesis testing problems we have discussed in this section and the previous sections are two-tailed tests. Like one-sample cases, two-sample problems can be formulated as one-tailed hypothesis tests.

9.5 THE PAIRED t TEST

Often, experiments in biomedical health sciences are designed so that the sample subjects (experimental units) are measured at baseline and after

treatment, or pre- and post-medical intervention. Examples of this sort of experiment are as follows:

1. To assess a weight loss program, the subject's body mass index is measured before he begins the program at baseline and again at the end of the program.
2. To evaluate a certain regimen of exercise program in reducing blood pressure, the subject's blood pressure is measured before he or she starts the program and at the end of the program.
3. To study the effect of beta carotene on reduction of serum cholesterol, the study subjects are instructed to drink a prescribed amount of beta carotene-rich juice for the duration of the clinical trial. Their serum cholesterol level is measured at baseline and at the end of the trial.
4. Periodontal diseases are caused by putative periodontopathic bacteria in periodontal pockets [6]. To evaluate the efficacy of periodontal treatment in removing periodontopathic bacteria, the number of porphyromonas gingivalis cells at baseline and after the treatment are compared.

In all of the examples described above, measurements are taken on the same subjects at two distinct time points. This type of study is known as **paired sample design**. In a paired sample design, we have a pair of observations for each subject. Each subject acts as his or her own control. Alternatively, investigators can form two study groups, one group of subjects representing those who are not on the weight loss program and another group of subjects representing those who are on the program. These two groups are compared to assess the efficacy of the weight loss program. This type of design is referred to as **cross-sectional design**. Subjects in a cross-sectional design are chosen to be as much alike as possible in terms of their prognostic variables, such as age, sex, or blood pressure. In general, studies with a paired sample design takes much more time to complete and tends to be more expensive than those with a cross-sectional design. But, the paired sample design has a definite advantage in a sense that the same confounding variables that influence the response at baseline will also be present at the end of the study. Therefore, any difference we observe is likely due to the treatment effect. In this section, we assume that the paired sample design is employed.

A study was conducted by an orthodontist to compare pre-treatment to post-treatment changes in patients undergoing fixed orthodontic therapy who have had buccinator release surgery. The alveolar and soft tissue changes in the mandible of the 13 subjects who are of the brachyfacial type were observed [7]. Table 9.5.1 below presents the measurement data on alveolar bone in the area of the symphysis for both pre-orthodontic treatment (X_{1i}) and post-orthodontic treatment (X_{2i}) based on their lateral cephalometric radiographs. Duration of fixed orthodontic treatment was approximately 30 months. The difference in alveolar bone area between pre- and post-treatment is denoted by $D_i = X_{2i} - X_{1i}$.

We assume that the alveolar bone area of the ith subject at baseline is normally distributed with mean μ_i and variance σ^2, and at the end of the treatment is also normally distributed with mean $\mu_i + \delta$ and variance σ^2. Of course, we can assume that the study subjects are statistically independent of each other. We can show that the difference $D_i = X_{2i} - X_{1i}$ is normally distributed with mean δ and variance σ_d^2, that is, $D_i \sim N(\delta, \sigma_d^2)$. Intuitively, if $\delta = 0$, then there is no treatment effect. If $\delta > 0$, then the treatment is associated with an increase in alveolar bone area. If $\delta < 0$, then the treatment is associated with a decrease in alveolar bone area. The hypothesis we wish to test is: $H_0: \delta = 0$ vs. $H_1: \delta \neq 0$. Since δ is the mean of the random variable representing the difference $D_i = X_{2i} - X_{1i}$, the hypothesis test can be considered a one-sample test. As we discussed in Chapter 8, the best test is based on the sample mean $\overline{D}$. The variance σ_D^2 is estimated by the sample variance given by

$$S_D^2 = \frac{\sum_{i=1}^{n}(D_i - \overline{D})^2}{n - 1}.$$

Then the test statistic is $t = \dfrac{\overline{D} - \delta}{S_D/\sqrt{n}}$, which follows a t distribution with the degrees of freedom $(n - 1)$. A test based on this statistic is referred to as a **paired t test**. Under the null hypothesis we have

$$t = \frac{\overline{D}}{S_D/\sqrt{n}} \sim t_{(n-1)}.$$

Thus, a paired t test will proceed just like a one-sample t test. From Table 9.5.1, we obtain the sample mean and sample variance; $\overline{D} = 11.44$, $S_D^2 = 82.47$ ($S_D = 9.08$). The value of the test statistic is given by

$$t = \frac{\overline{D}}{S_D/\sqrt{n}} = \frac{11.44}{9.08/\sqrt{13}} = 4.5427.$$

Because $t_{(12,0.975)} = 2.179 < 4.5427$, we reject H_0 at the significance level $\alpha = 0.05$. The p value is computed the same as the one-sample t test:

$$p = 2 \cdot P(4.5427 \leq t_{(12)}) < 2 \cdot P(4.318 \leq t_{(12)})$$
$$= 2(1 - 0.9995) = 0.001.$$

The p value is slightly smaller than 0.001. We can conclude that the alveolar bone area for the patients undergoing fixed orthodontic therapy, who have had buccinator release surgery, is statistically significantly larger.

Instead of defining the difference by $D_i = X_{2i} - X_{1i}$, we can subtract the follow-up measurements from baseline measurements so that we have $D_i = X_{1i} - X_{2i}$. Then the sample mean $\overline{D}$ will be -11.44 and the sample variance will remain the same $S_D^2 = 82.47$. The value of the test statistic will be $t = \dfrac{\overline{D}}{S_D/\sqrt{n}} = -4.5427 < t_{(12,0.025)} = -2.179$. By symmetry property of a t distribution, the p value is the same as before:

$$p = 2 \cdot P(4.5427 \leq t_{(12)})$$
$$= 2 \cdot P(t_{(12)} \leq -4.5427) < 0.001.$$

Table 9.5.1. Alveolar bone area (mm^2), pre- and post-treatment.

Subject	Pre-treatment (X_{1i})	Post-treatment (X_{2i})	$D_i = X_{2i} - X_{1i}$
1	57.16	62.65	5.49
2	50.38	72.01	21.63
3	70.67	79.17	8.50
4	89.53	122.12	32.59
5	62.18	62.01	−0.17
6	64.82	73.97	9.15
7	79.89	85.19	5.30
8	92.03	97.47	5.44
9	78.22	88.84	10.62
10	86.66	96.0	9.34
11	97.86	102.75	4.89
12	93.69	106.84	13.15
13	65.81	88.64	22.83

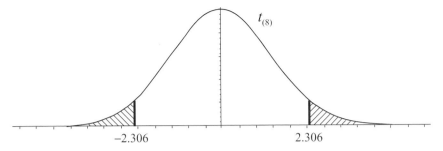

$t_{(8)}$

-2.306 2.306

Figure 9.5.1 Rejection and acceptance regions for the paired *t* test in Example 9.5.1.

Hence, the conclusion is the same as before, that is, we reject the null hypothesis.

Example 9.5.1. Agents with carbamide peroxide (CP) in various concentrations are widely prescribed for at-home tooth whitening. A study was conducted to evaluate the efficacy of a 10% CP with nine human subjects with maxillary anterior teeth. All of the study subjects underwent a professional prophylaxis and were given specific instructions regarding at-home use of a 10% CP tooth-whitening agent. They were required to use it for 2 weeks. Tooth shade index of their central incisors was measured at baseline and after the 2-week study period. It is assumed that the distribution of tooth shade index is normal. The following table summarizes the data. Would you be able to conclude that the 10% CP tooth-whitening agent is effective?

Subject	Baseline (X_{1i})	After 2-week Treatment (X_{2i})	$D_i = X_{2i} - X_{1i}$
1	14	21	7
2	16	15	-1
3	14	18	4
4	17	19	2
5	18	15	-3
6	11	18	7
7	15	22	7
8	13	16	3
9	12	14	2

Solution. We compute the sample mean and the sample SD of D_i from the data; $\overline{D} = 3.1111$, and $S_D = 3.5862$. The test statistic $t = \dfrac{\overline{D}}{S_D/\sqrt{n}}$ has a *t* distribution with the degrees of freedom

$n - 1 = 8$, and its observed value is obtained by

$$t = \frac{\overline{D}}{S_D/\sqrt{n}} = \frac{3.1111}{3.5862/\sqrt{9}} = 2.6026.$$

Because $t_{(8,0.975)} = 2.306 < t = 2.6026$, the null hypothesis H_0 is rejected. The *p* value is obtained by

$$p = 2 \cdot P(2.6026 \le t_{(8)}) < 2 \cdot P(2.449 \le t_{(8)})$$
$$= 2(1 - 0.98) = 0.04.$$

The *p* value is less than 0.04. We conclude that the 10% CP tooth-whitening agent is significantly effective at the significance level $\alpha = 0.05$. Rejection and acceptance regions for the paired *t* test are shown in Figure 9.5.1.

Example 9.5.2. Chronic leukemia involves an overgrowth of mature blood cells and is more common among patients who are 40–70 years of age. The most common treatment for leukemia is chemotherapy, which may involve one or a combination of antineoplastic drugs that destroy cancer cells. Researchers suspect that the treatment may lower the level of hemoglobin, the oxygen-carrying red pigment of the red blood corpuscles. Eight leukemia patients who underwent the treatment were selected to test the investigators' hypothesis. Each patient's hemoglobin was measured at baseline and at the end of the first course of the treatment. Determination of the hemoglobin content of the blood was done by using the Sahli method (g/100 ml). The following is the data the investigators collected. If the hemoglobin content is approximately normally distributed, would you conclude that the chemotherapy has a significant effect on the level of hemoglobin?

Subject	Baseline (X_i)	After Chemotherapy Treatment (Y_i)	$D_i = X_i - Y_i$
1	15.4	13.8	1.6
2	16.7	15.4	1.3
3	15.5	14.1	1.4
4	16.2	13.9	2.3
5	14.2	14.0	0.2
6	16.5	—	—
7	14.8	14.5	0.3
8	14.5	13.4	1.1

Solution. Two observations at two distinct time points were made for each subject. Thus, a paired t test is appropriate. The hypothesis to be tested is $H_0: \delta = 0$ vs. $H_1: \delta \neq 0$. The follow-up observation for subject number 6 is missing because the patient was unable to complete the treatment. Therefore, this patient is deleted from the study. Consequently, the sample size is $n = 7$. We compute the sample mean and the sample SD of the difference $D_i = X_i - Y_i$ from the data, and obtain $\overline{D} = 1.1714$ and $S_D = 0.7342$. The test statistic $t = \frac{\overline{D}}{S_D/\sqrt{n}}$ has a t distribution with the degrees of freedom $n - 1 = 6$, and its observed value is obtained by

$$t = \frac{\overline{D}}{S_D/\sqrt{n}} = \frac{1.1714}{0.7342/\sqrt{7}} = 4.2212.$$

Because $t_{(6,0.975)} = 2.447 < t = 4.2212$, the null hypothesis H_0 is rejected. The p value is obtained by:

$$p = 2 \cdot P(4.2212 \leq t_{(6)}) < 2 \cdot P(3.707 \leq t_{(6)})$$
$$= 2(1 - 0.995) = 0.01.$$

The p value is less than 0.01. We conclude that the leukemia treatment significantly lowers the hemoglobin level at the significance level $\alpha = 0.05$. The p value is depicted in Figure 9.5.2.

9.6 Z TEST FOR COMPARING TWO BINOMIAL PROPORTIONS

There are many problems in biomedical health sciences in which an observed difference between two sample proportions can be attributed to chance alone or in which the difference represents the true difference that exists between the corresponding population proportions. We illustrate some examples:

1. The Department of Public Health scientists suspect that the proportion of the chronic leukemia patients in an urban area is different from that in a rural area.
2. The proportion of patients who prefer to be treated by female dentists and physicians is higher than that of patients who prefer to be treated by male counterparts.
3. The proportion of impaired bone healing and/or necrosis during implant osteotomy is higher under prolonged exposure to high temperature than that under lower temperature.

Let p_1 be the proportion (probability) of the patients who experience impaired bone healing or necrosis during implant osteotomy as a result of prolonged exposure to high temperature and p_2 be the proportion of patients exposed to lower temperature. Then the hypothesis-testing problem can be stated as follows:

$$H_0: p_1 = p_2 \text{ vs. } H_1: p_1 \neq p_2,$$
$$H_0: p_1 \leq p_2 \text{ vs. } H_1: p_1 > p_2, \text{ or}$$
$$H_0: p_1 \geq p_2 \text{ vs. } H_1: p_1 < p_2.$$

Statisticians use two methods to compare two binomial proportions: a hypothesis-testing approach and a contingency table approach. The contingency table approach will be discussed in Chapter 10. Both methods yield the same p value.

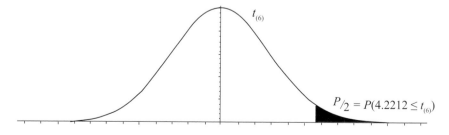

Figure 9.5.2 The p value for the paired t test in Example 9.5.2.

In this sense, the two methods are equivalent. In this section, we discuss the method of testing hypotheses. Our discussion is focused on the two-tailed test: H_0: $p_1 = p_2$ vs. H_1: $p_1 \neq p_2$. This is an extension of the one-sample test for a binomial proportion that we introduced in Section 8.7. By subtracting p_2 from both sides of the null and alternative hypotheses, we can state an equivalent hypothesis, H_0:$p_1 - p_2 = 0$ vs. H_1: $p_1 - p_2 \neq 0$. To test the hypothesis we take two random samples of size n_1 and n_2 from two independent populations whose unknown true proportions of our interest are p_1 and p_2, respectively. Let X_1 and X_2 be the number of events in the first and the second samples. As we discussed in Section 8.4, $\hat{p}_1 = \frac{X_1}{n_1}$ and $\hat{p}_2 = \frac{X_2}{n_2}$. It is reasonable to construct the significance test based on $\hat{p}_1 - \hat{p}_2$. Intuitively, if the sample difference $\hat{p}_1 - \hat{p}_2$ is very large or very small (a large negative value), the null hypothesis would be rejected. If it is very close to zero, then H_0 would be accepted, since it is an indication that the null hypothesis might be true. As before, we assume that the sample sizes are sufficiently large enough so that the normal approximation to the binomial distribution is valid. We can show that under H_0, $\hat{p}_1$ and $\hat{p}_2$ are approximately normally distributed with mean p and variance $\frac{pq}{n_1}$ and $\frac{pq}{n_2}$:

$$\hat{p}_1 \overset{\circ}{\sim} N\left(p, \frac{pq}{n_1}\right), \quad \text{and} \quad \hat{p}_2 \overset{\circ}{\sim} N\left(p, \frac{pq}{n_2}\right).$$

Furthermore, we can show that, since two samples are independent, the sample difference $\hat{p}_1 - \hat{p}_2$ is approximately normally distributed with mean 0 and variance $\frac{pq}{n_1} + \frac{pq}{n_2} = pq\left(\frac{1}{n_1} + \frac{1}{n_2}\right)$,

$$\hat{p}_1 - \hat{p}_2 \overset{\circ}{\sim} N\left(0, pq\left(\frac{1}{n_1} + \frac{1}{n_2}\right)\right).$$

By dividing $\hat{p}_1 - \hat{p}_2$ by the SD $\sqrt{pq\left(\frac{1}{n_1} + \frac{1}{n_2}\right)}$, we have

$$Z = \frac{\hat{p}_1 - \hat{p}_2}{\sqrt{pq\left(\frac{1}{n_1} + \frac{1}{n_2}\right)}} \overset{\circ}{\sim} N(0, 1).$$

A test based on this statistic is a Z test. To compute the test statistic, we have to estimate the proportion

p ($q = 1 - p$). The estimate is given by:

$$\hat{p} = \frac{X_1 + X_2}{n_1 + n_2} = \frac{n_1(X_1/n_1) + n_2(X_2/n_2)}{n_1 + n_2}$$
$$= \frac{n_1\hat{p}_1 + n_2\hat{p}_2}{n_1 + n_2}.$$

A simple algebraic manipulation shows that the estimate $\hat{p}$ is a weighted average of $\hat{p}_1$ and $\hat{p}_2$, and $\hat{q} = 1 - \hat{p}$. The sample mean associated with a larger sample size is given a greater weight. We have just reduced the two-sample test for comparing binomial proportions to a simple Z test.

Example 9.6.1. A study was done to compare the proportion of urban and suburban children in the United States who have early onset juvenile periodontitis (EOJP). Investigators randomly selected 130 urban children and 145 suburban children younger than 7 years of age and gave them a periodontal examination. The results of the examination indicated that 12 of the urban children and 16 of the suburban children had EOJP. The investigators hypothesized that there would be no difference in the proportion between the two populations. Given this information, what could you conclude?

Solution. Let p_1 and p_2 denote the proportion of urban and suburban children, respectively, with EOJP. The hypotheses of our interest is H_0: $p_1 = p_2$ vs. H_1: $p_1 \neq p_2$. From the given information, we have $n_1 = 130$, $n_2 = 145$, $X_1 = 12$, and $X_2 = 16$. Thus, the sample proportions are $\hat{p}_1 = \frac{12}{130} = 0.092$ and $\hat{p}_2 = \frac{16}{145} = 0.110$. The estimate $\hat{p}$ is given by $\hat{p} = \frac{X_1 + X_2}{n_1 + n_2} = \frac{12+16}{130+145} = 0.102$. So $\hat{q} = 1 - 0.102 = 0.898$. By replacing p and q by their estimates $\hat{p} = 0.102$ and $\hat{q} = 0.898$ in the denominator, the value of the test statistic is obtained by:

$$Z = \frac{\hat{p}_1 - \hat{p}_2}{\sqrt{pq\left(\frac{1}{n_1} + \frac{1}{n_2}\right)}}$$
$$= \frac{0.092 - 0.110}{\sqrt{(0.102)(0.898)\left(\frac{1}{130} + \frac{1}{145}\right)}} = -0.4924.$$

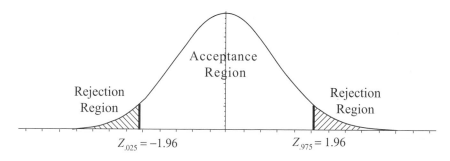

Figure 9.6.1   The rejection and acceptace regions for the test in Example 9.6.1.

Since $Z_{0.025} = -1.96 < -0.4924 < Z_{0.975} = 1.96$, we accept the null hypothesis at the significance level $\alpha = 0.05$. The p value is given by $p = 2 \cdot P(Z \leq -0.4924) > 2 \cdot P(Z \leq -0.50) = 0.6170$. The actual p value is slightly larger than 0.6170. We conclude that there is no statistically significant difference in the proportion of suburban children with EOJP and that for urban children with the p value a little larger than 0.6170. The rejection and acceptance regions for this test are illustrated in Figure 9.6.1.

Example 9.6.2. A study of comparative effects of two sedatives, Nembutal and diazepam, on anterograde amnesia was performed. The anterograde amnesia was assessed with the help of flash cards and a musical note to test the audiovisual memory of the patient during the surgical procedure [8]. Suppose that 46 of the 48 patients, who were exposed to IV sedation using Nembutal, experienced short-term memory loss, and 51 of the 62 patients, who were sedated with diazepam, experienced short-term memory loss. Anesthesiologists suspect that there is no difference in the proportion of patients who have a negative effect of amnesia between the two sedatives. Do the data support their suspicion? Test your hypothesis.

Solution. Let p_1 and p_2 denote the proportion of patients who experienced memory loss after being sedated using Nembutal and diazepam, respectively. The hypotheses of our interest is

$$H_0 : p_1 = p_2 \text{ vs. } H_1 : p_1 \neq p_2.$$

From the given data, we have the sample proportions $\hat{p}_1 = \frac{46}{48} = 0.9583$ and $\hat{p}_2 = \frac{51}{62} = 0.8226$.

The estimate $\hat{p}$ is obtained by $\hat{p} = \frac{X_1 + X_2}{n_1 + n_2} = \frac{46+51}{48+62} = 0.8818$ So $\hat{q} = 1 - 0.8818 = 0.1182$. By substituting p and q with their estimates $\hat{p} = 0.8818$ and $\hat{q} = 0.1182$ in the denominator, the value of the test statistic is computed:

$$Z = \frac{\hat{p}_1 - \hat{p}_2}{\sqrt{pq\left(\dfrac{1}{n_1} + \dfrac{1}{n_2}\right)}}$$

$$= \frac{0.9583 - 0.8226}{\sqrt{(0.8818)(0.1182)\left(\dfrac{1}{48} + \dfrac{1}{62}\right)}} = 2.1863$$

Since $Z_{0.975} = 1.96 < 2.1863$, we reject the null hypothesis at the significance level $\alpha = 0.05$. The p value is given by $p = 2 \cdot P(2.1863 \leq Z) < 2 \cdot P(2.18 \leq Z) = 0.0292$. The actual p value is slightly less than 0.0292. We conclude that the proportion of the Nembutal-sedated patients who lose their memory is significantly higher than that of the diazepam-sedated patients who experience a short-term memory loss, with the p value approximately equal to 0.0292.

9.7 THE SAMPLE SIZE AND POWER OF A TWO-SAMPLE TEST

9.7.1 Estimation of Sample Size

Determination of sample size for the one-sample Z test was presented in Section 8.6. When investigators design a research project, estimation of a sample size is one of the first key issues. We will introduce a method of sample size estimation for comparing two normal means, μ_1 and μ_2. Consider the case where we have equal sample sizes ($n = n_1 = n_2$) for two random samples for a two-sample Z test. The question investigators most frequently ask is "How large should n be for a two-sample Z test at the significance level $\alpha = 0.05$ in order to achieve the power of $1 - \beta$?" Assuming that the variances σ_1^2 and σ_2^2 are known, the required sample size n for each sample for a two-tailed Z test is given by

$$n = \frac{(\sigma_1^2 + \sigma_2^2) \cdot (Z_{1-\alpha/2} + Z_{1-\beta})^2}{(\mu_1 - \mu_2)^2},$$

where μ_1, σ_1^2 and μ_2, σ_2^2 are the mean and variance of the two independent normal populations, $N(\mu_1, \sigma_1^2)$ and $N(\mu_2, \sigma_2^2)$. As in the one-sample case, the researchers have to specify the amount of the mean difference $|\mu_1 - \mu_2|$ they wish the test to detect. For a one-tailed test, simply replace $Z_{1-\alpha/2}$ by $Z_{1-\alpha}$ in the formula. In many cases it is impractical to expect the two groups to have equal sample sizes. For instance, there may be twice as many non-smokers as there are smokers, the number of patients who floss their teeth daily is far less than those who do not floss, or there might be five times as many non-vegetarians as there are vegetarians. We wish to determine unequal sample sizes to achieve a predetermined level of power. Let $k > 0$ be some number such that $n_1 = k \cdot n_2$. The required sample sizes for a two-tailed Z test for achieving a power $1 - \beta$ are given as follows:

For sample size n_1 of first sample from $N(\mu_1, \sigma_1^2)$

$$n_1 = \frac{(\sigma_1^2 + k \cdot \sigma_2^2) \cdot (Z_{1-\alpha/2} + Z_{1-\beta})^2}{\delta^2}, \text{ and}$$

for sample size n_2 of second sample from $N(\mu_2, \sigma_2^2)$

$$n_2 = \frac{\left(\dfrac{\sigma_1^2}{k} + \sigma_2^2\right) \cdot (Z_{1-\alpha/2} + Z_{1-\beta})^2}{\delta^2}$$

where $\delta = (\mu_1 - \mu_2)$ and $k = \dfrac{n_1}{n_2}$. For a one-tailed test, replace $Z_{1-\alpha/2}$ by $Z_{1-\alpha}$ in the formula.

The mean difference $\delta = (\mu_1 - \mu_2)$ between μ_1 and μ_2 usually is prespecified by the investigators. This is the minimum amount of the difference they wish to detect using a significance test.

Example 9.7.1. Suppose we are interested in comparing two groups of patients with respect to plaque scores, which are represented in percentage. The first group will be given an antibacterial chlorhexidine mouthwash by the periodontists during periodontal treatments to determine if chlorhexidine is effective in reducing plaque scores. The second group will receive no chlorhexidine. In a small pilot study, we obtained $\overline{X}_1 = 18.4$, $S_1^2 = 72.2$, and $\overline{X}_2 = 22.2$, $S_2^2 = 86.1$. Determine an appropriate sample size for the future study using a two-tailed test at the significance level $\alpha = 0.05$ and for achieving a power of 90%. We may assume that plaque scores are normally distributed.

Solution. We have $Z_{0.975} = 1.96$, and $Z_{1-\beta} = Z_{0.90} = 1.282$. By substituting the sample data, $\overline{X}_1 = 18.4$, $S_1^2 = 72.2$, and $\overline{X}_2 = 22.2$, $S_2^2 = 86.1$, we get

$$
\begin{aligned}
n &= \frac{(\sigma_1^2 + \sigma_2^2) \cdot (Z_{1-\alpha/2} + Z_{1-\beta})^2}{(\mu_1 - \mu_2)^2} \\
&= \frac{(72.2 + 86.1) \cdot (1.96 + 1.282)^2}{(18.4 - 22.2)^2} = 115.22.
\end{aligned}
$$

The required sample size to achieve 90% power in a two-tailed test is $n = 116$ for each group.

Example 9.7.2. Investigators wish to perform a study to compare the effects of full mouth root planing with antibiotics on probing depth in smokers versus non-smokers. Two groups will be selected such that the first group is composed of non-smokers and the second group consists of smokers who smoke at least 10 cigarettes per day. At the end of the 6-month trial period, each subject's probing depths will be measured. Suppose that the distribution of probing depths is approximately normal. From a similar study reported in the literature, we get $S_1^2 = 3.5$ and $S_2^2 = 4.4$. The investigators wish to detect the mean difference of 1.2 mm. Let's assume there are three times as many non-smokers as there are smokers, that is, $n_1 = 3 \cdot n_2$ ($k = 3$). What are the required sample sizes if a two-tailed test with $\alpha = 0.05$ is planned to achieve 95% power?

Solution. Using $Z_{1-\beta} = Z_{0.95} = 1.645$, and by substituting the sample values, we get

$$n_1 = \frac{(\sigma_1^2 + k \cdot \sigma_2^2) \cdot (Z_{1-\alpha/2} + Z_{1-\beta})^2}{\delta^2}$$

$$= \frac{(3.5 + 3 \cdot 4.4) \cdot (1.96 + 1.645)^2}{(1.2)^2} = 150.72,$$

and

$$n_2 = \frac{\left(\dfrac{\sigma_1^2}{k} + \sigma_2^2\right) \cdot (Z_{1-\alpha/2} + Z_{1-\beta})^2}{\delta^2}$$

$$= \frac{\left(\dfrac{3.5}{3} + 4.4\right) \cdot (1.96 + 1.645)^2}{(1.2)^2} = 50.239.$$

We need 151 non-smokers and 51 smokers for the study.

9.7.2 The Power of a Two-Sample Test

Calculation of the power for a one-sample case was presented in Section 8.6 for both one-tailed and two-tailed tests. As defined in Section 8.6, the power of a test is the conditional probability of rejecting H_0, given that H_0 is false: $1 - \beta = P(\text{reject } H_0 \mid H_0 \text{ is false})$. The formula for computing the power of a two-tailed test at the significance level $\alpha = 0.05$ is expressed as follows.

Given the hypotheses H_0: $\mu_1 = \mu_2$ vs. H_1: $\mu_1 \neq \mu_2$ to compare two normal means, μ_1 and μ_2, the power of a two-tailed test at the significance level $\alpha = 0.05$ can be expressed

Power

$$= P\left(Z \leq -Z_{1-\alpha/2} + \frac{\delta \cdot \sqrt{k}}{\sqrt{(\sigma_1^2/n_1) + (\sigma_2^2/n_2)}}\right)$$

where $\delta = |\mu_1 - \mu_2|$ and $k = \dfrac{n_1}{n_2}$. For a one-tailed test, replace $Z_{1-\alpha/2}$ by $Z_{1-\alpha}$ in the formula.

We note that σ_1^2 and σ_2^2 are usually not known. Therefore, they have to be estimated from the data. Keep in mind that the power of a test depends on a number of factors, such as α, n_1, n_2, k, δ, σ_1^2 and σ_2^2.

Example 9.7.3. Suppose that a study is planned to compare the effectiveness of two brands of indirect bonding adhesives for ceramic brackets. The effectiveness of the materials is assessed by measuring the bond strength with shearing forces. For the experiment, 25 human teeth were extracted (maxillary incisors) and each will be used for brand A and brand B, that is, $n_1 = 25$ and $n_2 = 25$. Suppose the distribution of the bond strength is normal. From the manufacturer's brochure we have $\sigma_1 = 8.4$ and $\sigma_2 = 9.7$. If $\delta = 10$ (Newton), what is the power of a two-tailed test at the significance level $\alpha = 5\%$.

Solution. Since $n_1 = n_2 = 25$, $k = 1$, and $Z_{1-\alpha/2} = Z_{0.975} = 1.96$, using the formula given above

Power

$$= P\left(Z \leq -Z_{1-\alpha/2} + \frac{\delta \cdot \sqrt{k}}{\sqrt{(\sigma_1^2/n_1) + (\sigma_2^2/n_2)}}\right)$$

$$= P\left(Z \leq -1.96 + \frac{10 \cdot \sqrt{1}}{\sqrt{(8.4)^2/25) + (9.7^2/25)}}\right)$$

$$= P(Z \leq 1.9366) = 0.9736.$$

Hence, there is about 97.36% chance of detecting a significant difference using a two-tailed test at the significance level $\alpha = 5\%$. Using a one-tailed test,

Power

$$= P\left(Z \leq -Z_{1-\alpha} + \frac{\delta \cdot \sqrt{k}}{\sqrt{(\sigma_1^2/n_1) + (\sigma_2^2/n_2)}}\right)$$

$$= P\left(Z \leq -1.645 + \frac{10 \cdot \sqrt{1}}{\sqrt{(8.4)^2/25) + (9.7^2/25)}}\right)$$

$$= P(Z \leq 2.2516) = 0.9878.$$

There is about a 98.78% chance of detecting a significant difference at the significance level $\alpha = 5\%$.

Example 9.7.4. Acute chest syndrome is an acute pulmonic process in patients with sickle cell disease. Sickle cell diagnosis is made on the standard hemoglobin electrophoresis. Between January, 2001 and December, 2001, 28 boys and 22 girls were admitted to the pediatric ward. To compare the hemoglobin level (grams per deciliter) of two groups, pediatricians calculated the sample mean and sample variance of their hemoglobin, which is assumed to be normally distributed: $\overline{X}_1 = 8.1$, $S_1^2 = 4.0$ and $\overline{X}_2 = 9.3$, $S_2^2 = 5.3$. Estimate the power of a two-tailed test at the significance level $\alpha = 5\%$.

Solution. From the given information, we have $n_1 = 28$, $n_2 = 22$, and $k = \dfrac{n_1}{n_2} = \dfrac{28}{22} = 1.27$.

Thus,

Power

$$= P\left(Z \le -1.96 + \frac{|8.1 - 9.3| \cdot \sqrt{1.27}}{\sqrt{4.0/28) + 5.3/22}}\right)$$

$$= P\left(Z \le -1.96 + \frac{(1.2) \cdot \sqrt{1.27}}{\sqrt{4.0/28) + 5.3/22}}\right)$$

$$= P(Z \le 0.2230) = 0.5880.$$

Thus, a two-tailed test has about a 58.8% chance of detecting a significant difference.

9.8 THE F TEST FOR THE EQUALITY OF TWO VARIANCES

So far in this chapter, our discussions have been focused on comparisons of two independent normal means and two binomial proportions. In Section 8.8 we introduced the one-sample χ^2 test for the variance of a normal distribution. We now turn our attention to comparing the variances of two independent normal populations. The hypotheses of our interest is

$$H_0 : \sigma_1^2 = \sigma_2^2 \quad \text{vs.} \quad H_1 : \sigma_1^2 \ne \sigma_2^2$$

where σ_1^2 and σ_2^2 are the variances of two independent normal distributions, $N(\mu_1, \sigma_1^2)$ and $N(\mu_2, \sigma_2^2)$. Suppose that random samples of sizes n_1 and n_2 are taken from $N(\mu_1, \sigma_1^2)$ and $N(\mu_2, \sigma_2^2)$,

respectively. We obtain estimates S_1^2 and S_2^2 of σ_1^2 and σ_2^2. To test the hypothesis, it seems reasonable to compare the estimates in terms of the ratio, S_1^2/S_2^2. In fact, we can show that the statistics

$$F = \frac{S_1^2/\sigma_1^2}{S_2^2/\sigma_2^2}$$

has the F distribution with the degrees of freedom, $n_1 - 1$ and $n_2 - 1$. As usual, we denote

$$F = \frac{S_1^2/\sigma_1^2}{S_2^2/\sigma_2^2} \sim F_{(n_1-1, n_2-1)}.$$

The degrees of freedom $n_1 - 1$ is associated with the numerator S_1^2/σ_1^2, and $n_2 - 1$ is associated with the denominator S_2^2/σ_2^2. Along with the normal distribution, t distribution, and χ^2 distribution, the F distribution is an important distribution in the study of statistical inferences. Under the null hypothesis that $\sigma_1^2 = \sigma_2^2$, we get

$$F = \frac{S_1^2/\sigma_1^2}{S_2^2/\sigma_2^2} = \frac{S_1^2}{S_2^2} \sim F_{(n_1-1, n_2-1)}.$$

Recall from Section 8.8 that $\dfrac{(n-1)S^2}{\sigma^2}$ has the χ^2 distribution with $n - 1$ degrees of freedom. So the F distribution with the degrees of freedom, $n_1 - 1$ and $n_2 - 1$ is the ratio of two independent χ^2 distributions with degrees of freedom $n_1 - 1$ and $n_2 - 1$, respectively. Like the χ^2 distribution, the F distribution is positively skewed with a long tail on the right. See Figure 9.8.1 below.

The percentiles of the F distribution are provided in Table G in the Appendix. The first column in Table G lists the denominator degrees of freedom, the values in the second column indicate the probabilities, the numbers across the top of Table G are the numerator degrees of freedom, and the rest of the entry values in the table are the

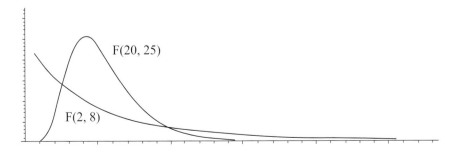

Figure 9.8.1 F densities with $F_{(2,8)}$ and $F_{(20,25)}$.

corresponding percentile points. Let δ_1 and δ_2 be the degrees of freedom. Then the $100 \times p^{th}$ percentile of $F_{(\delta_1, \delta_2)}$ is denoted by

$$P(F_{(\delta_1, \delta_2)} \leq F_{(\delta_1, \delta_2;p)}) = p.$$

Example 9.8.1.
(i) Find the upper 5th percentile of an F distribution with degrees of freedom 8 and 5.
(ii) Find the 90th percentile of an F distribution with degrees of freedom 25 and 30.

Solution.
(i) $P(F_{(8,5)} \leq F_{(8,5;0.95)}) = 4.818$.
(ii) $P(F_{(25,30)} \leq F_{(25,30;0.90)}) = 1.632$.

Table G provides only the upper percentile points of the F distribution. The lower percentile points of the F distribution can be derived from the corresponding upper percentile points by the following simple formula:

$$F_{(\delta_1, \delta_2;p)} = \frac{1}{F_{(\delta_2, \delta_1;1-p)}}.$$

The formula indicates that the lower p^{th} percentile of an F distribution with the degrees of freedom δ_1 and δ_2 is the reciprocal of the upper p^{th} percentile of an F distribution with the degrees of freedom δ_2 and δ_1. Remember the degrees of freedom are reversed.

Example 9.8.2. Find (i) $F_{(7,12;0.025)}$ and (ii) $P(F_{(18,16)} \leq 2.302)$.

Solution. Using the formula discussed above, we can write

(i) $F_{(7,12;0.025)} = \dfrac{1}{F_{(12,7;1-0.025)}} = \dfrac{1}{F_{(12,7;0.975)}}$

$= \dfrac{1}{4.666} = 0.2143$.

(ii) $P(F_{(18,16)} \leq 2.302) = 0.95$ from Table G in the Appendix.

We can now perform a significance test for the equality of two variances. It is helpful to keep in mind that the samples are drawn from two independent normal populations. As noted earlier, the test will be based on the ratio of the sample variances S_1^2/S_2^2. If S_1^2/S_2^2 is close to 1.0, it would be an indication that there is no difference between the variances, in which case H_0 will be accepted. On the other hand, if S_1^2/S_2^2 is very large or close to 0, then it would be an indication that the variances are different, in which case H_0 will be rejected. A test based on the statistic S_1^2/S_2^2 for testing the equality of two variances is called an F **test**. We formalize this heuristic argument below.

The F Test for the Equality of Two Normal Variances

For testing the hypothesis $H_0 : \sigma_1^2 = \sigma_2^2$ vs. $H_1 : \sigma_1^2 \neq \sigma_2^2$ at the significance level $\alpha = 0.05$, compute the value of the test statistic $F = \dfrac{S_1^2}{S_2^2}$.

Reject H_0 if $F < F_{(n_1-1, \ n_2-1,\alpha/2)}$ or $F > F_{(n_1-1, n_2-1,1-\alpha/2)}$.

Accept H_0 if $F_{(n_1-1, \ n_2-1,\alpha/2)} \leq F \leq F_{(n_1-1, n_2-1,1-\alpha/2)}$.

The p value of the test is given by the following:

If $F = S_1^2/S_2^2 \geq 1.0$, then $p = 2 \cdot P(F_{(n_1-1,n_2-1)} \geq F)$.
If $F = S_1^2/S_2^2 < 1.0$, then $p = 2 \cdot P(F_{(n_1-1,n_2-1)} < F)$.

The rejection and acceptance regions and the p value of the test are illustrated in Figures 9.8.2, 9.8.3, and 9.8.4.

Example 9.8.3. Direct bonding of orthodontic brackets to etched enamel is widely used by orthodontists and pediatric dentists. An investigation

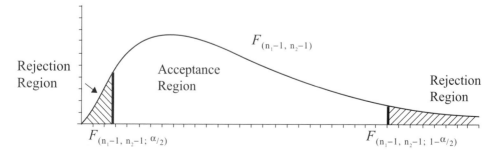

Figure 9.8.2 Rejection and acceptance regions of the F test.

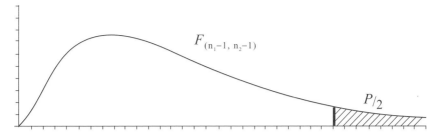

Figure 9.8.3 The p value of the F test when $F \geq 1$.

was performed to evaluate the shear bond strength of brackets fixed to enamel that has been etched for 15 or 60 seconds. For this investigation, 47 recently extracted human premolars were randomly divided into two groups. Group A, composed of 21 premolars, was etched for 15 seconds, and Group B composed of 26 premolars for 60 seconds. A 37% phosphoric acid solution was used for etching. The force required to dislodge the bracket was measured for each sample, and the respective variances were estimated by $S_1^2 = 18.92$ and $S_2^2 = 18.06$ [9]. Suppose the bond strength is normally distributed. Using the significance level $\alpha = 5\%$, test if there is a significant difference between the two variances.

Solution. Since $n_1 = 21$, and $n_2 = 26$, the degrees of freedom are 20 for the numerator and 25 for the denominator. The observed test statistic is

$$F = \frac{S_1^2}{S_2^2} = \frac{18.92}{18.06} = 1.0476.$$

The critical values are $F_{(n_1-1, \ n_2-1, 1-\alpha/2)} = F_{(20,25,0.975)} = 2.300$, and

$$F_{(n_1-1, n_2-1, \alpha/2)} = F_{(20,25,0.025)} = \frac{1}{F_{(25,20,0.975)}}$$

$$= \frac{1}{2.396} = 0.4174.$$

Because $F = 1.0476$ and $F_{(20,25,0.025)} = 0.4174 < F < F_{(20,25,0.975)} = 2.396$, we accept the null hypothesis. Let's compute the p value. Since $F = S_1^2/S_2^2 = 1.0476 > 1.0$, we have

$$p = 2 \cdot P(F_{(n_1-1,n_2-1)} > F)$$

$$= 2 \cdot P(F_{(20,25)} > 1.0476) \approx 1.0.$$

The p value is almost 1.0. Thus, we accept H_0 and conclude that there is no statistically significant difference in variance of the shear bond strength between 15- and 60-second etching.

Example 9.8.4. High levels of serum lipoprotein have been associated with an increased risk of coronary artery disease (CAD), but this association is not confirmed in older patients who are at least 65 years of age. To study the relation of lipoprotein as a coronary risk factor to type II diabetes mellitus and low-density lipoprotein cholesterol in these patients, 70 patients with CAD and 330 patients without CAD were examined and their lipoprotein levels (milligrams per deciliter) were recorded. Their sample SDs were $S_1 = 19.0$ and $S_2 = 19.4$ [10]. Assume that the levels of serum lipoprotein are normally distributed. Do these two groups have significantly different variances of levels of serum lipoprotein?

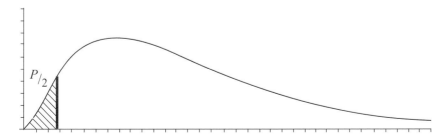

Figure 9.8.4 The p value of the F test when $F < 1$.

Solution. The hypothesis we wish to test is $H_0 : \sigma_1^2 = \sigma_2^2$ vs. $H_1 : \sigma_1^2 \neq \sigma_2^2$. Since $n_1 = 70$, and $n_2 = 330$, the degrees of freedom are 69 for the numerator and 329 for the denominator. Using $S_1 = 19.0$ and $S_2 = 19.4$, the observed test statistic can be calculated

$$F = \frac{S_1^2}{S_2^2} = \frac{(19.0)^2}{(19.4)^2} = 0.9592$$

The critical values are $F_{(n_1-1,\ n_2-1,1-\alpha/2)} = F_{(69,329,0.975)} = 1.363$ (approximated by linear interpolation explained below), and

$$F_{(n_1-1,n_2-1,\alpha/2)} = F_{(69,329,0.025)} = \frac{1}{F_{(329,69,0.975)}}$$

$$= \frac{1}{1.415}, \text{ by approximation}$$

$$= 0.7067.$$

Because $F = 0.9592$ and $F_{(69,329,0.025)} = 0.7067 < F < F_{(69,329,0.975)} = 1.363$, we accept the null hypothesis. Let's compute the p value. Since $F = S_1^2/S_2^2 = 0.9592 < 1.0$, we have

$$p = 2 \cdot P(F_{(n_1-1,n_2-1)} < F)$$

$$= 2 \cdot P(F_{(69,329)} < 0.9592) \approx 1.0.$$

Hence, there is no significant difference in variance between the patients with CAD and the patients without CAD.

Table G does not provide the corresponding percentile points to the degrees of freedom 69 and 329; therefore, we will first approximate $F_{(69,329,0.975)}$ by $F_{(70,\infty,0.975)}$. From the table we obtain $F_{(60,\infty,0.975)} = 1.388$, and $F_{(90,\infty,0.975)} = 1.313$. The distance between $F_{(60,\infty,0.975)}$ and $F_{(90,\infty,0.975)}$ is $1.388 - 1.313 = 0.075$. Since the degrees of freedom for the numerator of $F_{(70,\infty,0.975)}$ is 70, we get $(70 - 60)/(90 - 60) = 1/3$. To approximate $F_{(70,\infty,0.975)}$ one-third of the distance between $F_{(60,\infty,0.975)}$ and $F_{(90,\infty,0.975)}$; that is, 0.025 will be subtracted from $F_{(60,\infty,0.975)} = 1.388$. Thus, we have $F_{(70,\infty,0.975)} = F_{(60,\infty,0.975)} - 0.025 = 1.388 - 0.025 = 1.363$. The same argument was used to approximate $F_{(329,69,0.975)} = 1.415$.

Students often ask whether or not it makes a difference in the F test which sample appears in the numerator and which in the denominator, for example, $F = S_1^2/S_2^2$ or $F = S_2^2/S_1^2$. For a two-tailed test, it does not make any difference. To see this, consider

$$P(F_{(n_1-1,n_2-1,1-\alpha/2)} \leq S_1^2/S_2^2) = \alpha/2.$$

By taking the reciprocal of each side and reversing the direction of the inequality, we get

$$P\left(\frac{1}{F_{(n_1-1,n_2-1,1-\alpha/2)}} \geq S_2^2/S_1^2\right) = \alpha/2.$$

Since

$$\frac{S_2^2}{S_1^2} \sim F_{(n_2-1,n_1-1)},$$

we have $P(F_{(n_2-1,n_1-1,\alpha/2)} \geq S_2^2/S_1^2) = \alpha/2.$

9.9 EXERCISES

1 Explain why the sampling distribution of $\overline{X}_1 - \overline{X}_2$ is approximately normal for sufficiently large n_1 and n_2 even if the underlying distributions are not normal.

2 A group of dental students conducted a study to determine the effect of aging on pocket depth. A random sample of 18 young patients in their 20s and 30s and a sample of 24 senior citizens in their 60s or older were selected. Each subject's pocket depth was measured, and the sample means of the two samples are $\overline{X}_1 = 3.4$ mm and $\overline{X}_2 = 4.2$ mm. Suppose that the distribution of pocket depth is normal and that the variance of the younger group is known to be $\sigma_1^2 = 1.86$ and the variance of the senior citizens is $\sigma_2^2 = 2.02$. State a null and an alternative hypotheses, and perform the test at the significance level $\alpha = 5\%$.

3 A study was conducted to evaluate the efficacy of a bonding agent and epinephrine on the smooth muscle contraction of rat uterine muscle and carotid arteries. The contraction forces induced were recorded using a force displacement transducer. Sixteen rats each were assigned to either the bonding agent or the control (epinephrine), that is, $n_1 = n_2 = 16$. The specified dose level of 20 μl of both the bonding agent and epinephrine was applied. Suppose the contraction force is normally distributed and that $\sigma_1^2 = \sigma_2^2$ (the variances are equal). The researchers summarized their data as in the table.
a. How should the researchers formulate the hypotheses?

b. Complete the test at the significance level $\alpha = 0.05$.

c. What is the p value?

	Bonding Agent	Epinephrine
Sample size	$n_1 = 16$	$n_2 = 16$
Sample mean	$\overline{X}_1 = 81.2$	$\overline{X}_2 = 110.4$
Sample variance	$S_1^2 = 1223.6$	$S_2^2 = 2304.8$

4 Previous studies have demonstrated that enamel matrix derivative (EMD) has the ability to improve clinical parameters when used to treat intraosseous defects [11]. Twenty-three subjects with an intrabony defect were chosen. Suppose $n_1 = 12$ patients received EMD in conjunction with open flap debridement and $n_2 = 11$ were treated with open flap debridement alone. Hard tissue measurements were recorded during the initial and re-entry surgery 1 year later for the level of osseous depth. From the measurements they have recorded, the investigators calculated the sample mean and sample variance of the amount of decrease in osseous depth for both groups: $\overline{X}_1 = 4.28$ mm, $S_1^2 = 0.57$, $\overline{X}_2 = 2.65$ mm, and $S_2^2 = 0.21$. Assume the amount of decrease in osseous depth is normally distributed and that the population variances of the two groups are equal. Would you be able to conclude that the EMD with open flap debridement is significantly superior to the treatment without EMD?

5 Social phobia has in recent years been recognized as a considerable public health concern [12]. It was speculated by psychiatrists that socially phobic patients who are diagnosed as having chronic depression may have greater fear of social interaction than those who do not have chronic depression. Liebowitz social anxiety test was given to 16 socially phobic subjects who suffer from chronic depression (group I), and 21 socially phobic subjects who are not chronically depressed (group II). The investigators computed descriptive statistics from the social anxiety test scores: $\overline{X}_1 = 22.6$, $S_1^2 = 14.0$, $\overline{X}_2 = 20.1$, and $S_2^2 = 12.2$. If the distribution of Liebowitz social anxiety test scores are normally distributed, and the variances of the test scores for both populations are unequal, what can you conclude from the data?

a. State the appropriate hypothesis.

b. Perform the test by using the p value.

6 It has been suggested that smoking does not affect the risk of cardiovascular diseases in populations with low serum cholesterol levels. To determine whether cigarette smoking is an independent risk factor among men with low levels of serum cholesterol, a nationwide, multicentered study was conducted. At one of the study sites, Orange Crest Community Hospital, 25 smokers and 47 non-smokers signed the consent form to participate in the study. Their serum cholesterol measurements are summarized below. Suppose the distribution of serum cholesterol levels is approximately normal and the variance of the cholesterol levels for smokers is different from that for non-smokers. What can you conclude from the research data?

Serum Cholesterol (mg/dl)	Non-smokers	Current Smokers
Sample mean	$\overline{X}_1 = 209.1$	$\overline{X}_2 = 213.3$
Sample SD	$S_1 = 35.5$	$S_2 = 37.6$

7 A cephalometric study was conducted to assess long-term changes in the soft tissue profile following mandibular setback surgery. The study enrolled six patients operated with bilateral sagittal split osteotomy and rigid fixation. Lateral cephalograms were taken at two occasions: immediate pre-surgical and 2 months post-surgical [13]. One of the variables under observation was skeletal horizontal changes of pogonion (the most anterior point on the osseous contour of the chin). The sample mean and sample standard deviation of the difference between the two time points are $\overline{D} = -5.94$, and $S_D = 4.86$. Test an appropriate hypothesis to determine if the treatment has any significant effect.

8 Suppose we are interested in determining if oral hygiene instructions given by the periodontist during a periodontal examination are effective in reducing plaque scores. One group of 68 patients was given oral hygiene instructions (OHI) and the other group of 46 patients received no OHI. We wish to compare the proportion of patients who will have plaque score less than 20%. A periodontal exam was given to the subjects 6 months later. The results suggested that 24 patients in the first group that received OHI and 14 patients in the second group that did not receive OHI had plaque scores less than 20%. Is the OHI effective in helping patients reduce their plaque scores?

9 The following table shows the data collected by American Dental Association to evaluate the relationship between the use of ergonomic chairs and the incidence of backaches in dental offices. Test a hypothesis to determine if the use of ergonomic chair is effective.

		Backache		
		Yes	No	
Use of	Yes	17	68	85
Ergonomic Chair	No	28	70	98
		45	138	183

10 Suppose a study was designed to investigate the occurrence of enamel fracture upon the removal of the metal brackets versus ceramic brackets. Suppose that of 75 patients who had metal brackets, 9 had experienced enamel fracture upon removal of the brackets, and of 98 patients who had ceramic brackets, 16 had experienced enamel fracture. State an appropriate hypothesis and test if there is any significant difference in the proportion of cases in which an enamel fracture occurs between metal and ceramic brackets.

11 There are two competing glass ionomer orthodontic cements. The manufacturers provided the following data regarding the bond strength (megapascals) of their products: $\mu_A = 51.3$, $\sigma_A^2 = 62.5$, and $\mu_B = 55.6$, $\sigma_B^2 = 60.2$. An orthodontist wishes to compare these cements with respect to their bond strength. Using this information, he needs to determine the required sample size for a two-tailed test at the significance level $\alpha = 0.05$ for achieving a power of 85%. What is his required sample size?

12 A 4-week weight control program was developed by a team of nutrition scientists. To evaluate the efficacy of the program the investigators selected 11 subjects who have body mass index higher than 30. Subjects were given specific instructions to comply in order to control the variables that may affect their weight, such as physical exercise and snacks. The weight of each subject at baseline and at the end of the 4-week clinical trial was measured. Suppose the weight distribution is

known to be normal. State and test the hypothesis to determine if the program is effective.

Subject	Weight at Baseline (kg)	Weight After the Program (kg)
1	82.3	76.5
2	76.5	73.8
3	103.7	98.2
4	89.6	—
5	96.8	95.8
6	108.5	112.6
7	94.3	89.9
8	121.8	—
9	87.0	—
10	115.7	111.4
11	125.1	117.4

13 In the above problem, if Dr. Lee wants to perform a one-tailed test at $\alpha = 0.05$ for achieving a power of 90%, how many samples does he need?

14 The effectiveness of two intra-root canal medicaments were compared; medicament A and medicament B. The effectiveness was measured by the number of colony-forming units (CFU) produced when the root canals were cultured. Suppose that the CFU is approximately normally distributed and that the variances are known, $\sigma_A^2 = 75.5$ and $\sigma_B^2 = 80.7$. Thirty-one medicament A and 36 medicament B samples were tested, and their sample means were $\overline{X}_A = 68.4$ and $\overline{X}_B = 55.9$. What is the power of a two-tailed test at the significance level $\alpha = 0.05$?

15 Centric relation (CR) is defined as the relationship of the mandible to the maxilla with properly aligned condyles and discs in the most superior position against the eminentia. Restorative dentists have suggested using CR to provide a stable and reproducible position to reconstruct the dentition. Suppose a study was conducted to assess the effect of an anterior flat plane deprogramming appliance (Jig) in 40 subjects for whom CR records were obtained before and after the use of the appliance. Incisal overbite and overjet dimensions using the Panadent condylar path indicator were recorded from maximum intercuspation [14]. Assume that the overbite and overjet are statistically independent and that they are normally distributed. Suppose the sample mean and sample SD of overbite and overjet were computed from the records: $\overline{X}_1 = 4.14$ mm, $S_1 = 1.74$ and

$\overline{X}_2 = 3.33$ mm, $S_2 = 1.78$. Using a one-tailed test at the significance level $\alpha = 0.05$, estimate the power of the test.

16 Using Table G in the Appendix, find the following.

a. Find the upper 10th percentile of an F distribution with degrees of freedom 14 and 9.

b. Find the lower 10th percentile of an F distribution with degrees of freedom 14 and 9.

c. Find $P(F_{(20, \ 16)} \leq 2.185)$.

17 Suppose a study was to compare the level of frictional resistance generated between titanium and stainless steel brackets. The friction resistance was measured by an Instron Universal testing machine with a 10-pound load cell. The investigators tested 31 samples of titanium and 26 samples of stainless steel brackets and reported the sample means and sample standard deviations of kinetic friction, which is assumed to be normally distributed, as follows: $\overline{X}_1 = 118.3$, $S_1 = 64.8$ and $\overline{X}_2 = 84.0$, $S_2 = 74.9$. What would you conclude about the variances of the two groups? Test your hypothesis at the significance level $\alpha = 5\%$.

18 Black licorice contains glycyrrhizic acid, which is also found in chewing tobacco. Excessive ingestion of confectioner's black licorice can elevate blood pressure. To determine how much elevation in blood pressure the patients experience, a group of 125 subjects was selected and encouraged to ingest as much black licorice as possible in a day. Their blood pressure was measured before and 1 day after ingesting the licorice. The sample standard deviation of their blood pressure at baseline was 17.3 and that of the follow-up blood pressure was 2.3 mmHg higher. Was there a significant difference in the variances at baseline and follow-up?

19 Mineral trioxide aggregate (MTAD) is a root canal disinfectant that is a mixture of tetracycline, an acid and a detergent. A study was conducted to compare the antimicrobial activities of MTAD to that of sodium hypochloride (NaOCL). The following data indicate the zone of inhibition (millimeters) on plates inoculated with *Enterococcus faecalis* [15]. Suppose that the distribution of the zone of inhibition is normal. Perform a test to detect if there are any significant differences in mean and variance between MTAD and NaOCL.

Zone of Inhibition (mm)							
MTAD	35,	34,	35,	35,	34,	36,	35,	34
NaOCL	33,	34,	33,	34,	36,	35,	34,	36

9.10 REFERENCES

1. Caffesse, R., and Guinard, E. A. Treatment of localized gingival recessions. Part IV. Results after three years. *J. Periodont*: 1980, 51, 167–170.
2. Froes, J. A., et al. Smear layer influence on the apical seal of four different obturation techniques. *J. of Endodontics*: 2000, 26, 351–354.
3. Satterthwaite, F. W. An approximate distribution of estimates of variance components. *Biometrics Bulletin*: 1946, 2, 110–114.
4. Nagahara, K., et al. Prediction of the permanent dentition in deciduous anterior crossbite. *Angle Orthodontist*: 2001, 71, 390–396.
5. Dessein, P. H., et al. The acute phase response does not fully predict the presence of insulin resistance and dyslipidemia in inflammatory arthritis. *J Rheumotol*: 2002, 29, 462–466.
6. Nozaki, T., et al. A sensitive method for detecting porthyromonas gingivalis by polymerase chain reaction and its possible clinical application. *J Periodontol*: 2001, 72, 1228–1235.
7. Bernal, V. Evaluation of alveolar and soft tissue changes after buccinator release surgery in patients undergoing fixed orthodontic therapy. MA thesis. Loma Linda University, Loma Linda, CA. 2001.
8. Bashar, S. R., and Bastodkar, P. Private discussions. 2002.
9. Osorio, R., Toledano, M., and Garcia-Godoy, F. Bracket bonding with 15 or 60 second etching and adhesive remaining on enamel after debonding. *Angle Orthod*: 1999, 69, 45–49.
10. Solfrizzi, V., et al. Relation of lipoprotein as coronary risk factor to type II diabetes mellitus and low-density lipoprotein cholesterol in patients $\geq$ 65 years of age (The Italian longitudinal study on aging). *Am J cardiol*: 2002, 89, 825–829.
11. Froum, S. J., et al. A comparative study utilizing open flap debridement with and without enamel matrix derivative in the treatment of periodontal intrabony defects: a 12-month re-entry study. *J. Periondontol*: 2001, 72, 25–34.
12. Pellissolo, A., et al. Personality dimensions in social phobics with or without depression. *ACTA Psychiatr Scand*: 2002, 105, 94–103.
13. Mobarak, K. A., et al. Factors influencing the predictability of soft tissue profile changes following mandibular setback surgery. *Angle Orthod*: 2001, 71, 216–227.
14. Karl, P. J., and Foley, T. F. The use of a deprogramming appliance to obtain centric relation records. *Angle Orthod*: 1999, 69, 117–125.
15. Torabinejad, M., Shabahang, S., and Kettering, J. D. The antimicrobial effect of MTAD. Technical report. Loma Linda University, Loma Linda, CA. 2002.

Chapter 10

Categorical Data Analysis

10.1 INTRODUCTION

In Chapters 8 and 9, we presented the basic methods of testing hypotheses for continuous data, which is assumed to come from the underlying normal population, such as blood pressure, birth weight, gingival recession, bone resorption, shear bond strength, serum cholesterol level, and carbon monoxide in the air. Investigators often prefer to count the number of occurrences of an event in two or more mutually exclusive categories of a variable, instead of numerically measuring the variable. For instance:

1. The number of cancer patients who are in remission and those who have relapsed.
2. Patients who prefer fixed partial dentures over removable partial dentures.
3. Gingival index is classified as either 0 or 1.
4. Patients with elevated oral *Mutans streptococci* levels and those with low levels.
5. The effect of the use of various endodontic irrigants on interappointment pain can be categorized; free of interappointment symptoms, slight pain, or pain that requires palliative treatment, etc.

Our interest is in the number of observations that fall into each of the categories. A main goal of this chapter is to develop a statistical test that will allow us to determine whether or not there is an association between two variables, given the categorical data, which consists of frequency counts of observations occurring in the response categories. A statistic for testing hypotheses about categorical data is known to be approximately distributed as a χ^2 distribution. Recall that a χ^2 distribution was used in Section 8.8 to test a hypothesis about the variance σ^2 of the normal population.

This chapter discusses practical applications of a χ^2 test arising in biomedical health sciences when we encounter categorical data. We will in-

troduce the following topics: 2×2 contingency table, Fisher's exact test, $r \times c$ contingency table, Cochran-Mantel-Haenszel test, McNemar's test, kappa statistic, and χ^2 goodness-of-fit test.

10.2 2×2 CONTINGENCY TABLE

In this section we introduce 2×2 χ^2 contingency table techniques. These tables arise when there are two variables and each variable is studied at two levels. Such cases arise when we observe dichotomous or binary data. Each observation falls into exactly one of two categories or classes. To facilitate our discussion, let's consider an example.

Example 10.2.1. Hormone replacement therapy (HRT) is used by an increasing number of women to relieve menopausal problems. The past research showed a protective effect against bone loss and cardiovascular disease, but concern has been raised about an increased incidence of breast cancer after HRT use, especially after more than 10 years of use [1]. Breast cancer patients were interviewed regarding exogenous hormonal use. Suppose this represents a random sample of breast cancer patients in Southern California referred to the Department of Oncology at the Riverside County Hospital for treatment between 1985 and 2005 with a 100% follow-up. Of the 730 patients, 97 received hormone replacement therapy and 633 did not receive any HRT prior to diagnosis. A subsequent examination indicated that 70 of the patients who used HRT are estrogen-receptor (ER) positive, and 416 of those who did not use HRT are ER positive. The rest of the patients are ER negative.

In this example we are dealing with two variables: hormone replacement therapy status and ER status of each patient. Each subject is either a user or a non-user of HRT and is either ER positive or ER negative. Thus, the two variables define

Table 10.2.1. The 2×2 contingency table for the data in Example 10.2.1.

	ER Status		
HRT Status	Positive	Negative	
Users	70	27	$r_1 = 97$
Non-users	416	217	$r_2 = 633$
	$c_1 = 486$	$c_2 = 244$	$n = 730$

four categories. Each subject falls into exactly one of the four categories as illustrated in the 2×2 contingency table, Table 10.2.1.

The 2×2 contingency table contains four cells, with two rows and two columns. Each variable is arbitrarily assigned either to the rows or to the columns. In Table 10.2.1, HRT status is assigned to the rows and ER status is assigned to the columns. Let O_{ij} and E_{ij} denote the observed cell frequency and expected cell frequency, respectively, in row i and column j, where i and j are 1 and 2. Let

$$r_i = O_{i1} + O_{i2}$$

= number of observations in the ith row,

$$i = 1, 2$$

$$c_j = O_{1j} + O_{2j}$$

= number of observations in the jth column,

$$j = 1, 2.$$

The expected values of the cell frequencies are calculated by

$$E_{ij} = \frac{r_i \cdot c_j}{n} = \frac{(i^{\text{th}} \text{ row total}) \times (j^{\text{th}} \text{ column total})}{\text{grand total}}.$$

From Example 10.2.1 we have $O_{11} = 70$, $O_{12} = 27$, $O_{21} = 416$, $O_{22} = 217$, $r_1 = 97$, $r_2 = 633$, $c_1 = 486$, $c_2 = 244$, and the grand total $n = 730$. The expected cell frequencies are

$$E_{11} = \frac{(97)(486)}{730} = 64.578,$$

$$E_{12} = \frac{(97)(244)}{730} = 32.422,$$

$$E_{21} = \frac{(633)(486)}{730} = 421.42,$$

and

$$E_{22} = \frac{(633)(244)}{730} = 211.58.$$

The row and column sums, r_i and c_j, are also referred to as marginal row and marginal column to-

tal. The null hypothesis we wish to test by a 2×2 contingency table is that there is *no association* between the two variables; the alternative hypothesis is that there is an association. Two different sampling designs lead to 2×2 contingency tables.

1. All marginal totals, r_i and c_j, are free to vary.
2. One set of marginal totals is fixed and the other is free to vary.

In the first case, where all marginal totals are free to vary, the test of no association is equivalent to **a test of independence**. In the second case, where only one set of marginal totals is free to vary, the test of association is equivalent to **a test of homogeneity**. In a test of independence the grand total n is the only number that is under the investigator's control. As we have seen in Example 10.2.1, $n = 730$ breast cancer patients are randomly sampled, and each patient under study is classified by the two variables, X and Y. The cell frequencies, O_{ij}, as well as row and column totals, r_i and c_j, are not known in advance. In other words, these are random variables. The investigator wishes to compare the proportion of breast cancer patients in each group who have ER positivity. The null and alternative hypotheses can be stated as

H_0: X and Y are independent vs.

H_1: X and Y are not independent

(or there is an association between X and Y).

In Example 10.2.1, the null hypothesis is that the status of ER is independent of the status of HRT. The knowledge of the status of HRT does not help predict the status of ER.

Example 10.2.2. In spite of the fact that metal ceramic crowns have been frequently used in recent years, many patients seem to prefer the porcelain jacket crown. The main reason for their preference is superior esthetics, particularly in the anterior segment. Prosthodontists studied the survival rate of these two types of crowns. Over a 4-year period there were 368 patients who had metal ceramic crowns and 294 patients who had porcelain jacket crowns on the maxillary anterior segment at a dental school clinic, where they collected the data. The follow-up study showed that 330 patients with all-ceramic crowns and 251 patients with porcelain jacket crowns had their crowns still functioning

Table 10.2.2. The 2×2 contingency table for the crown data.

	Survival Time		
Type of Crown	Less than 5 yrs.	5 or more yrs.	
Metal ceramic	38	330	$r_1 = 368$
Porcelain	43	251	$r_2 = 294$
	$c_1 = 81$	$c_2 = 581$	$n = 662$

well beyond 5 years. The data is summarized in Table 10.2.2.

Let's consider the sampling design, in which one set of marginal totals is fixed by the investigators and the other set is random. In the above crown data, there are two independent samples: metal ceramic crowns and porcelain jacket crowns. Our goal is to compare the proportion of patients in each group whose crowns survived less than 5 years. The row totals are fixed at $r_1 = 368$ and $r_2 = 294$, and the number of cases where crowns failed within 5 years is a binomial random variable, given the fixed marginal row totals. See Table 10.2.3. For metal ceramic, 38 failed, and for porcelain, 43 failed within 5 years. Suppose p_{11} and p_{21} denote the proportion of crowns that fail within 5 years for metal ceramic and for porcelain, respectively. The null hypothesis of no association between two variables—type of crown (X) and survival time (Y)—is stated as $H_0 : p_{11} = p_{21}$. That is, H_0 : Proportion of metal ceramic crowns that fail in less than 5 years = proportion of porcelain jacket crowns that fail in less than 5 years.

As with Example 10.2.1, we have observed cell frequencies and row and column totals: $O_{11} = 38$, $O_{12} = 330$, $O_{21} = 43$, $O_{22} = 251$, $r_1 = 368$, $r_2 = 294$, $c_1 = 81$, $c_2 = 581$, and the grand total $n = 662$. The expected cell frequencies

are

$$E_{11} = \frac{(368)(81)}{662} = 45.027,$$

$$E_{12} = \frac{(368)(581)}{662} = 322.97,$$

$$E_{21} = \frac{(294)(81)}{662} = 35.973,$$

and

$$E_{22} = \frac{(294)(581)}{662} = 258.03.$$

A general 2×2 table with observed cell frequencies is illustrated in Table 10.2.4.

Using the notation in Table 10.2.4, the expected cell frequencies are obtained by

$$E_{11} = \frac{(r_1)(x_1 + x_2)}{r_1 + r_2},$$

$$E_{12} = \frac{(r_1)[(r_1 + r_2) - (x_1 + x_2)]}{r_1 + r_2},$$

$$E_{21} = \frac{(r_2)(x_1 + x_2)}{r_1 + r_2},$$

and

$$E_{22} = \frac{(r_2)[(r_1 + r_2) - (x_1 + x_2)]}{r_1 + r_2}.$$

Note that $E_{11} + E_{12} + E_{21} + E_{22} = r_1 + r_2 = n$. That is, the sum of all the cell frequencies is equal to the grand total. This should provide a quick and easy way to verify whether or not your calculations are correct. To test the hypothesis stated above, we wish to compare the observed frequency and expected frequency for each of the four cells in a 2×2 contingency table. If the observed values and the corresponding expected values for the cells are close, then H_0 will be accepted, and if they are sufficiently different, then H_0 will be rejected. It can be shown that the best way to compare the corresponding observed and expected cell frequencies

Table 10.2.3. Proportions associated with a 2×2 contingency table in which marginal row totals are fixed.

	Survival Time		
Type of Crown	Less than 5 yrs.	5 or more yrs.	
Metal ceramic	p_{11}	p_{12}	Fixed
Porcelain	p_{21}	p_{22}	Fixed
	Random	Random	n

Table 10.2.4. A general 2×2 contingency table with observed cell frequencies in which marginal row totals are fixed.

	Survival Time		
Type of Crown	Less than 5 yrs.	5 or more yrs.	
Metal ceramic	x_1	$r_1 - x_1$	r_1
Porcelain	x_2	$r_2 - x_2$	r_2
	$x_1 + x_2$	$(r_1 + r_2)$ $-(x_1 + x_2)$	$n = r_1 + r_2$

is to use the statistic

$$\frac{(O_{ij} - E_{ij})^2}{E_{ij}} \text{ for the } (i, j) \text{ cell.}$$

It is well-known in statistics that the sum of the above statistic for the cells is approximately χ^2 distributed with 1 degree of freedom,

$$\chi^2 = \sum_{i,j=1}^{2} \frac{(O_{ij} - E_{ij})^2}{E_{ij}} \overset{\circ}{\sim} \chi^2_{(1)}.$$

We may write the χ^2 statistic as

$$\chi^2 = \frac{(O_{11} - E_{11})^2}{E_{11}} + \frac{(O_{12} - E_{12})^2}{E_{12}}$$
$$+ \frac{(O_{21} - E_{21})^2}{E_{21}} + \frac{(O_{22} - E_{22})^2}{E_{22}} \overset{\circ}{\sim} \chi^2_{(1)}.$$

Because the distribution of the test statistic is approximately χ^2, this procedure is known as the χ^2 contingency table. The χ^2 test compares the observed frequency with the expected frequency in each category in the contingency table, given that the null hypothesis is true. The question here is whether or not the difference $O_{ij} - E_{ij}$ is too large to be attributed to chance. We reject H_0 when the sum is "large" and accept H_0, when the sum is "small." Note that we are approximating a continuous χ^2 distribution by discrete observations. The approximation is good for contingency tables with high degrees of freedom, but may not be valid for 2×2 tables that have only 1 degree of freedom. Therefore, statisticians use a continuity correction. With the continuity correction factor, the statistic $\frac{(|O_{ij} - E_{ij}| - 0.5)^2}{E_{ij}}$ rather than $\frac{(O_{ij} - E_{ij})^2}{E_{ij}}$ is computed for each cell. This test procedure is referred to as the χ^2 test, with Yates correction. The term 0.5 in the numerator is called the Yates

correction. From algebra, we see that the effect of this term is to decrease the value of the test statistic, and thus, as we have seen in Section 8.8, it increases the corresponding p value. This makes the test more conservative and less likely to reject the null hypothesis. While the Yates correction has been used extensively, many statisticians have questioned its validity, and some believe that the Yates correction makes the tests overly conservative and may fail to reject false H_0 [2]. When the sample size n is sufficiently large, the effect of the Yates correction is negligible. The test procedure is summarized below.

The χ^2 Test for a 2×2 Contingency Table with Yates Correction

1. Compute the value of the test statistic

$$\chi^2 = \sum_{i,j=1}^{2} \frac{(|O_{ij} - E_{ij}| - 0.5)^2}{E_{ij}}.$$

Under H_0, this statistic is approximately $\chi^2_{(1)}$.
2. Reject H_0 if $\chi^2_{(1,1-\alpha)} < \chi^2$ and accept H_0 if $\chi^2_{(1,1-\alpha)} \geq \chi^2$ at the significance level α.
3. The p value of the test is given by the area to the right of the value of the test statistic χ^2 under a $\chi^2_{(1)}$ distribution; $p = P(\chi^2 \leq \chi^2_{(1)})$.

The rejection and acceptance regions and the p value of the χ^2 test for a 2×2 contingency table are illustrated in Figure 10.2.1 and Figure 10.2.2.

Recall that when a χ^2 distribution was introduced in Chapter 8, we assumed that the underlying distribution is normal. As pointed out, we approximate a χ^2 distribution, which is continuous, by discrete observations. Thus the χ^2 test procedure for 2×2 contingency tables is valid only

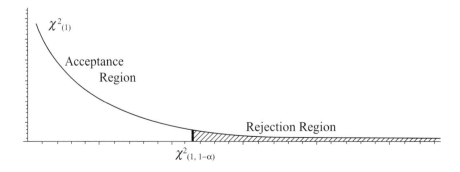

Figure 10.2.1 Rejection and aceptance regions of the χ^2 test for a 2×2 contingency table.

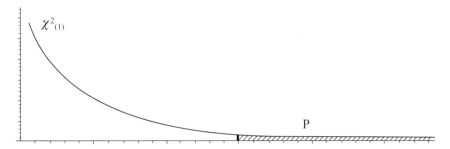

Figure 10.2.2   The p value of the χ^2 test for a 2×2 contingency table.

when the normal approximation to the binomial distribution is valid. This means that the χ^2 test procedure in this setting is meaningful and valid when the expected cell frequencies are at least 5 ($E_{ij} \geq 5$).

Example 10.2.3. Evaluate the data in Example 10.2.1 for statistical significance.

Solution. The observed and expected cell frequencies have been calculated. Note that the expected cell frequencies are much larger than 5, and hence we can use the test procedure given in this section. For each cell we need to compute $\dfrac{(|O_{ij} - E_{ij}| - 0.5)^2}{E_{ij}}$.

$$\frac{(|O_{11} - E_{11}| - 0.5)^2}{E_{11}} = \frac{(|70 - 64.578| - 0.5)^2}{64.578}$$
$$= 0.375$$

$$\frac{(|O_{12} - E_{12}| - 0.5)^2}{E_{12}} = \frac{(|27 - 32.422| - 0.5)^2}{32.422}$$
$$= 0.747$$

$$\frac{(|O_{21} - E_{21}| - 0.5)^2}{E_{21}} = \frac{(|416 - 421.420| - 0.5)^2}{421.420}$$
$$= 0.057$$

$$\frac{(|O_{22} - E_{22}| - 0.5)^2}{E_{22}} = \frac{(|217 - 211.58| - 0.5)^2}{211.58}$$
$$= 0.114.$$

The value of the test statistic is $\chi^2 = 0.375 + 0.747 + 0.057 + 0.114 = 1.293$. From Table F in the Appendix we get $\chi^2_{(1,0.95)} = 3.841 > \chi^2 = 1.293$. So we accept the null hypothesis at the significance level $\alpha = 0.05$ and conclude that the results are not significant. There is no statistically significant association between HRT and ER. The

p value is given by

$$p = P(\chi^2_{(1)} > 1.293) > P(\chi^2_{(1)} > 2.706) = 0.10.$$

The χ^2 test procedure is valid because all the E_{ij} are greater than 5.

Example 10.2.4. A study was conducted to examine the behavior of preschool children, each sedated with one of two drug regimens based on the patient's age, dental needs, and pre-operative clinical impression. Two hundred children whose ages range from 2 to 5 years were selected. The study subjects were randomly divided into two groups, and the groups received either chloral hydrate and hydroxyzine (A) or chloral hydrate, meperidine, and hydroxyzine (B). Their behavior after sedation was observed and classified as either quiet/sleeping or struggling. Suppose the data was summarized in the table below. What can you conclude about the association (homogeneity) between the variables from the data?

Drug Regimen	Behavioral Variable	
	Quiet/sleeping	Struggling
A	76	24
B	92	8

Solution. The marginal totals are $r_1 = r_2 = 100$, $c_1 = 168$, $c_2 = 32$, and the grand total $n = 200$. The expected frequency for each cell can be computed,

$$E_{11} = \frac{(100)(168)}{200} = 84.0,$$

$$E_{12} = \frac{(100)(32)}{200} = 16.0,$$

$$E_{21} = \frac{(100)(168)}{200} = 84.0$$

and

$$E_{22} = \frac{(100)(32)}{200} = 16.0.$$

All of the expected cell frequencies are greater than 5 ($E_{ij} > 5$), so that the test procedure described previously can be used. We now compute the test statistic χ^2,

$$\chi^2 = \frac{(|76 - 84| - 0.5)^2}{84} + \frac{(|24 - 16| - 0.5)^2}{16}$$
$$+ \frac{(|92 - 84| - 0.5)^2}{84} + \frac{(|8 - 16| - 0.5)^2}{16}$$
$$= 0.670 + 3.516 + 0.670 + 3.516 = 8.372.$$

Since $\chi^2 = 8.372 > \chi^2_{(1,0.95)} = 3.841$, the null hypothesis is rejected at the significance level $\alpha = 0.05$. The p value is obtained by $p = P(\chi^2_{(1)} > 8.372) < P(\chi^2_{(1)} > 7.879) = 1 - 0.995 = 0.005$. The results are highly significant. Thus, there is a statistically significant difference between the rate of quiet/sleeping behavior for the chloral hydrate and hydroxyzine group and the chloral hydrate, meperidine, and hyroxyzine group, with the second group having a higher rate.

Example 10.2.5. In many research projects, subjects are required to fill out survey questionnaires, such as a patient satisfaction survey. One of the main concerns in these situations is whether or not the subject's responses are consistent and reliable. A sample of 50 dental patients was selected at random to study their attitudes toward visiting dentists. To assess the reliability of his or her responses, each patient was required to fill out the same questionnaire a second time, a week after the first one. The questionnaires contain the identical questions, but in a different order. One of the survey questions was "Is visiting a dentist an anxiety provoking experience?" In the first questionnaire, 20 patients responded "Yes" to this question; in the second questionnaire, 24 people said "Yes." Fifteen (15) patients responded "Yes" to this question on both questionnaires. What can you say about the association between the two sets of responses on the question of dental anxiety? Use the significance level $\alpha = 0.05$.

Solution. The two variables of our interest are the "anxiety question" on the first questionnaire and the same "anxiety question" on the second questionnaire. The question can be answered either

"Yes" or "No." We can present the data described in the problem in a 2 × 2 table.

	First Questionnaire	
Second Questionnaire	Yes	No
Yes	15	24
No		
	20	50

The blank cells can easily be filled by simple algebra. We should keep in mind that the total sample size is $n = 50$. Some students may think the grand total is $n = 100$. After filling the blank cells, we obtain the following table.

	First Questionnaire		
Second Questionnaire	Yes	No	
Yes	15	9	24
No	5	21	26
	20	30	50

Computing the expected frequency for each cell, we get

$$E_{11} = \frac{(24)(20)}{50} = 9.6,$$
$$E_{12} = \frac{(24)(30)}{50} = 14.4,$$
$$E_{21} = \frac{(26)(20)}{50} = 10.4$$

and

$$E_{22} = \frac{(26)(30)}{50} = 15.6.$$

Since all of the $E_{ij} > 5$, the test procedure (10.2.2) can be used. We compute the test statistic χ^2,

$$\chi^2 = \frac{(|15 - 9.6| - 0.5)^2}{9.6} + \frac{(|9 - 14.4| - 0.5)^2}{14.4}$$
$$+ \frac{(|5 - 10.4| - 0.5)^2}{10.4} + \frac{(|21 - 15.6| - 0.5)^2}{15.6}$$
$$= 2.501 + 1.667 + 2.309 + 1.539 = 8.016.$$

Since $\chi^2 = 8.016 > \chi^2_{(1,0.95)} = 3.841$, the null hypothesis is rejected at $\alpha = 0.05$. The p value is obtained by $p = P(\chi^2_{(1)} > 8.016) < P(\chi^2_{(1)} > 7.879) = 1 - 0.995 = 0.005$.

The results are highly significant. There is a statistically significant association between the two questionnaires for the way in which the subjects have responded.

The χ^2 test procedure for 2×2 contingency tables is often used in exposure-disease relationships. For example, there are r_1 exposed subjects and r_2 unexposed subjects. The number of exposed subjects with the disease is x_1 and the number of unexposed subjects with the disease is x_2. When the grand total $n = r_1 + r_2$ is small, we might find some of the expected cell frequencies E_{ij} less than 5. What if at least one of the E_{ij} is less than 5? In such cases, it is not valid to use the procedure described in this section. Instead, we use a technique known as **Fisher's exact test**. This technique involves laborious computations, and thus it is not discussed in this text. Interested readers are referred to Fisher and Van Belle [3] and Rosner [4]. Most of the statistical software packages include a procedure to perform Fisher's exact test for a 2×2 contingency table.

Example 10.2.6. Candida species usually colonize in the oral cavity of denture wearers and may also colonize on their fingers because of frequent manual manipulation of the dentures. A study was performed to investigate the association between oral and fingertip candidal isolation in a group of denture wearers [5]. Oral rinse and fingerprints obtained from 25 healthy male complete denture wearers were microbiologically investigated for candidal growth, and isolated candida species were identified with a germ tube test and a commercially available yeast identification system. Candida species were isolated from the oral cavity of 15 subjects and fingertips of 11 subjects. Ten subjects had concomitant oral and fingertip candidal isolation, whereas 5 subjects had only oral candida. A 2×2 contingency table can be set up as follows.

	Fingertip Candida		
Oral Candida	Positive	Negative	
Positive	10	5	15
Negative	1	9	10
	11	14	25

The expected frequency for the cell $(2, 1)$ is $E_{21} = (10)(11)/25 = 4.4$. Since this expected cell frequency is less than 5, we can't use the χ^2 test procedure for a contingency table. Fisher's exact test must be used for this case. To avoid the use

of Fisher's exact test, the investigators should take sufficiently large samples so that all of the expected cell frequencies for a 2×2 contingency table will be at least 5.

10.3 $r \times c$ CONTINGENCY TABLE

In Section 10.2, our discussions were limited to nominal variables with two possible outcomes, and thus we have contingency tables with two rows and two columns. In this section we will extend the technique to situations in which there are two or more rows and columns. Two variables are assumed to have r ($r \geq 2$) levels and c ($c \geq 2$) levels, respectively. Therefore, the corresponding contingency table has r rows and c columns. It contains the total of rc cells. Table 10.3.1 illustrates a typical $r \times c$ contingency table. A typical $r \times c$ contingency table has more than two categories for one or both variables. Consider an example.

Example 10.3.1. Intrusive luxation has been defined as "displacement of the tooth deeper into the alveolar bone." Some researchers found intrusion to be the most common type of injury to the primary incisor region. The intruded primary incisor will in most cases re-erupt within 1–6 months without any pathological sequences. Complications associated with intrusion may affect the injured teeth or their permanent successors. As part of a retrospective study to analyze the major characteristics, the prognosis and sequelae of intrusion of primary incisors, 112 teeth have been classified into two categories according to the degree of intrusion (partial and complete), and the appearance of the pulp of these re-erupted teeth was evaluated radiographically and put into three categories: normal appearance, pulp canal obliteration, and arrest

Table 10.3.1. Observed frequencies for a $r \times c$ contingency table.

	Variable Y			Row Sum
Variable X	Level 1	Level 2	$\cdots$	Level c
Level 1	O_{11}	O_{12}	$\cdots$	O_{1c}	r_1
Level 2	O_{21}	O_{22}	$\cdots$	O_{2c}	r_2
$\cdots$	$\cdots$	$\cdots$	$\cdots$	$\cdots$	$\cdots$
Level r	O_{r1}	O_{r2}	$\cdots$	O_{rc}	r_r
Column sum	c_1	c_2	$\cdots$	c_c	n

Table 10.3.2. Radiographic appearance of the pulp of re-erupted teeth.

	Radiographic Appearance of the Pulp		
Degree of Intrusion	Normal Appearance	Pulp Canal Obliteration	Arrest of Dentin Apposition
Partial	27	24	8	59
Complete	11	33	9	53
	38	57	17	112

Table 10.3.3. Expected cell frequency for the data in Table 10.3.2.

	Radiographic Appearance of the Pulp		
Degree of Intrusion	Normal Appearance	Pulp Canal Obliteration	Arrest of Dentin Apposition
Partial	20.02	30.03	8.96
Complete	17.98	26.97	8.04

of dentin apposition [6]. The data is illustrated in the 2×3 contingency table (Table 10.3.2). How can we test for a relationship between the degree of intrusion and radiographic appearance of the pulp?

As with the 2×2 tables, there are two situations. In one case, we wish to test the null hypothesis

$$H_0 : \quad p_{11} = p_{12} = p_{13}$$
$$p_{21} = p_{22} = p_{23}$$

The alternative hypothesis is that the p_{ij}'s (i^{th} row, j^{th} column) are not all equal for at least one row. That is, $H_1 : p_{11}$, p_{12}, and p_{13} are not all equal, or p_{21}, p_{22}, and p_{23} are not all equal. In the first case, we are concerned with the null hypothesis that radiographic appearance of the pulp is independent of the degree of intrusion. In general, we state the null and alternative hypotheses as

H_0: Two variables (radiographic appearance and the degree of intrusion) are independent vs.

H_1: Two variables are not independent.

The analysis of an $r \times c$ contingency table is basically the same as that of a 2×2 table. The significance test is based on the difference between the observed and the expected cell frequencies in the table. In fact, the computation of the expected cell frequencies is the same as before:

$$E_{ij} = \frac{(r_i)(c_j)}{n}.$$

The corresponding expected cell frequencies for the data in Example 10.3.1 are presented in Table 10.3.3.

The sum of the expected cell frequencies across any row or column must equal the corresponding marginal row or column total, and the sum of all E_{ij} should equal the grand total. In some cases, due to the round-off error, the sum may

not be precisely equal. For example, the sum of the expected cell frequencies in the first row is $20.02 + 30.03 + 8.96 = 59.01$, which is not equal to the marginal total $r_1 = 59$.

We will compare the expected frequencies with the observed frequencies. We will again compute the sum of the differences $\frac{(O_{ij} - E_{ij})^2}{E_{ij}}$ over all the cells in the $r \times c$ table. If the sum is "small," we will accept the null hypothesis. If the sum is "large," we will reject it. Under H_0, the test statistic χ^2 for an $r \times c$ contingency table follows approximately a χ^2 distribution with the degrees of freedom $(r - 1)(c - 1)$. Empirical studies showed that the continuity correction for contingency tables larger than 2×2 does not improve the approximation of the test statistic by the χ^2 distribution. Thus, the correction factor is not usually used for the $r \times c$ tables. For the validity of the approximation, the χ^2 test procedure is recommended under the following conditions:

- No more than 20% of the cells have an expected cell frequency less than 5.
- No cells have an expected cell frequency less than 1.

We summarize the test procedure for an $r \times c$ contingency table. The rejection region and the p value are illustrated in Figure 10.3.1 and 10.3.2.

The χ^2 Test for an $r \times c$ Contingency Table

1. Compute the value of the test statistic

$$\chi^2 = \sum_{j=1}^{c} \sum_{i}^{r} \frac{(O_{ij} - E_{ij})^2}{E_{ij}}.$$

Under H_0, this test statistic is approximately $\chi^2_{((r-1)(c-1))}$

2. Reject H_0 if $\chi^2_{((r-1)(c-1), 1-\alpha)} < \chi^2$ and accept H_0 if $\chi^2_{((r-1)(c-1), 1-\alpha)} \geq \chi^2$ at the significance level α.

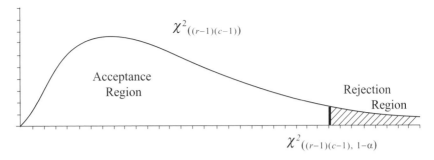

Figure 10.3.1 Rejection region of the χ^2 test for an $r \times c$ contingency table.

3. The p value of the test is given by the area to the right of the value of the test statistic χ^2 under a $\chi^2_{((r-1)(c-1))}$ distribution.

We will perform a statistical significance test for the data in Example 10.3.1. Table 10.3.3 shows that all the expected cell frequencies are > 5, so the test procedure given above can be applied. Since $r = 2$ and $c = 3$, we have $r \cdot c = 6$ cells. The test statistic χ^2 is approximately $\chi^2_{((2-1)(3-1))} = \chi^2_{(2)}$. We compute the test statistic as follows:

$$
\begin{aligned}
\chi^2 &= \sum_{j=1}^{c} \sum_{i}^{r} \frac{(O_{ij} - E_{ij})^2}{E_{ij}} \\
&= \frac{(O_{11} - E_{11})^2}{E_{11}} + \frac{(O_{12} - E_{12})^2}{E_{12}} \\
&\quad + \frac{(O_{13} - E_{13})^2}{E_{13}} + \frac{(O_{21} - E_{21})^2}{E_{21}} \\
&\quad + \frac{(O_{22} - E_{22})^2}{E_{22}} + \frac{(O_{23} - E_{23})^2}{E_{23}} \\
&= \frac{(27 - 20.02)^2}{20.02} + \frac{(24 - 30.03)^2}{30.03} \\
&\quad + \frac{(8 - 8.96)^2}{8.96} + \frac{(11 - 17.98)^2}{17.98} \\
&\quad + \frac{(33 - 26.97)^2}{26.97} + \frac{(9 - 8.04)^2}{8.04} = 7.920.
\end{aligned}
$$

Since $\chi^2_{(2,1-0.5)} = \chi^2_{(2,0.95)} = 5.991 < \chi^2 = 7.920$, we reject the null hypothesis and conclude that there is a statistically significant relationship between the degree of intrusion and the radiographic appearance of the pulp. The p value of the test is given by

$$
\begin{aligned}
p &= P\left(7.920 < \chi^2_{(2)}\right) < P\left(7.378 < \chi^2_{(2)}\right) \\
&= 0.025.
\end{aligned}
$$

10.4 THE COCHRAN-MANTEL-HAENSZEL TEST

Suppose that $n = 228$ implants placed in grafted maxillary sinuses have been followed for 5 years to evaluate the factors affecting the survival rate of implants. Patient's smoking habit (yes/no) and general oral hygiene (good/poor) were two of the primary variables on which the investigation was focused. The main goal of the study was to investigate the effect of oral hygiene on implant survival time. One potential confounding variable was patients' smoking habits, because active smoking is related to both oral hygiene and survival time of the implants. Therefore, it is important to control for active smoking before

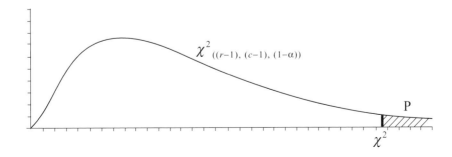

Figure 10.3.2 The p value of the χ^2 test for an $r \times c$ contingency table.

Table 10.4.1. Relationship between oral hygiene and implant survival rate among smokers.

Survival Time (Smokers)	Oral Hygiene		
	Good	Poor	
5 or more yrs.	12	13	25
Less than 5 yrs.	10	35	45
	22	48	70

Table 10.4.2. Relationship between oral hygiene and implant survival rate among non-smokers.

Survival Time (Non-smokers)	Oral Hygiene		
	Good	Poor	
5 or more yrs.	96	46	142
Less than 5 yrs.	6	10	16
	102	56	158

we study the relationship between oral hygiene and implant survival time. A statistical method was developed by Cochran [7] and Mantel and Haenszel [8] for examining this type of relationship between two categorical variables while controlling for another categorical variable. Table 10.4.1 and Table 10.4.2 display the data in a 2×2 table relating oral hygiene to implant survival rate for smokers and non-smokers, separately. Table 10.4.3 presents the combined data.

From the above tables we can estimate the odds ratio in favor of more than 5-year implant survival for the patients with good oral hygiene versus the patients with poor oral hygiene among smokers and non-smokers:

$$\hat{OR}_{\text{smokers}} = \frac{(12)(35)}{(10)(13)} = 3.2308$$

and

$$\hat{OR}_{\text{non-smokers}} = \frac{(96)(10)}{(6)(46)} = 3.4783$$

In both subgroups, the odds of an implant surviving more than 5 years is greater among

Table 10.4.3. Relationship between oral hygiene and implant survival rate among smokers and non-smokers.

Survival Time	Oral Hygiene		
	Good	Poor	
5 or more yrs.	108	59	167
Less than 5 yrs.	16	45	61
	124	90	228

Table 10.4.4. Relationship between oral hygiene and implant survival rate.

Survival Time	Oral Hygiene		
	Good	Poor	
Less than 5 yrs.	a_i	b_i	$a_i + b_i$
5 or more yrs.	c_i	d_i	$c_i + d_i$
	$a_i + c_i$	$b_i + d_i$	n_i

non-smokers than among smokers. Based on unstratified data in Table 10.4.3, we estimate the odds in favor of more than 5-year implant survival given by $\hat{OR} = (108)(45)/(16)(59) = 5.148$.

We have stratified the data into two subgroups according to a confounding variable to make the subjects within a stratum as homogeneous as possible. To facilitate the presentation of the Cochran-Mantel-Haenszel test method, we use the following notation for the ith 2×2 contingency table, in which the index i ranges from 1 to k. In this example of implant survival data, $i = 1$, and 2. See Table 10.4.4.

The test statistic is based on an overall comparison between the observed and expected cell frequencies in the $(1, 1)$ cell in each of the k subtables. As before, the expected cell frequency is obtained by

$$E_i = \frac{(a_i + b_i)(a_i + c_i)}{n_i}.$$

The observed and expected frequencies in the $(1, 1)$ cell are summed over all strata, that is,

$$O = \sum_{i=1}^{k} O_i, \quad \text{and} \quad E = \sum_{i=1}^{k} E_i.$$

The proposed test statistic is based on $(O - E)$. We need to calculate the variance $(\sigma_{O_i}^2)$ of O_i to assess if the difference is statistically significant.

$$\sigma_{O_i}^2 = \frac{(a_i + b_i)(c_i + d_i)(a_i + c_i)(b_i + d_i)}{n_i^2(n_i - 1)}.$$

The variance (σ_O^2) of $O = \sum_{i=1}^{k} O_i$ is then given by $\sigma_O^2 = \sum_{i=1}^{k} \sigma_{O_i}^2$. The test statistic is defined by

$$\chi_{CMH}^2 = \frac{(|O - E| - 0.5)^2}{\sigma_O^2} \overset{\circ}{\sim} \chi_{(1)}^2.$$

Under the null hypothesis that there is no association between the two dichotomous variables, the

Cochran-Mantel-Hanzsel test statistic is approximately χ^2 distributed with 1 degree of freedom. We summarize the Cochran-Mantel-Hanzsel test.

The Cochran-Mantel-Hanzsel Test

Evaluate the association between two dichotomous variables after controlling for confounding variables.

1. Compute the total number of observed subjects in the (1, 1) cell over all strata, and compute the corresponding expected cell frequency, $O = \sum_{i=1}^{k} O_i$, and $E = \sum_{i=1}^{k} E_i$.
2. Compute the variance (σ_O^2) of $O = \sum_{i=1}^{k} O_i$,

   where

   $$\sigma_O^2 = \sum_{i=1}^{k} \frac{(a_i + b_i)(c_i + d_i)(a_i + c_i)(b_i + d_i)}{n_i^2(n_i - 1)}.$$

3. The test statistics is defined by $\chi_{CMH}^2 = \frac{(|O - E| - 0.5)^2}{\sigma_O^2} \overset{\circ}{\sim} \chi_{(1)}^2$ under H_0.
4. Reject H_0 if $\chi_{(1,1-\alpha)}^2 < \chi_{CMH}^2$ and accept H_0 if $\chi_{(1,1-\alpha)}^2 \geq \chi_{CMH}^2$.
5. The p value of the test is given by $p = P(\chi_{CMH}^2 < \chi_{(1)}^2)$.

Example 10.4.1. Using the stratified data in Table 10.4.1 and Table 10.4.2, evaluate the relationship between oral hygiene and implant survival time.

Solution. Let O_1 equal the observed number of implants that survived more than 5 years for the patients who have good oral hygiene among smokers, and O_2 equal the observed number of implants that survived more than 5 years for the patients who have good oral hygiene among non-smokers. Then from the tables, we get $O_1 = 12$ and $O_2 = 96$. The corresponding expected cell frequencies are computed:

$$E_1 = \frac{(25)(22)}{70} = 7.857$$

and

$$E_2 = \frac{(142)(102)}{158} = 91.671.$$

The total observed and expected number of implants are

$$O = O_1 + O_2 = 12 + 96 = 108$$

and

$$E = E_1 + E_2 = 7.857 + 91.671 = 99.528$$

We can now calculate the variance,

$$\sigma_{O_1}^2 = \frac{(25)(45)(22)(48)}{70^2(70 - 1)} = 3.5138$$

and

$$\sigma_{O_2}^2 = \frac{(142)(16)(102)(56)}{158^2(158 - 1)} = 3.3112.$$

Thus, $\sigma_O^2 = \sigma_{O_1}^2 + \sigma_{O_2}^2 = 3.5138 + 3.3112 = 6.825$.

The value of the test statistics is

$$\chi_{CMH}^2 = \frac{(|O - E| - 0.5)^2}{\sigma_O^2} \overset{\circ}{\sim} \chi_{(1)}^2 \text{ under } H_0$$

$$= \frac{(|108 - 99.528| - 0.5)^2}{6.825} = 9.3118.$$

The p value is obtained by

$$p = P(\chi_{CMH}^2 < \chi_{(1)}^2)$$
$$= P(9.3118 < \chi_{(1)}^2) < P(7.879 < \chi_{(1)}^2)$$
$$= 0.005.$$

Since $\chi_{(1,0.95)}^2 = 3.841 \leq \chi_{CMH}^2 = 9.3118$, and the p value is less than 0.005, we reject the null hypothesis and conclude that there is a highly significant positive relationship between oral hygiene and implant survival rate, even after controlling for the confounding variable, which is smoking habits of the patients.

10.5 THE McNEMAR TEST

Let's consider an example to describe the **McNemar test**. Several techniques have been proposed to achieve root coverage to treat gingival recession defects, which represent a significant concern for patients and a therapeutic problem for clinicians. Suppose a clinical trial was performed to evaluate the effect of a connective tissue graft (CTG) in comparison to a guided tissue regeneration (GTR) procedure in the treatment of gingival recession. This clinical trial was designed to form matched pairs in which one member of each matched pair is randomly assigned to CTG and the

Table 10.5.1. Gingival recession treatment data.

Treatment	Soft Tissue Improvement		
	Yes	No	
CTG	101	51	152
GTR	92	60	152
	193	111	304

other member to GTR. The patients are matched on age, sex, oral hygiene standards, gingival health, probing depth, and other prognostic attributes. There were 304 patients, or 152 matched pairs. Six months after the treatment, patients were recalled and clinically significant improvement of the soft tissue conditions of the defects was recorded. The data are presented in a 2×2 contingency table, as shown in Table 10.5.1.

The proportion of soft tissue improvement for the treatment groups appears not that much different: $101/152 = 0.664$ for CTG and $92/152 = 0.605$ for GTR, respectively. What do these proportions tell us about the effectiveness of the treatments? Is it valid to use the 2×2 χ^2 contingency technique to compare the proportions? The χ^2 test with Yates correction cannot be used in this case because the two samples are not independent. Each matched pair is quite similar in clinical conditions, and thus they are not independent. In this type of situation, we use a statistical method known as the **McNemar test**, which takes the nature of matched pairs into account in the analysis. In this example, the matched pair constitutes the basic unit for the experiment so that the sample size is 152, instead of 304. We construct a 2×2 table by classifying the pairs according to whether or not members of that pair have clinically significant soft tissue improvement, as shown in Table 10.5.2.

Notice the chance that the member of treatment GTR of the pair improved, given that the member of treatment CTG of the pair improved, is $92/109 = 0.844$, while the chance that the

Table 10.5.2. Gingival recession treatment data for matched pairs.

Treatment CTG	Treatment GTR		
	Improvement	No Improvement	
Improvement	92	17	109
No improvement	14	29	43
	106	46	152

member of treatment GTR of the pair improved, given that the member of treatment CTG of the pair did not improve, is $14/43 = 0.326$. This suggests that the two samples are highly dependent on each other. If they are independent, then we would expect the probabilities to be approximately the same. We state the null hypothesis as follows:

H_0: There is no association between clinically significant improvement and the treatment.

H_1: An association exists between clinically significant improvement and the treatment.

In Table 10.5.2, for 92 matched pairs the outcomes of the two treatments, CTG and GTR, are "improvement" and for 29 pairs the outcomes of the two treatments are "no improvement." In other words, there are 121 pairs in which the outcomes of the treatments are the same. For the other $17 + 14 = 31$ pairs, the outcome of the patients of the matched pair is different.

Definition 10.5.1. (i) A matched pair in which the outcome is the same for both members of the pair is called a **concordant pair**. (ii) A matched pair, in which the outcomes are different for the members of the pair, is called a **discordant pair**.

In Table 10.5.2, there are 121 $(92 + 29)$ concordant pairs and 31 $(17 + 14)$ discordant pairs. The concordant pairs provide no information about differences between treatments and therefore will not be used. A test statistic is constructed based on the discordant pairs. There are two types of discordant pairs, as indicated in Table 10.5.2, where there are 14 discordant pairs in which only GTR patients improved, and 17 discordant pairs in which only CTG patients improved. Let b be the number of discordant pairs in which only the CTG patients of the pair improved, and c be the number of discordant pairs in which only the GTR patients of the pair improved. If the null hypothesis is true, then b and c should be approximately equal. If the difference between b and c is large, we would reject the null hypothesis if there is no association between the two variables. The McNemar test statistic is defined by

$$\chi_M^2 = \frac{[|b - c| - 1]^2}{(b + c)} \overset{\circ}{\sim} \chi_{(1)}^2.$$

The McNemar test statistics have an approximate χ^2 distribution with 1 degree of freedom. The basic setting for the McNemar test is that we deal with matched pairs in which two samples are correlated. When comparisons are made between two independent groups, significant differences may be observed that are not the result of the treatment. Two groups may not accurately reflect the relative effectiveness of the treatments because other clinical factors might be producing the observed differences in responses. One way to overcome this problem between the independent samples is to use matched pairs, achieved by pairing subjects as explained earlier. For the approximation to be valid, the total number of the discordant pairs should be at least 20, that is, $b + c \geq 20$. The test procedure is summarized below.

The McNemar Test for Matched Pairs

1. Count the number of discordant pairs b and c.
2. Evaluate the test statistic: $\chi_M^2 = \dfrac{[|b-c|-1]^2}{(b+c)}$
$\overset{\circ}{\sim} \chi_{(1)}^2$ under H_0.
3. Reject the null hypothesis if $\chi_{(1,1-\alpha)}^2 < \chi_M^2$ and accept H_0 if $\chi_{(1,1-\alpha)}^2 \geq \chi_M^2$.
4. The p value is obtained by $p = P(\chi_M^2 < \chi_{(1)}^2)$.

Example 10.5.1. Complete the significance test for the data in Table 10.5.2.

Solution. Because $b = 17$, $c = 14$, and $b + c = 31 > 20$, we may use the above test procedure. The value of the test statistic is

$$\chi_M^2 = \frac{[|b-c|-1]^2}{(b+c)} = \frac{[|17-14|-1]^2}{(17+14)}$$
$$= 0.1290.$$

The p value is obtained by

$$p = P\left(\chi_M^2 < \chi_{(1)}^2\right)$$
$$= P\left(0.129 < \chi_{(1)}^2\right) > P\left(2.706 < \chi_{(1)}^2\right)$$
$$= 0.10.$$

Since $\chi_{(1,0.95)}^2 = 3.841 \geq \chi_M^2 = 0.129$, and the p value is much larger than 0.10, we accept the null hypothesis at the significance level $\alpha = 0.05$, and conclude that there is no statistically significant difference in proportion of improved patients between CTG and GTR.

Example 10.5.2. A survey was taken by McCarthy and MacDonald [9] to investigate changes

Table 10.5.3. Infection control survey data for matched pairs.

First Survey	Second Survey		
	HBV Vaccine	No HBV Vaccine	
HBV vaccine	519	31	550
No HBV vaccine	57	181	238
	576	212	788

in infection control practices among dental professionals between 1994 and 1995. Their study was designed to measure changes in the proportion of dentists who reported the use of (i) basic barrier techniques, including the use of gloves, mask, and protective eyewear; (ii) hepatitis B virus vaccination (HBV) of dentists and clinical staff; (iii) heat sterilization of handpieces; and (iv) additional infection control precautions for patients with HIV/AIDS. A group of 788 dentists participated in both surveys taken in 1994 and 1995. Table 10.5.3 presents the survey data in a 2×2 table on compliance with the infection control recommendation for HBV vaccination of all clinical staff. Conduct a significance test at $\alpha = 0.05$.

Solution. Following the four steps described in the discussion above, we count the discordant pairs, $b = 31$ and $c = 57$. The value of the test statistic can be computed

$$\chi_M^2 = \frac{[|b-c|-1]^2}{(b+c)} = \frac{[|31-57|-1]^2}{(31+57)} = 7.102.$$

The p value is given by $p = P(\chi_M^2 < \chi_{(1)}^2) = P(7.102 < \chi_{(1)}^2) < P(6.635 < \chi_{(1)}^2) = 0.01$.

The critical value $\chi_{(1,0.95)}^2 = 3.841 < \chi_M^2 = 7.102$, and the p value is smaller than 0.01, so we reject the null hypothesis at the significance level $\alpha = 0.05$ and conclude that there is a statistically significant change in proportion of infection control compliance between 1994 and 1995, with a high compliance rate in 1995.

The McNemar test is often applied in social sciences. For example, researchers may attempt to compare the effectiveness of two teaching methods by pairing the subjects and to determine whether or not a particular political debate between two candidates was effective in changing viewers' preferences for them.

10.6 THE KAPPA STATISTIC

As we have seen in many examples for clinical studies, the response variables are qualitative: yes or no; survived or failed; tissue growth or no tissue growth; patient is cured or not cured; in remission or relapsed; and extreme pain, mild pain or no pain. In this section we will introduce Cohen's κ statistic (kappa statistic) [10] to measure the reliability of such data. Let X be the random variable representing a certain characteristic of subjects, for example, blood pressure. No matter how the blood pressure is measured and who measured it, it is measured unreliably in the sense that if the subject's blood pressure is measured again in similar conditions by the same experimenter or by a different experimenter, the second measurement will be different from the first measurement to some degree. In previous sections, the focus of our discussions was on tests of association between two categorical variables. Strictly speaking, there always will be some association between two variables. In the present section, we will discuss the issue of quantifying the extent to which two variables are associated. The question we ask is, How reliable or reproducible are they?

A χ^2 contingency table technique may be used for a test of association between first and second responses. However, the χ^2 test does not provide us with a quantitative measure of the degree of reliability (or reproducibility) between the two sets of responses. A good place to begin to measure reliability is concordant pairs in which both members in the pair produce the same responses. In Example 10.2.6 we have $15 + 21 = 36$ concordant pairs out of the total of 50 pairs. The rate of concordant responses is $36/50 = 0.72$. As with the χ^2 contingency table technique, we would like to compare this observed concordance rate, denoted p_0, with the expected concordance rate, denoted p_E, if the responses to the two separate questionnaires are statistically independent. The following table presents the relationship between survey responses in a 2×2 contingency table.

$$p_0 = \frac{\text{Total number of concordant pairs}}{\text{Total number of pairs}}$$
$$= \frac{O_{11} + O_{22}}{n}$$
$$p_E = \left(\frac{r_1}{n} \times \frac{c_1}{n}\right) + \left(\frac{r_2}{n} \times \frac{c_2}{n}\right).$$

As in the case of the χ^2 procedure, the better way to measure reliability is by the difference $p_0 - p_E$. If $p_0 - p_E = 0$, all the observed concordance could be attributed to chance alone. Cohen [10] proposed the following κ statistic to measure the degree of reliability.

$$\kappa = \frac{p_0 - p_E}{1 - p_E}$$

- If $p_0 < p_E$ (less than chance concordance), then $\kappa < 0$.
- If $p_0 = p_E$ (just chance concordance, that is, two questionnaires are completely independent), then $\kappa = 0$.
- If $p_0 > p_E$ (more than chance concordance), then $\kappa > 0$.
- If $p_0 = 1.0$ (perfect concordance), then $\kappa = 1.0$.

The following guidelines for the assessment of the κ statistic are given in various statistics literature:

- $0 \leq \kappa < 0.40$ suggests marginal reproducibility.
- $0.40 \leq \kappa \leq 0.75$ suggests good reproducibility.
- $0.75 < \kappa$ suggests excellent reproducibility.

For more discussions on the κ statistic, see Fleiss [11], Landis and Koch [12], Rosner [13], and Siegel and Castellan [14].

Example 10.6.1. An investigator selected 62 radiographs at random from patient charts. To assess the reliability of a dentist's ability to detect caries, these radiographs were shown to him at two separate times. After reviewing the radiographs, the dentist was asked to give dichotomous responses: caries present or caries absent. The dentist was not aware that he was reviewing the same radiographs twice. His responses are shown in Table 10.6.1. Evaluate the reliability of his measurements.

Table 10.6.1. Pocket depth measurement data.

	First Review	
Second Review	Caries Present	Caries Absent
Caries Present	20	5	25
Caries absent	14	23	37
	34	28	62

	Second Survey		
First Survey	Yes	No	
Yes	O_{11}	O_{12}	r_1
No	O_{21}	O_{22}	r_2
	c_1	c_2	n

Solution. The observed concordance rate is
$$p_0 = \frac{O_{11} + O_{22}}{n} = \frac{20 + 23}{62} = 0.6936 \text{ and the}$$
expected concordance rate is

$$p_E = \left(\frac{r_1}{n} \times \frac{c_1}{n}\right) + \left(\frac{r_2}{n} \times \frac{c_2}{n}\right)$$
$$= \left(\frac{25}{62} \times \frac{34}{62}\right) + \left(\frac{37}{62} \times \frac{28}{62}\right) = 0.4905.$$

We can now compute the κ statistic $\kappa = \frac{p_0 - p_E}{1 - p_E} = \frac{0.6936 - 0.4904}{1 - 0.4904} = 0.398\,7.$

Since $\kappa = 0.3987$, we conclude that the measurements of the dentist are marginally reproducible.

We discussed the κ statistic for 2×2 tables, but the concept can be extended to $r \times r$ contingency tables ($r > 2$) as illustrated in the following example.

Example 10.6.2. Dr. Dunford studied healing of a new root canal treatment. The evaluation of healing is done radiographically. He suspects that this type of measurement may not be highly reliable. To assess how reliable or reproducible radiographic readings are, Dr. Dunford had two other endodontists examine post-operative healing based on radiographs to determine a patient's condition in accordance with three categories: failing, partial healing, and complete healing. The endodontists evaluated 338 cases. Dr. Dunford's data is summarized in Table 10.6.2. Compute the κ statistic to measure the reproducibility between the two endodontists.

Solution. First, we need to compute the observed and expected concordance rates:

$$p_0 = \frac{O_{11} + O_{22} + O_{33}}{n} = \frac{52 + 107 + 86}{338}$$
$$= 0.724\,9.$$

Table 10.6.2. Radiographic data on root canal healing.

Second Endodontist	First Endodontist			
	Failing	Partial Healing	Complete Healing	
Failing	52	12	17	81
Partial healing	18	107	22	147
Complete healing	9	15	86	110
	79	134	125	338

$$p_E = \left(\frac{r_1}{n} \times \frac{c_1}{n}\right) + \left(\frac{r_2}{n} \times \frac{c_2}{n}\right) + \left(\frac{r_3}{n} \times \frac{c_3}{n}\right)$$
$$= \left(\frac{81}{338} \times \frac{79}{338}\right) + \left(\frac{147}{338} \times \frac{134}{338}\right)$$
$$+ \left(\frac{110}{338} \times \frac{125}{338}\right) = 0.3487.$$

We can compute the κ statistic $\kappa = \frac{p_0 - p_E}{1 - p_E} = \frac{0.7249 - 0.3487}{1 - 0.3487} = 0.577\,6.$

We get $\kappa = 0.578$, which suggests that there is a good reproducibility between the endodontists.

10.7 χ^2 GOODNESS-OF-FIT TEST

In the previous discussions we have conveniently assumed that the data came from a specific underlying probability distribution function, such as binomial or normal, and proceeded to estimate the unknown population parameters and to test hypotheses concerning the parameters. In this section we shall consider another application of the χ^2 technique in which an observed frequency distribution is compared with the underlying population distribution we assume to be true. Such a comparison is referred to as a χ^2 goodness-of-fit test. To illustrate the χ^2 goodness-of-fit test, we shall consider an example. The conventional method for the study of bonding failure has been the use of the shear bond strength test, in which a force is directed parallel to the base of the orthodontic bracket until the point of bonding failure occurs. Recently, a study was done using tensile bond strength to measure the bond strength of ceramic brackets to porcelain. The following table (see Table 10.7.1) shows the tensile strength (megapascals) of 50 samples of ceramic brackets bonded and then pulled off by an Instron machine. Let X be the random variable denoting the tensile strength.

Let's create 6 intervals (categories): $X \le 16.25$, $16.25 < X \le 17.20$, $17.20 < X \le 18.15$, $18.15 < X \le 19.10$, $19.10 < X \le 20.05$, and $20.05 < X$.

Table 10.7.1. Tensile strength of ceramic brackets.

20.2	16.0	18.2	16.8	16.5	19.0	20.2	18.6	19.1	18.7	18.4	18.1	19.1
19.2	20.3	18.3	16.2	19.9	18.6	20.6	16.4	21.0	18.0	17.1	19.3	19.4
19.1	19.8	17.3	18.1	17.3	17.6	20.0	18.9	19.7	19.6	18.7	20.6	19.3
17.9	18.0	15.8	17.1	17.4	16.8	16.4	15.3	18.1	18.3	18.0		

By counting the number of observed measurements in each category, we get $O_1 = 4$, $O_2 = 7$, $O_3 = 11$, $O_4 = 13$, $O_5 = 9$, and $O_6 = 6$. We would like to assume that these measurements came from a normal distribution. Recall that many statistical inferential procedures we discussed in the previous chapters were developed under the assumption of a normal distribution. The goodness-of-fit test is a technique that compares an observed number of measurements in each category with an expected number of measurements under the null hypothesis. From the data we can estimate the mean and variance and obtain $\overline{X} = 18.37$, and $S^2 = 1.92$. We state the null hypothesis as H_0: The underlying distribution from which the measurements came is $N(18.37, 1.92)$. (a normal distribution with $\mu = 18.37$ and $\sigma^2 = 1.92$)

We can also state it as $H_0 : X \sim N(18.37, 1.92)$. The next step is to estimate the expected cell frequencies for the 6 categories, assuming that the mean and SD of the hypothesized normal distribution are given by the sample mean and sample SD: $\overline{X} = 18.37$ and $S = 1.39$. The expected cell frequency is calculated by the following procedure, where n is the total sample size.

$$E_1 = n \cdot P(X \leq 16.25)$$
$$= n \cdot P\left(\frac{X - \mu}{\sigma} \leq \frac{16.25 - \mu}{\sigma}\right)$$
$$= n \cdot P\left(Z \leq \frac{16.25 - \mu}{\sigma}\right)$$
$$= 50 \cdot P\left(Z \leq \frac{16.25 - 18.37}{1.39}\right)$$
$$= 50 \cdot P(Z \leq -1.525)$$
$$= 50(1 - 0.9364) = 3.18.$$

Similarly, we obtain

$$E_2 = n \cdot P(16.25 < X \leq 17.20)$$
$$= 50(0.1136) = 5.68$$
$$E_3 = n \cdot P(17.20 < X \leq 18.15) = 11.87$$
$$E_4 = n \cdot P(18.15 < X \leq 19.10) = 13.15$$
$$E_5 = n \cdot P(19.10 < X \leq 20.05) = 9.35,$$

and

$$E_6 = n \cdot P(20.05 < X) = 5.67.$$

The observed and expected cell frequencies are given in the table below.

O_i	4	7	11	13	9	6
E_i	3.18	5.68	11.87	13.15	9.35	5.67

We use the same test statistic as before

$$\chi^2 = \frac{(O_1 - E_1)^2}{E_1} + \frac{(O_2 - E_2)^2}{E_2} + \frac{(O_3 - E_3)^2}{E_3}$$
$$+ \frac{(O_4 - E_4)^2}{E_4} + \frac{(O_5 - E_5)^2}{E_5} + \frac{(O_6 - E_6)^2}{E_6}.$$

Under the null hypothesis, this statistic follows approximately a χ^2 distribution with the degrees of freedom $c - 1 - k$, where $c =$ number of categories, and $k =$ number of the parameters estimated. In this example, $c = 6$, because we have created 6 categories, and $k = 2$, because we have estimated 2 parameters (mean and SD). We should note that the approximation is valid when no expected cell frequency is less than 1, and no more than 20% of the expected cell frequencies can be less than 5. In our example, all of the E_i's are greater than 1, and only 1 expected cell frequency (1 out of 6 expected cell frequencies) is less than 5.

$$\chi^2 = \frac{(4 - 3.18)^2}{3.18} + \frac{(7 - 5.68)^2}{5.68}$$
$$+ \frac{(11 - 11.87)^2}{11.87} + \frac{(13 - 13.15)^2}{13.15}$$
$$+ \frac{(9 - 9.35)^2}{9.35} + \frac{(6 - 5.67)^2}{5.67} = 0.616.$$

Under H_0, the test statistics has $\chi^2_{(c-1-k)} = \chi^2_{(6-1-2)} = \chi^2_{(3)}$. The critical value is $\chi^2_{(3, 1-\alpha)} = \chi^2_{(3, .95)} = 7.81$. Since $\chi^2 = 0.616 < \chi^2_{(3, 0.95)} = 7.81$, we accept the null hypothesis at the significance level $\alpha = 0.05$ and conclude that the normal distribution with mean 18.37 and standard deviation 1.39 provides an adequate fit to the tensile strength measurements.

The following should be noted:

1. Suppose that the null hypothesis was rejected in the above example. This does not necessarily mean that a normal distribution with different mean and SD will not fit the data.
2. The number of categories we decide to have is arbitrary, but a consideration must be given so that the approximation is valid. If we have too many categories, the expected cell frequencies will be small. Too many categories with the expected cell frequency less than 5 will violate the conditions for a valid approximation.
3. The concept of the χ^2 goodness-of-fit test procedure was explained in the context of a normal distribution, but it can be applied to any probability model. See Example 10.7.1 below.

We will summarize steps involved in a χ^2 goodness-of-fit test procedure.

1. Divide the data into c categories. The observations must be independent of each other.
2. Estimate the k parameters of the probability model using the data.
3. Count the observed cell frequencies, and calculate the corresponding expected cell frequencies using the hypothesized distribution.
4. Compute the test statistic $\chi^2 = \dfrac{(O_1 - E_1)^2}{E_1} + \dfrac{(O_2 - E_2)^2}{E_2} + \cdots + \dfrac{(O_c - E_c)^2}{E_c}$.
   Under H_0, the test statistic follows approximately a χ^2 distribution $\chi^2_{(c-1-k)}$ with the degrees of freedom $c - 1 - k$.

5. If $\chi^2_{(c-1-k,1-\alpha)} < \chi^2$, then reject H_0. If $\chi^2_{(c-1-k,1-\alpha)} \geq \chi^2$, then accept H_0.
6. The p value of the test is obtained by $P(\chi^2 < \chi^2_{(c-1-k)})$.

Example 10.7.1. Health-care satisfaction surveys conducted in the past indicated that a factor most significantly affecting the patient's overall perception of quality health care is waiting time in the clinic lobby. In order to understand the distribution of patient waiting time, an investigator decided to measure the length of time Dr. Brown's patients had to wait in his office. Suppose that Dr. Brown has 8 appointments each day he works. The investigator spent 100 days in Dr. Brown's office to observe patient waiting time. Since the patients in those surveys expressed that 15 minutes waiting time is tolerable, he recorded each appointment as either "on time" if a patient waited less than 15 minutes or "late" if a patient waited longer than 15 minutes. The patient waiting time data are displayed below. For each appointment, there are exactly two possible outcomes; either on time or late. Based on the data, test if the data came from a binomial distribution with $n = 8$.

No. of Late Appointments	No. of Days
0	14
1	7
2	9
3	17
4	12
5	13
6	25
7	3
8	0

Solution. We wish to test whether the data can be considered as having been observed from a binomial population with $n = 8$. Since the binomial probability p is not known, it needs to be estimated. Here, the probability $p = P$ (a patient waits longer than 15 minutes). In Section 6.2, we learned that the mean of the binomial distribution is $np = \overline{X}$. To estimate p, we will compute

$$\overline{X} = \frac{0 \cdot 14 + 1 \cdot 7 + 2 \cdot 9 + 3 \cdot 17 + 4 \cdot 12 + 5 \cdot 13 + 6 \cdot 25 + 7 \cdot 3 + 8 \cdot 0}{100} = \frac{360}{100} = 3.6.$$

We now have an equation $np = 3.6$. Solving the equation for p, we get

$$p = \frac{3.6}{n} = \frac{3.6}{8} = 0.45.$$

The null and alternative hypotheses are

H_0: The data are from a binomial distribution, $B(8, 0.45)$ vs.

H_1: The data are not from a binomial distribution with $n = 8$ and $p = 0.45$.

The possible values for the number of late appointments a day are 0, 1, 2, $\cdots$, 8. We will divide the data according to these values. Thus we have $c = 9$ categories. From Table B of the Appendix, we can obtain

No. of Late Appointments	Observed Freq.	Binomial Prob.	Expected Freq.
0	14	0.0084	0.84
1	7	0.0548	5.48
2	9	0.1570	15.70
3	17	0.2568	25.68
4	12	0.2627	26.27
5	13	0.1719	17.19
6	25	0.0703	7.03
7	3	0.0164	1.64
8	0	0.0017	0.17

The first two and the last two categories are combined to ensure the number of expected cell frequencies with values less than 5 is below 20% of the total number of categories. We now have

No. of Late Appointments	Observed Freq.	Expected Freq.
0 or 1	21	6.32
2	9	15.70
3	17	25.68
4	12	26.27
5	13	17.19
6	25	7.03
7 or 8	3	1.81

Calculate the test statistic

$$\chi^2 = \frac{(21 - 6.32)^2}{6.32} + \frac{(9 - 15.70)^2}{15.70}$$
$$+ \frac{(17 - 25.68)^2}{25.68} + \frac{(12 - 26.27)^2}{26.27}$$
$$+ \frac{(13 - 17.19)^2}{17.19} + \frac{(25 - 7.03)^2}{7.03}$$
$$+ \frac{(3 - 1.81)^2}{1.81}$$
$$= 95.381.$$

The critical value is $\chi^2_{(c-1-k, 1-\alpha)} = \chi^2_{(7-1-1, 0.95)} = \chi^2_{(5, 0.95)} = 11.070 < \chi^2 = 95.381$. Therefore, we reject the null hypothesis. The binomial distribution is not an adequate fit to the data.

10.8 EXERCISES

1 At the beginning of the last flu season, Orange County Community Hospital staff administered a flu vaccine. To determine if there is an association between the flu vaccine and contraction of the flu, 235 of the inoculated patients and 188 uninoculated subjects were randomly sampled. The investigators monitored the study subjects throughout the flu season and gathered the data shown in the table.

a. State the appropriate null hypothesis to test for an association between two variables.
b. Find the expected frequency for each cell.
c. Find the value of the test statistic.
d. What is the p value?
e. State the conclusion of the significance test.

	Contracted Flu		
Flu Vaccine	Yes	No	
Yes	43	192	235
No	51	137	188
	94	329	423

2 Alcohol consumption, like smoking, may be related to periodontal disease independent of oral hygiene status. To assess the relationship between alcohol consumption and severity of periodontal disease, 154 patients were chosen at random, and each patient was examined for gingival bleeding (yes/no) [15]. The patients were classified into two categories of alcohol consumption; fewer than five drinks a week and five or more drinks a week. The data is shown in table below. Perform an appropriate test to determine if there is an association between drinking and periodontal disease at the significance level $\alpha = 0.05$.

	Alcohol Consumption	
Gingival Bleeding	< 5 drinks	≥ 5 drinks
Yes	44	24
No	64	22

3 A study reviewed the outcome of 528 Branemark implants placed in the posterior region of the maxilla to investigate the relationship between smoking and implant failure [16]. Of the 528 implants, 89 were placed in smokers and 439 in non-smokers. Seventeen implants placed in the smoker's posterior maxilla and 48 implant placed in the non-smoker's posterior maxilla failed within a 5-year period. Is there a significant association between smoking habits and implant failure? Test an appropriate hypothesis at the significance level $\alpha = 0.05$.

4 Osteogenesis imperfecta is one of many genetic diseases. Suppose that an investigation was done to determine if there is any association between siblings being affected by osteogenesis imperfecta. Forty families, each with two children, were chosen at random for the study, and the children were thoroughly examined for the disease. The results of the dental exam showed that 12 of the first-born and 6 of the second-born children were affected by the disease. In 4 of the families, both the first- and second-born children were affected.

a. Construct a 2×2 contingency table.
b. Perform a significance test for association. If the χ^2 test procedure cannot be used, explain why. Discuss what technique can be applied to test the null hypothesis.

5 Assess the crown survival time data in Example 10.2.2 for statistical significance.

6 Many dental patients report that they experience dental anxiety and phobia. Dental researchers developed a video program that is designed to alleviate the patient's dental anxiety. To evaluate the effectiveness of the program, 160 patients have been selected in various dental clinics. Before and after the video program was shown to them, their anxiety level was classified into three categories: none, moderately anxious, and very anxious. The data are arranged in a 3×3 table, because both "before" and "after" have three categories. Perform a significance test for a relationship between *before* and *after*.

Before	After			
	None	Moderate	Very	
None	26	2	0	28
Moderate	7	62	18	87
Very	3	38	4	45
	36	102	22	160

7 Little attention has been given to the issue of obtaining informed consent for conscious sedation and general anesthesia from Spanish-speaking parents living in the United States. Clinicians are aware that the treatment of pediatric patients can only be as effective as the extent to which Spanish-speaking parents consent to the treatment. In a survey conducted with primarily Spanish-speaking parents of pediatric patients, the following two questions were included. Question 1: Language spoken at home (Spanish only, English only, both English and Spanish). Question 2: I prefer that the clinician who treats my child speak (Spanish only, English only, English and Spanish, no preference). The survey data are presented in the table below.

Language at Home	Clinician Speaks			
	Spanish only	English only	Both	No preference
Spanish only	78	23	64	46
English only	4	33	38	29
Both	43	57	64	48

a. State the null hypothesis to test for a relationship between the language spoken at home and the language parents prefer clinicians to speak.
b. Perform an appropriate test at the significance level $\alpha = 5\%$.
c. Compute the *p* value.

8 Each year, about 30, 000 new cases of oral cancer are diagnosed in the United States and about 9, 000 people die from the disease [17]. According to the National Cancer Institute, tobacco use is the most serious risk factor for oral cancer. A second major cause is chronic and/or heavy use of alcohol. The combination of tobacco and alcohol is particularly dangerous. Edwards [17] reported that smoking a pack of cigarettes a day increases the risk of oral cancer 4.5 times. Consuming up to six alcoholic drinks a day increases the risk 3.3 times and ingesting six to nine drinks a day increases the risk 15 times. Heavy use of alcohol and smoking combined increases the risk up to 100 times. Suppose a study was conducted with 492 randomly selected subjects, of whom 114 are heavy users of alcohol and 378 are not. Further investigations revealed that 46 of the 114 heavy users of alcohol and 110 of the 378 non-users of alcohol smoke at least one pack of cigarettes a day. There were 47 subjects diagnosed with oral cancer among the group of heavy alcohol users, while there were 74 subjects diagnosed with oral cancer among the non-alcohol group. The investigators learned that 35 subjects have oral cancer among those who smoke and drink alcohol, and 43 subjects have oral cancer among those who smoke but do not drink alcohol. Assess the relationship between oral cancer (Yes/No) and smoking (Yes/No), after controlling for alcohol consumption (Yes/No). Assess the relationship between the variables. What method would you use?

9 Discuss an example in biomedical health sciences where Cochran-Mantel-Hanszel method is appropriate.

10 Find a specific example where the McNemar test can be applied in your specialty area.

11 There are two tooth-numbering systems in use. The universal system is the most widely used system in the United States. The other system is the FDI system, developed by a committee from the Federation Dentaire Internationale. Suppose an investigator was interested in assessing whether the universal or FDI tooth-numbering system is easier for students to learn. The investigator has selected 264 students and formed 132 matched pairs according to several extraneous factors that might influence their ability to learn the tooth-numbering systems, such as the number of years in dental school, GPA, performance in clinical work, etc. Subjects in the same pair are randomly assigned to either the universal or FDI system. At the end of a tooth morphology course they were given a test to identify the teeth, using the system they learned to use [18]. The performance of the students was classified into 75% or more correct answers and less than 75% correct answers. Suppose that the test results showed that in 55 pairs both members of the pair scored 75% or better, in 24 pairs both members scored below 75%, and that 77 of the students who were assigned to the universal and 86 of the students who were assigned to FDI system scored at least 75%. Analyze the data for a statistical significance at the significance level $\alpha = 0.05$.

12 The probing depth equal to or greater than 6 mm is commonly used as the "yardstick" in determining periodontitis. It is not always easy to accurately measure the pocket depth and gingival recession due to soft tissues. To evaluate the reproducibility of measurements, 83 dental patients were randomly selected, and their pocket depth was measured by two periodontists. The measurements were classified into two categories, less than 6 mm and equal to or greater than 6 mm. Let X be the random variable describing the pocket depth. The data is illustrated in a 2×2 table. Compute the κ statistic.

Second Periodontist	First Periodontist		
	$X < 6$ mm	$X \geq 6$ mm	
$X < 6$ mm	41	5	46
$X \geq 6$ mm	8	29	37
	49	34	83

13 A dentist was asked to read radiographs and determine if she sees a rarefaction on the film. She was again asked to do the same 48 hours later. Her response to each radiograph was either yes, there is a rarefaction on film, or no, there is not. She was shown the same 143 radiographs. For 42 radiographs she indicated "yes," and for 51 radiographs she indicated "no" at both times. For 27 radiographs, she said "Yes" at initial reading but "No" 48 hours later. Evaluate the κ statistics for her readings.

14 From the tables shown in Example 10.2.5, measure the degree of reproducibility.

15 A table of random numbers is provided in Table A in the Appendix. This table is constructed in such a way that each digit, 0, 1, 2, $\cdots$, 9 is equally likely. In other words, they are observed with the equal probability of 0.10.
a. Construct a frequency table with the first 350 digits from Table A.
b. Find the expected cell frequency for each of the 10 digits.
c. Does the discrete uniform distribution adequately fit the data?

16 The past studies suggested that amalgam repair is a valid alternative to replacing damaged amalgam restorations [19]. However, many dentists believe that there is almost no cohesion between the application of fresh amalgam to previously placed amalgam, and thus they do not benefit from practicing the technique. A time-differentiated amalgam cohesion study was performed [20]. Seventy samples were prepared to test the bond between the aged amalgam surface and the fresh amalgam. The Instron machine was used to measure the shear strength of the specimens. The following data represent the peak load in megapascals. Test if a normal probability model fits the data adequately at the significance level $\alpha = 0.05$.

57.18	51.52	66.85	65.63	30.48	37.36	28.07	36.75	45.26	38.68
31.23	38.55	28.81	15.66	16.78	20.82	20.44	42.21	39.88	36.36
51.28	55.58	49.93	64.96	37.48	36.70	45.44	39.56	37.82	32.16
75.96	27.82	39.14	22.88	18.45	39.75	55.89	52.24	47.27	67.31
38.76	41.20	53.92	36.83	40.18	35.89	38.96	33.56	44.05	32.18
36.15	33.90	28.53	30.68	36.12	28.01	17.52	22.86	40.47	21.84
48.12	24.65	33.36	57.45	47.51	39.74	26.35	31.58	40.39	56.04

10.9 REFERENCES

1. Goldstein, F., et al. Postmenopausal hormone therapy and mortality. *N Engl J Med*: 1997, 336, 1769–1775.
2. Grizzle, J. E. Continuity correction in the χ^2 test for 2×2 tables. *The American Statistician*: 1967, 21, 28–32.
3. Fisher, L. D., and Van Belle, G. *Biostatistics: A Methodology for the Health Sciences.* John Wiley and Sons. 1993.
4. Rosner, B. *Fundamentals of Biostatistics.* Fourth edition, Duxbury Press. 1995.
5. Darwazeh, A. M., Al-Refai, S., and Al-Mojaiwel, S. Isolation of Candida species from the oral cavity and fingertips of complete denture wearers. *J Prosthet Dent*: 2001, 86, 420–423.
6. Holan, G., and Ram, D. Sequelae and prognosis of intruded primary incisors: A retrospective study. *Pediatr Dent*: 1999, 21, 243–248.
7. Cochran, W. G. Some methods for strengthening the common χ^2 tests. *Biometrics*: 1954, 10, 417–451.
8. Mantel, N., and Haenszel, W. Statistical aspects of the analysis of data from retrospective studies of disease. *J. Nat. Cancer Inst*: 1959, 22, 719–748.
9. McCarthy, G. M., and MacDonald, J. K. Improved compliance with recommended infection control practices in the dental office between 1994 and 1995. *Am J Infect Control*: 1998, 26, 24–28.
10. Cohen, J. A coefficient of agreement for nominal scales. *Educ Psychol Meas*: 1960, 20, 37–46.
11. Fleiss, J. *Statistical Methods for Rates and Proportions.* John Wiley & Sons. 1981.
12. Landis, J. R., and Koch, G. G. The measurement of observer agreement for categorical studies data. *Biometrics*: 1977, 33, 159–174.
13. Rosner, B. *Fundamentals of Biostatistics.* Fourth edition. Duxbury Press. 1995.
14. Siegel, S., and Castellan, N. J. *Nonparametric Statistics for the Behavioral Sciences.* Second edition. McGraw Hill. 1998.
15. Tezal, M., et al. The effect of alcohol consumption on periodontal disease. *J Periodontol*: 2001, 72, 183–189.
16. Bain, C. A., and Moy, P. K. The association between the failure of dental implants and cigarette smoking. *Int J Oral Maxillofac Implants*: 1993, 8, 609–615.
17. Edwards, *J. Oral cancer Access.* January, 2000.
18. Belfiglio, B., and Stevens, T. The Universal vs. the FDI Tooth Numbering System: A Learning Comparison. Loma Linda University student project. 2002.
19. Cowan, R. D. Amalgam repair—a clinical technique. *J Pros Dent*: 1983, 49, 49–51.
20. Kim, J., Lee, J., and Watkins, R. Cohesion of Newly Placed Amalgam to Different Aged Amalgam. Loma Linda University student project. 2001.

Chapter 11

Regression Analysis and Correlation

11.1 INTRODUCTION

The previous four chapters were devoted to two areas of statistical inference: confidence interval and hypothesis testing. In this chapter we will introduce another area of inferential statistics, known as regression analysis, which explores the nature of a relationship between two or more quantitative variables so that one variable can be predicted from the other(s). Simple linear regression, correlation, and multiple regression will be introduced. The primary goal of a simple linear regression is to establish a statistical relationship that makes it possible to predict one variable in terms of another. For example:

1. a study was conducted to predict family's dental and medical expenditures in terms of household income;
2. an investigation was done to study the relationship between weight loss and the number of days subjects have been on a $1,200$ kcal per day diet;
3. an analysis was performed to predict dental students' national board exam scores in terms of their GPA in basic science courses while in dental school;
4. a study was done to describe the relationship between drug potency and the assay response; and
5. a study was done to describe the relationship between height and weight of dentists; if Dr. Jackson is 5 feet 10 inches tall, how much is he expected to weigh?

In a simple regression problem, we are primarily interested in a statistical relationship between one **dependent variable** Y and one **independent variable** X. It is assumed that the values taken on by the random variable Y depend on a fixed value of X. In other words, the values of Y vary with changes in the values of X. In the above examples, Y represents a family's dental and medical

expenditures, weight loss, national board exam scores, and weight of the dentist. Independent variable X represents household income, the number of days on diet, dental school grade point average (GPA), and height of the dentist. Dependent variable Y is also called **response variable** or **outcome variable**. Independent variable X is also called **predictor variable**, **regressor variable**, or **explanatory variable**. The purpose of a regression analysis is to find a reasonable **regression equation** to predict the average value of a response variable Y that is associated with a fixed value of one independent variable X. We cannot predict precisely how much weight an individual subject will lose after having been on the diet program for 14 days, but given adequate data we can predict the average weight loss after 14 days. Similarly, we can predict students' average score on the national board exam given their GPA and the expected weight of the dentists in terms of their height. If more than one independent variable were used to predict the average value of a response variable, then we would need **multiple regression** (discussed later in this chapter). The dependent variable in regression is the variable that cannot be controlled. The score on the national board exam depends on the students' GPA, and the amount of weight loss depends on the number of days the individuals are on a diet. The determination of the dependent and independent variables is not always clear-cut and sometimes is an arbitrary decision made by researchers. For example, a different investigator may select height of the dentist as the dependent variable Y and weight as the independent variable X.

11.2 SIMPLE LINEAR REGRESSION

To study the statistical relationship between two variables, we first plot the independent and dependent variables on a scatter plot. The independent variable is plotted along the horizontal axis, and the dependent variable is plotted along the vertical axis. The scatter plots can aid us in determining the nature of the relationship. Figure 11.2.1 shows three scatter plots: A, B, and C.

Scatter Plot A

In many countries nowadays, people tend to drink greater amounts of soft drinks. Consumption of soft drinks affects dental health because of the potential risk of sugar and acid-containing drinks to cause caries and erosion. The factors that cause the erosion of tooth surface due to acidic soft drinks has been well documented [1]. Chung, et al. [1] investigated the influence of the high level of consumption of soft drinks on the behavior of dental materials and teeth with respect to erosion. Extracted human teeth were soaked in one of the popular carbonated drinks. The measurements of surface roughness of teeth samples were determined with a profilometer at various time points. This data is depicted in scatter plot A in Figure 11.2.1. Surface roughness (micrometers) is taken as the response or outcome variable Y, and the soaking time (hr) is taken as the independent or predictor variable X. The plot clearly suggests that there is a linear relation (a straight line) between surface roughness and soaking time, in the sense that the longer the soaking time, the greater tends to be the surface roughness, that is, there is a greater amount of erosion of the tooth surface. Figure 11.2.2 (A) indicates that the relationship is not perfectly linear, but it strongly suggests that a linear equation with a positive slope is a good fit.

Scatter Plot B

The Knoop's hardness of a widely used cement material was measured by using the conventional light curing method at various depths (millimeters) [2]. The relationship between hardness Y (the response variable) and depth X (the predictor variable) is plotted in scatter plot B in Figure 11.2.1. The plot suggests that there is a linear relationship between the two variables. Unlike scatter plot A, the slope of the equation in Figure 11.2.2 (B) is negative. The greater the depth, the smaller tends to be the Knoop's hardness of the composite ma-

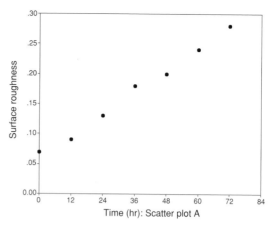

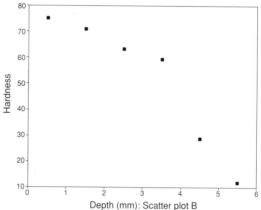

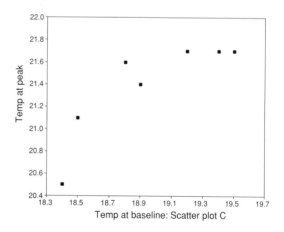

Figure 11.2.1   Three scatter plots.

terial cured by the conventional light. These data are slightly less linear than those in scatter plot A. Nevertheless, a straight line appears to provide an adequate fit. The plot indicates the general tendency by which the hardness varies with changes in depth.

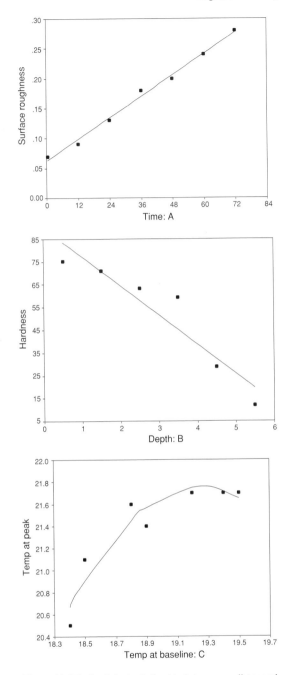

Figure 11.2.2 Statistical relationship between predictor and response variables.

Scatter Plot C

The vitality of bone tissue has been shown to be altered with temperatures above 47° C. Prolonged exposure to high temperature usually results in impaired bone healing and/or bone necrosis. The temperature during implant osteotomy can rise

over 100° C, which exceeds biologic tolerance for osseous repair. Consequently, heat-induced bone necrosis leads to implant failure. It has been shown in the dental literature [3] that proper irrigation is the most important factor in maintaining bone temperature within biologic tolerance. Hover et al. [4] investigated the effect of irrigation solutions on heat generation. Scatter plot C of Figure 11.2.1 represents the relationship between the maximum temperature during osteotomy and initial baseline temperature before osteotomy. The depth of the osteotomies was 4 mm. A chlorhexidine glycerine solution was one of the irrigation systems used on the study of reduction of heat generation during implant osteotomy. The data suggest that the relationship between the temperature at peak and the initial temperature is non-linear. It is non-linear (or curvilinear). The curve of the relation is drawn in Figure 11.2.2 (C). The plot suggests that as the initial temperature at baseline becomes higher, the maximum temperature during the osteotomy increases to a certain point, and then it levels off at about 21.7° C.

The scatter plot in Figure 11.2.3 represents the effect of sour toothpaste on tooth demineralization by testing micro-hardness of enamel using 14 extracted bovine incisors. It has been found that a low pH in the oral cavity leads to tooth demineralization. Due to the low pH of citric acid in the sour toothpaste, it was speculated that enamel demineralization will occur. Micro-hardness was measured before and after the treatment with the sour toothpaste [5]. The plot strongly suggests that

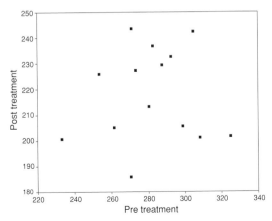

Figure 11.2.3 Scatter plot of pre- vs. post-treatment enamel hardness.

there is little or no linear relationship between pre- and post-treatments with respect to the micro-hardness. In fact, pre-treatment hardness does not seem to provide much help for predicting post-treatment hardness. There is no particular relation between the variables.

Based on the observed data, we like to estimate a mathematical model that describes the relationship between two variables. In statistics this procedure is known as regression analysis or curve fitting. A regression model is a formal expression of a statistical relationship between two variables. There are two basic questions we must keep in mind in any regression analysis.

1. What is the most appropriate model to use as a predicting equation: a straight line, a curvilinear, etc?
2. Given a specific model, how do we determine the particular equation that is "best" for the data?

The first question is usually addressed by inspecting the scatter plot of the data. We can determine the kind of model that best describes the overall pattern of the data by visual inspection. In this section the second question will be discussed in detail. Our discussions will primarily be focused on simple linear regression equations. Regression models may have more than one independent variable. Here are some examples:

1. In the study of a regression analysis to predict a family's dental and medical expenditure, the household income as well as the size of the family can be introduced as independent variables.
2. In the study of weight loss, we can use diet, physical exercise, and sex as explanatory variables in the model to predict the amount of weight loss.
3. A regression model can include GPA in basic sciences, dental admissions test (DAT) scores, and the number of hours spent for preparation as independent variables for predicting the national board exam scores.

For each of the above three applications one can think of many more independent variables, but only a limited number of predictor variables should be included in a regression model. The key issue, then, is choosing variables that are best for prediction of the response variable. Basically, this choice is made with consideration of the variables

that contribute to reducing the variation in the response variable Y.

11.2.1 Description of Regression Model

We consider a simple linear regression model that includes only one independent variable. The model can be stated as follows:

$$Y_i = \beta_0 + \beta_1 X_i + \varepsilon_i, \text{ where}$$

- Y_i is the value of the response variable at the ith level of the independent variable;
- parameters β_0 and β_1 are unknown regression coefficients whose values are to be estimated;
- X_i is a known constant, which is the value of the independent variable at the ith level; and
- ε_i represents an error term that is a random variable, assumed to be normally distributed with mean 0 and variance σ^2, that is, $\varepsilon_i \sim N(0, \sigma^2)$.

We assume that the errors at different levels of the predictor variable X_i are statistically independent. That is ε_i and ε_j are statistically independent. We also assume that the variance of the random error term ε_i is constant. Ignoring the error term and the indices for the variables in the model for an illustration, we have $Y = \beta_0 + \beta_1 X$. This is a familiar mathematical expression from an algebra course, which describes a straight line such as the line we have in Figure 11.2.2 (A). The parameter β_0 is called the Y-intercept, and β_1 is called the slope of a straight line. Recall that the intercept β_0 is the value of Y when X takes on the value 0. The slope β_1 is the amount of changes in Y for each one unit change in X. For a given linear equation, this rate of change is always constant. From the assumptions we have for the simple linear regression model regarding the random error term ε_i, the mean (or the expected value) of the response variable at the ith level of the independent variable is 0, denoted by $E(Y_i) = \beta_0 + \beta_1 X_i$, and the variance of Y_i is σ^2, denoted by $Var(Y_i) = \sigma^2$. Thus, the regression model assumes that the probability distributions of the responses Y_i have the same variance, irrespective of the levels of the independent variable X_i. This assumption of constant variability is known as **homoscedasticity**. In summary, the outcomes Y_i come from the population with a normal distribution with the mean given

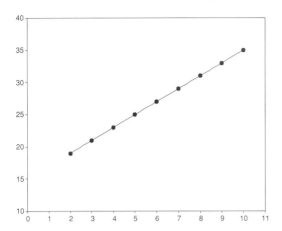

Figure 11.2.4   Perfect fit with $\sigma^2 = 0$.

by $E(Y_i) = \beta_0 + \beta_1 X_i$ and variance given by σ^2,

$$Y_i \sim N(E(Y_i) = \beta_0 + \beta_1 X_i, \sigma^2).$$

The expression $E(Y_i) = \beta_0 + \beta_1 X_i$ is called a **regression function.** If the value $X = 0$ in a regression model is meaningful, then the Y-intercept β_0 is the mean of the response variable Y when $X = 0$. Suppose we have a regression function $E(Y_i) = 7.8 + 2.5 \cdot X_i$. The mean value of the response at $X = 0$ is 7.8, and the slope $\beta_1 = 2.5$ indicates that one unit increase in X leads to a 2.5 unit increase in the mean of the distribution of the response variable Y. If $\sigma^2 = 0$, then every observation would fall right on the regression line as shown in Figure 11.2.4. As the variance increases, $\sigma^2 > 0$, the observations would be scattered about the regression line. See Figure 11.2.5.

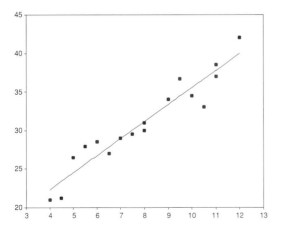

Figure 11.2.5   A regression equation with $\sigma^2 > 0$.

From $E(Y_i) = \beta_0 + \beta_1 X_i$ we can see that if $\beta_1 > 0$, a positive slope, then the mean response increases as X increases. On the other hand if $\beta_1 < 0$, a negative slope, then the mean response decreases as X increases. If $\beta_1 = 0$, then the mean response will be constant $E(Y_i) = \beta_0$, and hence there is no relationship between the mean response Y and the independent variable X. In a simple linear regression model we assume that the graph of the mean of the response variable $E(Y_i)$ for given values of the independent variable X_i is a straight line.

11.2.2 Estimation of Regression Function

The values of the regression coefficients β_0 and β_1 are usually not known, and therefore we need to estimate them from data. To estimate β_0 and β_1, we shall apply the **method of least squares**. The estimates of β_0 and β_1 will be denoted by b_0 and b_1. When the estimates are obtained, they will replace β_0 and β_1, and $\hat{Y}_i = b_0 + b_1 X_i$ will be referred to as a **fitted regression equation**. As in Figure 11.2.2, we could simply draw a straight line through the points, but this approach is somewhat arbitrary and subjective. Many such straight lines can be drawn from the scatter plot. With many points scattered on the graph, this approach of "eyeballing the data" could be imprecise in practice. We wish to determine a line that best fits the data, the best in the sense that the values b_0 and b_1 will be those that minimize the sum of the squares of the distance between the data points and the fitted regression line. To facilitate our discussion on the method of least squares, let's consider the following data, which represent the relationship between the average pre-clinic lab scores and perceptual aptitude test (PAT) scores of 15 dental students (Table 11.2.1).

Suppose we wish to develop a regression model by which the average pre-clinical scores of dental students can be predicted from the knowledge of their PAT scores. Figure 11.2.6 shows a fitted regression line drawn on the scatter plot of the data. The motivation behind the method of least squares is the following. Draw a vertical line from each data point to the regression line in Figure 11.2.6. The vertical distance between a data point and the

Table 11.2.1. Average pre-clinic lab score vs. PAT score of dental students.

PAT Score (X_i)	Ave. Preclinic Lab (Y_i)
13	2.96
14	3.02
15	3.08
16	3.10
17	3.14
18	3.32
19	3.37
20	3.35
21	3.51
22	3.34
23	3.67
24	3.19
25	—
26	3.43
27	3.76

fitted regression line is called a **residual**. The residuals are denoted by e_i as indicated in the figure,

$$e_i = Y_i - (b_0 + b_1 X_i).$$

The method of least squares yields the estimates b_0 and b_1 of the regression parameters that minimize the sum of squared distances of the data points from the regression line given by

$$Q = \sum_{i=1}^{n} e_i^2 = \sum_{i=1}^{n} [Y_i - (b_0 + b_1 X_i)]^2.$$

This method of estimating the regression coefficients β_0 and β_1 selects the straight line that comes as close as it can to all data points in the scatter plot.

It can be shown that the estimates are obtained by

$$b_1 = \frac{\sum_{i=1}^{n}(X_i - \overline{X})(Y_i - \overline{Y})}{\sum_{i=1}^{n}(X_i - \overline{X})^2}$$

$$= \frac{\sum_{i=1}^{n} X_i Y_i - \frac{\left(\sum_{i=1}^{n} X_i\right)\left(\sum_{i=1}^{n} Y_i\right)}{n}}{\sum_{i=1}^{n} X_i^2 - \frac{\left(\sum_{i=1}^{n} X_i\right)^2}{n}}$$

$$b_0 = \frac{1}{n}\left(\sum_{i=1}^{n} Y_i - b_1 \sum_{i=1}^{n} X_i\right) = \overline{Y} - b_1 \overline{X}$$

where

$$\overline{X} = \frac{1}{n}\sum_{i=1}^{n} X_i \quad \text{and} \quad \overline{Y} = \frac{1}{n}\sum_{i=1}^{n} Y_i.$$

We note that b_0 and b_1 obtained by the least squares method are minimum variance unbiased estimators.

Example 11.2.1. As part of a study to examine neuromuscular function, occlusal index, and centric relation-centric occlusion discrepancy of orthodontically treated patients, Kowalczyk [6] collected the following improved isometric masseter sEMG (surface electromyography) values of right anterior temporalis (R-AT) and left anterior temporalis (L-AT) of 23 patients. Estimate a regression function to predict left anterior temporalis given a value of right anterior temporalis.

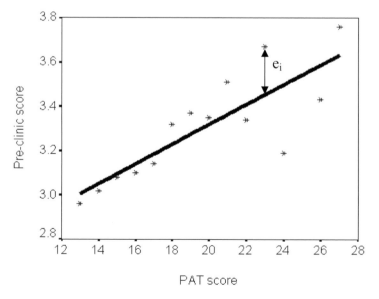

Figure 11.2.6 Vertical distance between the best fitted regression line and the data point.

Patient	R-AT	L-AT	Patient	R-AT	L-AT
1	61	60	13	110	95
2	180	185	14	49	20
3	190	180	15	75	88
4	115	90	16	103	102
5	200	185	17	145	170
6	155	80	18	245	220
7	185	190	19	100	150
8	48	77	20	160	120
9	75	75	21	160	190
10	70	65	22	101	120
11	142	110	23	15	40
12	98	50			

$$b_0 = \frac{1}{n}\left(\sum_{i=1}^{n} Y_i - b_1 \sum_{i=1}^{n} X_i\right)$$

$$= \frac{1}{23}[2,662 - (0.8589)(2,782)] = 11.850.$$

By substitution we obtain the fitted regression equation $\hat{Y}_i = 11.850 + 0.8589 X_i$.

If we are interested in the mean L-AT (or the predicted value) when the R-AT is $X = 125$, our estimate is $\hat{Y}_i = 11.850 + 0.8589(125) = 119.21$. The value of L-AT for any individual patient whose R-AT is 125 is not likely to be exactly 119.21 but either lower or higher because of the inherent variability in the response variable Y_i as represented by the error term ε_i. But bear in mind that the expected value of Y for a given value of $X = 125$ is 119.21. We note that the fitted regression line illustrated in Figure 11.2.7 has the smaller $Q = \sum_{i=1}^{n} e_i^2 = \sum_{i=1}^{n}[Y_i - (b_0 + b_1 X_i)]^2$ than any other arbitrary fitted regression lines.

Solution. The scatter plot in Figure 11.2.7 suggests that a straight line will be a good fit. Left anterior temporalis is the response variable Y_i and right anterior temporalis is the independent variable X_i. Using the method of least squares to estimate the regression coefficients β_0 and β_1, from the data presented in the table, we can calculate

$$b_1 = \frac{\sum_{i=1}^{n} X_i Y_i - \dfrac{\left(\sum_{i=1}^{n} X_i\right)\left(\sum_{i=1}^{n} Y_i\right)}{n}}{\sum_{i=1}^{n} X_i^2 - \dfrac{\left(\sum_{i=1}^{n} X_i\right)^2}{n}}$$

$$= \frac{384,857 - \dfrac{(2,782)(2,662)}{23}}{409,704 - \dfrac{(2,782)^2}{23}} = 0.8589.$$

11.2.3 Aptness of a Model

When a regression model is selected for an application, we cannot be quite certain whether or not the model is appropriate. Any one of the conditions for the simple linear regression model may not be satisfied. For example, the linearity of the

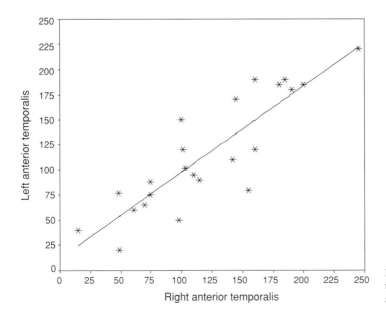

Figure 11.2.7 Scatter plot and the fitted regression model for right and left anterior temporalis.

regression function, normality of the error terms, or homoscedasticity may not be appropriate for the data we wish to fit. Therefore, it is important that we study the aptness of the model for our data. In this section we introduce some simple graphic techniques to examine the appropriateness of a model. At the beginning of Section 11.2 we defined the residual e_i, which is the difference between the observed value Y_i and the fitted value $\hat{Y}$:

$$e_i = Y_i - (b_0 + b_1 X_i) = Y_i - \hat{Y}_i.$$

The residual can be viewed as an observed error. The error term $\varepsilon_i = Y_i - (\beta_0 + \beta_1 X_i) = Y_i - E\{Y_i\}$ is the true unknown error in the regression model. We have stated that the error term ε_i is assumed to be statistically independent and normally distributed with mean 0 and the constant variance σ^2 (homoscedasticity). Hence, if the fitted model is appropriate for the data, it is reasonable to expect the observed residuals e_i to reflect these conditions assumed for the error term ε_i. A two-way plot of the residuals versus the values of the independent variable (or the fitted values of the response variable), known as the residual plot, is a useful tool for examining the aptness of a regression model. We will use the residual plots to check the following:

1. The regression function is linear.
2. The error terms have constant variance.
3. The error terms are statistically independent.
4. The error terms are normally distributed.
5. The model fits the data points except for a few outlier observations.

Linearity

The plot in Figure 11.2.8 (a) is the residual plot of the data in Example 11.2.1 against the independent variable X_i. This shows a typical situation in which the linear model is adequate. The residuals tend to fall around the horizontal $e_i = 0$, exhibiting no systematic patterns to stay above or below $e_i = 0$. If the linear regression model is not adequate, the residual plot would look like the plot shown in Figure 11.2.8 (b). The residuals tend to behave in a systematic fashion. They increase gradually and then decrease, staying above $e_i = 0$ in the middle of the range for the independent variable. This residual plot indicates that the linear regression model is not appropriate. An appropriate model has to be nonlinear.

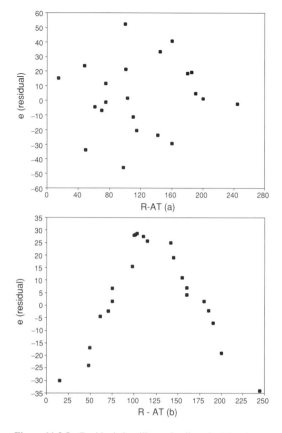

Figure 11.2.8   Residual plots illustrating linearity (a) and non-linearity (b).

Constant Error Variance

The scatter plots of the residuals against the independent variable (or against the fitted values) are useful for examining the adequacy of both the linear regression model and the homoscedasticity. The plot in Figure 11.2.8 (a) is an example of constant error term as well as appropriateness of the linearity of a model. Figure 11.2.9 illustrates an example of nonconstancy of error variance. The plot suggests there is a strong tendency that the larger the value of independent variable (X_i), the greater the spread of residuals. This indicates that the error variance (and therefore, the variance of the response variable) is greater for the larger values of R-AT. Of course, we could have a plot that shows that the spread of the residuals is greater for the smaller values of the independent variable and smaller for the larger values of R-AT. Either case is an indication of nonconstancy of error variance.

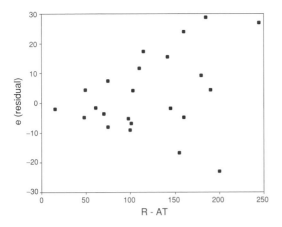

Figure 11.2.9 Residual plot illustrating nonconstancy of error variance.

Independence

When the error terms are statistically independent, we expect the residuals to randomly fluctuate around the horizontal line $e_i = 0$; some are positive and others are negative, as seen in Figure 11.2.8 (a). The residual plot in Figure 11.2.10 is an illustration of non-independence of error terms. The first half of the residuals for smaller values of X_i are above the line $e_i = 0$ (that is, $e_i > 0$), and the second half of the residuals for larger values of X_i are below the line $e_i = 0$ (that is, $e_i < 0$). Namely, positive residuals are associated with the smaller values of X_i and negative residuals are associated with the larger values of X_i. This type of a residual plot indicates a lack of independence of error terms.

Normality

The expression of the simple linear regression model assumes the normality of the error term ε_i. The normality assumption is justifiable because ε_i can be viewed as the term that represents the effects of many factors not included in the model that do influence the outcome variable. By central limit theorem, discussed in Section 6.2, the error term would be approximately normally distributed as the effects of factors become sufficiently large. The normality is the standard assumption, which greatly simplifies the theory of regression analysis. Small departures from normality are not considered as serious problems.

We have already introduced some graphic techniques to examine informally whether or not a particular set of data is drawn from a normal population: histograms, stem and leaf plots, and box plots. A box plot can be used to check the symmetry of the residuals and outliers. Another graphic method is a **normal probability plot of the residuals**. Residuals are plotted against their expected value under the normal distribution. Statistical software packages (e.g., Minitab, SPSS, SAS) can produce normal probability plots. The plot in Figure 11.2.11 is a normal probability plot of the data we discussed in Example 11.2.1. This plot is nearly straight, which suggests that the normality assumption is reasonable in this case. If the plot were substantially deviated from linearity, then the error term is not normal.

We remind the readers that the normal error regression model is assumed. Thus, the regression model implies that the outcome variable Y_i has the

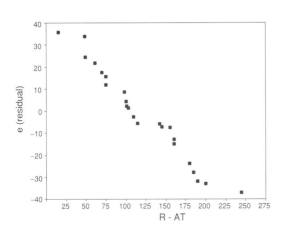

Figure 11.2.10 Non-independence of error terms.

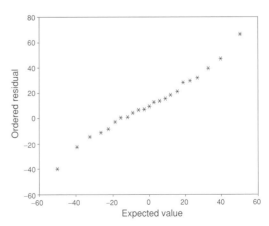

Figure 11.2.11 Normal probability plot of the data in Example 11.2.1.

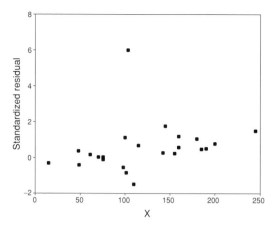

Figure 11.2.12   Residual plot with an outlier.

normal probability distribution. There are some rigorous methods used to study the normality of the data at hand, such as the χ^2 goodness-of-fit test discussed in Chapter 10.

Detection of Outliers

In Chapter 3 we discussed how outliers can be detected from box plots and stem and leaf plots. Residual outliers can be detected from residual plots against the independent variable X or $\hat{Y}$. Outliers can cause great difficulty in regression analysis. When the least squares method is used to estimate the regression function, a fitted line would be pulled toward the outliers. This could give us a misleading fit, especially if the outlier observation is due to an investigator's mistake. It is common practice to delete the outliers only if there is evidence that they are due to an error in reading, recording, calculating, or equipment malfunctioning. Sometimes standardized residuals are used in residual analysis. Standardized residual is defined by

$$\frac{e_i}{\sqrt{MSE}}$$

where MSE (mean squared error) is given by $MSE = \dfrac{\sum_{i=1}^{n} e_i^2}{n-2}$. MSE is also called residual mean square by some authors. Figure 11.2.12 shows a standardized residual plot against the independent variable. It shows that it contains one residual outlier at $X_i = 103$.

Frequently, a regression model is used to predict future events. In predicting future observations on the outcome variable, some caution must be exercised when the prediction is made pertaining to levels of the independent variable that fall outside its original range. It often occurs that the investigators want to predict the annual dental and medical expenditure for a family whose household income is far beyond the level they have observed. There is no guarantee the regression function that fits the past data well is also adequate over a much wider range of the independent variable. To illustrate this point further, let's consider the following example.

A regression equation for the body mass index (BMI) of past Miss Americas [7] is shown in Figure 11.2.13. Using the least squares method we have obtained the regression equation, $\hat{Y} = 97.148 - 0.040X_i$. This model will predict the BMI of 15.9 for Miss America for the year 2030. It is extremely unlikely that any Miss America would have BMI of 15.9, which can be considered as a health risk. We have not discussed inferences about regression coefficients in this chapter. There are many excellent textbooks on the topic. We refer interested readers to Kleinbaum et al. [8], Neter et al.[9], and Pagano and Gauvreau [10].

11.3 CORRELATION COEFFICIENT

So far, in this chapter, our discussion has been focused on a simple linear regression method of predicting one dependent variable from one independent variable. Instead of predicting the mean

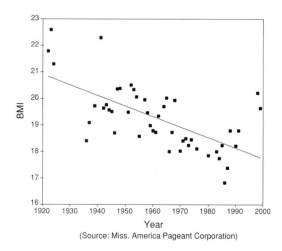

Figure 11.2.13   Regression function for body mass index of Miss America.

of one variable from another, investigators are often interested in measuring a relationship between two variables. Statisticians use a measure called the **correlation coefficient** to quantify the strength and direction of the relationship between two variables. There are several types of quantitative measures of correlation coefficient. In this section we will introduce the **Pearson product moment correlation coefficient**, or **Pearson correlation coefficient**. As usual, we will let X_i and Y_i denote two variables. In the regression analysis, the response variable Y_i is a random variable, but the independent variable X_i is not, though there are some situations where it is considered a random variable. In correlation analysis, both X_i and Y_i are random variables. We wish to determine the linear association that exits between these two random variables, X_i and Y_i. The most popular measure of linear association between two variables is the Pearson product moment correlation coefficient.

The Pearson sample correlation coefficient is denoted by r, and the population correlation coefficient is denoted by the Greek letter ρ (rho).

Definition 11.3.1. Let X_i and Y_i be a pair of random variables. Then the Pearson product moment correlation coefficient is defined by

$$r = \frac{\sum_{i=1}^{n}(X_i - \overline{X})(Y_i - \overline{Y})}{\sqrt{\sum_{i=1}^{n}(X_i - \overline{X})^2 \cdot \sum_{i=1}^{n}(Y_i - \overline{Y})^2}}$$

where n is the number of pairs of sample observations, and $\overline{X} = \frac{1}{n}\sum_{i=1}^{n} X_i$ and $\overline{Y} = \frac{1}{n}\sum_{i=1}^{n} Y_i$. It is computationally more convenient to use

$$r = \frac{\sum_{i=1}^{n} X_i Y_i - \frac{\left(\sum_{i=1}^{n} X_i\right)\left(\sum_{i=1}^{n} Y_i\right)}{n}}{\sqrt{\left(\sum_{i=1}^{n} X_i^2 - \frac{\left(\sum_{i=1}^{n} X_i\right)^2}{n}\right)\left(\sum_{i=1}^{n} Y_i^2 - \frac{\left(\sum_{i=1}^{n} Y_i\right)^2}{n}\right)}}.$$

Note that the denominator of the correlation coefficient r is always positive. If small values of X_i tend to be associated with small values of Y_i, and large values of X_i with large values of Y_i, then $(X_i - \overline{X})$ and $(Y_i - \overline{Y})$ will tend to have the same algebraic sign ($+$ or $-$). This implies that $(X_i - \overline{X})(Y_i - \overline{Y})$ in the numerator will tend to be positive, yielding a positive value of r. If small values of X_i tend to be associated with large values of Y_i, and vice versa, then $(X_i - \overline{X})$ and $(Y_i - \overline{Y})$ will tend to have opposite signs. This implies that $(X_i - \overline{X})(Y_i - \overline{Y})$ will tend to have negative signs, resulting in a negative value of r. The correlation coefficient r lies between -1 and $+1$ inclusive ($-1 \leq r \leq +1$).

- If $r = 1$, then we have perfect positive correlation between X and Y. Figure 11.3.1 (a) and Figure 11.3.1 (b) illustrate the cases with $r = 1$, in which there is perfect linear association between two variables. In both cases, small values of X are associated with small values of Y, and large values of X are matched with large values of Y. The slopes of the straight lines drawn through the sample points in Figure 11.3.1 (a) and (b) are different. The correlation coefficient does not measure the magnitude of the slope. We should stress that it is intended to measure only the linear relationship between X and Y.
- If $r = -1$, then we have perfect negative correlation between X and Y. Figure 11.3.1 (c) and Figure 11.3.1 (d) illustrate the cases with $r = -1$. In both (c) and (d), small values of X are associated with large values of Y, and large values of X are associated with small values of Y.
- If $r = 0$, then X and Y are uncorrelated. This means that there is no linear association between X and Y. Of course, there may be other associations between them, such as a quadratic relationship. Figure 11.3.1 (e) shows the correlation coefficient $r = 0.096$, which means there is hardly any linear association. Similarly, Figure 11.3.1 (f) shows the correlation coefficient

$r = 0.036$, which indicates there is virtually no linear association.

The Pearson sample correlation coefficient r is a point estimate of the unknown population correlation coefficient ρ. To compute the sample correlation coefficient, every observation X_i must be paired with the corresponding observation Y_i,

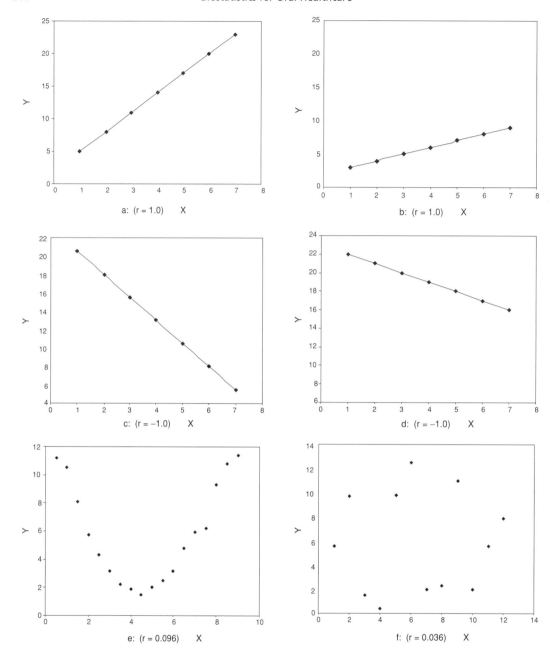

Figure 11.3.1   Different settings of correlation between X and Y.

so that the data consist of pairs of observations (X_i, Y_i).

Example 11.3.1. Twenty-five patient charts were randomly pulled from the patient database. Diastolic blood pressure (DBP) and systolic blood pressure (SBP) measurements of these 25 patients were recorded to study the relationship between the two variables. Calculate the correlation

coefficient r to evaluate the strength of the linear association between DBP and SBP. (See Table 11.3.1.)

Solution. Let X_i and Y_i be the systolic and diastolic blood pressure of the ith patient. From the above data we can calculate $\sum_{i=1}^{n} X_i = 3,184$, $\sum_{i=1}^{n} Y_i = 2,058$, $\sum_{i=1}^{n} X_i Y_i = 267,606$, $\sum_{i=1}^{n} X_i^2 = 412,926$, and $\sum_{i=1}^{n} Y_i^2 = 174,640$.

Table 11.3.1. Patient blood pressure data.

Patient No.	SBP	DPB	Patient No.	SBP	DBP
1	116	72	14	126	85
2	130	90	15	140	95
3	134	85	16	110	60
4	158	112	17	116	89
5	138	85	18	108	68
6	98	60	19	138	85
7	130	80	20	104	70
8	170	115	21	125	70
9	120	80	22	120	80
10	104	75	23	130	92
11	125	78	24	120	62
12	136	80	25	128	80
13	160	110			

with low DBP. The scatter plot of this relationship is displayed in Figure 11.3.2.

11.3.1 Significance Test of Correlation Coefficient

Our primary discussion in the previous section has been on the sample correlation coefficient r. If r is close to -1 or $+1$, there is a strong linear relationship. When r is close to 0, the association is weak or nonexistent. Since r is calculated from the data obtained from the sample, it is subject to chance. Frequently, statisticians are interested in determining whether or not there exists any correlation between two random variables X and Y.

By substituting these values in the formula, we get

$$r = \frac{\sum_{i=1}^{n} X_i Y_i - \frac{\left(\sum_{i=1}^{n} X_i\right)\left(\sum_{i=1}^{n} Y_i\right)}{n}}{\sqrt{\left(\sum_{i=1}^{n} X_i^2 - \frac{\left(\sum_{i=1}^{n} X_i\right)^2}{n}\right)\left(\sum_{i=1}^{n} Y_i^2 - \frac{\left(\sum_{i=1}^{n} Y_i\right)^2}{n}\right)}}$$

$$= \frac{267,606 - \frac{(3,184)(2,058)}{25}}{\sqrt{\left(412,926 - \frac{(3,184)^2}{25}\right)\left(174,640 - \frac{(2,058)^2}{25}\right)}} = 0.8836.$$

Since $r = 0.8836$, we can conclude that there is a strong linear association between SBP and DBP. Patients with high SBP tend to have high DBP, and those with low SBP are likely to be associated

This can be done by testing the hypotheses,

$$H_0 : \rho = 0 \quad \text{vs.} \quad H_0 : \rho \neq 0.$$

The null hypothesis states that there is no correlation between two variables X and Y in the underlying population. The alternative hypothesis means that there is a significant correlation between the variables in the population. As with other hypothesis tests we have discussed, the test procedure is naturally based on the sample correlation coefficient and involves finding the probability of obtaining r at least as extreme as the one we have just observed, given that the null hypothesis is true. When H_0 is rejected at a specified level of significance, then it means r is significantly different from 0, that is, much smaller or much larger than 0. When H_0 is accepted, then it means r is not significantly different from 0. The estimated standard error of r is given by

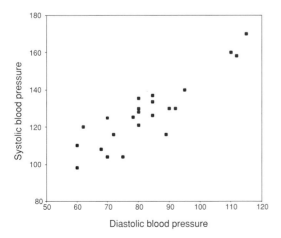

Figure 11.3.2 Scatter plot of the blood pressure data in Table 11.3.1.

$$SE(r) = \sqrt{\frac{1 - r^2}{n - 2}}.$$

The test statistic is defined by $t = \dfrac{r}{SE(r)} = \dfrac{r}{\sqrt{(1-r^2)/(n-2)}} = r\sqrt{\dfrac{n-2}{1-r^2}}$.

If we assume that X and Y are normally distributed, then the above test statistic t has a t distribution with the degrees of freedom $(n-2)$. We summarize the significance test for a correlation coefficient as follows.

To test the hypotheses $H_0 : \rho = 0$ vs. $H_0 : \rho \neq 0$, take the following steps.

1. Compute the sample correlation coefficient r from the sample data (X_i, Y_i), $i = 1, 2, \ldots, n$.
2. Compute the test statistic $t = r\sqrt{\dfrac{n-2}{1-r^2}} \sim t_{(n-2)}$.
3. Reject H_0 if $t < t_{(n-2,\ \alpha/2)}$ or $t_{(n-2,\ 1-\alpha/2)} < t$. Accept H_0 if $t_{(n-2,\ \alpha/2)} < t < t_{(n-2,\ 1-\alpha/2)}$.

Since the test defined above is a one-sample t test, the p value for the test is obtained in the same way as discussed in Chapter 8. That is,

if $t < 0$, then $p = 2\times$ (area to the left of t under a $t_{(n-2)}) = 2 \times P(t_{(n-2)} < t)$,

if $t \geq 0$, then $p = 2\times$ (area to the right of t under a $t_{(n-2)}) = 2 \times P(t \leq t_{(n-2)})$.

The rejection and acceptance regions are shown in Figure 11.3.3.

Example 11.3.2. Scaling and root planing are the most widely used techniques in periodontal therapy. These procedures are used to remove bacterial plaque and calculus from the surfaces of teeth. Despite the best efforts of clinicians to thoroughly root plane teeth, considerable amounts of calculus remain, even though the surface of teeth feel clinically smooth at the completion of scaling and root-planing procedures. Suppose a periodontist observed pocket depth and percentage of calculus after scaling was done with 12 patients, as presented in the table below. Perform a test of significance for the correlation coefficient for the data. We may assume both pocket depth and percentage of calculus are normally distributed.

Patient	Pocket Depth	% Calculus
1	5.5	26.3
2	4.5	32.4
3	3.2	20.8
4	8.5	30.6
5	2.5	9.7
6	5.0	12.3
7	6.0	25.7
8	3.0	14.5
9	4.0	14.6
10	6.5	18.4
11	4.8	25.6
12	7.5	41.8

Solution. We need to test $H_0 : \rho = 0$ vs. $H_0 : \rho \neq 0$. Using the formula above, we can calculate the sample correlation coefficient given by $r = 0.676$. By substituting $n = 12$ and $r = 0.676$, we have

$$t = r\sqrt{\frac{n-2}{1-r^2}} \sim t_{(10)}$$

$$= (0.676)\sqrt{\frac{12-2}{1-(0.676)^2}} = 2.9009.$$

From Table E in the Appendix

$$t_{(n-2,\,1-\alpha/2)} = t_{(10,0.975)} = 2.228$$

and

$$t_{(n-2,\,\alpha/2)} = t_{(10,0.025)} = -t_{(10,0.975)} = -2.228.$$

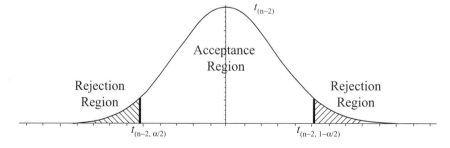

Figure 11.3.3 Rejection and acceptance regions of the significance test for a correlation coefficient.

Since $t = 2.9009 > t_{(10, 0.975)} = 2.228$, the null hypothesis is rejected at the significance level $\alpha = 0.05$. We can also compute the p value, $p = 2 \cdot P(2.9009 \geq t_{(10)})$. From Table E, we see that the p value is

$$2 \cdot P(2.932 \geq t_{(10)}) < p < 2 \cdot P(2.764 \geq t_{(10)}).$$

Or $2(0.0075) < p < 2(0.01)$. Thus, $0.015 < p < 0.02$. We conclude that there is a significantly higher percentage of calculus among the patients with deeper pocket depth.

11.4 COEFFICIENT OF DETERMINATION

In practice, the correlation coefficient r is a frequently used descriptive measure to represent the degree of linear association between two random variables X and Y. The **coefficient of determination** is another measure that is often used to describe the degree of linear association between X and Y. Before we formally introduce the coefficient of determination, we need to define a few more concepts. In regression analysis, the variation of the response variable Y_i is measured in terms of the deviations between Y_i and $\overline{Y}$, the sample mean of Y_i's. That is, $Y_i - \overline{Y}$. The sum of the squared deviation is defined by $SSTO = \sum_{i=1}^{n}(Y_i - \overline{Y})^2$. $SSTO$ stands for total sum of squares. If $SSTO = 0$, then every term $(Y_i - \overline{Y})^2 = 0$. This means every response Y_i is the same, or $Y_i = \overline{Y}$. The greater the value of $SSTO$, the greater the variation in the responses Y_i's. Using the fitted regression function $\hat{Y}_i$ we can decompose $SSTO$ as follows,

$$SSTO = \sum_{i=1}^{n}(Y_i - \overline{Y})^2$$
$$= \sum_{i=1}^{n}(Y_i - \hat{Y}_i)^2 + \sum_{i=1}^{n}(\hat{Y}_i - \overline{Y})^2.$$

The terms $\sum_{i=1}^{n}(Y_i - \hat{Y}_i)^2$ and $\sum_{i=1}^{n}(\hat{Y}_i - \overline{Y})^2$ are referred to as **error sum of squares** (SSE), and **regression sum of squares** (SSR), respectively;

$$SSE = \sum_{i=1}^{n}(Y_i - \hat{Y}_i)^2 \quad \text{and} \quad SSR = \sum_{i=1}^{n}(\hat{Y}_i - \overline{Y})^2.$$

The measure of variation in the data with the fitted regression model is the sum of the squared deviations, $SSE = \sum_{i=1}^{n}(Y_i - \hat{Y}_i)^2$. It is clear that if all observed responses fall on the fitted regression line, we get $Y_i - \hat{Y}_i = 0$, and thus $SSE = 0$. The other sum of the squared deviations $SSR = \sum_{i=1}^{n}(\hat{Y}_i - \overline{Y})^2$ is the sum of the squared deviations of the fitted values $\hat{Y}_i$ of its mean $\overline{Y}$. We see that $SSTO$ has two components, SSE and SSR; $SSTO = SSE + SSR$. Equivalently, we can write $SSR = SSTO - SSE$. Since $SSTO$, SSE, and SSR are all ≥ 0, we have $SSTO \geq SSE$. From the above expressions it can be seen that $SSTO$ measures the uncertainty in predicting the response Y_i when the independent variable X_i is not taken into account, and SSE measures the uncertainty in predicting Y_i when X_i is taken into consideration. Therefore, the difference $SSTO - SSE$ measures the effect of X_i in reducing the variation of Y_i.

Definition 11.4.1. The coefficient of determination, denoted r^2, is defined by

$$r^2 = \frac{SSTO - SSE}{SSTO} = 1 - \frac{SSE}{SSTO}.$$

Unlike the correlation coefficient, the coefficient of determination does not assume any negative values. In fact, $0 \leq r^2 \leq 1$. From the definition, we can interpret r^2 as representation of the proportion of reduction in total variation due to the use of the particular independent variable X_i in the regression model. The larger r^2 is, the greater the reduction in the total variation of the response variable Y_i. This means that the better prediction of Y_i can be made when r^2 is approximately 1. We make the following comments on the coefficient of determination r^2:

1. If $SSE = 0$ (all observations fall on the fitted line), then $r^2 = 1$. This is the case where all the variation in the outcome variable Y_i is explained by X_i.

2. If $SSR = SSTO - SSE = 0$, that is, $\hat{Y}_i - \overline{Y} = 0$, then $r^2 = 0$. This is the case where there is no linear association between X_i and Y_i, and the independent variable does not reduce any variation in Y_i with linear regression model.

3. The square root of r^2, $r = \pm\sqrt{r^2}$ is the correlation coefficient. If the slope of the fitted regression equation is positive, $r = +\sqrt{r^2}$. If the slope is negative, $r = -\sqrt{r^2}$.

Example 11.4.1. A study was conducted by endodontists to test the hypothesis that multiple sterilizations of endodontic nickel-titanium files will lead to a continuous decrease in the resistance of files to separation by torsion. Let the number of sterilization cycles be the independent variable X and torque at separation be the response variable Y. Suppose the researchers collected the following data. Compute the coefficient of determination and the correlation coefficient.

No. of Cycles	0	10	20	30	40
Torque		51.1	46.1	56.9	54.7	59.8

Solution. By the method of least squares, we obtain the fitted regression function

$$\hat{Y}_i = 48.52 + 0.26X_i.$$

By simple calculations, we get $SSTO = 112.97$ and $SSE = 45.37$. Thus,

$$r^2 = \frac{SSTO - SSE}{SSTO} = \frac{112.97 - 45.37}{112.97} = 0.5984.$$

The correlation coefficient is obtained as $r = \pm\sqrt{r^2} = \pm\sqrt{0.5984} = \pm0.7736$. Since the slope of the regression equation is positive, we take $r = 0.7736$. The coefficient of determination $r^2 = 0.5984$ indicates that the total variation in Y_i is reduced by about 59.8% by introducing the variable X_i (the number of sterilization cycles), and the correlation coefficient $r = 0.7736$ indicates

moderately strong linear association between the two variables X_i and Y_i.

The quantity $1 - r^2$ is called the **coefficient of nondetermination**. This is the amount of variation in the response variable that is not explained by the independent variable in the model. In the above example, the coefficient of nondetermination is $1 - r^2 = 1 - 0.5984 = 0.4016$. This means that 40.16% of the variation in torque at separation (Y) is not explained by the number of sterilization cycles (X).

Example 11.4.2. There is an increasing interest in starting orthodontic treatment in the mixed dentition stage rather than after all the permanent teeth have erupted. Orthodontists wish to predict the potential for a tooth size–arch length discrepancy in their growing patients. The need for developing a prediction model that utilizes jaw and tooth dimensions after eruption of the lower incisors arises because primary crowding is defined as a genetic discrepancy between jaw size and tooth dimension. Joe, Kim, and Oh [11] investigated a statistical relationship between the sum of the mandibular permanent incisors and the combined mesiodistal crown diameters of the maxillary and mandibular canine and premolars in a sample of Hispanic American subjects (see Figure 11.4.1). The dental casts of the maxillary and mandibular arches of 104 Hispanic American patients were randomly selected from the Orthodontic Department of the Loma Linda University School of Dentistry [11].

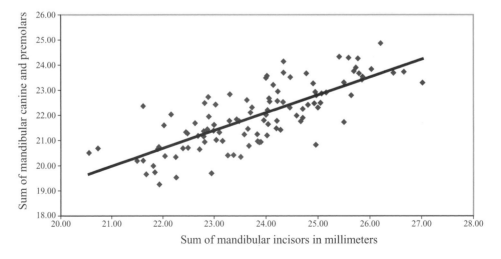

Figure 11.4.1 Regression model for the size of unerupted canines and premolars.

Using the least squares methods, we can establish a predictive regression function given by

$$\hat{Y}_i = 5.1169 - 0.7077 X_i.$$

By Definition 11.4.1, the coefficient of determination is $r^2 = 0.5884$. Discuss how you would interpret the value of $r^2 = 0.5884$.

Solution. See Exercise 14.

11.5 MULTIPLE REGRESSION

So far in this chapter we have discussed a simple linear regression in which there is only one independent variable and one response variable. While there are many problems in which the response variable can be predicted quite well in terms of only one independent variable, it is intuitively clear that the prediction should improve if we consider other independent variables, because they add more relevant information about the response variable. For example, we should be able to make a better prediction of the performance of dental and medical students on the national board exam if we consider not only their grade point average in basic science courses but also the number of hours they spent in preparation. In practical applications there are often two or more independent variables:

1. Prediction of blood pressure (Y), based on age (X_1) and the amount of weekly exercise (X_2)
2. Prediction of implant survival time (Y), based on age (X_1), bone height (X_2), and status of smoking (X_3)
3. Sales volume of toothpaste (Y) predicted from price (X_1), advertising expenditure (X_2), and quality of the product (X_3)

The general form of a multiple regression model with k independent variables and one response variable would have the form

$$Y_i = \beta_0 + \beta_1 X_{1i} + \beta_2 X_{2i} + \cdots + \beta_{ki} X_{ki} + \varepsilon_i.$$

This model is called a first-order regression model with k independent variables and one response variable. We will explain the multiple regression model with two independent variables. A multiple regression model with two independent variables

and one response variable would have the form

$$Y_i = \beta_0 + \beta_1 X_{1i} + \beta_2 X_{2i} + \varepsilon_i,$$

where

Y_i is the response in the ith trial or the outcome of the ith subject,

X_{1i} and X_{2i} are the values of the two independent variables in the ith trial,

β_0, β_1 and β_2 are regression parameters, and

ε_i is the error term.

Similar to those for a simple linear regression model, the following assumptions for a multiple regression model are made:

1. The error terms ε_i are independent and normally distributed with $\mu = 0$ and variance σ^2.
2. The values of the response variable Y_i are independent and normally distributed with $Y_i = \beta_0 + \beta_1 X_{1i} + \beta_2 X_{2i}$ and the constant variance σ^2; that is, $Y_i \sim N(\beta_0 + \beta_1 X_{1i} + \beta_2 X_{2i}, \sigma^2)$.
3. There is a linear relationship between the independent variables and the dependent variable.
4. The independent variables are not correlated. This is called **non-multicolinearity** assumption.

The simple linear regression model with one independent variable is a straight line, but the regression model with two independent variables X_{1i} and X_{2i} is a plane. The parameter β_0 is the Y-intercept of the regression plane. The parameters β_0, β_1, and β_2 are called **partial regression coefficients**. The parameter β_1 indicates the change in the mean response per unit increase in X_1 when X_2 is held constant, and the parameter β_2 indicates the change in the mean response per unit increase in X_2 when X_1 is held constant. The partial regression coefficients β_0, β_1, and β_2 need to be estimated by b_0, b_1, and b_2 using the least squares method. That is, use the least squares method to obtain the values b_0, b_1, and b_2, that minimize the sum

$$Q = \sum_{i=1}^{n} e_i^2 = \sum_{i=1}^{n} [Y_i - (b_0 + b_1 X_{1i} + b_2 X_{2i})]^2.$$

Example 11.5.1. Dental school administrators are interested in developing a regression model to predict students' performance on the national board exam. A few months prior to the national board exam, students are given a mock board exam to assess their strengths and weaknesses so that they can be better prepared for the board exam. Seventeen fourth-year students were randomly selected. Their science grade point average and mock board scores are recorded for the regression analysis. Given the following data, obtain the multiple regression model.

Student	Sci. GPA	Mock Score	NB Score
1	3.20	55.0	76
2	2.51	55.5	76
3	3.21	67.7	91
4	2.45	49.3	77
5	3.55	66.1	83
6	3.23	54.8	82
7	2.43	63.8	87
8	3.02	67.0	87
9	2.81	51.4	81
10	3.03	48.2	77
11	3.35	55.7	80
12	2.95	52.8	77
13	2.36	53.2	77
14	3.24	64.7	88
15	3.62	67.2	91
16	2.12	39.9	67
17	3.02	57.3	82

Solution. The national board exam score (Y_i) is the response variable, and the two independent variables are science grade point average (X_{1i}) and mock board score (X_{2i}). We can use the statistics software package (SPSS) to obtain the least squares estimates. The multiple regression equation is given by $\hat{Y}_i = 38.690 + 0.696X_{1i} + 0.917X_{2i}$. This fitted regression equation indicates that the national board exam score increases by 0.696 per 1 unit increase in science GPA when the independent variable X_2 is held fixed, and increases by 0.917 per 1 unit increase in mock board score with the independent variable X_1 held constant.

In a multiple regression model, as in a simple linear regression model, the strength of the relationship between the response variable and independent variables is measured by a **multiple correlation coefficient**, denoted by R. The multiple correlation coefficient R with two independent variables is defined by

$$R = \sqrt{\frac{r_{x_1 y}^2 + r_{x_2 y}^2 - 2 \cdot r_{x_1 y} \cdot r_{x_2 y} \cdot r_{x_1 x_2}}{1 - r_{x_1 x_2}^2}}$$

where $r_{x_1 y}$ is the correlation coefficient between X_1 and Y, $r_{x_2 y}$ is the correlation coefficient between X_2 and Y, and $r_{x_1 x_2}$ is the correlation coefficient between X_1 and X_2.

Let's evaluate the multiple correlation coefficient in the above example. We use Definition 11.3.1 to compute the correlation coefficients $r_{x_1 y}$, $r_{x_2 y}$, and $r_{x_1 x_2}$ and get $r_{x_1 y} = 0.599$, $r_{x_2 y} = 0.916$, and $r_{x_1 x_2} = 0.610$.

Substituting these values in the formula, we have

$$R = \sqrt{\frac{r_{x_1 y}^2 + r_{x_2 y}^2 - 2 \cdot r_{x_1 y} \cdot r_{x_2 y} \cdot r_{x_1 x_2}}{1 - r_{x_1 x_2}^2}}$$

$$= \sqrt{\frac{(0.599)^2 + (0.916)^2 - 2(0.599)(0.916)(0.610)}{1 - (0.610)^2}}$$

$$= 0.918.$$

The values of R range between 0 and $+1$. The closer R is to $+1$, the stronger the relationship; the closer to 0, the weaker the relationship. The multiple correlation coefficient R is always larger than the individual correlation coefficients. In this example, with $R = 0.918$, there is a strong relationship among the variables. As with a simple linear regression model, we have the **coefficient of multiple determination**, denoted R^2, which represents the amount of variation in the response variable explained by the regression model. Similarly, $1 - R^2$ is the amount of variation in response that is not explained by the model. We have $R^2 = (0.918)^2 = 0.843$, and $1 - R^2 = 1 - 0.843 = 0.157$. The above multiple regression equation, based on science GPA and mock board score, has the ability to predict the average national board exam scores well.

The coefficient of multiple determination R^2 depends on the number of pairs of observations n and the number of the independent variables k, so that statisticians often present an adjusted R^2 (adjusted for n and k), denoted R_{adj}^2. The formula for an adjusted R_{adj}^2 is given by

$$R_{adj}^2 = 1 - \left[\frac{(1 - R^2)(n - 1)}{n - k - 1}\right].$$

Since $n = 17$ and $k = 2$ in Example 11.5.1, we

obtain

$$R_{adj}^2 = 1 - \left[\frac{(1 - R^2)(n - 1)}{n - k - 1} \right]$$

$$= 1 - \left[\frac{(1 - 0.843)(17 - 1)}{17 - 2 - 1} \right] = 0.821.$$

The adjusted R_{adj}^2 is always smaller than the coefficient of multiple determination R^2. When n and k are approximately equal, then the denominator of R_{adj}^2 is small. Therefore, the value of R_{adj}^2 can be artificially large, not because of the strong relationship among the variables, but because of sampling error.

11.6 LOGISTIC REGRESSION

In our discussions of a simple linear regression model $Y_i = \beta_0 + \beta_1 X_i + \varepsilon_i$, we assume that the response variable Y is continuous and, in particular, normally distributed. Our focus was to predict the mean of the corresponding response to a given set of values for the independent variable X. There are many situations where the response variable is dichotomous rather than continuous. Here are some examples.

1. In a study to determine the prevalence and risk factors for gingival enlargement in nifedipine-treated patients, periodontists also observed whether or not inflammation of the gingiva is present. We let the dichotomous random variable Y take on the value 1 if inflammation is present and the value 0 if inflammation is absent.
2. One hundred fifty patients were treated with a bilateral sagittal split osteotomy over the last 5 years. During the follow-up examination, presence of nerve dysfunction was recorded. The response variable $Y = 1$ if nerve dysfunction is present, and $Y = 0$ if nerve damage is absent.
3. Clinicians and researchers studied the effect of pacifier sucking on the prevalence of posterior crossbite among young children. If the study subject has posterior crossbite, then $Y = 1$, and if not, then $Y = 0$.
4. After bone marrow transplantation with total body irradiation, children show continuous growth impairment. Bone density is often reduced in long-term survivors of childhood malignancies. Children treated for childhood

cancers also exhibit both acute and long-term complications in the oral cavity and in dental and craniofacial development [12]. The dichotomous response variable $Y = 1$, if there is an evidence for arrested root development with v-shaped roots, premature apical closure, microdontia, enamel disturbances, and aplasia. The response variable $Y = 0$, if there is no evidence.

A linear regression approach is based on the assumption that the response variable is normally distributed. However, the dichotomous response variables that we illustrated do not satisfy this normality assumption. Therefore, we are forced to use a technique known as **logistic regression**, which allows us to study the relationship between a response variable with two possible outcomes and one or more independent variables. Independent variables in logistic regression models can be either continuous or discrete.

11.6.1 The Logistic Regression Model

As we discussed in Section 5.2, the mean of the binary random variable is the proportion of times that it assumes the value 1. That is, $P(Y = 1) = p$. Similar to a simple regression model, one may attempt to fit a model of the form

$$p = \beta_0 + \beta_1 X.$$

The response variable Y has been replaced by the proportion p, which represents the probability of taking on values between 0 and 1. On the other hand, the right-hand side $\beta_0 + \beta_1 X$ could be less than 0 or greater than 1. To circumvent this difficulty, we often use the logistic transformation of p as the response variable;

$$p = \frac{e^{\beta_0 + \beta_1 X}}{1 + e^{\beta_0 + \beta_1 X}}.$$

Regardless of the values of X, the right-hand side of the above equation assumes values between 0 and 1, which is the required range of p. Recall that the odds in favor of an event when the event occurs with the probability p are given by $p/(1 - p)$. As we described in the first example in Section 11.6, let p be the probability that inflammation of the gingiva is present (or the probability of success).

Then the odds in favor of inflammation of the gingiva are

$$\frac{p}{1-p} = \frac{e^{\beta_0+\beta_1 X}/(1+e^{\beta_0+\beta_1 X})}{1/(1+e^{\beta_0+\beta_1 X})} = e^{\beta_0+\beta_1 X}.$$

By taking the natural logarithm of both sides of the equation, we obtain

$$\ln\left(\frac{p}{1-p}\right) = \ln(e^{\beta_0+\beta_1 X}) = \beta_0 + \beta_1 X.$$

This logit transformation is also denoted by *logit*(p). Instead of having Y as a response variable in the model, we have the logarithm of the odds in favor of inflammation of gingiva. In the above equation, we assume that there is a linear relationship between $\ln[p/(1-p)]$ and a explanatory variable X. The statistical technique of fitting a model given in this section is known as logistic regression.

11.6.2 Fitting the Logistic Regression Model

To fit the logistic regression model to a set of data we need to estimate the unknown parameters β_0 and β_1. The method we introduced in Section 11.2 for estimating the unknown parameters in simple linear regression was the least squares method. However, the least squares method assumes that the response variable is normally distributed. When the least squares method is applied to a model with a dichotomous response variable, the estimators of the parameters no longer possess the same desirable statistical properties. Thus, the method of maximum likelihood estimation is used to fit a logistic regression. The method of maximum likelihood estimation will not be presented

here, since it is beyond the scope of our discussion. Readers who are interested in studying it are referred to an excellent text by Hosmer and Lemeshow [13]. Consider the following example.

Example 11.6.1. Halitosis is an offensive odor of the breath resulting from local and metabolic conditions. Sonis [14] states that the known causes of halitosis are food retention, periodontal infection, caries, acute necrotizing gingivitis, and mucosal infection. Extraoral and systemic causes of halitosis include smoking, alcohol ingestion, pulmonary or bronchial disease, metabolic defects, diabetes mellitus, sinusitis, and tonsillitis [14]. Suppose a study was conducted to investigate a relationship between bleeding index (BI) and halitosis. Investigators used the Halimeter to quantify the strength of halitosis. Bleeding index is the response variable represented by a dichotomous variable Y. We let $Y = 0$ if there is no evidence of bleeding in gingiva, and $Y = 1$ if there is an evidence of bleeding. Table 11.6.1 presents the halitosis and BI data for $n = 63$ patients.

Let p be the probability that there is an evidence of bleeding in gingiva. The estimated logistic regression function is

$$\ln\left(\frac{\hat{p}}{1-\hat{p}}\right) = \hat{\beta}_0 + \hat{\beta}_1 X = -0.3898 + 0.0035X.$$

The estimated coefficient $\hat{\beta}_1 = 0.0035$ implies that for each unit increase in halitosis, on the average the logarithm of the odds that the patient has an evidence of bleeding in gingiva is increased by 0.0035. When the logarithm of the odds increases, the probability p increases as well. In Table 11.6.2 we summarize the output from the SAS Proc Logistic.

Table 11.6.1. Halitosis and BI data.

Halitosis	141	131	94	140	104	112	219	135	94	93	97	133	300	101
BI	1	0	1	1	0	0	0	1	0	1	1	1	1	1
Halitosis	98	129	86	91	163	102	95	116	119	82	73	89	103	108
BI	0	1	1	0	1	0	0	0	1	1	1	1	0	0
Halitosis	94	113	164	72	116	116	93	105	156	125	248	256	109	126
BI	0	1	0	0	1	1	0	1	1	1	0	1	0	0
Halitosis	175	130	151	139	157	120	92	97	119	114	131	119	123	93
BI	0	0	1	1	0	0	0	0	1	1	1	1	0	0
Halitosis	92	84	89	105	78	94	140							
BI	1	0	0	0	1	1	0							

Table 11.6.2. Analysis of maximum likelihood estimates.

Parameter	df	$\hat{\beta}_i$	Standard error SE $(\hat{\beta}_i)$	χ^2	$Pr > \chi^2$	Exp(Est)
Intercept	1	-0.3898	0.7808	0.2493	0.6176	0.6772
Halitosis	1	0.0035	0.0061	0.3237	0.5694	1.0035

The estimated odds ratio relating BI to halitosis is 1.0035. Table 11.6.2 shows the p values corresponding to the significance test for the regression coefficients β_0 and β_1 are 0.6176 and 0.5694. These p values indicate that the tests are not significant. Since the null hypotheses are accepted, we conclude that there is no relationship between the probability $p = P(Y = 1)$ and halitosis.

11.7 MULTIPLE LOGISTIC REGRESSION MODEL

Similar to the multiple regression model discussed in Section 11.5, it is intuitive that inclusion of more than one independent variable in the logistic regression model would likely improve our ability to predict the probability p. Suppose in Example 11.6.1 we let $X_1 =$ halitosis and $X_2 =$ the number of times the subjects floss their teeth. The logistic regression model containing two independent variables would have the following form.

$$\ln\left(\frac{p}{1-p}\right) = \beta_0 + \beta_1 X_1 + \beta_2 X_2.$$

In general, if Y is a binary response variable with the probability of success $p = P(Y = 1)$, and X_1, $X_2, \cdots, X_k$ are k independent variables, then the multiple logistic regression can be expressed as

$$\ln\left(\frac{p}{1-p}\right) = \beta_0 + \beta_1 X_1 + \beta_2 X_2 + \cdots + \beta_k X_k.$$

Any of the available statistical software packages, such as SAS, can be used to produce a table as shown in the previous section to fit a multiple logistic regression model. For further discussions on multiple logistic regression and interpretations of regression parameters, readers are referred to Hosmer and Lemeshow [13] and Kleinbaum et al. [8].

11.8 EXERCISES

1 Twenty students were selected at random from the fourth-year class in dental school. Consider the following scores on independent variable X_i and dependent variable Y_i. The independent variable is the student's score in a basic science course, and the dependent variable is the student's score in clinic. Construct the scatter plot. What can you say about the relationship between the two variables from the scatter plot?

X_i	Y_i	X_i	Y_i	X_i	Y_i	X_i	Y_i	X_i	Y_i
74	88	84	92	77	61	96	78	89	93
86	90	68	75	80	82	91	86	69	73
89	85	60	65	73	77	83	78	75	86
78	80	85	80	76	77	66	78	91	84

2 Eighteen patient records were chosen randomly to determine the relationship between age and systolic blood pressure (SBP). Based on the data in the table below, does a straight line (linear regression) appear to be applicable?

Age	SBP	Age	SBP	Age	SBP	Age	SBP
55	148	36	120	32	118	37	130
71	160	58	134	42	138	82	168
65	152	67	143	58	140	65	146
43	128	79	158	28	118		
25	110	47	128	30	127		

3 A study was conducted by Rhee and Nahm [15] to establish a statistical relationship between the shape of the labial crowns of the incisors and crowding. Plaster cast models of 15 untreated male patients whose Little's irregularity index is normal were evaluated. The table below presents part of the data Rhee and Nahm [15] collected. Suppose upper incisor irregularity index (UIRI) is the response variable Y_i and upper central incisor mesiodistal width ratio (UIR) is the independent variable X_i.

a. Draw a scatter plot for the data.
b. Find $\sum_{i=1}^{n} X_i$, $\sum_{i=1}^{n} X_i^2$, $\sum_{i=1}^{n} Y_i$, and $\sum_{i=1}^{n} X_i Y_i$.
c. Estimate the regression function.
d. Use the fitted regression line to predict the UIRI for a patient whose UIR value is 145.

Patient	UIR (X_i)	UIRI (Y_i)
1	139.97	11.7
2	141.17	11.7
3	142.51	11.25
4	141.02	13.61
5	140.91	16.61
6	132.94	8.47
7	135.41	12.84
8	143.26	12.84
9	130.1	14.1
10	149.62	14.1
11	139.33	15.27
12	130.1	10.26
13	139.84	10.26
14	160.94	17.68
15	134.66	10.84

4 It is well-known in implant dentistry that as the tightening torque increases, the screw elongation (abutment screw) increases within the design limit. Suppose that Dr. Kirk investigated and collected the following data to establish a statistical relationship between screw elongation and tightening torque. Find the best fitting curve for the data using the least squares method.

Torque (Nmm)	Elongation (μm)
5	1.0
10	2.0
15	3.7
20	5.5
25	8.0
30	9.0
32	9.5

5 An investigation was conducted by endodontists to assess total carbohydrate concentration, as well as the noncollagenous protein content, in human dental pulp. Pulps were obtained from eight premolars and homogenized in saline solution. The following data were collected by the investigators [16]. Develop an appropriate regression function to predict the protein content in dental pulp.

Total wt. pulp (mg)	Protein (μg/mg)
12.5	46.93
10.6	42.73
9.0	44.40
14.8	47.84
15.1	36.68
18.0	30.25
14.0	48.66
6.8	63.77

6 In Exercise 5, examine the aptness of the regression model.
a. Is linearity appropriate?
b. Is there any graphic evidence of non-constant error variance?
c. Are independence of error terms adequate?
d. Are there any residual outliers?

7 Using the data in Exercise 5, estimate the population correlation coefficient ρ between the total weight of pulp and the amount of protein.

8 Compute the correlation coefficient r for the data in Exercise 2 by letting X_i = age, and Y_i = SBP. If you now exchange X_i and Y_i, that is, if you let X_i = SBP, and Y_i = age, and calculate the correlation coefficient r. Would you expect the correlation coefficient r to be the same? Explain why?

9 A researcher selected nine sets of identical twins to determine whether there is a relationship between the first-born and second-born twins in the IQ scores. Is there a strong association in the IQ score between identical twins? The following table presents their IQ scores.

	1	2	3	4	5	6	7	8	9
I[st] born	112	127	105	132	117	135	122	101	128
2nd born	118	120	100	128	102	133	125	104	114

10 A research project was conducted to determine the effect of physical exercise on the level of low-density lipoprotein (LDL) cholesterol. The following data on the amount of weekly exercise and LDL-cholesterol are collected. Would you suggest there is a strong enough association between the variables to conclude that physical exercise is beneficial for lowering LDL-cholesterol?

15 Water samples were tested for fluoride ion concentration using an Orion 720A ion meter and

	1	2	3	4	5	6	7	8	9	10	11
Exercise (hr.)	3.0	1.5	0.5	4.2	2.5	2.0	4.75	5.0	1.75	3.25	2.25
LDL (mg/dl)	96.0	136.4	168.8	102.1	145.0	98.6	104.3	124.5	147.3	120.4	130.6

11 Perform a one-sample t test for a correlation coefficient for the data in Exercise 10.

12 An investigation was conducted to evaluate the effect of water and saliva contamination on the bond strength of metal orthodontic brackets cemented to etched (10% polyacrylic acid) human premolar enamel. The bonding agent used was an experimental light-cured glass ionomer. The following table shows the shear bond strength (megapascals) for water and saliva contamination measured after aging for 5 minutes. The probability distribution of bond strength is assumed to be normal. Let water be the independent variable (X) and saliva be the outcome variable (Y).

a. Compute the sample correlation coefficient and give an appropriate interpretation.

b. Perform a significance test for a correlation coefficient at the significance level $\alpha = 0.05$.

c. Calculate the p value.

	1	2	3	4	5	6	7
Water (X_i)	4.5	3.6	5.6	2.2	4.9	6.5	4.0
Saliva (Y_i)	6.1	4.9	5.5	3.0	4.3	7.9	6.1

13 Oral stereognosis was analyzed in a group of edentulous subjects rehabilitated with complete removable dentures. From the patient charts we have observed their age (X) and duration of edentulism (Y). We are interested in evaluating any linear association between the variables and how much variability in the response variable Y is reduced by including the age variable in the regression model. Calculate r^2 and r.

fluoride ion electrode. The electrode is known to have a sensitivity of 0.02 ppm and measures in millivolts [17]. The following table shows the relationship between fluoride concentration in parts per million (independent variable) and an electrode in millivolts (response variable) for 5 samples. Is a simple linear regression adequate? If not, why?

ppm	0.02	0.10	0.50	1.00	10.00
mV	180.6	156.8	119.2	101.6	42.3

11.9 REFERENCES

1. Chung, K. H., Hong, J., and Park, Y. K. Observations of the Effect of the Soft Drinks on Restorative Margin. Student table clinic. Loma Linda University. 2001.

2. Lautt, A., Welebir, M., and Willardsen, J. Analysis of Hardness for Varying Light and Product Types. Student table clinic. Loma Linda University. 2001.

3. Tehemar, S. Factor affecting heat generation during implant site preparation: A review of biologic observations and future considerations. *Int. J of Oral & Max Impl*: 1999, 14, 127–135.

4. Hover, S., Jeffery, J., and Peter, M. Effect of Different Irrigation Systems on Heat Generation During Implant Osteotomy. Student table clinic. Loma Linda University. 2002.

5. Hutchingson, S., Tan, J., and Tomarere, A. Effects of Sour Toothpaste on Tooth Demineralization. Student table clinic. Loma Linda University. 2001.

6. Kowalczyk, M. Post-Treatment Evaluation of Isometric Function of the Elevator Muscles. Master's thesis. Loma Linda University. 2000.

7. Miss America Pageant Corporation. Available at: www.missamerica.org. May, 2000.

8. Kleinbaum, D. G., Kupper, L. L., Muller, K. E., and Nizam, A. Applied Regression Analysis and Other Multivariable Methods. Third edition. Duxbury Press. 1998.

Age	63	50	75	86	61	78	82	69	53	56	73	59
Duration (yr)	12.0	13.5	3.0	1.0	8.5	4.0	3.5	4.3	10.0	9.0	2.5	5.0

14 How would you interpret the coefficient of determination we obtained in Example 11.4.2.

9. Neter, J., Wasserman, W., and Kutner, M. H. *Applied Linear Statistical Models*. Third edition. Richard D. Irwin, Inc. 1990.

10. Pagano, M., and Gauvreau, K. *Principles of Biostatistics*. Second edition. Duxbury Press. 2000.

11. Joe, S., Kim, S., and Oh, J. Prediction of the Size of Unerupted Canines and Premolars in a Hispanic American Population. Student project. Loma Linda University. 2001.

12. Dahllöf, G., Jönsson, A., Ulmner, M., and Uuggare, J. Orthodontic treatment in long-term survivors after pediatric bone marrow transplantation. *Am J Orthod Dentofacial Orthop*: 2001, 120, 459–465.

13. Hosmer, D. W., and Lemeshow, S. *Applied Logistic Regression*. John Wiley & Sons. 1989.

14. Sonis, S. T. *Dental Secrets*. Second edition. Hanley & Belfus, Inc. 1999.

15. Rhee, S. H., and Nahm, D. S. Triangular-shaped incisor crowns and crowding. *Am J Orthod Dentofacial Orthop*: 2000, 118, 624–8.

16. Mendez, C., and Zarzoza, I. A Study of Noncollagenous Protein Content in Human Dental Pulp. Student project. Loma Linda University, Loma Linda, CA. 2002.

17. Wiggins, J. The Effect of Activated Carbon Water Filtration Systems on Community Fluoridated Water. Student research project. Loma Linda University. 2002.

Chapter 12

One-way Analysis of Variance

12.1 INTRODUCTION

Chapter 9 introduced a two-sample t test for comparing the population means of two independent normal distributions. The t test is an efficient method of testing the significance of the difference between two population means. In many practical applications, however, it is necessary to compare three or more population means. Let us consider several examples:

1. We want to decide whether there is a difference in the effectiveness of four commercial denture cleansers in eliminating oral pathogens. We must decide whether the observed differences among the four sample means can be attributed to chance, or whether there are real differences among the means of the four populations.
2. We may want to determine, based on the sample data, whether there is a difference in the effectiveness of three teaching methods being used in American dental and medical schools. We might want to ask whether an observed difference in the effectiveness of the teaching methods is really due to the differences of the methods and not due to the instructors or to the intelligence and motivation of the students who are being taught.
3. Doctors want to determine whether there is a statistically significant difference among the population means of the blood pressure of three groups of patients who have received different treatments for their hypertension.
4. Individuals who met certain inclusion criteria have been randomly assigned to four different diet programs that are designed to help reduce body weight. Subjects' body weight, body mass index (BMI), and blood pressure measurements have been taken at the baseline as well as at the end of the clinical trial. Investigators want to test the null hypothesis that the population

means of the baseline BMI measurements of the four groups are identical. This can be stated as

H_0: $\mu_1 = \mu_2 = \mu_3 = \mu_4$ vs.

H_1: At least one of the population means is different from one of the other three means.

In this chapter, we will introduce the statistical method known as the **analysis of variance** (ANOVA), which is an extension of the two-sample t test to three or more samples. Some may ask, if the ANOVA is involved in comparing the population means, why is it not called the analysis of means? Actually, the acronym is justifiable. We will see later that the means are compared by using the estimates of variance. Regression models, introduced in Chapter 11, describe the nature of the statistical relationship between the mean response and the levels of the independent variable. Like regression models, ANOVA models are concerned with the statistical relation between a dependent variable and one or more independent variables. Unlike the regression models, however, the independent variables in ANOVA models may be qualitative, such as sex, type of treatment, hair color, and cause of tooth extraction. In this chapter, we shall focus on the one-way ANOVA, where there is only one independent variable.

12.2 FACTORS AND FACTOR LEVELS

A **factor** is an independent variable to be studied in the ANOVA models. In the first example in the introduction, which compares the effectiveness of four denture cleansers, the factor being investigated is denture cleanser. In the second example comparing three teaching methods, the factor under investigation is teaching method. Some studies are **single-factor** studies, where only one factor is of concern. The four examples illustrated above are all single-factor studies. Sometimes, two or more factors are being investigated simultaneously. These are called **multi-factor** studies. The one-way ANOVA model deals with single-factor studies. Statisticians often talk about a factor **level**, or a particular category of a factor. For instance, in the third example, one particular hypertensive treatment is a factor level. In that study, the factor "hypertensive treatment" has three levels.

There are two types of factors: fixed and random. A fixed factor refers to a factor whose levels are the only ones of interest. Examples of fixed factors are smoking habit (heavy smoking, light smoking, passive smoking, non-smoking), age (young, middle-aged, old), and medication for severe cancer pain (morphine, oxycodone, fentanyl, hydromorphone methadone). In a study in which smoking habit is a factor, investigators are only interested in four levels of the factor—heavy smoking, light smoking, passive smoking, and non-smoking. A random factor refers to a factor whose levels are considered as a sample from a population of levels, such as subjects, clinicians, or time points. The one-way ANOVA, when the factor under investigation is fixed, is called a **one-way ANOVA fixed effects model**. When the factor under study is random, it is called a **one-way ANOVA random effects model**.

12.3 STATEMENT OF THE PROBLEM AND MODEL ASSUMPTIONS

The main problem in the one-way ANOVA fixed-effects model is to determine whether k ($k > 2$) population means are equal or not. The different populations correspond to different factor levels. Given k population means, the hypotheses we wish to test may be stated as

$H_0:\ \mu_1 = \mu_2 = \cdots = \mu_k$ vs.
H_1 : not all k means are equal. Alternatively, H_1 : $\mu_i \neq \mu_j$ for some pair i and j, where $i \neq j$.

The following assumptions must be met for one-way ANOVA fixed effects model to be valid.

1. Independent samples are taken from each of the k populations.

2. The populations from which the samples are taken must be normally distributed.
3. The variances of the populations must be equal, that is, $\sigma_1^2 = \sigma_2^2 = \cdots = \sigma_k^2 = \sigma^2$. This assumption is also referred to as **homogeneity of variance**.

These assumptions provide the theoretical justification for using the ANOVA model. The real world problems are unlikely to satisfy these assumptions exactly. In general, ANOVA models can be applied even if the above assumptions are not completely satisfied as long as they are not egregiously violated. The normality assumption does not have to be met exactly if we have large enough samples of size 20 or more from each population. However, the consequences of large deviation from normality could be quite severe. The assumption of the equality of variances can also be mildly violated without serious consequences if the sample sizes are large enough. A violation of the independence assumption can lead to serious mistakes in statistical inference. Thus, special care must be taken to ensure that the observations are independent. The F test for one-way ANOVA is known to be robust with respect to violation of the equality of variance assumption [1] if the number of observations for each treatment level is the same, the populations are normally distributed, and the ratio of the largest variance to the smallest variance is no greater than 3.0.

Suppose an ANOVA is performed and the null hypothesis $H_0 : \mu_1 = \mu_2 = \cdots = \mu_k$ is rejected. What does this tell us? We know that at least one population mean μ_j is different from some of the other means. The problem is to find out where the differences occur. If $k = 3$ and the null hypothesis $H_0 :\ \mu_1 = \mu_2 = \mu_3$ is rejected, then we want to determine whether the differences are between μ_1 and μ_2, between μ_1 and μ_3, between μ_1 and $\frac{\mu_2 + \mu_3}{2}$, etc. We can answer this question using one of the multiple comparison procedures described later in this chapter.

12.4 BASIC CONCEPTS IN ANOVA

An observation can be thought of as a combination of the effects of the independent variable of interest, the characteristics of patient subjects or experimental units, chance variation in the subject's response, and environmental and other extraneous conditions that are beyond the investigator's control. As mentioned, the ANOVA procedure is dependent on estimates of variance. We are interested in comparing the means of k populations that are assumed to be independent and normally distributed with the same variance. Therefore, the procedure begins by taking a random sample of size n_1 from the first population, which is $N(\mu_1, \sigma_1^2)$, a random sample of size n_2 from the second population, which is $N(\mu_2, \sigma_2^2)$, $\cdots$, and a random sample of size n_k from the kth population, which is $N(\mu_k, \sigma_k^2)$. It is not necessary that the numbers of observations in each sample are equal. Let Y_{ij} denote the jth observation in the ith group. The following model is assumed to hold:

$$Y_{ij} = \mu + \alpha_i + \epsilon_{ij}$$

where

μ = constant representing the grand mean of the population means,

α_i = constant representing the treatment effect of ith population, which is equal to $\mu_i - \mu$, and

ϵ_{ij} = the error term associated with Y_{ij}, which is equal to $Y_{ij} - \mu - \alpha_i$.

The observation Y_{ij} is the sum of three unknown parameters; μ, α_i, and ϵ_{ij}. These unknown parameters can be estimated from the sample data. The error term ϵ_{ij} is assumed to be normally distributed with mean 0 and variance σ^2, that is, $\epsilon_{ij} \sim N(0, \sigma^2)$. From the model stated above, it is easy to see that an observation Y_{ij} is also normally distributed with mean $\mu + \alpha_i$ and variance σ^2. The term α_i is constrained in the model so that the sum of the α_i's over all groups is 0, that is, $\sum_{i=1}^{n} \alpha_i = 0$. Note that $\mu_1 = \mu + \alpha_1$, $\mu_2 = \mu + \alpha_2$, $\cdots$, $\mu_k = \mu + \alpha_k$. Equivalently, $\alpha_1 = \mu_1 - \mu$, $\alpha_2 = \mu_2 - \mu$, $\cdots$, $\alpha_k = \mu_k - \mu$. If $\mu_1 = \mu_2 = \cdots = \mu_k = \mu$, then $\alpha_1 = \alpha_2 = \cdots = \alpha_k = 0$. Therefore, the null hypothesis $H_0 : \mu_1 = \mu_2 = \cdots = \mu_k$ is equivalent to testing the hypothesis that all population treatment effects α_i's are equal to zero. The alternative hypothesis is that at least one of the treatment effects is not zero. The hypotheses can be expressed as: $H_0 :$ all $\alpha_i = 0$ versus $H_1 :$ at least one $\alpha_i \neq 0$. The k sample data is displayed in Table 12.4.1. The sample sizes n_1, n_2, $\cdots$, n_k are not necessarily equal. Let $N = \sum_{i=1}^{k} n_i$ denote the total number of all the observations in k samples. Let

Table 12.4.1. Samples drawn from k independent populations.

Group 1	Group 2	$\cdots$	Group k
Y_{11}	Y_{21}	$\cdots$	Y_{k1}
Y_{12}	Y_{22}	$\cdots$	Y_{k2}
$\vdots$	$\vdots$	$\vdots$	$\vdots$
Y_{1,n_1}	Y_{2,n_2}	$\cdots$	Y_{k,n_k}
n_1	n_2	$\cdots$	n_k
$\overline{Y}_1$	$\overline{Y}_2$	$\cdots$	$\overline{Y}_k$
S_1	S_2	$\cdots$	S_k

$\overline{Y}_1$, $\overline{Y}_2$, $\cdots$, $\overline{Y}_k$ be the k treatment means, and S_1, S_2, $\cdots$, S_k be the k sample standard deviations (SDs). The grand mean, $\overline{\overline{Y}}$, is obtained by summing all the observations in the table and dividing by $N = \sum_{i=1}^{k} n_i$. Note that the grand mean can be viewed as a weighted average of the k sample means.

$$\overline{\overline{Y}} = \frac{\sum_{i=1}^{k} \sum_{j=1}^{n_i} Y_{ij}}{N}$$

$$= \frac{n_1 \overline{Y}_1 + n_2 \overline{Y}_2 + \cdots + n_k \overline{Y}_k}{n_1 + n_2 + \cdots + n_k}.$$

12.5 *F* TEST FOR COMPARISON OF k POPULATION MEANS

One of the assumptions we make in the ANOVA is that the population variance in each of the k groups has the same value σ^2. Two different measures of variability can be estimated. One is the variation of the individual observations around their population means, and the other the variation of the population means around the grand mean. The first estimate is called the **within-group variability**, and the second estimate is called **between-group variability**. If the variability within the k different populations is small relative to the variability among their respective means, this indicates that the population means are different. We will describe how an F test is used to test the null hypothesis, $H_0 : \mu_1 = \mu_2 = \cdots = \mu_k$.

The deviation of an individual observation Y_{ij} from the grand mean $\overline{\overline{Y}}$ can be written as

$$Y_{ij} - \overline{\overline{Y}} = \left(Y_{ij} - \overline{Y}_i \right) + (\overline{Y}_i - \overline{\overline{Y}}).$$

The first term $\left(Y_{ij} - \overline{Y}_i\right)$ represents the deviation of an individual observation from the ith group mean, and the second term $(\overline{Y}_i - \overline{\overline{Y}})$ represents the deviation of a group mean from the grand mean. If the above decomposition is squared and the squared deviations are summed over all $N = \sum_{i=1}^{k} n_i$ observations, we can obtained the following expression:

$$\sum_{i=1}^{k}\sum_{j=1}^{n_i}\left(Y_{ij} - \overline{\overline{Y}}\right)^2 =$$

$$\sum_{i=1}^{k}\sum_{j=1}^{n_i}\left(Y_{ij} - \overline{Y}_i\right)^2 + \sum_{i=1}^{k}\sum_{j=1}^{n_i}\left(\overline{Y}_i - \overline{\overline{Y}}\right)^2.$$

Definition 12.5.1.
1. The **total sum of squares** (SSTO) is defined by $SSTO = \sum_{i=1}^{k}\sum_{j=1}^{n_i}(Y_{ij} - \overline{\overline{Y}})^2$.
2. The **within-groups sum of squares** (SSW) is defined by $SSW = \sum_{i=1}^{k}\sum_{j=1}^{n_i}\left(Y_{ij} - \overline{Y}_i\right)^2$.
3. The **between-groups sum of squares** (SSB) is defined by $SSB = \sum_{i=1}^{k}\sum_{j=1}^{n_i}(\overline{Y}_i - \overline{\overline{Y}})^2$.

Using the definition, the expression $\sum_{i=1}^{k}\sum_{j=1}^{n_i}(Y_{ij} - \overline{\overline{Y}})^2$ can be written as $SSTO = SSW + SSB$. It is easy to see that $SSW = SSTO - SSB$. Note that SSW is also referred to as **error sum of squares** and SSB as **treatment sum of squares**. We can derive the following identities that may appear to be complicated but computationally more convenient:

$$SSTO = \sum_{i=1}^{k}\sum_{j=1}^{n_i}Y_{ij}^2 - \frac{Y_{..}^2}{N},$$

where $Y_{..} = \sum_{i=1}^{k}\sum_{j=1}^{n_i}Y_{ij}$ denotes the grand total sum of all observations in k samples.

$$SSB = \sum_{i=1}^{k}n_i\overline{Y}_i^2 - \frac{\left(\sum_{i=1}^{k}n_i\overline{Y}_i\right)^2}{N},$$

$$SSW = \sum_{i=1}^{k}(n_i - 1)S_i^2.$$

Before we can proceed, we need to discuss the degrees of freedom associated with these sums of squares. The number of degrees of freedom associated with SSB (between-groups sum of squares) is $(k - 1)$, which is one less than the number of treatment means. The ith treatment level has $(n_i - 1)$ degrees of freedom. Thus, there

are $(n_1 - 1) + (n_2 - 1) + \cdots + (n_k - 1) = N - k$ degrees of freedom associated with SSW (within-groups sum of squares). If the sample sizes are equal, $n_1 = n_2 = \cdots = n_k = n$, then there are $k(n - 1)$ degrees of freedom associated with SSW. The number of degrees of freedom assigned with $SSTO$ (total sum of squares) is $N - 1$, one less than the total number of observations in the k samples. We discussed above that $SSTO = SSW + SSB$. The same relationship holds for their respective degrees of freedom, that is, $(N - 1) = (N - k) + (k - 1)$. We define a new term, called **mean square** (MS). The concept of mean square is the same as variance. A mean square is obtained by simply dividing a sum of squares by its degrees of freedom.

Between-groups mean square: $MSB = \dfrac{SSB}{(k - 1)}$.

Within-groups mean square: $MSW = \dfrac{SSW}{(N - k)}$.

The null hypothesis of equality of k population means, $H_0 : \mu_1 = \mu_2 = \cdots = \mu_k$, is tested based on the following F statistic, which is the ratio between MSB and MSW as follows:

$$F = \frac{MSB}{MSW}.$$

As discussed in Section 10.8, the null hypothesis will be rejected if the value of the F statistic is large. If it is small, the null hypothesis will be accepted. Under the null hypothesis, the test statistic $\dfrac{MSB}{MSW}$ follows an F distribution with the numerator degrees of freedom $(k - 1)$ and the denominator degrees of freedom $(N - k)$. The F test procedure for one-way ANOVA can be summarized.

For testing the hypotheses $H_0 : \mu_1 = \mu_2 = \cdots = \mu_k$ vs. H_1 : at least one mean is different from the others at the significance level α, and the following steps must be taken.

1. From the data compute the degrees of freedom, sum of squares (SSB and SSW), and mean squares (MSB and MSW) using the above formulas.
2. Compute the value of the test statistic $F = \dfrac{MSB}{MSW} \sim F_{(k-1, N-k)}$ under H_0.
3. Reject H_0 if $F > F_{(k-1, N-k; 1-\alpha)}$ and accept H_0 if $F \leq F_{(k-1, N-k; 1-\alpha)}$. The critical value $F_{(k-1, N-k; 1-\alpha)}$ can be found in the F table (Table G).

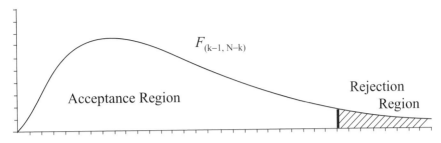

Figure 12.5.1 The rejection and acceptance regions for the F test for one-way ANOVA.

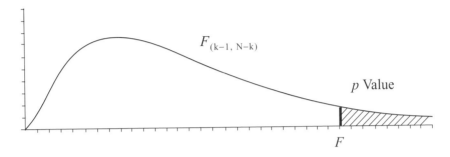

Figure 12.5.2 The p value of the F test for one-way ANOVA.

4. The p value is given by the area to the right of the calculated F value under an F distribution with the degrees of freedom $k - 1$ and $N - 1$. That is, p value $= P(F < F_{(k-1, N-k)})$.

The rejection and acceptance regions for the F test are displayed in Figure 12.5.1. The exact p value of the test is also shown in Figure 12.5.2. The statistical results of the one-way ANOVA are usually presented in an ANOVA table, as shown in Table 12.5.1. We present the following examples to illustrate one-way ANOVA procedures.

Example 12.5.1. The bonding of composite resin to enamel gained particular popularity in orthodontics, where benefits to patients include improved esthetics, caries and decalcification control, decreased periodontal insult, and simpler plaque control. For the last two decades bonding

metal brackets to enamel has been acceptable clinical practice, with much success and patient satisfaction [2]. Blount, Streelman, and Tkachyk [2] investigated if the use of bonded orthodontic brackets and/or bonded composite is a viable alternative to the traditional mandibular canine rest seat technique. The advantages are leaving healthy, vital abutment teeth unprepared, which contributes to added strength and longevity and is less costly than creating cast test seats. Their goal was to evaluate the strength of four different types of bonded rest seats (smooth enamel bond, roughened bond, ceramic brackets, stainless steel brackets) as compared to rest seats cut into maxillary canines, which is the control group. Seventy-five intact mandibular and maxillary canines were collected after extraction. Following bonding, the rest seats were loaded to failure in a Universal testing

Table 12.5.1. One-way ANOVA table.

Source of Variation	df	Sum of Squares	Mean Square	F value	p value
Between	$k - 1$	SSB	$\dfrac{SSB}{(k-1)}$	$\dfrac{SSB/(k-1)}{SSW/(N-k)}$	$P(F < F_{(k-1, N-k)})$
Within	$N - k$	SSW	$\dfrac{SSW}{(N-k)}$		
Total	$N - 1$	$SSTO$			

Table 12.5.2.　Peak load data in kilograms.

	Factor Levels				
	Control	Roughened Bond	Smooth Enamel Bond	Ceramic Bracket	Stainless Steel Bracket
Observations (kg) (Y_{ij})	47.39　42.73 31.07　45.61 36.25　49.06 40.21　46.54 49.31　40.01 42.33　30.31 42.11	10.92　14.02 22.60　19.00 14.76　21.13 12.67　12.20 19.41　16.27 21.54　17.03 31.92　29.41 16.52　16.73 8.21　14.29 19.20	25.27　19.38 8.54　12.34 13.73　10.23 22.20　8.78 12.46	39.54　43.87 35.15　23.42 31.38　26.80 40.71　29.56 34.44　33.97 30.87　35.29 30.04　36.32 29.56　28.82 25.77　24.74 33.35　35.34 18.76	7.08　8.56 7.87　25.11 19.73　9.17 11.79　12.42 12.61　17.18 14.14　19.38 5.60
Sample size	$n_1 = 13$	$n_2 = 19$	$n_3 = 9$	$n_4 = 21$	$n_5 = 13$
Sample mean	$\overline{Y}_1 = 41.764$	$\overline{Y}_2 = 17.781$	$\overline{Y}_3 = 14.770$	$\overline{Y}_4 = 31.795$	$\overline{Y}_5 = 13.126$
Sample SD	$S_1 = 6.207$	$S_2 = 5.901$	$S_3 = 6.066$	$S_4 = 6.041$	$S_5 = 5.800$
Grand mean	$\overline{\overline{Y}} = 24.694$	$(\sum_{i=1}^{5} n_i = 75)$			

machine and the peak load (maximum dislodging force) in kilograms for each specimen was recorded as shown in Table 12.5.2.

The notation $Y_i.$ is the sum of all observations in the ith sample. That is, $Y_i. = \sum_{j=1}^{n_i} Y_{ij}$. The grand total sum of all observations in k samples is denoted by $Y.. = \sum_{i=1}^{k} \sum_{j=1}^{n_i} Y_{ij} = 1852.03$. The grand mean is $\overline{\overline{Y}} = \dfrac{1852.03}{75} = 24.694$. We now compute SSB and SSW.

The value of the test statistic is given by

$$F = \frac{MSB}{MSW} = \frac{1,632.2234}{35.9576}$$
$$= 45.3930 \sim F_{(4,70)} \text{ under } H_0.$$

From the F table in the Appendix, we find that

$$F_{(4,70;0.999)} < F_{(4,60;0.999)} = 5.307 < F = 45.3930.$$

So the p value $= P(F < F_{(k-1,N-k)}) = P(45.3930 < F_{(4,70)}) < 0.001$. Therefore, we reject

$$SSB = \sum_{i=1}^{k} n_i \overline{Y}_i^2 - \frac{\left(\sum_{i=1}^{k} n_i \overline{Y}_i\right)^2}{N}$$

$$= 13(41.764)^2 + 19(17.781)^2 + 9(14.770)^2 + 21(31.795)^2 + 13(13.126)^2$$
$$- \frac{[13(41.764) + 19(17.781) + 9(14.770) + 21(31.795) + 13(13.126)]^2}{75}$$
$$= 54,114.660 - 47,585.7665 = 6,528.8935.$$

$$SSW = \sum_{i=1}^{k} (n_i - 1)S_i^2$$

$$= 12(6.207)^2 + 18(5.901)^2 + 8(6.066)^2 + 20(6.041)^2 + 12(5.800)^2 = 2,517.030.$$
$$SSTO = SSW + SSB = 2,517.030 + 6,528.8935 = 9,045.9235.$$

Since $k - 1 = 5 - 1 = 4$ and $N - k = 75 - 5 = 70$,

$$MSB = \frac{SSB}{(k-1)} = \frac{6,528.8935}{4} = 1,632.2234$$

$$MSW = \frac{SSW}{(N-k)} = \frac{2,517.030}{70} = 35.9576.$$

the null hypothesis that all the treatment means are equal and conclude that at least one mean is different. These results are summarized in an ANOVA table, Table 12.5.3.

Example 12.5.2. An investigation was conducted to compare the efficacy of three types of

Table 12.5.3. One-way ANOVA table.

Source of Variation	df	Sum of Squares	Mean Square	F value	p value
Between	4	6,528.8935	1,632.2234	45.3930	$p < 0.001$
Within	70	2,517.030	35.9576		
Total	74	9,045.9235			

commercially available toothpastes against the bacteria responsible for caries, gingivitis, and periodontitis. The introduction of fluoride into dentifrices was a milestone in dental science. Despite its great effects, scientists have been continually looking to improve dental care by investigating new agents that could help further decrease the rate of dental disease [3]. The study also included chlorhexidine, which has been the "gold standard" antimicrobial agent when compared with other products made for plaque control. Marsh [4] has shown that chlorhexidine can reduce dental plaque, caries, and gingivitis in humans. Table 12.5.4 displays the summary of the data that represent the zones of microbial inhibition produced by the four treatments against *Lactobacillus salivarious*.

The degrees of freedom are $(k - 1) = 4 - 1 = 3$ and $(N - k) = 41 - 4 = 37$. We now compute SSB, SSW, MSB, and MSW.

$$SSB = 10(7.368)^2 + 11(6.779)^2 + 9(6.412)^2 + 11(6.572)^2$$
$$- \frac{[10(7.368) + 11(6.779) + 9(6.412) + 11(6.572)]^2}{41}$$
$$= 1,893.5042 - 1,883.3538 = 10.1504.$$
$$SSW = 9(1.892) + 10(1.927) + 8(1.843) + 10(2.013)$$
$$= 71.1720.$$
$$SSTO = SSW + SSB = 71.1720 + 10.1504$$
$$= 81.3224.$$
$$MSB = \frac{SSB}{(k - 1)} = \frac{10.1504}{3} = 3.3835,$$
$$MSW = \frac{SSW}{(N - k)} = \frac{71.1720}{37} = 1.9236.$$

Table 12.5.4. Zone of inhibition data in square centimeters.

Toothpaste	n_i	Mean of Zone of Inhibition $(\overline{Y}_i)$	Sample Variance (S_i^2)
Group A	10	7.368	1.892
Group B	11	6.779	1.927
Group C	9	6.412	1.843
Group D (chlorhexidine)	11	6.572	2.013

The value of the F test statistic is given by

$$F = \frac{MSB}{MSW} = \frac{3.3835}{1.9236}$$
$$= 1.7589 \sim F_{(3,37)} \text{ under } H_0.$$

From the F table in the Appendix, we find that

$$F_{(3,60;0.95)} = 2.758 < F_{(3,37;0.95)} < F_{(3,30;0.95)}$$
$$= 2.922.$$

Since the value of the test statistic $F = 1.7589 < F_{(3,37;0.95)}$, F falls in the acceptance region.

The p value $= P(F < F_{(k-1,N-k)})$
$$= P(1.7589 < F_{(3,37)}) > P(2.177 < F_{(3,60;0.90)})$$
$$= 0.10.$$

Therefore, we accept the null hypothesis that there are no significant differences among all the treatment means. These results are summarized in an ANOVA table (Table 12.5.5).

Suppose the null hypothesis $H_0 : \mu_1 = \mu_2 = \cdots = \mu_k$ is rejected. Which population means are different? This question will be addressed in the next section.

Example 12.5.3. In the pharmaceutical sciences the investigators are often interested in comparing three or more assay methods. Specifically, suppose that 12 tablets were selected at random for the comparison of three assay methods, four tablets for each assay. The results of assays comparing the three analytical methods are displayed in Table 12.5.6.

Test the equality of the three treatment means (that is, $H_0 : \mu_A = \mu_B = \mu_C$ vs. $H_1 :$ not all means are equal). From the above data, we obtain $\overline{Y}_A = 311.40$, $\overline{Y}_B = 308.0$, $\overline{Y}_C = 308.78$, $S_A = 1.517$, $S_B = 1.095$, $S_C = 1.615$, and the grand mean $\overline{\overline{Y}} = 309.39$. One can mimic the steps discussed in the preceding examples to complete the test.

Table 12.5.5. One-way ANOVA table.

Source of Variation	df	Sum of Squares	Mean Square	F value	p value
Between (model)	3	10.1504	3.3835	1.7589	$p > 0.10$
Within (error)	37	71.1720	1.9236		
Total	40	81.3224			

Table 12.5.6. Comparing three assay methods.

Method A	Method B	Method C
312.2	308.4	309.8
310.5	309.2	310.5
309.8	306.6	307.3
313.1	307.8	307.5

12.6 MULTIPLE COMPARISONS PROCEDURES

When $k = 2$, the F test statistic for one-way ANOVA is equivalent to the square of the corresponding t test statistic used for testing the equality of two means. Why can we not use the t test comparing two means at a time to compare three or more population means? When two means are compared at a time, the rest of the population means under investigation are not being considered. When all possible pairwise comparisons are made, the probability of rejecting the null hypothesis when it is true is increased, since there are many more t tests being performed. The likelihood of finding some significant differences by chance alone is greater. For example, for the comparison of $k = 3$ treatment means, three separate t tests are required. For the comparison of $k = 10$ means, we need to perform $\binom{10}{2} = 45$ two-sample t tests. This suggests that at the significance level of $\alpha = 0.05$, we may find about two comparisons that are significant by chance, since $(0.05)(45) = 2.25$. To protect ourselves against finding false significant differences due to making too many pairwise comparisons, several statistical procedures have been suggested. These procedures are referred to as **multiple comparisons procedures**.

12.6.1 Least Significant Difference Method

We first describe a procedure known as Fisher's least significant difference (LSD) method for

comparing two specific group means among the k group means; $H_0 : \mu_i = \mu_j$ vs. $H_1 : \mu_i \neq \mu_j$ $(i \neq j)$. The test statistic is given as follows:

$$t = \frac{\overline{Y}_i - \overline{Y}_j}{S\sqrt{(\frac{1}{n_i} + \frac{1}{n_j})}} \sim t_{(N-k)} \quad \text{under the null} \atop \text{hypothesis, where}$$

$$S^2 = \frac{\sum_{i=1}^{k}(n_i - 1)S_i^2}{N - k},$$

the pooled estimate of the variance, which is the same as the MSW discussed in the preceding section. For a two-tailed test at the significance level of α, we reject H_0 if $t < t_{(N-k,\alpha/2)}$ or $t > t_{(N-k,1-\alpha/2)}$, and accept H_0 if $t_{(N-k,\alpha/2)} \leq t \leq t_{(N-k,1-\alpha/2)}$. The p value of the test is computed;

if $t < 0$, $p = 2 \cdot P(t_{(N-k)} < t)$
$\qquad = 2 \cdot$ {area to the left of the value
$\qquad\qquad t$ under a t distribution with df
$\qquad\qquad N - k$},

if $t \geq 0$, $p = 2 \cdot P(t_{(N-k)} > t)$
$\qquad = 2 \cdot$ {area to the right of the value t
$\qquad\qquad$ under a t distribution with df
$\qquad\qquad N - k$}.

If $N - k = 70$, the critical values for the LSD procedure are given by

$$t_{(N-k,\alpha/2)} = t_{(70,0.025)} = -1.9944$$

and

$$t_{(N-k,1-\alpha/2)} = t_{(70,0.925)} = 1.9944.$$

12.6.2 Bonferroni Approach

One of the simplest and most widely used multiple comparison procedures is the approach proposed by Bonferroni. The basic idea of the Bonferroni approach is the modification of the significance level. This method is applicable whether the sample size n_i for each group is equal or unequal. Suppose we want to make a pairwise comparison between any two treatment means among k means in

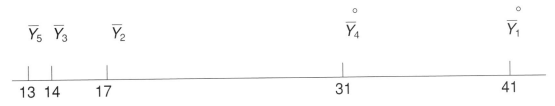

Figure 12.6.1 Results of Bonferroni approach.

one-way ANOVA. The hypothesis to be tested is $H_0 : \mu_i = \mu_j$ vs. $H_1 : \mu_i \neq \mu_j$ $(i \neq j)$. Let α be the specified significance level.

1. Compute the sample means $\overline{Y}_i$ and the pooled estimate of the SD obtained by

$$S = \sqrt{\frac{\sum_{i=1}^{k}(n_i - 1)S_i^2}{N - k}}.$$

2. Compute the test statistic $t = \dfrac{\overline{Y}_i - \overline{Y}_j}{S\sqrt{\left(\frac{1}{n_i} + \frac{1}{n_j}\right)}} \sim$

   $t_{(N-k)}$ under the null hypothesis.
3. Let c be the number of pairwise comparisons to be made, that is, $c = \binom{k}{2}$. Let $\alpha^* = \dfrac{\alpha}{c}$.
   Reject H_0 if $t < t_{(N-k,\alpha^*/2)}$ or $t > t_{(N-k,1-\alpha^*/2)}$.
   Accept H_0 if $t_{(N-k,\alpha^*/2)} \leq t \leq t_{(N-k,1-\alpha^*/2)}$.

The above procedure is basically the same as the two-sample t test with equal variances, which was introduced in Section 9.3. The difference is that the estimate S^2 of the variance is the pooled estimate from all k samples rather than two samples that are involved for the comparison. Instead of using the significance level α, we have the adjusted significance level $\alpha^* = \dfrac{\alpha}{c}$ proposed by Bonferroni.

Example 12.6.1. In Example 12.5.1, the null hypothesis $H_0 : \mu_1 = \mu_2 = \cdots = \mu_k$ was rejected. We apply the Bonferroni approach to detect which of the k population means are different. The test was performed at the significance level $\alpha = 0.05$. We have $k = 5$ groups, $N = 75$, and $N - k = 70$. Thus, the number of pairwise comparisons to be made is $c = \binom{k}{2} = 10$, and $\alpha^* = \dfrac{\alpha}{c} = \dfrac{0.05}{10} = 0.005$. Therefore, we perform the t test between each pair of groups using the adjusted significance level $\alpha^* = 0.005$. The critical values are given by $t_{(N-k,\alpha^*/2)} = t_{(70,0.0025)}$ and $t_{(N-k,1-\alpha^*/2)} = t_{(70,0.9975)}$. From the t table (Table E) in the Appendix, we find $t_{(70,0.9975)} = 2.8987$ and $t_{(70,0.0025)} = -2.8987$. We let A = control, B = roughened bond, C = smooth enamel bond, D = ceramic bracket, and E = stainless steel bracket. The results of these significance tests show that there are no significant differences between the pairs (B, C), (B, E), and (C, E), but significant differences exist in all other pairwise comparisons; that is, one treatment mean is significantly different from the other treatment mean. This is displayed in the above figure (Figure 12.6.1). The summary of the results using the Bonferroni method is presented in Table 12.6.1. The first column of the table indicates the specific groups being

Table 12.6.1. Pairwise comparisons of the data in Example 12.5.1.

Groups Compared	Mean Difference $(\overline{Y}_i - \overline{Y}_j)$	Value of the Test Statistic	p value
(A, B)	23.983	$t = 10.4848$	$p < 0.0005$
(A, C)	26.994	$t = 9.6821$	$p < 0.0005$
(A, D)	9.969	$t = 4.7117$	$p < 0.0005$
(A, E)	28.638	$t = 12.1760$	$p < 0.0005$
(B, C)	3.011	$t = 1.2410$	$p > 0.30$
(B, D)	−14.014	$t = -7.3828$	$p < 0.0005$
(B, E)	4.655	$t = 2.1572$	$p > 0.04$
(C, D)	−17.025	$t = -7.1270$	$p < 0.0005$
(C, E)	1.644	$t = 0.6323$	$p > 0.60$
(D, E)	18.669	$t = 8.3333$	$p < 0.0005$

compared, the second column the difference between the sample means $(\overline{Y}_i - \overline{Y}_j)$, the third column the test statistic, and the last column the corresponding p value.

For the data in Example 12.5.1, the critical values for the least significant difference (LSD) procedure are given by $t_{(N-k,\alpha/2)} = t_{(70,0.025)} = -1.9944$ and $t_{(N-k,1-\alpha/2)} = t_{(70,0.925)} = 1.9944$. Given $\alpha = 0.05$, the rejection regions using LSD are defined by $t < -1.9944$ and $t > 1.9944$, while the rejection regions using the Bonferroni approach are defined by $t < -2.8987$ and $t > 2.8987$. Thus, there are comparisons between pairs of groups for which the LSD would find a significant difference but the Bonferroni approach would not. We should note that one disadvantage of the adjusted significance level is that it is so much smaller than the α level that none of the pairwise tests will be rejected. Consequently, the power of the test procedure will be low. Some other procedures that are more powerful have been suggested by Scheffé and Tukey.

12.6.3 Scheffé's Method

In most situations, the multiple comparisons procedures are applied if pairs of group means are being compared. However, in some other cases, we are interested in all possible contrasts involving more complicated comparisons. Scheffé's method is widely used in this type of comparison. We first define a linear contrast.

Definition 12.6.1. A **linear contrast** (L) is any linear combination of the individual group means such that the sum of the coefficients c_i is zero.

$$L = \sum_{i=1}^{k} c_i \mu_i \quad \text{where} \quad \sum_{i=1}^{k} c_i = 0.$$

Since an unbiased estimator of the population mean μ_i is $\overline{Y}_i$, an unbiased estimator of the above linear contrast $L = \sum_{i=1}^{k} c_i \mu_i$ is given by

$$\hat{L} = \sum_{i=1}^{k} c_i \overline{Y}_i \quad \text{where} \quad \sum_{i=1}^{k} c_i = 0.$$

The simplest example of a linear contrast is the mean difference used in the Bonferroni approach:

$$\hat{L} = \overline{Y}_1 - \overline{Y}_2$$

where $c_1 = 1, c_2 = -1$, and $c_3 = c_4 = c_5 = 0$ $\left(\sum_{i=1}^{5} c_i = 0\right)$.

It can be shown that the estimated variance of the linear contrast given in the above expression is

$$S^2(\hat{L}) = S^2 \sum_{i=1}^{k} \frac{c_i^2}{n_i},$$

where S^2 is the pooled estimate of the variance and n_i is the number of observations in the ith sample.

Example 12.6.2. Here are several examples of linear contrasts.

1. $L = \mu_1 - \mu_2$
2. $L = \mu_3 - \mu_5$
3. $L = \dfrac{\mu_1 + \mu_2}{2} - \dfrac{\mu_3 + \mu_4}{2}$
4. $L = \dfrac{\mu_1 + \mu_2}{2} - \mu_3$
5. $L = \mu_1 - \dfrac{\mu_2 + \mu_3 + \mu_4 + \mu_5}{4}$

Linear contrasts are often used in drug development. Suppose a new drug at two different dosage levels is being compared with a placebo. μ_1 and μ_2 denote the mean response for dosage level 1 and level 2, respectively, and μ_3 denotes the mean response for placebo. The investigators will consider $L = \dfrac{\mu_1 + \mu_2}{2} - \mu_3$ to compare the overall effect of the drug with the placebo effect.

To apply Scheffé's multiple comparisons procedure to test the hypothesis $H_0 : \sum_{i=1}^{k} c_i \mu_i = 0$ vs. $H_0 : \sum_{i=1}^{k} c_i \mu_i \neq 0$, follow the steps described below:

1. Compute the test statistic $t = \dfrac{\hat{L}}{S\sqrt{\sum_{i=1}^{k} \dfrac{c_i^2}{n_i}}}$.

2. Find the critical values defined by
$$-\sqrt{(k-1)F_{k-1,N-k;1-\alpha}}$$
and $\sqrt{(k-1)F_{k-1,N-k;1-\alpha}}$.

3. Reject H_0 if $t < -\sqrt{(k-1)F_{k-1,N-k;1-\alpha}}$ or $t > \sqrt{(k-1)F_{k-1,N-k;1-\alpha}}$.

Example 12.6.3. Suppose we wish to make a comparison of bond (roughened bond and smooth enamel) and bracket (ceramic and stainless steel) with respect to their peak load from the data presented in Table 12.5.2. The linear contrast we have is

$$L = \frac{\mu_2 + \mu_3}{2} - \frac{\mu_4 + \mu_5}{2}$$

where $c_1 = 0$, $c_2 = c_3 = 1/2$, and $c_4 = c_5 = -1/2$. Thus, $\sum_{i=1}^{5} c_i = 0$. To test the hypotheses

$$H_0 : \frac{\mu_2 + \mu_3}{2} - \frac{\mu_4 + \mu_5}{2} = 0 \quad \text{vs.}$$

$$H_0 : \frac{\mu_2 + \mu_3}{2} - \frac{\mu_4 + \mu_5}{2} \neq 0$$

we need to compute

$$\hat{L} = \frac{\overline{Y}_2 + \overline{Y}_3}{2} - \frac{\overline{Y}_4 + \overline{Y}_5}{2}$$

$$= \frac{17.781 + 14.770}{2} - \frac{31.795 + 13.126}{2}$$

$$= -6.185.$$

$$\sum_{i=1}^{5} \frac{c_i^2}{n_i} = 0 + \frac{(0.5)^2}{19} + \frac{(0.5)^2}{9}$$

$$+ \frac{(-0.5)^2}{21} + \frac{(-0.5)^2}{13}$$

$$= 0.07207.$$

Since $S^2 = MSW = 35.9576$ from Example 12.5.1, $S = \sqrt{35.9576} = 5.9965$, the value of the test statistic is obtained by

$$t = \frac{\hat{L}}{S\sqrt{\sum_{i=1}^{k} \frac{c_i^2}{n_i}}} = \frac{-6.185}{(5.9965)\sqrt{0.07207}}$$

$$= -3.8414.$$

From the F table, using $\alpha = 0.05$, we get the critical values:

$$-\sqrt{(k-1)F_{k-1,N-k;1-\alpha}} = -\sqrt{(4)F_{4,70;0.95}}$$

$$= -\sqrt{(4)2.508}$$

$$= -3.1673$$

and

$$\sqrt{(k-1)F_{k-1,N-k;1-\alpha}} = 3.1673.$$

Because

$$t = -3.8414 < -\sqrt{(k-1)F_{k-1,N-k;1-\alpha}}$$

$$= -3.1673,$$

the null hypothesis H_0 is rejected at the significance level of $\alpha = 5\%$. We conclude that on the average the brackets tend to have significantly higher peak load than the bonds.

As illustrated in Example 12.6.2, Scheffé method can be used to compare pairs of treatment means, since a difference between two means is a special case of a linear contrast. Using the Scheffé method, the null hypothesis is rejected if $t < -3.1673$ or $t > 3.1673$, while using the Bonferroni multiple comparisons procedure, the null hypothesis is rejected if $t < -2.8987$ or $t > 2.8987$. Therefore, Bonferroni method will find significant differences more often than does Scheffé method when only pairwise comparisons are being made.

12.6.4 Tukey's Procedure

One of the best known and widely used multiple comparisons procedures is Tukey's method. When Tukey's multiple comparisons procedure is used for testing pairwise mean differences, the test is commonly referred to as **Tukey's honestly significant difference** (HSD) test. The Tukey's HSD method is applicable when the sample sizes for the k groups are equal ($n_1 = n_2 = \cdots = n_k = n$) and pairwise comparisons of the means are of primary focus. This method is based on the **studentized range distribution**. Suppose we have n independent observations $Y_1, Y_2, \cdots, Y_n$ from a normal distribution with mean μ and variance σ^2. Then the range, w, of this observations is denoted $w = \text{Max}(Y_i) - \text{Min}(Y_i)$. Let S^2 be an estimate of the variance σ^2. Then the ratio $\frac{w}{S}$ is known as the **studentized range**, and is denoted by $q(k, \upsilon) = \frac{w}{S}$. The studentized range depends on k and υ, the degrees of freedom associated with the estimate S^2. Many statistics textbooks ([5], [6]) include a table of percentiles of the studentized range distribution for performing the Tukey's HSD test. The test statistic, denoted by q, is given by

$$q = \frac{\overline{Y}_i - \overline{Y}_j}{\sqrt{\frac{MSW}{n}}} \sim q_{k,N-k}, \quad \text{under the null hypothesis}$$

where N ($N = kn$) is the total number of observations.

For the Tukey's method, we assumed that the sample sizes are equal for each of the k groups. The Tukey's multiple comparisons procedure for unequal sample sizes is called the **Tukey-Kramer** method. The **Student-Newman-Keuls**

Biostatistics for Oral Healthcare

(SNK) multiple comparisons procedure is an often-used method by investigators, which is an alternative to the Tukey's procedure. The SNK procedure is also based on the studentized range distribution, but the numerator degrees of freedom k in $q_{k,N-k}$ is modified such that k replaced by $k^* =$ number of treatment means in the range of means being compared. For example, if a comparison is being made between the second largest and the fourth largest means, then $k^* = 3$. If the comparison is being made between the largest and fourth largest, then $k^* = 4$. Other multiple comparisons procedures have been developed and proposed, such as Dunn-Šidàk test and Dunnett's method. Dunnett's procedure is applicable only when several treatment means are being compared with a single control mean. No comparisons between the treatment means are allowed. Readers, who are interested in studying the test procedures suggested by Dunn-Šidàk and Dunnett, are referred to Kirk [7] and Forthofer and Lee [8].

12.7 ONE-WAY ANOVA RANDOM EFFECTS MODEL

As we mentioned earlier in this chapter, there are situations in which the factor levels are considered as a random sample from a population of factor levels or treatments. In the present section, we shall introduce the one-way ANOVA random effects model in which the factor under study is considered random. The mathematical form of one-way ANOVA random effects models looks the same as the one for fixed effect models stated in Section 12.3:

$$Y_{ij} = \mu + \alpha_i + \epsilon_{ij}$$

where

Y_{ij} = the jth observation in the ith factor level or i^{th} treatment
α_i = independent random variables that are assumed to follow a normal distribution,
$\alpha_i \sim N(0, \sigma_B^2)$
ϵ_{ij} are independent $N(0, \sigma^2)$
α_i and ϵ_{ij} are independent random variables, $i = 1, 2, \cdots, k$ and $j = 1, 2, \cdots, n_i$.

Recall that the factor level means α_i are constant for the fixed effect model but are random variables

Table 12.7.1. CA 19-9 data.

Replicate	Subject				
	1	2	3	4	5
1	27	101	48	187	45
2	38	76	39	104	63
3	15	68	22	88	74
4	43	88	37	134	33
5	31	92	33	158	66
6	40	65	24	141	49

for the random effects model. Before we can further explain the model, consider an example.

Example 12.7.1. A tumor marker for pancreatic cancer is known as CA 19-9 and is measured by a blood test. CA 19-9 is often used to monitor treatment progress of previously diagnosed pancreatic cancer patients. Physicians rely on this blood test in conjunction with periodic CT scans to determine whether the cancer is in remission or continuing to grow [9]. Suppose that blood samples were drawn from five patients who were diagnosed with pancreatic cancer within the last 2 years. Table 12.7.1 shows the blood test results of CA 19-9 levels from a laboratory. Each subject has six measurements (replicates).

The underlying mean of the ith subject is obtained by $\mu + \alpha_i$, where α_i has a normal distribution with mean 0 and variance σ_B^2. Thus, for example, the first subject would have the underlying mean $\mu + \alpha_1$, and the third subject would have the underlying mean $\mu + \alpha_3$. The variability of $\mu + \alpha_i$ is represented by σ_B^2. The more the different patients vary in their mean CA 19-9 levels, the larger is the value of σ_B^2. If all patients have the same mean level of CA 19-9, we will have the variance $\sigma_B^2 = 0$. The variance σ_B^2 represents the between-subject variation. The term ϵ_{ij} represents the variability associated with the replicates of different subjects. The above model assumes that all ϵ_{ij} have the same variance σ^2, which represents the within-subject variation. This implies that the replicates from the ith subject are normally distributed with mean $\mu + \alpha_i$ and variance σ^2. Hence, the variance of Y_{ij} in this random effects model is the sum of two variance components, σ_B^2 and σ^2. In Example 12.7.1, we are primarily interested in the mean CA 19-9 level of all patients, that is, in effect their variability rather than the mean levels

Table 12.7.2. ANOVA table for one-way random effects model.

Source of Variation	df	Sum of Squares	Mean Square	F value	p value
Between (Model)	4	43,970.76	10,992.69	28.53	< 0.0001
Within (Error)	25	9,632.90	385.32		
Total	29	53,603.66			

of the five subjects. Therefore, the hypotheses of our interest is: $H_0 : \sigma_B^2 = 0$ vs. $H_1 : \sigma_B^2 > 0$.

If the null hypothesis H_0 is true, then there is no between-subject variability and therefore, all $\mu + \alpha_i$ are equal. If H_1 is true, then $\sigma_B^2 > 0$ implies that they are different and that there is a difference between the means for the subjects. A test procedure employing an F statistic will be used to test the hypothesis. Here are the steps to be taken.

1. Compute the value of the test statistic $F = \dfrac{MSB}{MSW} \sim F_{(k-1, N-k)}$ under the null hypothesis H_0, where

$$MSB \text{ (between MS)} = \frac{\sum_{i=1}^{k} n_i (\overline{Y}_i - \overline{\overline{Y}})^2}{k-1},$$

$$MSW \text{ (within MS)} = \frac{\sum_{i=1}^{k} \sum_{j=1}^{n_i} (Y_{ij} - \overline{Y}_i)^2}{N-k}.$$

$\overline{Y}_i$ and $\overline{\overline{Y}}$ were defined in Section 12.4, and $N = \sum_{i=1}^{k} n_i$.

2. Reject H_0, if $F > F_{(k-1, N-k; 1-\alpha)}$ and accept H_0, if $F \leq F_{(k-1, N-k; 1-\alpha)}$.

3. The p value is obtained by

$$p = P(F < F_{(k-1, N-k)})$$
$$= \text{the area to the right of the calculated}$$
$$\text{value } F \text{ under an } F_{(k-1, N-k)} \text{) distribution.}$$

From the data displayed in Table 12.7.1, we can compute the means:

$$\overline{Y}_1 = 32.33, \quad \overline{Y}_2 = 81.67, \quad \overline{Y}_3 = 33.83,$$

$$\overline{Y}_4 = 135.33, \quad \overline{Y}_5 = 55.00, \quad \text{and} \quad \overline{\overline{Y}} = 67.63,$$

With $k = 5$, $n_1 = n_2 = \cdots = n_5 = n = 6$, and

$N = \sum_{i=1}^{k} n_i = 30$, we obtain

$$SSB = \sum_{i=1}^{k} n_i (\overline{Y}_i - \overline{\overline{Y}})^2 = 43,970.76$$

$$SSW = \sum_{i=1}^{k} \sum_{j=1}^{n_i} (Y_{ij} - \overline{Y}_i)^2 = 9,632.90$$

$$MSB = \frac{SSB}{4} = 10,992.69$$

$$MSW = \frac{SSW}{25} = 385.316$$

The value of the test statistic is $F = \dfrac{MSB}{MSW} = \dfrac{10,992.69}{385.316} = 28.529$.

From the F table in the Appendix, we get $F_{(k-1, N-k; 1-\alpha)} = F_{(4, 25; 0.95)} = 2.759$. Since $F_{(4, 25; 0.95)} = 2.759 < F = 28.529$, we reject the null hypothesis. We conclude that $\sigma_B^2 > 0$, which means that the mean levels of CA 19-9 of the subjects are significantly different. The $p = P(F < F_{(k-1, N-k)}) < 0.0001$. The results can be summarized in Table 12.7.2.

12.8 TEST FOR EQUALITY OF k VARIANCES

At the beginning of this chapter we learned that the ANOVA models require the k populations ($k > 2$) to have equal variances. The F test for the equality of two variances was discussed in Section 9.8. This section will introduce two formal statistical procedures available for testing whether or not three or more populations have the same variance.

12.8.1 Bartlett's Test

The Bartlett test requires the populations under study are normally distributed and can be used for equal or unequal sample sizes. Suppose that there are k independent normal populations and that random samples of size n_i are drawn from each of the k populations. The hypothesis we wish to test is:

$$H_0 : \sigma_1^2 = \sigma_2^2 = \cdots = \sigma_k^2 \quad \text{vs.}$$
$$H_1 : \text{ not all } \sigma_i^2 \text{ are equal.}$$

It would seem quite intuitive to construct a test statistic based on their sample variances to study whether or not the variances σ_i^2 are equal. Let $S_1^2, S_2^2, \cdots, S_k^2$ be the sample variances estimated from the samples taken from k independent normal populations. The degrees of freedom associated with S_i^2 is $(n_i - 1)$. The total sum of the degrees of freedom is $\sum_{i=1}^{k}(n_i - 1) = N - k$, where $N = \sum_{i=1}^{k} n_i$. As discussed in Section 12.5, the mean square MSW is the weighted average of the sample variances:

$$MSW = \frac{\sum_{i=1}^{k}(n_i - 1)S_i^2}{N - k}.$$

We define the weighted geometric average of the sample variances S_i^2, denoted by GMS (geometric mean square), as follows:

$$GMS = \left\{ (S_1^2)^{(n_1-1)}(S_2^2)^{(n_2-1)} \cdots (S_k^2)^{(n_k-1)} \right\}^{1/(N-k)}.$$

It can be shown that $GMS \leq MSW$ or $1 \leq \frac{MSW}{GMS}$. If the ratio $\frac{MSW}{GMS}$ is close to 1, it is an indication that the population variances are equal. If the ratio $\frac{MSW}{GMS}$ is large, it indicates that the variances are not equal. Bartlett has shown that for large samples (i.e., large n_i), a function of

$$\log \frac{MSW}{GMS} = \log MSW - \log GMS \overset{\circ}{\sim} \chi^2_{(k-1)}$$
$$\text{under } H_0,$$

that is, a function of $\log MSW - \log GMS$ is approximately χ^2 distributed with degrees of freedom $(k-1)$ when the population variances are equal. To perform the Bartlett test, the following steps are to be taken:

1. Compute the MSW and GMS from the sample data.

2. Compute the test statistic $B = \dfrac{(N-k)}{C}$ $\times \{\log MSW - \log GMS\} \overset{\circ}{\sim} \chi^2_{(k-1)}$ under H_0,

where $C = 1 + \dfrac{1}{3(k-1)} \left\{ \left(\sum_{i=1}^{k} \dfrac{1}{n_i - 1} \right) - \dfrac{1}{N-k} \right\}.$

Alternatively, the test statistic B can be expressed as

$$B = \frac{1}{C} \left\{ (N-k) \cdot \log MSW - \sum_{i=1}^{k}(n_i - 1) \cdot \log S_i^2 \right\}.$$

3. Reject the null hypothesis if $B > \chi^2_{(k-1,1-\alpha)}$ and accept the null hypothesis if $B \leq \chi^2_{(k-1,1-\alpha)}$.

The χ^2 approximation is adequate if all sample sizes $n_i \geq 5$.

Example 12.8.1. Obesity is a serious health hazard. Obese patients are more likely to have hypertension and coronary artery disease than patients who are not overweight. Obese patients also have increased mortality from all causes, including cancer [10]. Investigators conducted a 16-week clinical trial to compare the effectiveness of four diet programs designed to help reduce the body weight for obese subjects. The four diet programs are (i) strictly vegetarian diet, (ii) vegetarian diet with snacks, (iii) regular diet A, and (iv) regular diet B. Subjects in regular diet A group are required to eat their normal meals, mixed with vegetable and fruits, and those in regular diet B group are required to eat their normal meals, but have 30-minutes of physical exercise a day. All subjects admitted into the clinical trial had BMI index ≥ 32 at the baseline. The table below (Table 12.8.1) displays the summary data of the amount of weight loss in pounds at the end of the weight loss study. Are the variances (σ_i^2) equal? Test at 5% significance level.

Solution. We need to test the hypothesis

$$H_0 : \sigma_1^2 = \sigma_2^2 = \sigma_3^2 = \sigma_4^2 \quad \text{vs.}$$
$$H_1 : \text{ not all } \sigma_i^2 \text{ are equal.}$$

Since $n_1 = 22$, $n_2 = 30$, $n_3 = 25$, and $n_4 = 27$, $(N - k) = 104 - 4 = 100$. Using the Bartlett's procedure and Table 12.8.1, we can obtain the

Table 12.8.1. Weight loss data.

Treatment Group	Sample Size n_i	Mean Wt. Loss $\overline{Y}_i$	Sample SD S_i
Strict vegetarian	22	18.28	5.11
Vegetarian with snack	30	15.63	3.90
Regular diet A	25	10.02	3.05
Regular diet B	27	14.47	4.22

constant C by substitution:

$$C = 1 + \frac{1}{3(k-1)} \left\{ \left(\sum_{i=1}^{k} \frac{1}{n_i - 1} \right) - \frac{1}{N-k} \right\}$$

$$= 1 + \frac{1}{3(3)} \left\{ \left(\sum_{i=1}^{k} \frac{1}{n_i - 1} \right) - \frac{1}{100} \right\}$$

$$= 1.0169.$$

The $\log MSW = \log \left[\frac{(21)(5.11)^2 + (29)(3.90)^2 + (24)(3.05)^2 + (26)(4.22)^2}{100} \right] = 1.2242,$

$$\sum_{i=1}^{k} (n_i - 1) \cdot \log S_i^2 = (21) \log(5.11)^2 + (29) \log(3.90)^2 + (24) \log(3.05)^2 + (26) \log(4.22)^2$$

$$= 119.798.$$

We can now compute the test statistic

$$B = \frac{1}{C} \left\{ (N-k) \cdot \log MSW - \sum_{i=1}^{k} (n_i - 1) \cdot \log S_i^2 \right\}$$

$$= \frac{1}{1.0169} \{ (100)(1.2242) - 119.798 \} = 2.5784.$$

From the χ^2 probability table in the Appendix, we get $\chi^2_{(k-1,1-\alpha)} = \chi^2_{(3,0.95)} = 7.815$.

Since the value of the test statistic $B = 2.5784 < \chi^2_{(3,0.95)} = 7.815$, the null hypothesis is accepted. We conclude that the four population variances are equal at the significance level $\alpha = 0.05$. The p value of the test is $P(2.5784 < \chi^2_{(3)}) > P(6.251 < \chi^2_{(3)}) = 0.10$.

The Bartlett's test is known to be sensitive to departures from normality. Therefore, if the population deviates substantially from normality, it is not recommended that the Bartlett's method be applied for testing variance homogeneity. If the population is not normally distributed, the actual significance level may differ quite a bit from the specified α. When any of the sample sizes n_i is less than four, the χ^2 approximation to the distribution of the Bartlett's test statistic B should not be used.

12.8.2 Hartley's Test

There is a simple test for homogeneity of variances due to Hartley if the sizes n_i of samples drawn from normal populations are equal ($n_1 = n_2 = \cdots = n_k = n$), that is, if the sample variances S_i^2 have the same degrees of freedom, $n_1 - 1 = n_2 - 1 = \cdots = n_k - 1$. The Hartley's test statistic is based on the largest and smallest sample variances:

$$H = \frac{Max(S_i^2)}{Min(S_i^2)}.$$

It is quite intuitive that the values of the test statistic H close to 1 would suggest the null hypothesis

$$H_0 : \sigma_1^2 = \sigma_2^2 = \cdots = \sigma_k^2$$

is true. On the other hand, the values of the test statistic H greater than 1 would suggest that the null hypothesis is false. The distribution of the test statistic H, when the null hypothesis H_0 holds, is provided in some textbooks [5]. The critical values can be found using the percentiles of the H distribution in Neter, et al. [5], and

reject H_0 if $H > H_{(k,n-1;1-\alpha)}$ and

accept H_0 if $H \leq H_{(k,n-1;1-\alpha)}$.

One great advantage of the Hartley's test is its simplicity for computing the test statistic. The Hartley's procedure strictly requires the sample sizes to be equal. If the sample sizes are unequal but reasonably close to each other, then it can still be used as an approximation. It is suggested that the average of the sample sizes will be used for the

c. Do the six group means significantly differ? Use the significance level $\alpha = 0.05$.
d. Present the results in an ANOVA table.

Group	Number of Hours per Week										
Endodontists	28	34	40	35	29	30	42	40	34	32	32
Hygienists	34	40	24	30	38	35	36	32	29	30	
Orthodontists	42	28	31	36	30	38	29	31	32	26	34	30
Pediatric dentists	34	37	28	40	33	27	33	38	36	34	26
Periodontists	37	28	27	38	33	31	26	34	40	40	35
Prosthodontists	41	33	24	27	35	34	32	29	30	40	32

degrees of freedom. Like the Bartlett's test, the Hartley's test is quite sensitive to departures from normality. When the departures from normality are substantial, the Hartley's test should not be used. Unlike the Hartley's test, the Bartlett's procedure does not require equal sample sizes, thus it is more flexible than the Hartley's. A drawback of the Bartlett's test is that the computation for the test statistic is far more complicated.

12.9 EXERCISES

1 What statistical method is used to compare three or more population means?

2 Name three tests you would use to compare the population means if the one-way ANOVA rejects the null hypothesis.

3 In the list item number 3 described in Section 12.1, what is the factor under investigation? How many levels are there in the study?

4 A survey was taken with 66 dental professionals. Each subject was required to indicate the number of hours they spend per week in patient contact. The survey data by specialty area is displayed in a table below.
a. Compute the sample means and the sample SDs for each group.
b. Compute the sums of squares.

5 The following is an ANOVA table with missing values.
a. Fill in the blanks to complete the table.
b. Calculate the approximate p value for the F statistic.

Source of Variation	df	Sum of Squares	Mean Square	F value
Between		1080.59		
Within	60			
Total	84	1884.45		

6 Table 12.9.1 presents descriptive statistics for systolic blood pressure data of subjects who participated in a hypertension reduction study. Hypertensive patients were randomly assigned to five different study groups: Group A = vegetarian diet, Group B = low-sodium meals with vegetables, Group C = regular meals with hypertensive medications, Group D = regular meals and regular exercise, and Group E = control.
a. Are there any significant differences among the five groups with regard to their mean systolic blood pressure? Test the null hypothesis at the significance level $\alpha = 0.05$.
b. Construct a one-way ANOVA table.
c. If the null hypothesis is rejected, use Fisher's least significant difference method for comparing pairs of group means.

Table 12.9.1. Systolic blood pressure at the end of the study.

	Group A	Group B	Group C	Group D	Group E
Sample size (n_i)	41	36	44	39	46
Sample mean ($\overline{Y}_i$)	123.8	129.5	131.3	127.9	144.7
Sample SD (S_i)	6.45	5.89	6.91	5.77	7.13

7 In a linear contrast given by $L = \dfrac{\mu_1 + \mu_2}{2} - \dfrac{\mu_3 + \mu_4}{2}$ for Example 12.6.2, what are the coefficients c_i's?

8 In Exercise 6 above, contrast between groups with vegetable diet (Group A and Group B) and groups with regular meals. What can you conclude from the results?

9 From Table 12.9.1, conduct multiple comparisons procedures using Bonferroni's method and Scheffe's method.

10 From Table 12.5.5, show if the assumption of the homogeneity of variances is satisfied for a one-way ANOVA model.

11 From the community hospital and clinics around the city, the ages of dentists, nurses, and physicians are recorded as shown in the table below. At $\alpha = 0.05$, test if the variances are equal. You may assume that the distribution of the ages is normal.

methods. What can you conclude from the information presented in the following table?

	n_i	$\overline{Y}_i$	S_i^2
Class A	29	82.8	24.3
Class B	31	76.6	29.2
Class C	32	79.1	19.6

12.10 REFERENCES

1. Box, G. E. P. Some theorems on quadratic forms applied in the study of analysis of variance problems: I. Effect of inequality of variance in the one-way classification. *Annals of Mathematical Statistics*; 1954, 25, 290–302.
2. Blount, C., Streelman, S., and Tkachyk, D. An Evaluation of Bonded Orthodontic Brackets and Composites as Rest Seats. A student project. Loma Linda University. 2000.
3. Baek, S., Lane, A., and Lena, D. Antimicrobial Efficacy of Commercially Available Toothpastes. A student project. Loma Linda University. 2001.
4. Marsh, P. D. Microbiological aspects of the chemical control of plaque and gingivitis. *J Dent Res*; 1992, 71: 1431–1438.

Ages																	
Dentists	29	57	62	44	47	34	37	31	40	56	49	52	43	39	45	34	
Nurses	44	23	27	35	55	41	38	49	57	33	26	38	49	60	25	34	47	46
Physicians	39	47	41	58	68	60	54	47	35	49	50							

12 Given the data in Exercise 11, would you consider using the Hartley's test for the equality of variance? If not, give a reason why you would not use it.

13 At the beginning of a school year, 92 students were randomly assigned to three classes being taught by three different instructional methods. Suppose that the students in these classes are even, with respect to their ability and motivation, and that the instructors have been carefully calibrated. At the end of the school year, students were given an identical examination to evaluate the teaching

5. Neter, J., Wasserman, W., and Kutner, M. H. (1990). *Applied Linear Statistical Models*. Richard D. Irwin, Inc. 1998.
6. Kleinbaum, D. G., et al. *Applied Regression Analysis and Other Multivariate Methods*. Third edition. Duxbury Press. 1997.
7. Kirk, R. *Statistics: An Introduction*. Fourth edition. Harcourt Brace & Company. 1999.
8. Forthofer, R. N., and Lee, E. S. *Introduction to Biostatistics: A Guide to Design, Analysis, and Discovery*. Academic Press. 1995.
9. www.pathology.jhu.edu/pancreas/
10. Zollo, A. J. *Medical Secrets*. Third edition. Hanley & Belfus, Inc. 2001.

Chapter 13

Two-way Analysis of Variance

13.1 INTRODUCTION

In Chapter 12, the use of the analysis of variance (ANOVA) technique was restricted to one independent variable with two or more levels. There are many situations in which two different variables are used to define treatment groups. We will discuss the use of ANOVA techniques in cases in which there are two independent variables (factors) and one dependent variable. In a high-density lipoprotein (HDL) research project, investigators want to study the effects of smoking habit and body mass index (BMI). They want to consider the effects of one variable after controlling for the effects of the other variable. Suppose they have created two categories for BMI: low (27 or lower) and high (higher than 27). The data resulting from this research project can be arranged in a 2×2 contingency table (Table 13.1.1). Factor A, representing smoking habit, has 2 levels, and factor B, representing BMI, also has 2 levels. This type of data involving two independent variables is analyzed using a statistical procedure known as **two-way ANOVA**, which is an extension of the one-way ANOVA. Smoking habit and BMI are the two independent variables, and HDL cholesterol level is the dependent variable. The investigators' goal is to determine whether smoking habit or BMI independently influences HDL and whether these two factors jointly have some influence on HDL. In case of the former, we say that smoking habit and BMI have **main effects**. In case of the latter, we say that smoking habit and BMI have an **interaction effect**. The investigators want to test the effects of smoking habit and BMI on high-density lipoprotein.

To conduct this research, four groups of subjects are required. These groups are often referred to as **treatment groups** or **treatment combinations**.

Group 1:   Smokers with low BMI
Group 2:   Smokers with high BMI
Group 3:   Non-smokers with low BMI
Group 4:   Non-smokers with high BMI

The two-way ANOVA enables us to test three hypotheses. We can test the effects of each of the two factors (smoking habit and BMI), and the effect of the interaction between the two factors. If there is a difference between smokers with high BMI and non-smokers with low BMI in HDL, we say there is the interaction effect of smoking and BMI. Smoking affects the HDL differently in different BMI status. The three hypotheses can be illustrated as follows:

1. Are there any differences in mean HDL between smokers and non-smokers?

   H_0: There is no difference in the mean of HDL between smokers and non-smokers, vs.

   H_1: There is a difference in the means of HDL between smokers and non-smokers.

   If the alternative hypothesis is true, the means for the treatment groups might look like that in Table 13.1.2. Note that the HDL level is lower for smokers regardless of their BMI status.

2. Are there any differences in mean HDL between low and high BMI?

   H_0: There is no difference in the mean of HDL between subjects with low and high BMI, vs.

   H_1: There is a difference in the mean of HDL between subjects with low and high BMI.

   If the alternative hypothesis is true, the means for the treatment groups might look like that shown in Table 13.1.3. The HDL level is much lower for the high-BMI groups regardless of their smoking habit.

3. Are there any differences in mean HDL due to neither smoking nor BMI alone, but due to the combination of both factors?

Table 13.1.1. 2×2 contingency table for HDL.

	BMI	
Smoking Habit	Low	High
Yes		
No		

Table 13.1.2. Means for treatment groups: difference due to smoking habit.

	BMI	
Smoking Habit	Low	High
Yes	34	30
No	52	48

H_0: There is no interaction effect on HDL between smoking and BMI status, vs.

H_1: There is an interaction effect on HDL between smoking and BMI status.

If the alternative hypothesis is true, the means for the treatment groups might look as shown in Table 13.1.4.

Definition 13.1.1. An **interaction effect** between two factors is defined as one in which the effect of one factor depends on the level of the other factor.

Throughout the discussion, we will assume that the treatment groups have equal samples. Having the equal number of observations for treatment combinations makes the analysis fairly

Table 13.1.3. Means for treatment groups: difference due to BMI.

	BMI	
Smoking Habit	Low	High
Yes	45	20
No	52	26

Table 13.1.4. Means for treatment groups: difference due to the interaction between smoking and BMI.

	BMI	
Smoking Habit	Low	High
Yes	47	30
No	32	48

straightforward. It is essential that each treatment group has more than one observation. If only one smoker who has BMI higher than 27 is observed, then we would not be able to determine the HDL level for another subject in the same treatment group. In other words, we would not be able to determine the variability in the HDL level among the patients under the same conditions. A major reason for requiring at least two observations per treatment combination is to enable us to estimate σ^2. This will be discussed in the next section. Unequal sample sizes are more complicated and will not be presented. Interested readers are referred to Neter, Wasserman, and Kutner [1] and Kleinbaum et al. [2].

13.2 GENERAL MODEL

To illustrate the meaning of the model, let us consider a simple two-factor study in which the effects of smoking habit and BMI on systolic blood pressure (SBP) are of interest. The dependent variable in this study is SBP. As before, let smoking habit be factor A with two levels (yes = smoker and no = non-smoker) and BMI be factor B with three levels instead of two (low = less than 27, medium = between 27 and 31, and high = greater than 31). We are interested in the effects of smoking and BMI on the level of SBP. The data collected by investigators is presented in Table 13.2.1.

A two-way ANOVA model is given by

$$Y_{ijk} = \mu + \alpha_i + \beta_j + (\alpha\beta)_{ij} + \epsilon_{ijk}$$

where

Y_{ijk} = SBP of the kth subject in the ith smoking group and j^{th} BMI group

μ = a constant

α_i = a constant representing the effect of smoking

β_j = a constant representing the effect of BMI

$(\alpha\beta)_{ij}$ = a constant representing the interaction effect between smoking and BMI

ϵ_{ijk} = an error term, assumed to be independent normal with mean 0 and variance σ^2, that is,

$$\epsilon_{ijk} \sim N(0, \sigma^2), \qquad i = 1, 2, \cdots, r;$$
$$j = 1, 2, \cdots, c;$$
$$k = 1, 2, \cdots, n$$

Table 13.2.1. Systolic blood pressure data.

Smoking	BMI			Row Average
	Low ($j = 1$)	Medium ($j = 2$)	High ($j = 3$)	
Yes ($i = 1$)	135, 141, 139, 143, 134 Mean = 138.4	147, 136, 144 141, 148 Mean = 143.2	148, 154, 155 146, 160 Mean = 152.6	144.7
No ($i = 2$)	121, 124, 128 122, 125 Mean = 124.0	131, 124, 135 126, 122 Mean = 127.6	147, 151, 148 153, 154 Mean = 150.6	134.1
Column average	131.2	135.4	151.6	139.4

These terms are subject to the restriction: $\sum_{i=1}^{r} \alpha_i = 0$, $\sum_{j=1}^{c} \beta_j = 0$

$$\sum_{i=1}^{r} (\alpha\beta)_{ij} = 0 \quad \text{for all } j,$$

and

$$\sum_{j=1}^{c} (\alpha\beta)_{ij} = 0 \quad \text{for all } i.$$

The SBP data in Table 13.2.1 indicates that $r = 2$, $c = 3$, and $n = 5$, since there are 2 levels of factor A, 3 levels of factor B, and 5 subjects are assigned to each treatment combination. Thus,

$$\alpha_1 + \alpha_2 = \beta_1 + \beta_2 + \beta_3 = 0,$$

and

$$(\alpha\beta)_{1j} + (\alpha\beta)_{2j} = (\alpha\beta)_{i1} + (\alpha\beta)_{i2} + (\alpha\beta)_{i3} = 0.$$

From the model described above, the SBPs Y_{ijk} are independent normal with mean $\mu + \alpha_i + \beta_j + (\alpha\beta)_{ij}$ and variance σ^2. To facilitate the discussion we introduce some notation:

$$\overline{Y}_{ij} = \frac{\sum_{k=1}^{n} Y_{ijk}}{n}$$

$$= \text{the (sample) mean SBP for the } i^{\text{th}} \text{ row (level) and } j^{\text{th}} \text{ column (level)}$$

$$\overline{Y}_{i.} = \frac{\sum_{j=1}^{c} \sum_{k=1}^{n} Y_{ijk}}{cn}$$

$$= \text{the (sample) mean SBP for the } i^{\text{th}} \text{ row}$$

$$\overline{Y}_{.j} = \frac{\sum_{i=1}^{r} \sum_{k=1}^{n} Y_{ijk}}{rn}$$

$$= \text{the (sample) mean SBP for the } j^{\text{th}} \text{ column}$$

$$\overline{Y}_{..} = \frac{\sum_{i=1}^{r} \sum_{j=1}^{c} \sum_{k=1}^{n} Y_{ijk}}{rcn}$$

$$= \text{the overall mean}$$

From Table 13.2.1, we have the six cell means: $\overline{Y}_{11} = 138.4$, $\overline{Y}_{12} = 143.2$, $\overline{Y}_{13} = 152.6$, $\overline{Y}_{21} = $

124.0, $\overline{Y}_{22} = 127.6$, and $\overline{Y}_{23} = 150.6$. The two row means are $\overline{Y}_{1.} = 144.7$ and $\overline{Y}_{2.} = 134.1$, and the three column means are $\overline{Y}_{.1} = 131.2$, $\overline{Y}_{.2} = 135.4$, and $\overline{Y}_{.3} = 151.6$. The overall mean is given by $\overline{Y}_{..} = 139.4$. We may recognize whether or not interactions are present by examining

- whether the difference between the mean SBP for any two levels of factor B (BMI) is the same for all levels of factor A (smoking status). Note in Table 13.2.1 that the mean SBP increases by 9.4 for smokers but by 23.0 for non-smokers between medium BMI and high BMI.
- whether the difference between the mean SBP for any two levels of factor A (smoking status) is the same for all levels of factor B (BMI). Note that the difference in mean SBP between smokers and non-smokers for medium BMI is 15.6 but that for high BMI group is only 2.0.
- whether the mean blood pressure curves for different factor levels are parallel or not. The curves of the mean responses in a graph as in Figure 13.2.1, which are not parallel, indicate the presence of the interaction effects of the two factors. If, instead, the curves of the mean responses for the different factor levels are essentially parallel as in Figure 13.2.2, then there are no interaction effects between the two factors.

13.3 SUM OF SQUARES AND DEGREES OF FREEDOM

We need to test whether or not the effects are real effects or simply represent only random variations. To perform such tests, a breakdown of the total sum of squares is required. The deviation of an individual observation from the overall mean can be decomposed reflecting the factor A main effect, the factor B main effect, and the interaction effect

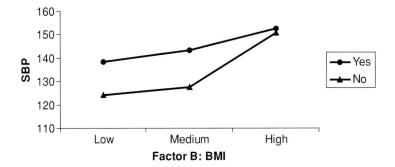

Figure 13.2.1 Effects of smoking and BMI, with interaction effect.

between the two factors as follows:

$$Y_{ijk} - \overline{Y}_{..} = (\overline{Y}_{ij} - \overline{Y}_{..}) + (Y_{ijk} - \overline{Y}_{ij})$$
$$= (\overline{Y}_{i.} - \overline{Y}_{..}) + (\overline{Y}_{.j} - \overline{Y}_{..})$$
$$+ (\overline{Y}_{ij} - \overline{Y}_{i.} - \overline{Y}_{.j} + \overline{Y}_{..}) + (Y_{ijk} - \overline{Y}_{ij})$$

$$(13.3.1)$$

- The term on the left-hand side of equation (13.3.1), $Y_{ijk} - \overline{Y}_{..}$, is the **total deviation**.
- The first term on the right-hand side, $\overline{Y}_{i.} - \overline{Y}_{..}$, represents the deviation of the mean of the ith row from the overall mean and is the **factor A main effect** or **row effect**.
- The second term on the right-hand side, $\overline{Y}_{.j} - \overline{Y}_{..}$, represents the deviation of the mean of the jth column from the overall mean and is the **factor B main effect** or **column effect**.
- The third term on the right-hand side, $\overline{Y}_{ij} - \overline{Y}_{i.} - \overline{Y}_{.j} + \overline{Y}_{..} = (\overline{Y}_{ij} - \overline{Y}_{i.}) - (\overline{Y}_{.j} - \overline{Y}_{..})$, represents the deviation of the column effect in the ith row from the overall column effect $\overline{Y}_{.j} - \overline{Y}_{..}$ and is the **interaction effect**.
- The last term on the right-hand side, $Y_{ijk} - \overline{Y}_{ij}$, represents the deviation of an individual observation from the mean of the treatment group to which the observation belongs and is the **error term**. This term describes **within-group variability**.

When we square equation (13.3.1) and sum over all cases, we obtain: $SSTO = SSTR + SSE$ where

$$SSTO = \sum_{i=1}^{r}\sum_{j=1}^{c}\sum_{k=1}^{n}(Y_{ijk} - \overline{Y}_{..})^2,$$

$$SSTR = n\sum_{i=1}^{r}\sum_{j=1}^{c}(\overline{Y}_{ij} - \overline{Y}_{..})^2$$

$$SSE = \sum_{i=1}^{r}\sum_{j=1}^{c}\sum_{k=1}^{n}(Y_{ijk} - \overline{Y}_{ij})^2$$

SSTR, called **treatment sum of squares,** represents the variability between rc treatment means. *SSE* represents the variability within treatments and is the **error sum of squares**. From the data in Table 13.2.1, we obtain the following sums of squares:

$$SSTO = (135 - 139.4)^2 + (141 - 139.4)^2$$
$$+ (139 - 139.4)^2 + \cdots + (154 - 139.4)^2$$
$$= 3,919.2$$
$$SSTR = 5[(138.4 - 139.4)^2 + (143.2 - 139.4)^2$$
$$+ (152.6 - 139.4)^2 + (124.0 - 139.4)^2$$
$$+ (127.6 - 139.4)^2 + (150.6 - 139.4)^2]$$
$$= 3,457.6$$

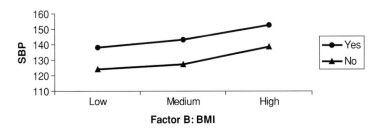

Figure 13.2.2 Effects of smoking and BMI, with no interaction effect.

$$SSE = (135 - 138.4)^2 + (141 - 138.4)^2$$
$$+ (139 - 138.4)^2 + (143 - 138.4)^2 + \cdots$$
$$+ (151 - 150.6)^2 + (148 - 150.6)^2$$
$$+ (153 - 150.6)^2 + (154 - 150.6)^2$$
$$= 461.6$$

From the relationship $SSTO = SSTR + SSE$, we can derive

$$SSTR = SSTO - SSE$$

and

$$SSE = SSTO - SSTR. \qquad (13.3.2)$$

Hence, $SSTR$ and SSE can easily be obtained from the other two sums of squares. Notice that we can test whether or not the six treatment means are equal by using the one-way ANOVA technique ($H_0 : \mu_1 = \mu_2 = \mu_3 = \mu_4 = \mu_5 = \mu_6$ vs. H_1 : not all treatment means are equal). If they are equal, then neither of the two factors has any significant effect. In order to test factor effects we need to further decompose the treatment sum of squares as follows.

One can obtain a decomposition of $SSTR$. This is known as an orthogonal decomposition in statistics.

$$SSTR = SSA + SSB + SSAB \qquad (13.3.3)$$

where

SSA = factor A sum of squares
$= nc \sum_{i=1}^{r} (\overline{Y}_{i\cdot} - \overline{Y}_{\cdot\cdot})^2$

SSB = factor B sum of squares
$= nr \sum_{j=1}^{c} (\overline{Y}_{\cdot j} - \overline{Y}_{\cdot\cdot})^2$

$SSAB$ = interaction sum of squares
$= n \sum_{i=1}^{r} \sum_{j=1}^{c} (\overline{Y}_{ij} - \overline{Y}_{i\cdot} - \overline{Y}_{\cdot j} + \overline{Y}_{\cdot\cdot})^2.$

The above decomposition is called an orthogonal decomposition. Factor A sum of squares SSA measures the (estimated) variability of factor A level means $\overline{Y}_{i\cdot}$ (i.e., row average) about the overall mean $\overline{Y}_{\cdot\cdot}$. The larger the variability, the greater will be the value of SSA. Factor B sum of squares SSB measures the (estimated) variability of factor B level means $\overline{Y}_{\cdot j}$ (i.e., column average) about the overall mean $\overline{Y}_{\cdot\cdot}$. The interaction sum of squares $SSAB$ measures the variability of interactions $\overline{Y}_{ij} - \overline{Y}_{i\cdot} - \overline{Y}_{\cdot j} + \overline{Y}_{\cdot\cdot}$ for the cr treatment groups. These three sums of squares provide relevant information about the main effects of factors A and B, and the interaction effect between factor

A and factor B. We present the following identities for computational purposes:

$$SSTO = \sum_{i=1}^{r} \sum_{j=1}^{c} \sum_{k=1}^{n} Y_{ijk}^2 - \frac{Y_{\cdot\cdot\cdot}^2}{nrc},$$

where $Y_{\cdot\cdot\cdot} = \sum_{i=1}^{r} \sum_{j=1}^{c} \sum_{k=1}^{n} Y_{ijk}$

$$SSTR = \frac{\sum_{i=1}^{r} \sum_{j=1}^{c} Y_{ij\cdot}^2}{n} - \frac{Y_{\cdot\cdot\cdot}^2}{nrc},$$

where $Y_{ij\cdot} = \sum_{k=1}^{n} Y_{ijk}.$

$$SSA = \frac{\sum_{i=1}^{r} Y_{i\cdot\cdot}^2}{nc} - \frac{Y_{\cdot\cdot\cdot}^2}{nrc},$$

where $Y_{i\cdot\cdot} = \sum_{j=1}^{c} \sum_{k=1}^{n} Y_{ijk}$

$$SSB = \frac{\sum_{j=1}^{c} Y_{\cdot j\cdot}^2}{nr} - \frac{Y_{\cdot\cdot\cdot}^2}{nrc},$$

where $Y_{\cdot j\cdot} = \sum_{i=1}^{r} \sum_{k=1}^{n} Y_{ijk}$

$$SSE = \sum_{i=1}^{r} \sum_{j=1}^{c} \sum_{k=1}^{n} Y_{ijk}^2$$
$$- \frac{\sum_{i=1}^{r} \sum_{j=1}^{c} Y_{ij\cdot}^2}{n}.$$

The interaction sum of squares can be obtained by simple formulas

$$SSAB = SSTO - SSA - SSB - SSE$$

or

$$SSAB = SSTR - SSA - SSB.$$

From Table 13.2.1, we can calculate the sums of squares SSA and SSB using the above identities:

$$SSA = \frac{\sum_{i=1}^{r} Y_{i\cdot\cdot}^2}{nc} - \frac{Y_{\cdot\cdot\cdot}^2}{nrc}$$
$$= \frac{(2,171)^2 + (2,011)^2}{5(3)} - \frac{(4,182)^2}{5(2)(3)}$$
$$= 853.33$$

$$SSB = \frac{\sum_{j=1}^{c} Y_{\cdot j\cdot}^2}{nr} - \frac{Y_{\cdot\cdot\cdot}^2}{nrc}$$
$$= \frac{(1,312)^2 + (1,354)^2 + (1,516)^2}{5(2)}$$
$$- \frac{(4,182)^2}{5(2)(3)} = 2,320.8$$

Thus,

$$SSAB = SSTR - SSA - SSB$$
$$= 3,457.6 - 853.33 - 2,320.8 = 283.47$$

From (13.3.2) and (13.3.3), we get

$$SSTO = SSTR + SSE$$
$$= SSA + SSB + SSAB + SSE$$
$$3,919.2 = 853.33 + 2320.8 + 283.47 + 461.6$$

We note that the large part of the total variation is associated with the effects of factor B (BMI).

We have discussed in Section 12.5 how the degrees of freedom for one-factor ANOVA are divided between the sums of squares. The degrees of freedom for two-factor ANOVA is determined as follows: In case of n observations for each treatment group, we have a total of $N = nrc$ observations. The number of treatment groups is rc. Therefore, the degrees of freedom associated with $SSTO$, $SSTR$, and SSE are given by $nrc - 1$, $rc - 1$, and $nrc - rc = rc(n - 1)$. Corresponding to the decomposition of the treatment sum of squares $SSTR = SSA + SSB + SSAB$, the degrees of freedom $rc - 1$ associated with $SSTR$ can be broken down to $(r - 1)$ degrees of freedom associated with SSA, $(c - 1)$ with SSB, and $(rc - 1) - (r - 1) - (c - 1) = (r - 1)(c - 1)$ with $SSAB$ (the interaction sum of squares), respectively.

The mean squares are obtained in the similar way by dividing the sum of squares by their associated degrees of freedom. We get

$$MSTR = \frac{SSTR}{rc - 1}, \qquad MSA = \frac{SSA}{r - 1},$$
$$MSB = \frac{SSB}{c - 1}, \qquad MSAB = \frac{SSAB}{(r - 1)(c - 1)},$$
$$MSE = \frac{SSE}{rc(n - 1)}$$

Example 13.3.1. From the SBP data in Table 13.2.1, we obtain the degrees of freedom associated with the sums of squares and their corresponding mean squares.

$SSTO$: $nrc - 1 = (5)(2)(3) - 1 = 29$
$SSTR$: $rc - 1 = (2)(3) - 1 = 5$
SSA: $r - 1 = 2 - 1 = 1$
SSB: $c - 1 = 3 - 1 = 2$
$SSAB$: $(r - 1)(c - 1) = (2 - 1)(3 - 1) = 2$
SSE: $rc(n - 1) = (2)(3)(5 - 1) = 24$

$$MSTR = \frac{3,457.6}{5} = 691.52,$$
$$MSA = \frac{853.33}{1} = 853.33,$$
$$MSB = \frac{2,320.8}{2} = 1,160.4,$$
$$MSAB = \frac{283.47}{2} = 141.74,$$
$$MSE = \frac{461.6}{24} = 19.233$$

We note that unlike the sum of squares, which are additive, that is, $SSTR = SSA + SSB + SSAB$, the sum of mean squares (MSA, MSB, and $MSAB$) is not equal to $MSTR$. That is, $691.52 \neq 853.33 + 1,160.4 + 141.74$.

The two-way ANOVA model was stated in the previous section, and it was discussed that the assumptions for the two-way ANOVA are essentially the same as those for the one-way ANOVA. We will restate the assumptions below:

1. The populations from which the observations are made (or the samples are drawn) must be normally distributed or approximately normally distributed.
2. The populations must be statistically independent.
3. The variances of the populations must be equal.
4. The treatment groups must have equal numbers of observations.

The third assumption, the homogeneity of the variance, is often overlooked in practice by the researchers. We have seen the ANOVA techniques being applied to situations where the normality assumption is not satisfied. Keep in mind that the populations under consideration must be at least approximately normally distributed. When the observations are not normally distributed, there are some techniques available in statistics that will allow us to obtain observations that are normally distributed, such as a logarithmic transformation. These techniques will not be discussed. As with the one-way ANOVA, the results of the two-way ANOVA can be summarized as shown in Table 13.3.1.

13.4 *F* TESTS

We mentioned earlier that the two-way ANOVA enables us to test three hypotheses. As in the

Table 13.3.1. Two-way ANOVA table.

Source of Variation	df	Sum of Squares	Mean Squares
Between treatments	$rc - 1 = 5$	3,457.6	$691.52 = \dfrac{3,457.6}{5}$
Factor A	$r - 1 = 1$	853.33	$853.33 = \dfrac{853.33}{1}$
Factor B	$c - 1 = 2$	2,320.8	$1,160.4 = \dfrac{2,320.8}{2}$
$A * B$ interaction	$(r - 1)(c - 1) = 2$	283.47	$141.74 = \dfrac{283.47}{2}$
Error (Residual)	$rc(n - 1) = 24$	461.6	$19.233 = \dfrac{461.6}{24}$
Total	$nrc - 1 = 29$	3,919.2	

one-way ANOVA, the test statistics are based on the ratio of appropriate mean squares (MS), which follow the F distribution. Thus, the tests are called F tests. Usually, the two-factor ANOVA begins with a test to determine whether or not these two factors interact. We state the hypotheses to test if two factors interact.

Test for Interactions

H_0: all $(\alpha\beta)_{ij} = 0$ vs. H_1: not all $(\alpha\beta)_{ij}$ equal 0

The test statistic is given by $F = \dfrac{MSAB}{MSE}$.

The values of the test statistic being close to 1 (i.e., the values of $MSAB$ are almost equal to the values of MSE) would indicate that there are no interaction effects. On the other hand, the "large" values of F would indicate the existence of interactions. When H_0 holds, it is known that the above test statistic is distributed as $F_{[(r-1)(c-1),\ rc(n-1)]}$, the F distribution with the degrees of freedom, $(r - 1)(c - 1)$ and $rc(n - 1)$. Here are the steps to be taken to perform the test at the significance level α.

1. Compute the test statistic $F = \dfrac{MSAB}{MSE}$.
2. Reject the null hypothesis if

   $F > F_{[(r-1)(c-1), rc(n-1):\ 1-\alpha]}$.

   Accept the null hypothesis if

   $F \leq F_{[(r-1)(c-1),\ rc(n-1):\ 1-\alpha]}$.

   where $F_{[(r-1)(c-1),\ rc(n-1):\ 1-\alpha]}$ is a critical value of the test that is the $(1 - \alpha)$100th percentile point.
3. The corresponding p value is given by $p = P(F \leq F_{[(r-1)(c-1),rc(n-1)]})$.

Test for Main Effects of Factor A

To test for main effects of factor A, we state the hypotheses H_0: $\alpha_1 = \alpha_2 = \cdots = \alpha_r = 0$ vs. H_1: not all α_i equal 0.

The test statistic is given by $F = \dfrac{MSA}{MSE}$

The "large" values of F indicate the existence of main effects. When H_0 holds, the test statistic is distributed as $F_{[(r-1),\ rc(n-1)]}$, the F distribution with the degrees of freedom, $(r - 1)$ and $rc(n - 1)$. Here are the steps to be taken to perform the test at the significance level α.

1. Compute the test statistic $F = \dfrac{MSA}{MSE}$.
2. Reject the null hypothesis if

   $F > F_{[(r-1),\ rc(n-1):\ 1-\alpha]}$.

   Accept the null hypothesis if

   $F \leq F_{[(r-1),\ rc(n-1):\ 1-\alpha]}$.

   where $F_{[(r-1),\ rc(n-1):\ 1-\alpha]}$ is a critical value of the test that is the $(1 - \alpha)$100th percentile point.
3. The corresponding p value is given by

   $p = P(F \leq F_{[(r-1),\ rc(n-1)]})$.

Test for Main Effects of Factor B

To test for main effects of factor B, we state the hypothesis H_0: $\beta_1 = \beta_2 = \cdots = \beta_c = 0$ vs. H_1: not all β_j equal 0.

The test statistic is given by $F = \dfrac{MSB}{MSE}$

Similar to the test for the factor A main effect, the "large" values of F indicate the existence of main effects. When H_0 holds, the test statistic is distributed as $F_{[(c-1),\ rc(n-1)]}$, the F distribution with the degrees of freedom, $(c - 1)$ and

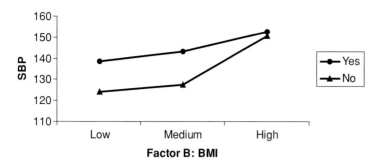

Figure 13.4.1 Interaction effects between two factors—SBP data.

$rc(n-1)$. The steps to perform the test at the significance level α are:

1. Compute the test statistic $F = \dfrac{MSB}{MSE}$.

2. Reject the null hypothesis if

$$F > F_{[(c-1),\ rc(n-1):\ 1-\alpha]}.$$

Accept the null hypothesis if

$$F \leq F_{[(c-1),\ rc(n-1):\ 1-\alpha]}.$$

where $F_{[(c-1),\ rc(n-1):\ 1-\alpha]}$ is a critical value of the test which is the $(1-\alpha)100$th percentile point.

3. The corresponding p value is given by

$$p = P(F \leq F_{[(c-1),\ rc(n-1)]}).$$

Example 13.4.1. We shall perform the above F tests, using the blood pressure data in Table 13.2.1. Let the significance level be specified by $\alpha = 0.05$.

Interaction effects: We obtain the value of the test statistic

$$F = \frac{MSAB}{MSE} = \frac{141.74}{19.233} = 7.370.$$

Since the risk of committing a type I error is fixed at $\alpha = 0.05$, we get

$$F_{[(r-1)(c-1),\ rc(n-1):\ 1-\alpha]}$$
$$= F_{[2,24:\ 0.95]} = 3.407 \text{ by linear interpolation,}$$

but one may simply approximate it by taking $F_{[2,\ 25:\ 0.95]} = 3.385$, which is found in Table G of the Appendix. The test statistic $F = 7.370 > F_{[2,\ 24:\ 0.95]} = 3.407$. Hence, we reject H_0 and conclude that there exist statistically significant interaction effects between smoking and BMI. We now compute the p value of the test.

$$p = P(F \leq F_{[(r-1)(c-1),\ rc(n-1)]})$$
$$= P(7.370 \leq F_{[2,\ 24]}) < P(6.598 \leq F_{[2,\ 25]})$$
$$= 0.005.$$

So the p value is less than 0.005, and as Figure 13.4.1 shows, the test is significant.

Main effects of factor A: We compute the value of the test statistic

$$F = \frac{MSA}{MSE} = \frac{853.33}{19.233} = 44.368.$$

The critical value is obtained by $F_{[(r-1),\ rc(n-1):\ 1-\alpha]} = F_{[1,24:\ 0.95]} = 4.264$. Since $F_{[1,\ 24:\ 0.95]}$ is not provided in Table G in the Appendix, one can approximate it by $F_{[1,\ 25:\ 0.95]} = 4.242$. The test statistic $F = 44.368 > F_{[1,\ 24:\ 0.95]} = 4.264$. Hence, we reject H_0 and conclude that there exist statistically significant main effects of factor A (smoking). The p value of the test is

$$p = P(44.368 \leq F_{[1,\ 24]}) < P(13.88 \leq F_{[1,\ 25]})$$
$$= 0.001.$$

Main effects of factor B: The test procedure for main effects of factor B is quite similar to that for factor A. We compute the value of the test statistic

$$F = \frac{MSB}{MSE} = \frac{1,160.4}{19.233} = 60.334.$$

The critical value is obtained by $F_{[(c-1),rc(n-1):1-\alpha]} = F_{[2,24:0.95]} = 3.407$. The test statistic $F = 60.334 > F_{[2,\ 24:\ 0.95]} = 3.407$. Hence, we reject H_0 and conclude that there exist statistically significant main effects of factor B (BMI). The p value of the test is

$$p = P(60.334 \leq F_{[2,\ 24]}) < P(9.223 \leq F_{[2,\ 25]})$$
$$= 0.001.$$

The results of the two-factor ANOVA indicate that smoking and BMI have significant interaction effects on systolic blood pressure, and furthermore, the individual factors have significant main effects as well.

Table 13.4.1. Two-way ANOVA table.

Source of Variation	df	SS	MS	F	p value
Smoking	1	853.33	853.33	44.368	< 0.001
BMI	2	2,320.8	1,160.4	60.334	< 0.001
Smoking*BMI	2	283.47	141.74	7.370	< 0.005
Error	24	461.6	19.233		
Total	29	3,919.2			

We summarize the above results in the two-way ANOVA table (Table 13.4.1).

Example 13.4.2. A study was performed to evaluate the effectiveness of two different systems of light cure polymerization for composite resins in orthodontic bracket bonding. In this study, conventional tungsten halogen light system was compared to a recently developed system using plasma light. Bonding strength, measured in megapascals, was tested at 2 minutes, 10 minutes, and 15 minutes after bonding. The summary of the data is presented in the following ANOVA table. Complete the table. What conclusions can you draw from the table?

Source of Variation	df	SS	MS	F	p value
Factor A (Light cure)		0.075			
Factor B (Time)		45.603			
Light*time interaction		3.336			
Error (Residual)	18	24.480			
Total					

Solution. We will leave this as an exercise. See Exercise 9.

In summary the following steps are to be taken by the investigators to perform a two-way ANOVA:

1. State the hypotheses.
2. Compute the sums of squares and the appropriate mean squares by dividing the *SS* by the associated degrees of freedom.
3. Compute the value of the test statistic, *F*.
4. Find the critical value for each *F* test, using the significance level $\alpha = 0.05$.
5. Summarize the results in an ANOVA table.
6. Make the decisions and draw conclusions.

There are many experimental designs for ANOVA. The most popular ones are randomized factorial designs, randomized block designs, Latin square designs, nested designs, and repeated measures designs. We will introduce repeated measures design in the following section. Readers who wish to study other designs are referred to an excellent book by Neter et al. [1].

One may ask, "what do we do when the assumptions of normality and the homogeneity of variances are seriously violated?" Although the F test is robust with respect to the deviations from the normality assumption, non-parametric procedures are advisable if the sample sizes are equal and the homogeneity of variances can't be assumed. For example, when the observations greatly deviate from the normal distribution and the variances for different samples are considerably different, non-parametric ANOVA procedures, such as Kruskal-Wallis and Friedman rank tests, should be considered. These non-parametric tests will be introduced in Chapter 14.

13.5 REPEATED MEASURES DESIGN

In clinical trials in dental and medical research projects, it is common practice to make a sequence of observations from each subject over time. The crossover design we discussed in Chapter 2 is an example of this in which investigators observe subjects' responses from successive treatment periods. The term **repeated measures design** is used to refer to such situation in which measurements of the same variable are made on each subject on two or more different points in time. Some examples of repeated measures design are as follows:

1. Pulse rates are measured every 15 minutes to assess a patient's anxiety level while waiting in the clinic lobby.
2. Daily level of insulin is recorded by subjects with diabetes mellitus.
3. Periodontal/implant patients are recalled every 3 months to observe their bony dehiscence.
4. Tooth shade is measured at baseline and 3 and 7 days after treatment with a tooth-whitening agent.
5. The same 10 individuals are used to investigate the effect of three different drugs over a period of time.

13.5.1 Advantages and Disadvantages

The major advantage of the repeated measures design is the fact that fewer subjects are required than in a design in which different subjects are used for each treatment in the study. Suppose, for example, three treatments are under investigation. If a different sample of 10 subjects is used for each of the three treatments, a total of 30 subjects would be required. However, if we can make observations on the same subjects for each treatment or point in time, that is, if a repeated measures design is employed, only 10 subjects would be required. This is a very attractive feature if the subjects are difficult to recruit. Another advantage is that in a repeated measures design, equivalent pretreatment measures are not a matter of concern because each individual serves as his or her own control.

A major disadvantage is the risk of withdrawal from the study if the subjects require multiple tests over a long period of time. The other disadvantage is that the order in which treatment levels are administered must be controlled. A subject's response to a treatment received last in a sequence may be different from the response that would have occurred if the treatment had been received first in the sequence. The problem of the order effect can be solved by randomizing the sequence of treatments for each subject. Investigators should also be alert for carryover effect. The carryover effect can be eliminated by allowing a sufficient length of time between treatments.

In statistics, the repeated measures design is referred to as a randomized block design, with each subject designated as a block. The simplest repeated measures design is the one in which one additional variable, referred to as a factor, is considered. This design is called a single-factor repeated measures design. When the treatment and subject effects are additive (that is, there is no interaction between treatments and subjects), we have the following model for the fixed-effect additive single-factor repeated measures:

$$Y_{ij} = \mu + \alpha_i + \beta_j + \epsilon_{ij}$$

This model is very similar to the one discussed in Section 13.2. An example of a repeated measures design is presented in the following.

Table 13.5.1. L values at three time points.

Subject	Baseline	3-day	7-day
1	70.4	71.6	72.5
2	74.0	76.2	75.3
3	73.5	74.5	75.0
4	64.5	64.5	64.9
5	74.5	74.6	75.3
6	68.4	69.5	70.8
7	70.0	71.9	69.4
8	67.8	68.7	70.8
9	71.0	70.2	71.9
10	68.9	72.4	72.0

Example 13.5.1. Ten subjects were recruited for a tooth-whitening study. The subjects were instructed to use Whitestrips once a day for 20 min. per day. Investigators measured the individual's L value at the baseline, 3, and 7 days to evaluate the effectiveness of the whitening product. Is there a difference in the mean L value among the three time points? (See Table. 13.5.1.)

Solution. The hypotheses to be tested are H_0 : $\mu_{BL} = \mu_{3Day} = \mu_{7Day}$ vs. H_1: Not all μs are equal.

We need to calculate *SSTO, SSB, SSTR,* and *SSE* as follows:

$$SSTO = (70.4^2 + 74.0^2 + 73.5^2 + \cdots + 72.0^2)$$
$$- (2, 135^2/30)$$
$$= 294.39$$

$$SSB = \frac{214.5^2 + 225.5^2 + 223.0^2 + \cdots + 213.3^2}{3}$$
$$- (2, 135^2/30)$$
$$= 268.25$$

$$SSTR = \frac{703.0^2 + 714.1^2 + 717.9^2}{10}$$
$$- (2, 135^2/30)$$
$$= 11.97$$

$$SSE = 294.39 - 268.25 - 11.97$$
$$= 14.17$$

Using the significance level $\alpha = 0.05$, the critical value is 3.555 ($F_{(2, 18; 0.95)} = 3.555$). We reject the null hypothesis and conclude that the mean L value is statistically significantly different among the three time points, with the p value less than 0.005. The results of the calculation are presented in Table 13.5.2.

Table 13.5.2. ANOVA table for Example 13.5.1.

Source of Variation	df	SS	MS	F	p value
Treatments	2	11.97	5.985	7.605	< 0.005
Blocks	9	268.25	29.806		
Error	18	14.17	0.787		
Total	29	294.39			

13.6 EXERCISES

1 What are the assumptions for the two-way ANOVA?

2 What are between-group variance and within-group variance?

3a. Explain what interaction effects and main effects are.

b. Explain how you can recognize interaction effects without preparing an ANOVA table.

4 In Section 13.2, what is the factor under investigation? How many levels are there in the study?

a. Compute the sample means and the sample standard deviations for each group.

b. Compute the sums of squares.

c. Do the six group means significantly differ? Use the significance level $\alpha = 0.05$.

d. Present the results in an ANOVA table.

5 What is the difference between one-way and two-way ANOVA?

6 Final exam scores in the biostatistics course for hygiene students, dental students, and residents are given. At the significance level $\alpha = 0.05$, can you conclude that there is a difference in the mean score of the three groups?

Exam Score								
Hygiene	83	88	68	84	74	94	75	80	71
Dental	77	92	48	82	79	85	66	73	82
Residents	98	84	79	88	95	82	76	94	89

7 How many independent variables are there in two-way ANOVA?

8 The following income data for physicians is reported. Four physicians in each treatment group are randomly selected. Is there any sex difference? Perform a two-way ANOVA at $\alpha = 0.05$.

	Location							
Sex	San Bernardino				Riverside			
Female	123	354	275	327	224	250	155	285
Male	265	402	160	312	245	268	508	146

9a. Complete the ANOVA table presented in Example 13.4.2.

b. What conclusions can you draw from the table?

10 Medical research was done to assess the effectiveness of diet (vegetarian and non-vegetarian) and physical exercise on hypertension. The investigators created three categories for physical exercise according to the amount of time spent in physical activities: low, medium, and high. Twenty-eight subjects were randomly assigned to each treatment group. Summary of the SBP data is presented in the following table. Would you use a two-way ANOVA? If not, why?

Diet	Physical Exercise		
	Low	Med	High
Vegetarian	$\overline{X} = 1.30.5$	$\overline{X} = 126.7$	$\overline{X} = 121.4$
	$S = 12.9$	$S = 13.8$	$S = 12.7$
Non-vegetarian	$\overline{X} = 139.2$	$\overline{X} = 135.7$	$\overline{X} = 133.8$
	$S = 13.7$	$S = 29.4$	$S = 10.2$

13.7 REFERENCES

1. Neter, J., Wasserman, W., and Kutner, M. H. *Applied Linear Statistical Models.* Third edition. Richard D. Irwin, Inc. 1990.
2. Kleinbaum, D. G., Kupper, L. L., Muller, K. E., and Nizam, A. *Applied Regression Analysis and Other Multivariable Methods.* Third edition. Duxbury Press. 1998.

Chapter 14

Non-parametric Statistics

14.1 INTRODUCTION

Statistical procedures discussed in the previous chapters assumed that the samples were drawn from a known population, such as the normal or at least approximately normal, whose mathematical form of distribution function is known. It was stressed throughout the discussions that the normality assumption is necessary for the method of testing hypotheses to be valid. Statistical procedures based on the assumption of the known underlying distributions are referred to as **parametric statistics**. The results of a parametric method depend on the validity of these assumptions. For the statistical tests in which the population from which the samples are drawn is not normally distributed, statisticians developed alternative procedures based on less stringent assumptions, referred to as **non-parametric statistics** or **distribution-free statistics**. Non-parametric tests can be used in place of their parametric counterparts, such as Z test, t test, and F test, when the normality assumption is untenable in practical applications. There are some advantages as well as disadvantages in the use of nonparametric statistics.

Advantages of non-parametric methods are as follows.

1. They can be used without the normality assumption.
2. They can be used with nominal or ordinal data.
3. Hypothesis testing can be performed when population parameters, such as mean μ and standard deviation σ are not involved.
4. The computations are lighter in most cases and the procedures are easier to understand.
5. Because they deal with ranks rather than the actual observed values, non-parametric techniques are less sensitive to the measurement errors than parametric techniques and can use ordinal data rather than continuous data.

For these reasons, nonparametric statistical methods are quite popular and extensively used in practice.
Disadvantages of non-parametric methods are the following.

1. They tend to use less information than the parametric methods.
2. They are less sensitive than the parametric tests. Thus the larger differences are needed to reject the null hypothesis.
3. They are less efficient than their parametric counterparts. Roughly, this means that larger sample sizes are required for non-parametric tests to overcome the loss of information.

If the underlying population is normally distributed (or approximately normal) or if the central limit theorem can be appropriately applied, then the parametric methods are preferred. However, if the parametric assumption is not met, the researcher should be able to use the non-parametric methods as valuable tools for data analysis. It is usually difficult to tell from a small sample whether the sample is taken from a normal population. Non-parametric procedures should be used when the researcher has any doubt about normality assumption. Even if the assumption of normality is reasonable, non-parametric methods can still be used. We shall introduce the non-parametric test procedures that are most popular and widely applied in journal articles in biomedical sciences. Readers will realize that non-parametric statistical methods often involve less computational work and are easier to apply than other statistical methods. We note that much of the theory behind the non-parametric methods can be developed rigorously using hardly any mathematics beyond college algebra.

14.2 THE SIGN TEST

The sign test is known to be the oldest non-parametric test procedure. It can be applied to compare paired samples. The test is useful for testing whether one random variable in a pair (X, Y) tends to be larger than the other random variable in the pair. It is often used for biomedical research in which quantitative measurements are not feasible, but it is possible to determine the order for each pair (X_i, Y_i) of the observations. The assumptions required by the sign test are (a) the random variable under consideration has a continuous distribution, (b) the paired samples (X_i, Y_i) are independent, and (c) the measurement scale is at least ordinal within each pair. The test does not make any assumptions about the mathematical form of the distribution. The populations from which the samples are drawn are not necessarily statistically independent. The null hypothesis of the sign test is

$$H_0 : P(X_i < Y_i) = P(X_i > Y_i) = \frac{1}{2}$$

(The median of X_i is equal to the median of Y_i for all i),

where X_i may represent the observation before the treatment and Y_i may represent the observation after treatment. That is, X_i and Y_i can be viewed as two observations for a matched pair. Each pair of sample data is represented by either

- a plus sign $(+)$ if the first value X_i is greater than the second value Y_i of the pair, or
- a minus sign $(-)$ if the first value X_i is smaller than the second value Y_i of the pair, or
- if the two values are equal, in which case the pair is deleted from the data.

Similarly, the null hypothesis can be stated as

$$H_0 : \mu_1 = \mu_2 \text{ (the two means are equal)}.$$

Either $H_0 : P(X_i < Y_i) = P(X_i > Y_i) = 1/2$ or $H_0 : \mu_1 = \mu_2$; the sign test is a non-parametric procedure designed to test if X_i and Y_i have the same location parameter. When the null hypothesis is true, we would expect that the number of pairs (X_i, Y_i) in which $X_i < Y_i$ is equal to the number of pairs (X_i, Y_i) in which $X_i > Y_i$. In other words, if H_0 is true, we expect the number of plus signs and the number of minus signs to be about the same. The null hypothesis is rejected if too few or too many plus (minus) signs are observed. The test

Table 14.2.1. Weekly new patient data.

Week	Barton	Colton	Sign
1	4	2	+
2	1	0	+
3	3	3	
4	1	2	−
5	3	2	+
6	4	2	+
7	3	4	−
8	4	1	+
9	2	0	+
10	2	2	
11	3	1	+
12	1	2	−

statistic T is defined by

$$T = \text{total number of plus signs}.$$

That is, T equals the number of pairs (X_i, Y_i) in which X_i is larger than Y_i. The following examples describe the test procedure. Example 14.2.1 deals with a small sample problem and Example 14.2.2 a large sample problem with $n \geq 30$.

Example 14.2.1. An implant specialist has two offices in adjacent communities, Barton and Colton. In terms of the patient volume, the two offices have been about the same for a number of years. He has been advertising for the Barton office in the local newspaper. To determine the effectiveness of the advertisement, he had his office managers record the new patients each week in both offices for the 12-week period while the advertisement appeared in the paper. From Table 14.2.1, perform a hypothesis test to determine whether the advertisement is effective at the significance level $\alpha = 0.05$.

Solution. Let μ_1 and μ_2 denote the mean numbers of new patients per week at the offices in Barton and Colton, respectively. The implant specialist suspects that the advertisement would attract more new patients. We may state the hypotheses as $H_0 : \mu_1 = \mu_2$ vs. $H_1 : \mu_1 > \mu_2$.

Since two pairs, week 3 and week 10, have the same number of new patients, they will be deleted from the data. Thus, the sample size for the sign test is $n = 10$. Let the test statistic T be the number of plus signs. Then $T = 7$. From the table of binomial probabilities (Table B in the Appendix), we find the p value for $n = 10$, and $\alpha = 0.05$,

$$p = P(X = 7) + P(X = 8) + P(X = 9)$$
$$+ P(X = 10)$$
$$= 0.1172 + 0.0440 + 0.0098 + 0.0010$$
$$= 0.1720.$$

Because the p value is $0.1720 > 0.05$, we accept the null hypothesis and cannot conclude on the basis of the data that the advertisement is effective in producing a statistically significantly larger number of new patients.

When the number of sample pairs n is sufficiently large such that $npq \geq 5$, we can use the normal approximation to the binomial distribution.

Example 14.2.2. A manufacturer of toothbrushes has developed two types of mechanical toothbrushes, A and B. Thirty-nine subjects were randomly selected to determine acceptability of the toothbrush products by the consumers. Subjects were instructed to use both A and B for 4 days each. At the end of the study, subjects assigned a score 0 (unacceptable) or 1 (acceptable) to each product. The manufacturer's data is presented in Table 14.2.2. Is there any difference in consumer acceptability between A and B? Let p_1 and p_2 be the proportion of consumer acceptance for A and B. Perform a significance test at $\alpha = 0.05$. That

Table 14.2.2. Consumer response to mechanical toothbrush.

Subj No.	A	B	A − B	Subj No.	A	B	A − B
1	0	1	−1	21	1	0	1
2	0	1	−1	22	1	0	1
3	0	0	0	23	0	1	−1
4	1	0	1	24	1	0	1
5	1	1	0	25	1	0	1
6	0	1	−1	26	1	0	1
7	1	0	1	27	1	0	1
8	1	0	1	28	0	1	−1
9	1	0	1	29	0	0	0
10	0	1	−1	30	1	0	1
11	1	0	1	31	1	0	1
12	1	0	1	32	1	0	1
13	0	1	−1	33	0	1	−1
14	1	0	1	34	0	1	−1
15	1	0	1	35	1	0	1
16	1	0	1	36	1	0	1
17	1	0	1	37	1	0	1
18	0	1	−1	38	1	0	1
19	1	1	0	39	1	0	1
20	1	0	1				

is, test the hypotheses

$$H_0 : p_1 = p_2 = \frac{1}{2} \quad \text{vs.} \quad H_1 : p_1 > p_2$$

Solution. Because there are four pairs in which the scores are equal, that is, $A - B = 0$, these will be deleted from the samples. So the sample size $n =$ total number of " $+$ " and " $-$ " $= 39 - 4 = 35$. The test statistic is $T =$ total number of plus signs $= 25$. Because $n = 35$ is large enough, the normal approximation to the binomial distribution can be used. Under the null hypothesis, $\mu = np = \dfrac{n}{2}$ and $\sigma^2 = npq = \dfrac{n}{4}$.

The statistic $Z = \dfrac{T - \dfrac{n}{2}}{\sqrt{n/4}} \overset{\circ}{\sim} N(0, 1)$.

$$Z = \frac{(25 - 0.5) - \dfrac{35}{2}}{\sqrt{35/4}} = 2.3664.$$

The value 0.5 in the numerator is a continuity correction. The p value is obtained by

$$p = P(2.3664 < Z) = 0.0089 < 0.05.$$

Thus we conclude that the consumer acceptance for toothbrush A is statistically significantly different than that for toothbrush B. In fact, the acceptance level for A is significantly higher with the p value of 0.0089.

14.3 THE WILCOXON RANK SUM TEST

The sign test considers only the sign (plus or minus), not the magnitude of the differences of the sample values. The **Wilcoxon rank sum test**, which considers the magnitude of the differences via ranks, was developed to test the null hypothesis that there are no differences in two treatments. That is, the two samples come from identical populations. The test does not require that the two independent populations follow normal distributions. It requires only that the samples are from continuous distributions to avoid ties. In practice, however, we will sometimes observe ties, and the ties will not prevent us from using the test. The test statistics are based on the ranks of observations rather than their actual numerical values, and hence this procedure is appropriate for a wide variety of situations in biomedical sciences as well as social sciences. The test is also known as the **Mann-Whitney U**

Table 14.3.1. Amount of mercury released from amalgam fillings (µg)

X_i (10%)	.29	.52	.70	.51	.54	.58	1.58	.60	1.18	.67	.98	.77	.72
Rank	2	7	13	6	8	9.5	23	11	20	12	19	16	14
Y_j (15%)	1.23	.37	2.10	2.29	1.28	.44	1.76	.96	.08	.39	.93	.58	.76
Rank	21	3	25	26	22	5	24	18	1	4	17	9.5	15

test and is widely used as a non-parametric alternative to the two-sample t test for independent samples. The null and alternative hypotheses can be stated as follows:

$H_0 : P(X > Y) = 1/2$ (X and Y have the same distribution)

vs.

$H_1 : P(X > Y) \neq 1/2$ (X and Y have different distributions),

or

$H_1 : P(X > Y) > 1/2$ (observations from population X are likely to be larger than those from population Y),

or

$H_1 : P(X > Y) < 1/2$ (observations from population Y are likely to be larger than those from population X)

In the Wilcoxon rank sum test, the observed values from both samples are combined and then ranked. If the first sample has n_1 observations and the second sample has n_2 observations, the combined sample will be ranked from 1 to N, where $N = n_1 + n_2$. The test statistic is the sum of the ranks for the first sample (X_i), denoted W_X, or the sum of the ranks for the second sample (Y_j), denoted W_Y. In practice, it does not matter which sum we prefer to use. The sum of the first N integers is equal to $(N)(N + 1)/2$. This formula enables us to obtain W_X from W_Y and vice versa. Since it is easier to work with a smaller sample size, let n_1 be the smaller of the two sample sizes. Without loss of generality, we assume that the first sample has size n_1. The test can be performed with small samples (less than 10 samples), but we assume that both n_1 and n_2 are at least 10 so that the normal approximation can be used. Steps leading to the Wilcoxon rank sum test are:

1. Compute $Z = \dfrac{W_X - \mu_W}{\sigma_W}$, where $W_X = $ sum of the ranks of the first sample

$$\mu_W = \frac{(n_1)(n_1 + n_2 + 1)}{2}$$

and

$$\sigma_W = \sqrt{\frac{(n_1 \cdot n_2)(n_1 + n_2 + 1)}{12}}$$

2. Find the critical values. For the significance level $\alpha = 0.05$, use the z values of -1.96 and 1.96.

3. Reject the null hypothesis if $Z = \dfrac{W_X - \mu_W}{\sigma_W} < -1.96$ or $Z = \dfrac{W_X - \mu_W}{\sigma_W} > 1.96$. Accept the null hypothesis if $-1.96 \leq Z = \dfrac{W_X - \mu_W}{\sigma_W} \leq 1.96$.

The next examples illustrate the Wilcoxon rank sum test.

Example 14.3.1. To determine if at-home bleaching products for teeth cause mercury to be released from amalgam fillings, the facial surface of 26 posterior teeth were prepared and amalgam was then condensed into the preparation and carved. One day later, 13 teeth samples each were put into 10% and 15% carbamide peroxide. A week later the amount of mercury released was measured. Let X represent the measurements of mercury released for the first sample in 10% carbamide peroxide and Y the second sample in 15% carbamide peroxide. Table 14.3.1 presents the data.

Notice that one measurement value 0.58 from the first sample is tied with the same value in the second sample. The average rank $\dfrac{9 + 10}{2} = 9.5$ is assigned to the tied observations. We compute the sum of the ranks of the first sample

$$W_X = 2 + 7 + 13 + 6 + 8 + 9.5 + 23 + 11$$
$$+ 20 + 12 + 19 + 16 + 14 = 160.5$$

The mean μ_W and the SD σ_W are obtained by

Table 14.3.2. Attachment levels of 30 study subjects.

Subject No.	1	2	3	4	5	6	7	8
PLA (X)	5.2	5.8	4.3	5.0	5.5	4.7	4.8	4.2
ePTFE (Y)	5.8	6.0	5.6	4.4	5.6	5.0	4.8	5.4
Subject No.	9	10	11	12	13	14	15	16
PLA (X)	5.1	5.7	5.5	4.5	4.0	4.9	4.1	4.2
ePTFE (Y)	5.9	5.6	5.6	5.7	4.4	5.7		

substitution,

$$\mu_W = \frac{(n_1)(n_1 + n_2 + 1)}{2} = \frac{(13)(13 + 13 + 1)}{2}$$
$$= 175.5$$

$$\sigma_W = \sqrt{\frac{(n_1 \cdot n_2)(n_1 + n_2 + 1)}{12}}$$
$$= \sqrt{\frac{(13 \cdot 13)(13 + 13 + 1)}{12}} = 19.5$$

The value of the test statistic is

$$Z = \frac{W_X - \mu_W}{\sigma_W} = \frac{160.5 - 175.5}{19.5} = -0.7692$$

Since $Z = -0.7692$ is between -1.96 and 1.96, we accept the null hypothesis and conclude that there is no statistically significant difference in mercury released between 10% and 15% carbamide peroxide at the significance level $\alpha = 0.05$.

Example 14.3.2. A study was performed to assess periodontal regenerative techniques in intrabony defects utilizing a bioabsorbable, polylactic acid (PLA) barrier or the non-resorbable, expanded polytetrafluoroethylene (ePTFE) barrier [1]. Thirty patients each with one radiographically evident intrabony periodontal lesion of probing depth ≥ 6 mm participated in a 12-month controlled clinical trial. The subjects were randomly divided into two groups. The test group of $n_1 = 16$ subjects received a PLA barrier, and the control group of $n_2 = 14$ subjects received a ePTFE barrier. The attachment level of the subjects was measured when the clinical trial ended, as shown in Table 14.3.2. Perform a significance test at $\alpha = 0.05$.

Solution. The Wilcoxon rank sum test is chosen to test

H_0 : attachment level for the test group is not different from that for the control group,

Table 14.3.3. Observations from two populations are ranked.

X	Y	Rank	X	Y	Rank	X	Y	Rank
4.0		1	4.8		10.5		5.6	21.5
4.1		2	4.9		12		5.6	21.5
4.2		3		5.0	13.5		5.6	21.5
4.2		4	5.0		13.5		5.7	25
4.3		5	5.1		15		5.7	25
	4.4	6.5	5.2		16	5.7		25
	4.4	6.5		5.4	17		5.8	27.5
4.5		8	5.5		18.5	5.8		27.5
4.7		9		5.5	18.5		5.9	29
	4.8	10.5		5.6	21.5		6.0	30

H_1 : attachment level for the control group is larger than that for the test group.

There are six groups of tied observations in Table 14.3.2. The average of the ranks that would have been assigned is assigned to the tied observations within each group, as shown in Table 14.3.3. The statement of the alternative hypothesis H_1 is one-tailed test. The sum of the ranks assigned to Y is

$$W_Y = 6.5 + 6.5 + 10.5 + 13.5 + 17 + 21.5$$
$$+ 21.5 + 21.5 + 21.5 + 25 + 25$$
$$+ 27.5 + 29 + 30 = 276.5$$

The mean μ_W and the SD σ_W are obtained by substitution,

$$\mu_W = \frac{(16)(30 + 1)}{2} = 248$$

and

$$\sigma_W = \sqrt{\frac{(16 \cdot 14)(30 + 1)}{12}} = 24.06.$$

The value of the test statistic is $Z = \dfrac{W_Y - \mu_W}{\sigma_W} = \dfrac{276.5 - 248}{24.06} = 1.1845$

Table D in the Appendix shows that $P(1.1845 < Z) > 0.1170$. Since this p value is larger than $\alpha = 0.05$, a decision should be made not to reject the null hypothesis. We conclude that there is no statistically significant difference in attachment level between the test and control groups.

14.4 THE WILCOXON SIGNED RANK TEST

The Wilcoxon signed rank test is also designed to test that two treatments are the same, or the hypothesis that two population distributions are identical. This test can be used in place of the t test for dependent samples, without the assumption of the usual normal distributions. Thus, the test is referred to as the **Wilcoxon matched pairs test for dependent samples**. In dentistry, such matched pairs can occur from obtaining repeated measures on the same subjects at baseline and at follow-up examinations, or obtaining pairs of subjects who are matched based on their prognostic variables such as age, smoking status, oral health, probing depth, or bone density. The Wilcoxon signed rank test is based on the ranks of the absolute differences between the paired observations rather than the numerical values of the differences. As a result, the Wilcoxon test is appropriate for the observations that represent ordinal data. A matched pair (X_i, Y_i) is a single observation on a bivariate random variable. In the sign test discussed in Section 14.2, the matched pairs of the data were reduced for analysis to a plus, a minus, or zero in case of ties. The Wilcoxon signed rank test also reduces the matched pair (X_i, Y_i) to a single observation by taking the difference

$$D_i = X_i - Y_i(\text{or } D_i = Y_i - X_i) \text{ for}$$
$$i = 1, 2, \cdots, n$$

These differences $D_i, i = 1, 2, \cdots, n$, will constitute a sample of single observations. Unlike the sign test, which merely considers whether D_i has a positive or a negative sign or zero, the Wilcoxon signed rank test takes the magnitude of the positive differences relative to the negative differences. In this section, we assume that the distribution of the differences D_i is **symmetric**. This assumption was not made for the sign test. The distribution of a random variable is said to be symmetric with respect to some constant c, if $P(X \leq c - x) = P(X \geq c + x)$ for all x. All normal distributions and t distributions are symmetric. So is the binomial distribution if $p = 1/2$. The Wilcoxon signed rank test will be described to test

H_0 : Treatment A and treatment B are equivalent.

1. Compute the difference $D_i = X_i - Y_i$ for matched pairs.

2. Rank all of the D_i without regard to sign. That is, rank the absolute values $|D_i|$.
3. Affix the sign of the difference to each rank. This indicates which ranks are associated with positive D_i or negative D_i.
4. Compute $T^+ = $ the sum of the ranks R_i^+ of the positive D_i, and $T^- = $ the sum of the ranks R_i^- of the negative D_i.

When two observations of any pair are equal, that is, $D_i = X_i - Y_i = 0$, such pairs will be deleted from the analysis and thus the sample size will be reduced accordingly. When two or more D_i are tied, the average rank is assigned to each of the differences. If the sum of the positive ranks T^+ is different (much smaller or much larger) from the sum of the negative ranks T^-, we would conclude that treatment A is different from treatment B, and therefore, the null hypothesis H_0 will be rejected. That is, H_0 is rejected if either $T^+ = \sum R_i^+$ or $T^- = \sum R_i^-$ is too small. Without loss of generality, the test statistic is defined by $T^+ = \sum R_i^+$, which is approximately normally distributed with

$$\text{Mean} = \mu = \frac{n(n+1)}{4}$$

and

$$\text{Variance} = \sigma^2 = \frac{n(n+1)(2n+1)}{24}$$

$$\text{Thus, } Z = \frac{T^+ - \mu}{\sigma}$$
$$= \frac{T^+ - n(n+1)/4}{\sqrt{n(n+1)(2n+1)/24}} \overset{\circ}{\sim} N(0, 1)$$

For small samples ($n \leq 10$), the critical values can be found by referring to the table for Wilcoxon signed rank test included in many statistics textbooks [2, 3]. In this section, we will illustrate the test procedure assuming the number of matched pairs is larger than 10 so that the test can be performed by normal approximation. Keep in mind that the approximation improves as the sample size becomes larger.

Example 14.4.1. To evaluate the effectiveness of a teeth-whitening gum, 12 subjects who met the inclusion–exclusion criteria were selected for a 4-week clinical trial. The subjects were provided with specific instructions for using the gum. Their compliance was checked weekly. A chromameter was used to measure the shade of their teeth at the baseline and at the end of the 4-week period. Let X_i and Y_i denote the chromameter measurements

Table 14.4.1. The whitening gum data.

Subject	BL (X_i)	4-wk (Y_i)	$D_i = Y_i - X_i$	$|D_i|$	Rank	Signed Rank (R_i)
1	44.3	50.5	6.2	6.2	12	12
2	55.3	55.4	0.1	0.1	1	1
3	49.4	54.7	5.3	5.3	11	11
4	51.2	51.5	0.3	0.3	2	2
5	53.6	56.7	3.1	3.1	10	10
6	52.7	54.9	2.2	2.2	8	8
7	53.7	53.2	−0.5	0.5	3	−3
8	47.9	45.1	−2.8	2.8	9	−9
9	54.3	55.7	1.4	1.4	6	6
10	51.7	52.5	0.8	0.8	4.5	4.5
11	56.5	55.7	−0.8	0.8	4.5	−4.5
12	55.5	54.0	−1.5	1.5	7	−7

Note: BL, baseline.

at the baseline and at the end of the study, respectively. The chromameter measurements for the 12 subjects are displayed in the second and third columns in Table 14.4.1. Test the hypotheses at the significance level $\alpha = 0.05$:

H_0 : No difference in the shade of teeth before and after the use of the whitening gum

H_1 : Difference exists in the shade of teeth before and after the use of the whitening gum.

Solution. Following the steps described above, the differences, ranks, and signed ranks are displayed in Table 14.4.1.

1. The differences between the baseline measurement and the 4-week measurement for the subjects are in fourth column. For example, $D_1 = Y_1 - X_1 = 50.5 - 44.3 = 6.2, \cdots,$ $D_{12} = Y_{12} - X_{12} = 54.0 - 55.5 = -1.5.$
2. Take the absolute value of the differences, that is,

$$|Y_1 - X_1| = |6.2| = 6.2, \cdots, |Y_{12} - X_{12}|$$
$$= |-1.5| = 1.5.$$

3. Rank the absolute differences from lowest to highest. In the case of a tie, assign the average rank. For example, the rank 12 is assigned to the first subject. The tenth and eleventh subjects are tied, thus the average rank of 4.5 is assigned to both.
4. Give each rank a "+" or "−" sign according to the signs of the differences D_i, as shown in the last column of Table 14.4.1.
5. Find the sum of the positive ranks: $T^+ = \sum R_i^+ = 12 + 1 + 11 + 2 + 10 + 8 + 6 + 4.5 = 54.5.$

6. The mean and variance of T^+ are given by

$$\mu = \frac{12(12 + 1)}{4} = 39.0,$$

and

$$\sigma^2 = \frac{12(12 + 1)(2 \cdot 12 + 1)}{24} = 162.5.$$

7. The value of the test statistic is $Z = \frac{T^+ - \mu}{\sigma} = \frac{54.5 - 39}{\sqrt{162.5}} = 1.2159.$
8. Since $-1.96 < Z = 1.2159 < 1.96$, the null hypothesis H_0 is not rejected. The p value is

$$p = 2 \cdot P(1.2159 < Z) > 2(0.1131)$$
$$= 0.2262 > 0.05 \text{ from Table D in the Appendix.}$$

9. We conclude there is no significant difference in the shade of teeth before and after the use of the whitening gum. So the whitening gum is not effective.

Example 14.4.2. A split-mouth study was conducted to compare the clinical and radiographic healing results in intrabony periodontal defects 12 months after guided tissue regeneration (GTR) therapy with two different bioresorbable barriers [4]. The study comprised 22 healthy patients with one pair of contralaterally located intrabony defects with a probing pocket depth of at least 6 mm and radiographic evidence of angular bone loss of at least 4 mm.

The two defects of each patient were randomized for treatment either with polylactic acid (PLA) membranes or with polylactin-910 (PG-910) membraines. Suppose the investigators measured gingival recession of each subject 12 months

Table 14.4.2. Gingival recession data (mm).

Subject	PLA	PG-910	Subject	PLA	PG-910
1	2.1	1.5	12	2.6	1.6
2	1.7	1.8	13	2.3	2.1
3	1.1	1.6	14	2.2	1.1
4	1.4	1.4	15	1.4	1.3
5	1.8	1.2	16	1.7	1.2
6	2.4	1.6	17	1.6	1.8
7	2.5	2.0	18	1.7	1.7
8	1.9	1.9	19	2.3	1.5
9	2.0	1.1	20	2.5	1.4
10	1.8	1.2	21	2.0	1.8
11	1.9	1.2	22	2.4	2.2

after the therapy, as shown in Table 14.4.2. Do the two treatments, PLA and PG-910, have different effects?

Solution. Let X_i and Y_i be the pair of observations on gingival recession for i^{th} patient. Since (X_i, Y_i) form matched pairs, the Wilcoxon signed rank test is appropriate for this case. The computed results with $D_i = X_i - Y_i$ are showed in the following table. There are three pairs in which $D_i = X_i - Y_i = 0$. Thus the sample size is reduced to $n = 22 - 3 = 19$. The sum of the positive ranks is:

$$T^+ = \sum R_i^+ = 11 + 11 + 14.5 + 8 + 16$$
$$+ 11 + 13 + 17 + 4.5 + 18.5 + 1.5 + 8$$
$$+ 14.5 + 18.5 + 4.5 + 4.5$$
$$= 176.0$$

Subj.	X_i	Y_i	D_i	Signed rank (R_i)
1	2.1	1.5	0.6	11
2	1.7	1.8	−0.1	−1.5
3	1.1	1.6	−0.5	−8
4	1.4	1.4	0	•
5	1.8	1.2	0.6	11
6	2.4	1.6	0.8	14.5
7	2.5	2.0	0.5	8
8	1.9	1.9	0	•
9	2.0	1.1	0.9	16
10	1.8	1.2	0.6	11
11	1.9	1.2	0.7	13
12	2.6	1.6	1.0	17
13	2.3	2.1	0.2	4.5
14	2.2	1.1	1.1	18.5
15	1.4	1.3	0.1	1.5
16	1.7	1.2	0.5	8
17	1.6	1.8	−0.2	−4.5
18	1.7	1.7	0	•
19	2.3	1.5	0.8	14.5
20	2.5	1.4	1.1	18.5
21	2.0	1.8	0.2	4.5
22	2.4	2.2	0.2	4.5

The mean and variance of T^+ are given by

$$\mu = \frac{19(19 + 1)}{4} = 95.0,$$

and

$$\sigma^2 = \frac{19(19 + 1)(2 \cdot 19 + 1)}{24} = 617.5$$

The value of the test statistic is $Z = \dfrac{T^+ - \mu}{\sigma} = \dfrac{176 - 95}{\sqrt{617.5}} = 3.2596.$

Since $Z = 3.2596 > 1.96$, the null hypothesis is rejected. The p value is obtained by

$$p = 2 \cdot P(3.2596 < Z) < 0.0012$$

We conclude that the gingival recession treated with PLA is statistically significantly greater with $p < 0.0012$.

14.5 THE MEDIAN TEST

The median test is a statistical procedure for testing whether two independent populations (treatments) differ in central tendencies when the populations are far from normally distributed. The hypotheses can be stated

H_0 : Two treatments are from populations with the same median.

H_1 : The populations of two treatments have different medians.

Intuitively, if the null hypothesis is true, we expect that about half of each sample observation to be below the combined median and about half to be above. The key to the median test is to combine the samples and count the number of observations from each sample that falls below or above the median of the combined data. Let n_1 and n_2 be the number of samples drawn from two populations and N be the size of the combined sample. The data can be put in a 2×2 contingency table shown below.

	Treatment A	Treatment B	Combined
No. of observations ≤ combined median	a	b	$a + b$
No. of observations > combined median	c	d	$c + d$
Total	n_1	n_2	$N = n_1 + n_2$

Table 14.5.1. Bone height data for smokers and non-smokers.

	Smokers	Non-smokers	Combined
No. of observations ≤ the median	19	21	40
No. of observations > the median	8	32	40
Total	$n = 27$	$m = 53$	$N = 80$

Example 14.5.1. Of 80 randomly chosen implant patients, 27 were smokers and 53 were non-smokers. Their bone heights were measured to determine whether there is a significant difference in bone height between smokers and non-smokers. All the measurements for both groups were combined and the median of the combined data was determined. Table 14.5.1 shows the number of patients in each group whose bone height is below or above the median. Test if the two groups have the same median.

Solution. Here the combined sample size is $N = n + m = 27 + 53 = 80$. As can be seen below, none of the expected cell frequencies is less than 5. Thus the χ^2 contingency table technique can be used. The expected cell frequencies are

$$E_{11} = E_{21} = \frac{40 \cdot 27}{80} = 13.5$$

and

$$E_{12} = E_{22} = \frac{40 \cdot 53}{80} = 26.5$$

The value of the test statistic is given by

$$\chi^2 = \frac{(|19 - 13.5| - 0.5)^2}{13.5} + \frac{(|21 - 26.5| - 0.5)^2}{26.5}$$
$$+ \frac{(|8 - 13.5| - 0.5)^2}{13.5}$$
$$+ \frac{(|32 - 26.5| - 0.5)^2}{26.5}$$
$$= 5.5905$$

The test statistic χ^2 is approximately χ^2-distributed with 1 degree of freedom. The critical value is $\chi^2_{(1,0.95)} = 3.841$. Because $\chi^2 = 5.5905 > \chi^2_{(1,0.95)} = 3.841$, we reject the null hypothesis and conclude that the median bone height of nonsmokers is significantly higher than that for smokers at the significance level $\alpha = 0.05$.

When applying the χ^2 test to a 2×2 contingency table, it is computationally more convenient to use the following formula.

$$\chi^2 = \frac{N(|ad - bc| - N/2)^2}{(a + b)(c + d)(a + c)(b + d)}$$

Applying this formula to the data in Example 14.5.1, we should be able to obtain the same value for the test statistic $\chi^2 = 5.5905$:

$$\chi^2 = \frac{N(|ad - bc| - N/2)^2}{(a + b)(c + d)(a + c)(b + d)}$$
$$= \frac{80(|19 \cdot 32 - 21 \cdot 8| - 80/2)^2}{(19 + 21)(8 + 32)(19 + 8)(21 + 32)}$$
$$= 5.5905.$$

The median test discussed in this section can be extended to examine whether three or more samples came from populations having the same median. Suppose from each of c (≥ 3) populations a random sample of size n_i is taken, $i = 1, 2, \cdots, c$. The grand median is determined from the combined sample of $N = n_1 + n_2 + \cdots + n_c$. The combined sample of N observations is arranged in a $2 \times c$ contingency table as follows.

	Treatment 1	Treatment 2	$\cdots$	Treatment c	Combined
No. of obs ≤ the median	O_{11}	O_{12}	$\cdots$	O_{1c}	r_1
No. of obs > the median	O_{21}	O_{22}	$\cdots$	O_{2c}	r_2
Total	n_1	n_2	$\cdots$	n_c	N

The $r \times c$ contingency table was discussed in Section 10.3. The test statistic is obtained by a formula expressed in a more convenient form:

$$\chi^2 = \frac{N^2}{r_1 \cdot r_2} \sum_{i=1}^{c} \frac{O_{1i}^2}{n_i} - \frac{N \cdot r_1}{r_2} \overset{\circ}{\sim} \chi^2_{(c-1)}$$

Example 14.5.2. A study was performed to evaluate in-vitro the effectiveness of two light-emitting diode (LED) curing lights and one quartz tungsten halogen on the tensile bond strength of orthodontic brackets at 10-second curing time. Fifteen samples were prepared for each of the three treatments (two LED's and halogen), and the shear bond strength of orthodontic brackets bonded to extracted human teeth cured by the treatments were measured (in Newtons), as shown in the table below [5]. Do the three groups come from populations with the same median? Test at the significance level $\alpha = 0.05$.

Sample	1	2	3	4	5	6	7	8
LED 1	80	80	107	96	59	82	90	87
LED 2	119	92	75	93	69	101	103	105
Halogen	101	92	68	118	107	131	132	113

Sample	9	10	11	12	13	14	15
LED 1	93	106	100	62	82	109	84
LED 2	109	84	110	73	86	127	93
Halogen	109	117	126	112	98	125	126

Solution. Since there are three groups, each with 15 samples, we have $k = 3$, $n_1 = n_2 = n_3 = 15$, the combined sample $N = n_1 + n_2 + n_3 = 45$. It is easy to determine that the grand median is 100. By counting the frequencies below and above the combined sample median from each group, we can construct the following 2×3 contingency table.

	LED1	LED2	Halogen	Combined
No. of obs $\leq$ the median	12	8	3	23
No. of obs $>$ the median	3	7	12	22
Total	15	15	15	45

The value of the test statistic is given by

$$\chi^2 = \frac{N^2}{r_1 \cdot r_2} \sum_{i=1}^{c} \frac{O_{1i}^2}{n_i} - \frac{N \cdot r_1}{r_2}$$

$$= \frac{45^2}{23 \cdot 22} \left(\frac{12^2}{15} + \frac{8^2}{15} + \frac{3^2}{15} \right) - \frac{45 \cdot 23}{22}$$

$$= 10.850$$

It exceeds the critical value $\chi^2_{(2, 0.95)} = 5.99$, therefore the null hypothesis is rejected. The p value is slightly less than 0.005.

14.6 THE KRUSKAL-WALLIS RANK TEST

The one-way ANOVA technique used the F test to compare the means of three or more populations. For the ANOVA procedure to be valid, the population distributions must be normal or approximately normal and the variances must be equal. When these assumptions are not satisfied, a non-parametric test known as the **Kruskal-Wallis test** may be employed to test whether the treatment means are equal. This test is based on the ranks of the observations. The only assumption required about the population distributions is that they are independent, continuous and of the same shape. That is, the populations must have the same variability or skewness. It is recommended that at least five samples should be drawn from each population. This test is also called the **Kruskal-Wallis one-way ANOVA by ranks**.

Suppose that k $(k \geq 3)$ population means are being compared and we wish to test

$$H_0 : \mu_1 = \mu_2 = \cdots = \mu_k \quad \text{vs.}$$

$$H_1 : \text{ not all } \mu_i \text{ are equal}$$

Let $n_1, n_2, \cdots, n_k$ be the number of samples taken from the k populations. It is not required that the sample sizes are equal. Let $N = n_1 + n_2 + \cdots + n_k$ be the sum of the k samples. All N observations are ranked from 1 to N. Let $\overline{R}_i$ be the mean of the ranks for the ith group. The Kruskal-Wallis test statistic is defined by

$$\chi^2_{KW} = \frac{12}{N(N+1)} \left(n_1 \overline{R}_1^2 + n_2 \overline{R}_2^2 + \cdots + n_k \overline{R}_k^2 \right) - 3(N+1)$$

The test statistic is known to be approximately a χ^2 random variable with $(k-1)$ degrees of freedom. Thus,

$$\text{Reject } H_0 \text{ if } \chi^2_{KW} > \chi^2_{(k-1, 1-\alpha)}$$

and

$$\text{accept } H_0 \text{ if } \chi^2_{KW} \leq \chi^2_{(k-1, 1-\alpha)}.$$

Example 14.6.1. Studies have shown that composite resins soften in the presence of alcohol. To assess the effect of ethanol concentrations on four composite resins, eight samples of each composite resin were prepared and subjected to wine for 15 days at a specific temperature. At the end of the 15-day period, the hardness test was accomplished using the Knoops hardness index [6]. The

Table 14.6.1. Knoops hardness data for four composite resins.

Composite A	53.5	51.6	52.2	50.4	52.3	52.8	49.2	48.8
Rank	19	15	16	13	17	18	12	11
Composite B	23.9	23.6	22.3	18.7	19.8	19.7	24.8	22.0
Rank	7	6	5	1	3	2	8	4
Composite C	45.4	42.4	53.8	50.6	54.9	56.9	62.2	55.2
Rank	10	9	20	14	21	23	26	22
Composite D	64.4	61.8	61.4	70.1	70.0	69.8	69.6	67.9
Rank	27	25	24	32	31	30	29	28

resulting hardness data, along with their ranks in a combined sample, is presented in Table 14.6.1. Test H_0 : There is no difference among the four composite resins in the effect of ethanol concentrations.

Solution. After ranking all 32 observations from 1 to 32, the mean of the ranks for each composite material can be computed:

$$\overline{R}_1 = (19 + 15 + 16 + 13 + 17 + 18$$
$$+ 12 + 11)/8 = 15.125$$
$$\overline{R}_2 = (7 + 6 + 5 + 1 + 3 + 2 + 8 + 4)/8 = 4.5$$
$$\overline{R}_3 = (10 + 9 + 20 + 14 + 21 + 23$$
$$+ 26 + 22)/8 = 18.125$$
$$\overline{R}_4 = (27 + 25 + 24 + 32 + 31 + 30$$
$$+ 29 + 28)/8 = 28.25$$

The value of the test statistic is obtained as

$$\chi^2_{KW} = \frac{12}{N(N + 1)} \left(n_1 \overline{R}_1^2 + n_2 \overline{R}_2^2 + \cdots + n_k \overline{R}_k^2 \right)$$
$$- 3(N + 1)$$
$$= \frac{12}{32(32 + 1)} [8 \cdot (15.125)^2 + 8 \cdot (4.5)^2 + 8$$
$$\times (18.125)^2 + 8 \cdot (28.25)^2] - 3(32 + 1)$$
$$= 26.054.$$

The critical value from the χ^2 table is $\chi^2_{(k-1,1-\alpha)} = \chi^2_{(4-1,0.95)} = 7.81$. Since $\chi^2_{KW} = 26.054 > \chi^2_{(3,0.95)} = 7.81$, we reject the null hypothesis and conclude that there is statistically significant difference in mean hardness among the four composite materials after having been soaked in wine for 15 days at the significance level $\alpha = 0.05$.

The Kruskal-Wallis test does not require the sample sizes to be equal. In the above example, we could have $n_1 = 8$, $n_2 = 6$, $n_3 = 11$, and $n_4 = 7$. If the sample sizes are small enough that the χ^2

approximation is not appropriate, we can use a special table to perform the test. However, we recommend that the sample sizes be at least 5 so that the approximation can be applied. When ties occur between two observations within the treatment group or different treatment groups, each observation is assigned the mean of the ranks for which they are tied. Tied observations influence the variance of the sampling distribution, and thus the test statistic needs to be corrected for ties. As in Example 14.6.1, when the Kruskal-Wallis test is significant, it indicates at least one of the treatment groups is different from the others. A procedure is needed to determine which treatment groups are different. We need to test $H_0 : \mu_i = \mu_j$ vs. $H_1 : \mu_i \neq \mu_j$. This is a pairwise test that tests the significance of individual pairs of differences. The test statistic is based on $|\overline{R}_i - \overline{R}_j|$, which is approximately normally distributed. Similar to the multiple comparison procedures introduced in Section 12.6, comparisons must be made among k treatment groups. We reject the null hypothesis if

$$|\overline{R}_i - \overline{R}_j| \geq z_{1-\alpha/k(k-1)} \sqrt{\frac{N(N + 1)}{12} \left(\frac{1}{n_i} + \frac{1}{n_j} \right)}.$$

Comparisons to be made are:

$$|\overline{R}_1 - \overline{R}_2| = |15.125 - 4.5| = 10.625$$
$$|\overline{R}_1 - \overline{R}_3| = |15.125 - 18.125| = 3.0$$
$$|\overline{R}_1 - \overline{R}_4| = |15.125 - 28.25| = 13.125$$
$$|\overline{R}_2 - \overline{R}_3| = |4.5 - 18.125| = 13.625$$
$$|\overline{R}_2 - \overline{R}_4| = |4.5 - 28.25| = 23.75$$
$$|\overline{R}_3 - \overline{R}_4| = |18.125 - 28.25| = 10.125$$

For $\alpha = 0.05$ and $k = 4$ treatment groups, we obtain $z_{1-\alpha/k(k-1)} = z_{1-0.05/4(4-1)} = z_{0.9968} = 2.73$ from the normal table. Because $|\overline{R}_i - \overline{R}_j| > z_{1-\alpha/k(k-1)} = z_{0.9968} = 2.73$, all of the comparison tests are significant.

Table 14.7.1. Cleanliness data for left-handed patients.

	1	2	3	4	5	6	7	8	9	10	11	12
A	2 (1)	5 (3)	3 (2)	3 (3)	3 (2)	1 (1)	2 (1)	4 (3)	2 (1)	3 (2)	2 (1)	1 (1)
B	4 (3)	1 (1)	4 (3)	2 (2)	2 (1)	4 (3)	5 (3)	1 (1)	4 (2)	1 (1)	4 (2)	3 (2)
C	3 (2)	2 (2)	2 (1)	1 (1)	4 (3)	2 (2)	3 (2)	3 (2)	5 (3)	4 (3)	5 (3)	5 (3)

14.7 THE FRIEDMAN TEST

The Kruskal-Wallis rank test for k *independent* samples was discussed in the preceding section. In the present section, we will introduce the **Friedman test for k-related samples** to determine whether the k samples have been drawn from the sample population. This test is also known as the **Friedman two-way analysis of variance by ranks**. To facilitate the discussion, consider a study comparing four teaching methods in dental education. The researcher may select 20 groups of four students. Each group consists of four matched subjects in terms of age, IQ, motivation, and GPA. Subjects in the same group are randomly assigned to one of the four teaching methods; later, their performance is evaluated. Within the group, the performance of the subjects is ranked 1 to 4. In case of ties, the average rank is assigned. The test is based on the ranks of the subjects who were taught by a specific teaching method. When there are no ties in the data, the test statistic is given by

$$F_r = \left[\frac{12}{Nk(k+1)} \sum_{i=1}^{k} R_i^2 \right] - 3N(k+1)$$

where

N = number of groups
k = number of treatments
R_i = sum of the ranks for i^{th} treatment

When the number of groups N and/or the number of treatments k is large, the distribution of the test statistic F_r is approximately $\chi^2_{(k-1)}$ with $(k-1)$ degrees of freedom. When ties occur, we need to make an adjustment. Thus, the expression of the test statistic is slightly more complicated:

$$F_r = \frac{12 \sum_{i=1}^{k} R_i^2 - 3N^2 k(k+1)^2}{Nk(k+1) + \dfrac{Nk - (U+V)}{(k-1)}},$$

where

U = number of untied observations in the data
V = sum of $(\tau)^3$,
τ denotes the size of the ties.

For example, if two scores in the same group are tied, $\tau = 2$. We present an example each with no ties and with ties.

Example 14.7.1. Investigators were interested in evaluating left-handed patients' ability to clean teeth in all four quadrants of their teeth using three newly designed toothbrushes. Twelve left-handed subjects have been recruited for the study. Each subject was instructed to use one of the three toothbrushes for 1 week. At the end of the week investigators examined the subjects and the cleanliness of their teeth was rated by a prespecified scoring system ranging from score 1 (worst) to score 5 (best). From the data tabulated in the following table, what conclusion can we draw? The numbers in the parentheses in Table 14.7.1 indicate the ranks.

Solution. There are $N = 12$ matched samples with $k = 3$ treatments. The rank sums are given by $R_1 = 21$, $R_2 = 24$, and $R_3 = 27$. There are no ties in the data. Thus the test statistic is

$$F_r = \left[\frac{12}{Nk(k+1)} \sum_{i=1}^{k} R_i^2 \right] - 3N(k+1)$$

$$= \frac{12}{12 \cdot 3(3+1)} (21^2 + 24^2 + 27^2)$$
$$\quad - 3 \cdot 12(3+1)$$

$$= 1.5.$$

The critical value $\chi^2_{(2,0.95)} = 5.99$ and $F_r < \chi^2_{(2,0.95)}$, thus the test is not significant. We conclude that there is no statistically significant difference among the three toothbrushes.

Example 14.7.2. Table 14.7.2, summarizes the data for the 20 matched samples for the study of four teaching methods in dental education. Using

Table 14.7.2. Matched data for teaching methods in dental education.

Groups	Method A Scores (Rank)	Method B Scores (Rank)	Method C Scores (Rank)	Method D Scores (Rank)
1	78 (3)	82 (4)	67 (1)	75 (2)
2	74 (2)	85 (4)	62 (1)	84 (3)
3	84 (4)	79 (3)	73 (2)	68 (1)
4	76 (2.5)	76 (2.5)	74 (1)	80 (4)
5	87 (4)	74 (2)	86 (3)	69 (1)
6	58 (1)	76 (3)	66 (2)	79 (4)
7	78 (1.5)	83 (3)	85 (4)	78 (1.5)
8	78 (2)	88 (3)	77 (1)	90 (4)
9	86 (4)	74 (3)	68 (1)	73 (2)
10	84 (3)	88 (4)	76 (1)	79 (2)
11	63 (2)	66 (3)	71 (4)	58 (1)
12	75 (2)	63 (1)	79 (4)	77 (3)
13	79 (2)	84 (3)	72 (1)	92 (4)
14	87 (4)	72 (1)	79 (2)	80 (3)
15	91 (3.5)	91 (3.5)	86 (1)	88 (2)
16	78 (3)	70 (2)	65 (1)	83 (4)
17	76 (4)	74 (3)	62 (1)	65 (2)
18	87 (2.5)	83 (1)	92 (4)	87 (2.5)
19	63 (2)	75 (4)	68 (3)	56 (1)
20	85 (3)	81 (2)	88 (4)	80 (1)
R_i	55	55	42	48

the Friedman test, we wish to test if there is any difference in the teaching methods. The number of matched samples is $N = 20$, the number of treatments $k = 4$, and the rank sums are $R_1 = 55$, $R_2 = 55$, $R_3 = 42$, and $R_4 = 48$. There are four sets of ties in groups 4, 7, 15, and 18. Only two scores in each group are tied. Hence, $\tau = 2$ for each tied pair. Since 8 observations resulted in ties, we have $U = 72$ untied observations among the total of 80 observations. We can now compute the value of the test statistic:

$$F_r = \frac{12 \sum_{i=1}^{k} R_i^2 - 3N^2 k(k+1)^2}{Nk(k+1) + \frac{Nk - (U+V)}{(k-1)}}$$

$$= \frac{12(55^2 + 55^2 + 42^2 + 48^2) - 3 \cdot 20^2 \cdot 4(4+1)^2}{20 \cdot 4(4+1) + \left[\frac{20 \cdot 4 - (72 + 2^3 + 2^3 + 2^3 + 2^3)}{(4-1)}\right]}$$

$$= 3.6122$$

Since the critical value $\chi^2_{(3,0.95)} = 7.81$ and $F_r < \chi^2_{(3,0.95)}$, the test is not significant. We conclude there is no statistically significant difference in the effectiveness of the four teaching methods at the significance level $\alpha = 0.05$.

Suppose the test in Example 14.7.2 was significant. It would then indicate that at least one of the teaching methods is different from the others. The test would not tell us which one is different. We need to perform multiple comparisons test between the treatments. The multiple comparisons procedure is based on the sum of ranks for individual treatments. For comparing i^{th} and j^{th} teaching methods, the null hypothesis will be rejected if

$$\left| R_i - R_j \right| \geq z_{1-\alpha/k(k-1)} \sqrt{\frac{Nk(k+1)}{6}}$$

This procedure is very similar to the multiple comparisons procedure discussed in Section 14.6.

14.8 THE PERMUTATION TEST

The permutation test is used when we have the paired observations for each subject or the observations are made for matched pairs. Paired observations (X, Y) occur in either case. As a non-parametric procedure, the advantage of the permutation test is that neither normality nor homogeneity of variances is assumed. For example consider the following.

1. To compare the effectiveness of two treatments for hypertension associated with acute post-streptococcal glomerulonephritis (PSGN), eight subjects have been recruited for a clinical trial. Subjects were given one treatment for 3 weeks, and after a 4-week washout period, they were given the other treatment for 3 weeks. Subjects' blood pressure levels were compared to evaluate the effectiveness of the treatments.
2. To evaluate the impact of two types of implant loading—the immediate loading and delayed loading—on survival time, 16 patients were accepted into a clinical trial. Eight matched pairs were formed according to their prognostic variables, such as age, sex, bone height, smoking status, and oral hygiene conditions. Within each pair, one patient was randomly assigned to the immediate loading and the other to the delayed loading. The survival time of the implants was followed to complete the study. The null hypothesis is H_0 : two treatments are equivalent (or there is no difference).

Biostatistics for Oral Healthcare

Table 14.8.1. Survival time of implants (in month).

Loading	Pairs							
	1	2	3	4	5	6	7	8
Delayed (X_i)	118	96	127	134	105	66	113	140
Immediate (Y_i)	110	103	112	120	89	54	82	142
$d_i = X_i - Y_i$	+8	−7	+15	+14	+16	+12	+31	−2

The first step is to calculate the difference between the paired observations $d_i = X_i - Y_i$ for the ith subject or the ith matched pair. The difference d_i would be positive but just as likely to be negative if H_0 is true, since we made the random assignment. Under H_0, every observed difference will be equally likely to have had the opposite sign. If we have $n = 8$ pairs, assuming H_0 is true, we would have $2^n = 2^8 = 256$ outcomes that are equally likely. The test statistic is based on the sum of the differences: $D = \sum_{i=1}^{n} d_i$. To complete the test, we need to define the rejection region. If H_0 is false, then either $D = \sum_{i=1}^{n} d_i$ is very small or very large. In the case of the two-tailed test with the significance level $\alpha = 0.05$, the rejection region would consist of 5% of the 256 outcomes. That is, $(256)(0.05) = 12.8$ extreme values. In other words, the largest 6 and the smallest 6 constitute the rejection region. If H_0 is true, the chance that we observe 1 of these 12 extreme cases is $12/256 = 0.0469$. To further illustrate the permutation test, consider the following example.

Example 14.8.1. From eight matched pairs of 16 implant patients, the survival time data was collected as shown in Table 14.8.1. Assume that the normality assumption is not met.

The differences in descending order of absolute values are

$$+31, +16, +15, +14, +12, +8, -7, -2$$

The sum is obtained by $D = \sum_{i=1}^{n} d_i = 31 + 16 + 15 + 14 + 12 + 8 - 7 - 2 = 87.0$. Table 14.8.2 shows 6 most extreme positive sums to perform the test. These 6 outcomes are in the rejection region. As we can easily see, the observed outcome, $+31, +16, +15, +14, +12, +8, -7, -2$, which yields the sum $\sum_{i=1}^{n} d_i = 87.0$, falls in the rejection region. Hence, we reject the null hypothesis and conclude that the delayed loading results in significantly longer survival times at the significance level $\alpha = 0.05$.

If the number of pairs is large, the permutation test can be extremely tedious and time consuming. For example, if $n = 12$, the number of possible outcomes is $2^{12} = 4096.0$. Therefore, the rejection region contains $(4096)(0.05) = 204.8$ extreme values. When the sample size n is large enough for easy computation, it is recommended to use the Wilcoxon signed rank test instead of the permutation test. It turns out that the Wilcoxon signed rank test is the permutation test based on ranks.

14.9 THE COCHRAN TEST

The McNemar test for two related samples presented in Section 10.5 can be extended for use in comparing more than two related samples. This extension is known as the Cochran test for k

Table 14.8.2. Six most extreme positive sums for Example 14.8.1.

Outcomes								$D = \sum_{i=1}^{n} d_i$
+31	+16	+15	+14	+12	+8	+7	+2	105
+31	+16	+15	+14	+12	+8	+7	−2	101
+31	+16	+15	+14	+12	+8	−7	+2	91
+31	+16	+15	+14	+12	−8	+7	+2	89
+31	+16	+15	+14	+12	+8	−7	−2	87
+31	+16	+15	+14	+12	−8	+7	−2	85

Table 14.9.1. A layout for the Cochran test for k-related samples.

Block	Treatment 1	2	$\cdots$	k	Row Sum
1	X_{11}	X_{12}	$\cdots$	X_{1k}	r_1
2	X_{21}	X_{22}	$\cdots$	X_{2k}	r_2
$\cdots$	$\cdots$	$\cdots$	$\cdots$	$\cdots$	$\cdots$
b	X_{b1}	X_{b2}	$\cdots$	X_{bk}	r_b
Col. sum	c_1	c_2	$\cdots$	c_k	N = Total

Table 14.9.2. Endodontic file data.

	File A	File B	File C	r_i
1	1	1	0	2
2	1	0	1	2
3	1	1	1	3
4	0	1	1	2
5	0	1	1	2
6	1	0	0	1
7	1	1	0	2
8	1	1	0	2
9	1	1	0	2
10	1	1	0	2
11	0	1	1	2
12	1	1	0	2
c_j	9	10	5	$N = 24$

(≥ 3) related samples. The Cochran test provides a method for testing whether or not k matched sets of frequencies differ from each other. In biomedical applications, k typically represents the number of treatments. There are situations in biomedical sciences in which each of k treatments is applied independently to each of b subjects (sometimes, referred to as blocks in statistics), and the outcome response is recorded by investigators as either "cured" or "not cured," or "success" or "failure." These responses are represented by either 1 (success) or 0 (failure). The sample data can be presented in a table with k columns and b rows. Let r_i ($i = 1, 2, \cdots, k$) be the row sum, and c_j ($j = 1, 2, \cdots, b$) be the column sum. Each entry of the table X_{ij} is either 0 or 1. (See Table 14.9.1).

The hypotheses can be stated

H_0 : The k treatments are equally effective
H_1 : The k treatments are not equally effective (there is a difference in effectiveness)

By letting $p_{ij} = P(X_{ij} = 1)$, the hypotheses can be restated $H_0 : p_{i1} = p_{i2} = \cdots = p_{ik}$ for each $i = 1, 2, \cdots, k$ vs. H_1 : Not all p_{ij} are equal.

The test statistic is given by

$$Q = \frac{(k-1)\left[k \sum_{j=1}^{k} c_j^2 - \left(\sum_{j=1}^{k} c_j\right)^2\right]}{k \sum_{i=1}^{b} r_i - \sum_{i=1}^{b} r_i^2}$$

where

c_j = total number of success in the jth column
r_i = total number of successes in the ith row.

If the null hypothesis is true and if the number, b, of subjects is not too small, the test statistic is approximately χ^2 distributed with degrees of freedom $k - 1$. Note that this test is sometimes known as the Cochran Q test.

Example 14.9.1. An investigation was conducted to assess the reliability of endodontic files. Suppose that an endodontic file is considered *success* if it is used at least 10 times and *failure* if it becomes deformed or broken before it is used 10 times. Assume that there are three types of files being used by most endodontists. To compare the reliability of these files, 12 endodontists were selected at random and each recorded the results of the files they had tested. Table 14.9.2 summarizes the data from the 12 endodontists who participated in the study (0 = failure, 1 = success). Are the three files equally reliable?

Solution. There are three treatments, $k = 3$, and $b = 12$ subjects. Note that the responses are dichotomized observations. Since each of the 12 subjects tested all three files, we have three related samples. The Cochran test is an appropriate approach for the problem.

The test statistic is given by

$$Q = \frac{(k-1)\left[k \sum_{j=1}^{k} c_j^2 - \left(\sum_{j=1}^{k} c_j\right)^2\right]}{k \sum_{i=1}^{b} r_i - \sum_{i=1}^{b} r_i^2}$$

$$= \frac{(k-1)\left(k \sum_{j=1}^{k} c_j^2 - N^2\right)}{kN - \sum_{i=1}^{b} r_i^2}$$

By making substitutions, we get

$$Q = \frac{(3-1)[3(9^2 + 10^2 + 5^2) - 24^2]}{3 \cdot 24 - 50} = 3.8182.$$

Since $Q = 3.8182 < \chi^2_{(2, 0, .95)} = 5.99$, the null hypothesis is accepted. Thus, we conclude that there

Table 14.9.3. Clinic competency ratings of 10 residents.

	Rater A	Rater B	Rater C	Rater D	Row sum
1	1	1	0	1	3
2	1	1	0	1	3
3	1	1	1	1	4
4	1	1	0	1	3
5	1	1	0	1	3
6	0	1	1	1	3
7	1	1	0	1	3
8	1	1	0	1	3
9	1	0	1	0	2
10	1	1	0	1	3
Col. sum	9	9	3	9	$N = 30$

is no statistically significant difference in reliability among the three endodontic files.

Example 14.9.2. Parkview Medical Center has 10 residents who are undergoing training under the supervision of four attending physicians. At the end of the year residents' clinical competency is evaluated by the four supervisors, either $0 =$ unacceptable or $1 =$ acceptable as shown in Table 14.9.3. Is there any supervisor bias in the evaluation?

Solution. There are 10 subjects who were evaluated by all four raters, and each response is a dichotomous variable (either 0 or 1); the Cochran test is applicable. By making appropriate substitutions, we obtain the value of the test statistic

$$
\begin{aligned}
Q &= \frac{(k-1)\left(k \sum_{j=1}^{k} c_j^2 - N^2\right)}{kN - \sum_{i=1}^{b} r_i^2} \\
&= \frac{(4-1)[4(9^2 + 9^2 + 3^2 + 9^2) - 30^2]}{4 \cdot 30 - 92} \\
&= 11.5714.
\end{aligned}
$$

Since $Q = 11.5714 > \chi^2_{(3, 0, .95)} = 7.81$, the null hypothesis is rejected. Thus, we conclude that there is a statistically significant rater bias with $p < 0.01$ from the χ^2 table in the Appendix.

14.10 THE SQUARED RANK TEST FOR VARIANCES

In most of the practical problems, the usual standard of comparison for several treatments is based on the population means or other measures of location of the populations. In some other situations, the variances of the treatments may be the focus of an investigation. The squared rank test provides a method to test the equality of variances without the assumption of normality. We shall first discuss the two-sample case when the sample sizes are at least 10. For the small sample case with no ties, the readers are referred to Conover [2]. Let $X_1, X_2, \cdots, X_{n_1}$ denote n_1 observations from population A, and $Y_1, Y_2, \cdots, Y_{n_2}$ denote n_2 observations from population B. To perform the squared rank test,

1. calculate the sample means $\overline{X}$ and $\overline{Y}$.
2. calculate the absolute deviations of the observations from the mean

$$
U_i = \left| X_i - \overline{X} \right| \text{ for } i = 1, 2, \cdots, n_1, \quad \text{and}
$$
$$
V_j = \left| Y_j - \overline{Y} \right| \text{ for } j = 1, 2, \cdots, n_2.
$$

3. combine the absolute deviations and assign the ranks from 1 to $N = n_1 + n_2$.
4. compute the value of the test statistic

$$
T = \frac{\sum_{i=1}^{n_1} [R(U_i)]^2 - n_1 \cdot \overline{R^2}}{\sqrt{\dfrac{n_1 \cdot n_2}{N(N-1)} \sum_{i=1}^{N} R_i^4 - \dfrac{n_1 \cdot n_2}{(N-1)} \left(\overline{R^2}\right)^2}}
$$

where $R(U_i) =$ the rank of the absolute deviation U_i

$$
\overline{R^2} = \frac{1}{N} \left\{ \sum_{i=1}^{n_1} [R(U_i)]^2 + \sum_{j=1}^{n_2} [R(V_j)]^2 \right\}
$$

= average of the squared ranks of both samples

$$
\sum_{i=1}^{N} R_i^4 = \sum_{i=1}^{n_1} [R(U_i)]^4 + \sum_{j=1}^{n_2} [R(V_j)]^4
$$

Under the null hypothesis, the above test statistic is approximately normally distributed. The test can be performed using the normal probability table in the Appendix.

Example 14.10.1. Periodontal probing has become increasingly more important as a diagnostic tool to determine the presence and severity of periodontal disease. Since the accuracy and reliability of probing is critical, a study was conducted to evaluate two types of probes: the hand-held probe with visual measurement recording and the pressure-controlled electronic probe with direct

Table 14.10.1. Periodontal probing: hand-held vs. computer.

Hand-held X_i	Computer Y_j	Absolute Deviation		Rank $R(U_i)$	Rank $R(V_j)$	Squared Rank	
		$U_i = |X_i - \overline{X}|$	$V_j = |Y_j - \overline{Y}|$			$[R(U_i)]^2$	$[R(V_j)]^2$
4.5	6.7	1.5	0.2	13.5	5	182.25	25.0
6.0	5.2	0	1.7	1	16.5	1.0	272.25
5.0	7.4	1.0	0.5	11.5	8	132.25	64.0
7.5	7.0	1.5	0.1	13.5	3	182.25	9.0
9.0	6.4	3.0	0.5	21	8	441.0	64.0
8.0	6.8	2.0	0.1	18.5	3	342.25	9.0
2.5	5.3	3.5	1.6	22	15	484.0	225.0
7.0	9.4	1.0	2.5	11.5	20	132.25	400.0
6.5	6.2	0.5	0.7	8	10	64.0	100.0
4.0	7.0	2.0	0.1	18.5	3	342.25	9.0
	8.6		1.7		16.5		272.25
	7.3		0.4		6		36.0
$\overline{X} = 6.0$	$\overline{Y} = 6.9$						

computer data capture. Suppose the data indicates that the samples are not from normal populations. From the data in Table 14.10.1, can we conclude that there is no difference in the precision level between the two types of probe?

Solution: From Table 14.10.1, we find that $n_1 = 10$, $n_2 = 12$, and $N = n_1 + n_2 = 22$. We can compute

$$\sum_{i=1}^{10}[R(U_i)]^2 = 2,303.5, \quad \sum_{j=1}^{12}[R(V_j)]^2 = 1,485.5$$

$$\overline{R^2} = \frac{1}{N}\left\{\sum_{i=1}^{10}[R(U_i)]^2 + \sum_{j=1}^{12}[R(V_j)]^2\right\}$$

$$= \frac{1}{22}(2,303.5 + 1,485.5)$$

$$= 172.23$$

$$\sum_{i=1}^{N} R_i^4 = \sum_{i=1}^{10}[R(U_i)]^4 + \sum_{j=1}^{12}[R(V_j)]^4$$

$$= 768,514.38 + 379,221.13$$

$$= 1,147,735.51$$

We can compute the value of the test statistic by substitution

$$T = \frac{2,303.5 - 10 \cdot 172.23}{\sqrt{\frac{10 \cdot 12}{22(22-1)}(1,147,735.51) - \frac{10 \cdot 12}{(22-1)}(172.23)^2}}$$

$$= 1.6207.$$

The calculated value $T = 1.6207 < z_{0.975} = 1.96$. Thus, the null hypothesis is not rejected and we conclude that there is no statistically significant difference in the variance between hand-held and computerized probes.

If there are more than two variances to be compared, the squared rank test can easily be modified to test the equality of several variances: $H_0 : \sigma_1^2 = \sigma_2^2 = \cdots = \sigma_k^2$ vs. H_1 : not all σ_i^2 are equal. From each observation in each sample, subtract its sample mean and then take the absolute value of the difference to get $|X_{ij} - \overline{X_i}|$, $i = 1, 2, \cdots, k$ and $j = 1, 2, \cdots, n_i$. Let the pooled sample size be denoted by $N = n_1 + n_2 + \cdots + n_k$. Combine all N absolute values and rank them from 1 to N, assigning the average rank if there are ties. Like the two-sample case, we now compute the sum of the squares of the rank for each of the k samples and let these sums be denoted by $T_1, T_2, \cdots, T_k$.

The test statistic is given by

$$T^* = \frac{1}{K}\left[\sum_{i=1}^{k}\frac{T_i^2}{n_i} - N \cdot (\overline{T})^2\right]$$

where $\overline{T} = \frac{1}{N}\sum_{i=1}^{k} T_i$ = the average of all the squared ranks

$$K = \frac{1}{N-1}\left[\sum_{i=1}^{k}\sum_{j=1}^{n_i} R_{ij}^4 - N \cdot (\overline{T})^2\right],$$

$\sum_{i=1}^{k}\sum_{j=1}^{n_i} R_{ij}^4$ is the sum taken after every rank is raised to the fourth power.

Table 14.10.2. Number of bacteria species in dentin samples.

	(A)	(B)	(C)		(A)	(B)	(C)
1	27	18	11	6	18	19	26
2	32	21	12	7	35	26	14
3	24	22	16	8	31	28	18
4	20	18	23	9	30	20	32
5	26	24	13	10	25	34	30

We note that if there are no ties in the data, $\overline{T}$ and K can be simplifies as follows:

$$\overline{T} = \frac{N(N+1)(2N+1)(8N+11)}{180},$$

$$K = \frac{(N+1)(2N+1)}{6}$$

If the null hypothesis is true, the test statistic T^* is approximately χ^2 with $(k-1)$ degrees of freedom. At this point the hypothesis test will proceed as if it is a usual χ^2 test, so the null hypothesis is rejected if $T^* > \chi^2_{(k-1,1-\alpha)}$. When we reject the null hypothesis, multiple comparisons procedure will be used to compare the ith and j^{th} populations. In such a case, the variances of the ith and j^{th} populations are said to be different if

$$\left| \frac{T_i}{n_i} - \frac{T_j}{n_j} \right| > t_{(N-k,1-\alpha/2)} \left[K \cdot \frac{(N-1-T^*)}{N-k} \right]^{1/2}$$
$$\times \left[\frac{1}{n_i} + \frac{1}{n_j} \right]^{1/2}$$

Example 14.10.2. Ten single-rooted human teeth were inoculated with saliva and incubated for 7 days. After 7 days, dentin samples were taken at coronal (A), midroot (B), and apex (C). These samples were cultured for anaerobic bacteria, and the number of species in each sample was reported. It is known that the samples do not follow a normal distribution. Test the hypotheses $H_0 : \sigma_A^2 = \sigma_B^2 = \sigma_C^2$ vs. $H_1 :$ variances are not equal.

Solution. From the data in Table 14.10.2, the sample means are obtained; $\overline{X}_A = 26.8$, $\overline{X}_B = 23.0$, $\overline{X}_C = 19.5$. Following the steps described above, we compute the sum of the squares of the rank of the each of the three samples: $T_A = 2,695.0$, $T_B = 2,158.0$, and $T_C = 4,598.0$. The average of

all the squared ranks is

$$\overline{T} = (2,695 + 2,158 + 4,598)/30 = 315.03$$

Hence,

$$N \cdot (\overline{T})^2 = 30 \cdot (315.03)^2 = 2,977,317.027$$

$$K = \frac{1}{N-1} \left[\sum_{i=1}^{k} \sum_{j=1}^{n_i} R_{ij}^4 - N \cdot (\overline{T})^2 \right]$$

$$= \frac{1}{30-1} [5,268,365 - 2,977,317.027]$$

$$= 79,001.654$$

We can now compute the test statistic

$$T^* = \frac{1}{K} \left[\sum_{i=1}^{k} \frac{T_i^2}{n_i} - N \cdot (\overline{T})^2 \right]$$

$$= \frac{1}{79001.654} (3306159.3 - 2977\,317.027)$$

$$= 4.1625 < \chi^2_{(2,0.95)} = 5.99.$$

The null hypothesis of no difference in variance is accepted.

14.11 SPEARMAN'S RANK CORRELATION COEFFICIENT

A measure of correlation between two variables X and Y was introduced in Section 11.3. The Pearson product moment correlation coefficient ρ ranges from -1 to $+1$. To test the hypothesis that $H_0 : \rho = 0$, we require that samples are drawn from normal populations. **Spearman rank correlation coefficient** is an alternative to the Pearson correlation coefficient when the normality assumption is not appropriate. This non-parametric equivalent can be used when the data can be ranked. The computations for the Spearman rank correlation coefficient is simpler than the Pearson correlation coefficient because they involve ranking the samples. If both samples have the same ranks, then ρ will be $+1$. If the ranks of the two samples are completely opposite, then ρ will be -1. Suppose we have two sets of data that are paired as (X_1, Y_1), $(X_2, Y_2), \cdots, (X_n, Y_n)$, These pairs of observations may represent height (X_i) and weight (Y_i) of n patients. Let $R(X_i)$ be the rank of ith subject's height as compared to the heights of other subjects. Similarly, let $R(Y_i)$ be the rank of ith subject's weight

Table 14.11.1. Bone height (mm) and implant failure time (in month) data.

	1	2	3	4	5	6	7	8	9	10
Bone ht. (X_i)	5.4	3.5	7.0	8.2	6.8	6.4	8.2	2.7	6.5	4.6
Survival time (Y_i)	110	86	113	132	120	92	135	71	106	93
Rank $R(X_i)$	4	2	8	9.5	7	5	9.5	1	6	3
Rank $R(Y_i)$	6	2	7	9	8	3	10	1	5	4
$U = R(X_i) - 5.5$	-1.5	-3.5	2.5	4.0	1.5	-0.5	4.0	-4.5	0.5	-2.5
$V = R(Y_i) - 5.5$	0.5	-3.5	1.5	3.5	2.5	-2.5	4.5	-4.5	-0.5	-1.5
$U \cdot V$	-0.75	12.25	3.75	14.0	3.75	1.25	18.0	20.25	-0.25	3.75

$U \cdot V = [R(X_i) - 5.5] \cdot [R(Y_i) - 5.5]$

as compared to the weights of other subjects. If there are no ties, the Spearman rank correlation coefficient is defined by

$$\rho = \frac{\sum_{i=1}^{n} \left[R(X_i) - \frac{n+1}{2} \right] \left[R(Y_i) - \frac{n+1}{2} \right]}{n(n^2 - 1)/12}$$

If there are many ties, the Spearman rank correlation coefficient is given by

$$\rho = \frac{\sum_{i=1}^{n} [R(X_i) \cdot R(Y_i)] - n \cdot \left(\frac{n+1}{2} \right)^2}{\sqrt{\sum_{i=1}^{n} [R(X_i)]^2 - n \cdot \left(\frac{n+1}{2} \right)^2} \cdot \sqrt{\sum_{i=1}^{n} [R(Y_i)]^2 - n \cdot \left(\frac{n+1}{2} \right)^2}}$$

This can be viewed as the Pearson correlation coefficient computed on the ranks of X_i and Y_i and their average ranks. If only a moderate number of ties are involved, the first formula, which is less cumbersome, may be used.

Example 14.11.1. Suppose that 10 patients received titanium implants. To study the relationship between the bone height at the time of implant placement and the implant survival rate, investigators carefully measured the subject's bone height and followed implant failure time of each patient in the study. The data is presented in Table 14.11.1. Assuming that both the bone height and survival time data are not normally distributed, determine the Spearman rank correlation coefficient.

Solution. Since there are 10 subjects in the study, we have $\frac{n+1}{2} = \frac{10+1}{2} = 5.5$. Since there are only two ties in the bone height measurements, we

will use the first formula.

$$\rho = \frac{\sum_{i=1}^{n} \left[R(X_i) - \frac{n+1}{2} \right] \left[R(Y_i) - \frac{n+1}{2} \right]}{n(n^2 - 1)/12}$$

$$= \frac{\sum_{i=1}^{n} [R(X_i) - 5.5][R(Y_i) - 5.5]}{10(10^2 - 1)/12}$$

$$= \frac{76.0}{10(10^2 - 1)/12} = 0.9212$$

Bone height and implant survival time have a very high Spearman rank correlation coefficient of 0.9212.

14.12 EXERCISES

1 In order to determine the effect of chlorhexidine on the salivary *Streptococcus mutans* (SM) levels, 18 subjects were recruited into a clinical study. Each subject submitted a saliva sample that was tested to establish a baseline (BL) colony count. Subjects were instructed to rinse twice daily with 0.12% chlorhexidine mouthrinse over a 2-week period. Four weeks after the end of the period, another saliva sample was taken from the subjects to investigate the recolonization trends. Saliva samples were tested using a commercially available strip test. The value of 0 is given to a sample with less than 3, 000 colony-forming units per milliliter

(CFU/ml), and 1 to a sample with greater than 3, 000 (CFU/ml). Data is summarized in the table below. Perform an appropriate test to determine if chlorhexidine is effective in reducing the salivary SM.

Subj no.	BL	4-wk	Subj no.	BL	4-wk
1	1	0	19	1	0
2	1	1	20	1	0
3	0	0	21	1	1
4	1	0	22	1	0
5	1	0	23	0	1
6	1	1	24	1	0
7	1	0	25	0	1
8	0	1	26	1	0
9	1	0	27	1	0
10	1	0	28	1	0
11	1	0	29	1	0
12	0	0	30	0	1
13	1	0	31	0	1
14	1	0	32	1	0
15	0	1	33	0	1
16	0	1	34	0	1
17	1	0	35	1	0
18	1	1	36	1	0

2 HGH Corporation has made a substantial quality improvement on their top selling medical product. The company's marketing department wants to find out if there is any difference in consumer preference scores between old and new improved products. If you were the company's marketing scientist, what would be your conclusion based on the following data.

Original product:	71,	82,	84,	69,	88,	93,
	56,	78,	80,	79,	56,	88,
	90,	72,	77,	81		
Improved product:	85,	66,	98,	67,	79,	81,
	82,	95,	88,	87,	79,	92,
	82,	93,	87,	94		

3 A major consumer complaint about adhesive bandages is that they come off when moistened. A pharmaceutical company has developed two types of adhesive bandage: type A and type B. The company needs to determine which one stays on longer. They selected 17 college students and asked them to apply both types of bandage to the same area. The following data indicates the number of hours

the bandages stayed on the skin. Is there a difference between A and B?

Subject	1	2	3	4	5	6	7	8	9
Type A	33	14	42	33	23	20	28	19	22
Type B	37	26	35	31	23	38	43	33	42

Subject		10	11	12	13	14	15	16	17
Type A		18	49	31	29	21	30	39	27
Type B		35	45	40	32	34	43	28	38

4 Investigators prepared 12 samples of each of two sealants, A and B. Their goal is to compare bond strength, which was measured in Newtons using an Instron machine. State the hypotheses and perform a significance test at $\alpha = 0.05$.

X_i (Sealant A)				Y_i (Sealant B)			
8.15	9.32	7.16	9.01	11.46	13.96	17.65	17.05
9.65	8.04	6.47	7.54	12.01	18.74	15.55	13.04
10.14	6.55	6.45	11.23	9.00	8.42	16.65	10.46

5 Two different formulations of a tablet of a new drug are to be compared with regard to rate of dissolution. Fourteen tablets of formulation A and 12 tablets of formulation B are tested, and the percent of dissolution after 15 min. in the dissolution apparatus is observed. From the results tabulated below, perform a significance test to determine whether they came from populations having the same median.

Formulation A	68	84	81	85	75	74	79
	80	65	90	77	72	69	78
Fromulation B	80	63	79	74	71	61	69
	65	80	72	76	75		

6 The following data represent blood protein levels (g/100 ml) for the comparison of four drugs. All four drugs were tested on each subject in random order. What conclusion can you draw regarding their median?

Patient	1	2	3	4	5	6	7	8	9	10	11	12
Drug A	9.3	6.6	8.1	7.2	6.3	6.6	7.0	7.7	8.6	8.1	9.0	8.3
Drug B	9.2	8.2	9.9	7.3	7.0	9.1	9.0	8.9	8.3	8.3	8.8	6.0
Drug C	7.4	7.1	6.2	6.1	8.0	8.2	7.5	6.8	6.7	8.4	7.7	7.5
Drug D	6.0	5.8	4.9	6.5	6.3	7.2	6.9	8.1	6.4	7.2	6.6	7.4

7 Eleven patients were randomly selected to evaluate four different alginate flavorings for patient preference. All four of them were used for each subject and patients were asked to rank them from 1 (worst) to 4 (best). Given the following data, perform an appropriate test to determine if there are any differences in patient preference among the four flavorings?

	1	2	3	4	5	6	7	8	9	10	11
Strawberry	3	2	3	2	3	2	2	2	3	1	2
Chocolate	2	2	4	1	1	3	1	1	2	2	1
Mint	1	3	2	4	2	3	4	4	4	3	3
Pineapple	4	4	1	3	4	4	3	3	1	4	4

8 There are 10 football teams in the Pacific Coast Conference. All 10 teams played a non-conference game at the start of the season. Four football fans were selected from third-year dental school class. They predicted the outcome of the games, and the results of their predictions were tabulated with 0 = wrong prediction and 1 = correct prediction. Perform an appropriate test to determine if there is any consistency in their ability to predict the outcome of the games?

	John	Dave	Melissa	Sam
Team 1	0	0	1	1
2	1	1	1	1
3	1	1	0	1
4	0	1	1	1
5	0	0	0	0
Team 6	0	1	0	0
7	1	0	1	1
8	0	0	1	1
9	1	0	1	0
10	1	0	0	1

9 The data tabulated in the table below represent the measurement (in millimeters) of the length of maxillary central incisors using a manual caliper and a computerized device. Suppose the measurements are not normally distributed. Are the measurements done by a computerized device more precise?

	1	2	3	4	5	6	7
Manual	10.0	10.4	11.1	10.9	10.6	9.8	9.7
Computer	10.3	10.2	9.8	10.6	10.7	10.3	10.2

	8	9	10	11	12	13
Manual	10.5	11.2	10.8	9.1		
Computer	9.9	10.0	10.2	10.1	10.1	9.9

10 Fifteen patients were selected at random from a clinic to study the relationship between blood pressure and the amount of weekly exercise. The amount of exercise represents the average daily exercise in minutes. Compute the Spearman rank correlation coefficient.

Patient	SBP	Exercise	Patient	SBP	Exercise
1	146	25	8	148	35
2	134	30	9	139	28
3	152	15	10	175	0
4	129	45	11	126	37
5	168	10	12	120	40
6	115	35	13	116	40
7	155	28	14	138	22
			15	140	15

14.13 REFERENCES

1. Weltman, R. et al. Assessment of guided tissue regeneration procedures in intrabony defects with bioabsorbable and non-resorbable barriers. *J. Periodontol*: 1997, 68: 582–591.
2. Conover, W. J. *Practical Nonparametric Statistics*. Second edition. John Wiley & Sons, Inc. 1980.
3. Siegel, S., and Castellan, N. J. *Nonparametric Statistics for the Behavioral Sciences*. Second edition. McGraw Hill. 1988.
4. Christgau, M. et al. GTR therapy of intrabony defects using 2 different bioresorbable membranes: 12-month results. *J Clin Periodontol*: 1998, 25: 499–509.
5. Kavanaugh, J. A Comparison of Three LED Curing Lights Measured by Tensile Bond Strength. MA thesis. Loma Linda University. 2003.
6. Hernandez, Y., Poh, A., and Robinson, J. The Effects of Alcohol on Composite Resins. Student project. Loma Linda University. 2003.

Chapter 15

Survival Analysis

15.1 INTRODUCTION

In clinical trials in dentistry and medicine, success is usually measured in terms of the lifetime, which is a continuous variable, that a certain desirable condition is maintained, such as survival of implants or remission of cancer. In many situations, however, it is inconvenient or impossible for investigators to observe the precise failure time or the time of death of all members of a random sample. For example, in dental implant follow-up studies to determine the lifetime distribution (i.e., survival function) after the implants have been placed, patients failed to visit the clinic for follow-up examinations or contact with some patients was lost for a variety of reasons. In medical studies, patients could be lost for follow-up before their death (or relapse) or the studies have been terminated before the investigators had an opportunity to observe the death of every subject in the study sample. Those patients for whom implant failure time or relapse time is not observed are said to yield **incomplete** or **censored** observations. A sample that contains censored observations is referred to as **censored data** in survival analysis. The key variable in this section is time-related lifetime or survival time. Survival time is defined as the time to the occurrence of a certain event, such as the failure of an implant, death of a patient, relapse, or development of a disease. These times are subject to random variations.

To illustrate survival data containing censored observations, consider the following implant failure times in months for nine patients: 12^+, 24, 68, 68^+, 68^+, 98, 120^+, 144^+, 144^+. Six censored observations and 3 uncensored (or complete) observations are included in the data. The "+" sign indicates the observations that have been censored for various reasons. The failure time measurement of 12^+ indicates that the patient's implant was known to be functioning for 12 months after its place-

ment, but that the patient was lost to follow-up or withdrawn from the studies. The investigators have no knowledge as to how much longer the implant would have provided its intended service had the subject remained in the study. The three uncensored observations indicate that the investigators did observe the implant failure times at 24, 68, and 98 months.

Many studies in biomedical sciences are designed to evaluate whether a new treatment or a new procedure will perform better than the one currently being used or compare two or more treatment options to provide more effective and better quality health care with most desirable outcomes. The readers should keep in mind that censored data occurs naturally in biomedical research projects. Not all patients have the implants placed at the same time. Patients enter the clinical trial for a newly developed treatment at different time points. Situations such as loss of patients to follow-up, withdrawal from the study, or termination of the study for data analysis give rise to survival data that is censored. Analysis of survival data was used in 13.7% of the articles published in *The International Journal of Oral & Maxillofacial Implants* between 1986 and 2002. It is reported that survival analysis was used in 32% of the papers in *The New England Journal of Medicine* [1]. The statistical methods of data analysis discussed in the previous sections are not appropriate for the type of survival data obtained from measuring the length of lifetime. In this chapter, special methods needed to analyze survival times will be discussed.

15.2 PERSON-TIME METHOD AND MORTALITY RATE

A concept often used in epidemiology is **person-years on observation,** which is defined by the number of failures (or deaths) per 100 person-years

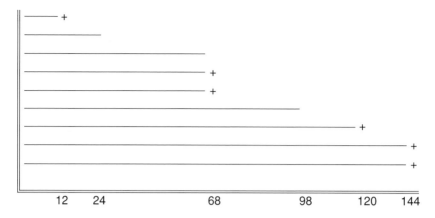

Figure 15.1.1 Censored data with nine patients arranged in ascending order ("+" sign represents a censored observation).

under observation during the study period. To describe this method, consider the data illustrated in Figure 15.1.1. The first patient remained in the study for 12 months before being withdrawn from the study, contributing the value of 12 to the calculation of the total time the investigators spent on observations. The implant failure of the second patient was observed by the investigators after 24 months. From the figure it is clear that the investigators observed the failure time of one patient after 68 months, and two patients were lost to follow-up at 68 months. Thus, each of the three patients contributed the value of 68 months to the total time on observation. Implant failure was observed for the sixth patient at 98 months. The seventh patient was censored at 120 months. The last two patients were censored when the study was terminated at 144 months. The total time on observation is calculated by adding individual contributions as follows:

$$\text{Total time} = 12 + 24 + (68 \times 3) + 98$$
$$+ 120 + (144 \times 2) = 746 \text{ (months)}$$

Dividing 746 months by 12 yields 62.167 person-years. The investigators spend a total of 62.167 person-years observing the 9 patients during the study period. During the period, three implants failed. This gives $3 \div 62.167 = 0.0483$ or 4.83 failures per 100 person-years on observation. There are a few problems with using this method:

1. The method inherently assumes the constant failure rate (or survival rate) over any fixed time interval within the study period, which is unrealistic in most cases. This is the most serious problem.

2. The same value of 100 years for the total time on observation will be obtained by observing 10 patients for 10 years or by observing 100 patients for 1 year.

3. The censored observation 12^+ could have been a complete observation if the patient had not withdrawn from the study, increasing the number of failures from three to four if the patient had not withdrawn.

Mortality rate is a standard method used by investigators in epidemiology and biomedical sciences that is designed to compare incidents of death or failure occurring in different populations. Mortality rate is defined by dividing the number of subjects who died in a given time period by the number of subjects at risk of dying in the same period. The mortality rate depends heavily on *when* the data analysis is performed. If it is calculated at the very early stage of the study when there are no occurrences of death, the mortality rate will be zero (0%). If the study period is long enough and the calculation is done at the end of the study when all subjects at risk have died, the mortality rate will be 100%. Thus the typical approach taken in oncology research is 2- or 5-year mortality rate in which only those subjects who have been in the study for 2 or 5 years are used in the data. The shortcoming of this approach is that the contributions from the censored subjects who withdrew, for example, 4 years after entering the clinical trial are completely ignored. The approach is generally accepted when a large number of subjects is being followed, provided the proportion of censored observations is at a manageable level.

Table 15.2.1. Interval failure rate for 894 implants.

Interval (month)	No. of Implants at Beginning of Interval	No. of Implant Failed during Interval	Interval Failure Rate (%)
0–12	894	13	1.5
12–24	702	12	1.7
24–36	445	9	2.0
36–48	189	5	2.6
48–60+	88	3	3.4

The concept of **interval failure rate** discussed in implant literature is similar to that of mortality rate. Table 15.2.1 shows typical success rate data that represent survival times of 894 implants placed by utilizing a variety of prosthodontic designs. Like the calculations for mortality rate, interval failure rate for the first interval is calculated by dividing the number of failures in the interval by the number of implants at the beginning of the interval, that is, $13/894 = 0.015$ (1.5%). Interval failure rates for other intervals are calculated likewise. The five interval failure rates given in Table 15.2.1 are equivalent to mortality rates calculated for five distinct time periods. Since there are 894 implants at the beginning of the first interval, 13 of which failed in the interval and 702 implants are still functioning at the beginning of the second interval, the number of censored implants during the first interval is $894 - 13 - 702 = 179$. These 179 implants have been censored at various time points during the first interval (0–12 months). Note that the failure time contributions from these censored implants have been ignored in the calculation of the interval failure rate. The methods that take uncensored (i.e., complete) as well as censored observations into consideration—actuarial life table analysis, Kaplan-Meier product limit estimator, and piecewise exponential extimator—are discussed in the following sections.

15.3 LIFE TABLE ANALYSIS

One of the primary goals of survival analysis is to estimate the survival function, denoted $S(t)$. In the above example, $S(t)$ represents the probability of dental implants successfully providing intended services for at least t months or patients remaining in remission for at least t weeks. Whether it is t months or t weeks, the time unit is immaterial for the discussion. The survival function is also referred to as survival probability, cumulative survival rate, or survival curve. In engineering and physical sciences, it is called system reliability or reliability function. The life table analysis is one of the oldest techniques developed for studying the survival experience of a population. It has been widely used by actuaries in the insurance industry, demographers, and medical researchers.

Let the time axis be partitioned into a fixed sequence of interval, $I_1, I_2, \cdots, I_k$. These intervals are usually, but not necessarily, of equal length. In most of the applications in implant dentistry, the length of each interval is one year. In Figure 15.3.1 below, $t_0 = 0, t_1 = 12, t_2 = 24, \cdots, t_5 = 60$.

It is necessary to introduce some notation to facilitate the discussion.

Let
d_i = No. of implants failed during the interval I_i;
w_i = No. of implants withdrawn during the interval I_i;
p_i = probability of surviving through I_i, given that it is functioning at the beginning of I_i; and
$q_i = 1 - p_i$ = probability of failure during I_i, given that it is functioning at the beginning of I_i.

From the summary of survival data presented in Table 15.3.1,

$$n_0 = 894, \quad n_1 = 702, \quad n_2 = 445, \quad n_3 = 189, \quad n_4 = 88$$
$$d_1 = 13, \quad d_2 = 12, \quad d_3 = 9, \quad d_4 = 5, \quad d_5 = 3$$
$$w_1 = 179, \quad w_2 = 245, \quad w_3 = 247, \quad w_4 = 96, \quad w_5 = 85$$

In survival analysis, it is said that $n_0 = 894$ are at risk of failing at the beginning of interval I_1, $n_1 = 702$ are at risk of failing at the beginning

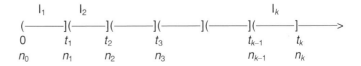

Figure 15.3.1 A sequence of time intervals.

Table 15.3.1. Implant survival data.

Months Since Implant Placement	No. of Implants Functioning at Beginning of Interval (n_i)	No. of Implant Failed during Interval (d_j)	No. of Implants Withdrawn or Lost to Follow-up
0–12	894	13	179
12–24	702	12	245
24–36	445	9	247
36–48	189	5	96
48–60+	88	3	85

of interval I_2, etc. The life table method gives an estimate for each p_i, the probability of survival during each time interval I_i, and then multiplies the estimates together to obtain an estimate of the survival function $S(t)$. The probability p_i can be estimated by using

$$p_i = 1 - \frac{d_i}{n_i} \quad \text{if there were no withdrawals in } I_i (w_i = 0).$$

If there were withdrawals, then it is assumed that on the average, these implants that were censored during interval I_i were at risk for half the length of the interval. Therefore, the **effective sample size,** n_i^*, can be defined by

$$n_i^* = n_i - \frac{1}{2} w_i.$$

Hence, estimates are given by $\widehat{q}_i = \frac{d_i}{n_i^*}$, and $\widehat{p}_i = 1 - \frac{d_i}{n_i^*}$. The actuarial estimate of the survival function is

$$\widehat{S}(t_k) = \widehat{p}_1 \widehat{p}_2 \cdots \widehat{p}_k.$$

From the discussions in this section, we know that the values of the survival function $\widehat{S}(t_k)$ in different samples will be different due to inherent uncertainty. The estimate of the variance of $\widehat{S}(t_k)$ is

obtained by Greenwood's formula [2] as follows:

$$\widehat{Var}[\widehat{S}(t_k)] = [\widehat{S}(t_k)]^2 \cdot \sum_{i=1}^{k} \frac{d_i}{n_i^*(n_i^* - d_i)}.$$

The standard error of $\widehat{S}(t_k)$ is given by

$$SE[\widehat{S}(t_k)] = [\widehat{S}(t_k)] \cdot \sqrt{\sum_{i=1}^{k} \frac{d_i}{n_i^*(n_i^* - d_i)}}.$$

Table 15.3.2 presents a life table analysis based on the implant survival data in Table 15.3.1.

The actuarial life table method assumes that all withdrawals during a given interval occur on the average at the midpoint of the interval. If the length of the intervals is small, a violation of this assumption may not be serious. However, if the length of the intervals is large, then it may introduce a considerable amount of bias. Many withdrawals could occur in a interval that do not occur at the midpoint. The second assumption is that probability of survival in one particular interval is statistically independent of the probability of survival in any other intervals.

15.4 HAZARD FUNCTION

The survival function is defined as the probability that an implant (or a subject) survives at least a specified time period. In this section, the concept of

Table 15.3.2. Life table analysis of implant survival data.

Interval I_i	Effective Sample Size n_i^*	Probability of Failure $\widehat{q}_i$	Probability of Surviving $\widehat{p}_i$	Cumulative Survival Rate $\widehat{S}(t_i)$
0–12	894 − (179/2) = 804.5	13/804.5 = 0.016	0.984	0.984
12–24	702 − (245/2) = 579.5	12/579.5 = 0.021	0.979	0.963
24–36	445 − (247/2) = 321.5	9/321.5 = 0.028	0.972	0.936
36–48	189 − (96/2) = 141.0	5/141.0 = 0.035	0.965	0.904
48–60	88 − (85/2) = 45.5	3/45.5 = 0.066	0.934	0.844

the hazard function will be introduced. The probability distribution of survival times can be characterized by three functions, one of which is known as the hazard function. Given a set of data, the users of statistics would like to calculate the mean and standard deviation. Investigators have learned that the problem with survival time data is that the mean survival time depends on *when* the data is analyzed. The unique feature of survival data is that the subjects typically join the study at different time points, may withdraw from the study, or may be lost to follow-up. Thus, the value of the average survival time will change as time elapses until the point at which the lifetimes of all of the implants in the study have been observed. In survival analysis, it is often unrealistic to expect a set of data without any censored observations. However, there is a procedure that gives a reasonable estimate of mean survival time when the sample size is fairly large. The procedure, called the *hazard function,* is defined as the probability that an implant fails in a time interval between t and $t + \Delta t$, given that the implant has survived until time t. In statistics, this concept is known as the conditional probability. In engineering, the term *instantaneous failure rate* and in epidemiology, the term *force of mortality* are more commonly used. The hazard function is a measure of the likelihood of failure as a function of the age of the individual implants. The hazard function reflects the risk of failure per unit time during the aging process of the implant. It plays an important role in the study of survival times. In practice, when there are no censored observations, the hazard function is estimated as the proportion of implants failing in an interval per time unit, given that they have survived to the beginning of the interval:

$$\widehat{h}(t) = \frac{\text{number of implants failing in the interval beginning at time } t}{(\text{number of implants functioning at } t) \cdot (\text{width of the interval})}$$

$$= \frac{\text{number of implants failing per time unit in the interval}}{\text{number of implants functioning at } t}$$

In actuarial sciences, the hazard function, $\widehat{h}(t)$, is defined by

$$\widehat{h}(t) = \frac{\text{number of implants failing per time unit in the interval}}{(\text{number of implants functioning at } t) - (\frac{1}{2})(\text{number of implant failures in the interval})}$$

When failure times are observed, and if it is reasonable to assume that the shape of a survival curve follows what is known as an exponential distribution, the hazard function can be expressed as given

below and the mean survival time is obtained by taking its reciprocal:

$$\widehat{h} = \frac{\text{number of implant failures}}{(\text{sum of failure times}) + (\text{sum of censored times})}$$

To illustrate the hazard rate, consider a simple example.

Example 15.4.1. A prosthodontist has collected the following time data (in month) from 16 patients who had received implant-supported fixed partial dentures that were cement retained. Failures were defined by complications such as porcelain fracture, cement washout, implant failure, and loose central screws. There are 4 uncensored and 12 censored observations in the data displayed in the following table. The sums of failure times and censored observations are as follows:

Sum of failure times $= 16.5 + 12.0 + 5.5 + 14.5 = 48.5$

Sum of censored times $= 35 + 34 + 27 + 27 + 25 + 23 + 22 + 15 + 14 + 11 + 7 + 5.5 = 245.5$

Patient No.	Date of Treatment	Date of Failure	Survival Time
1	1/14/00	6/2/01	16.5
2	1/31/00		35.0+
3	3/2/00		34.0+
4	5/3/00	4/30/01	12.0
5	7/28/00	1/16/01	5.5
6	9/25/00		27.0+
7	10/4/00		27.0+
8	11/30/00		25.0+
9	1/30/01		23.0+
10	3/5/01		22.0+
11	6/26/01	9/15/02	14.5
12	9/27/01		15.0+
13	11/2/01		14.0+
14	2/4/02		11.0+
15	5/31/02		7.0+
16	7/17/02		5.5+

The hazard rate is: $\widehat{h} = \dfrac{4}{48.5 + 245.5}$
$= 0.0136.$

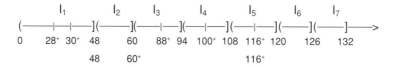

Figure 15.5.1 Display of survival data for porcelain-faced crowns.

So the mean survival time of the survival data in Example 15.4.1 is estimated to be

$$\overline{X} = \frac{1}{\hat{h}} = \frac{1}{0.0136} = 73.5 \text{ (months)}.$$

15.5 KAPLAN-MEIER PRODUCT LIMIT ESTIMATOR

The Kaplan-Meier product limit estimator [3] has become the most commonly used approach to survival analysis in biomedical sciences. The Kaplan-Meier estimator is similar to the actuarial life table analysis except the intervals I_i are determined by the time points at which failures are observed. Because failures occur at random, the lengths of the intervals I_i are random variables. Consider the following example to illustrate the Kaplan-Meier method. Porcelain-faced crowns placed in anterior maxilla were studied retrospectively. A 11-year study resulted in survival data consisting 15 samples. These 15 observations in month are displayed in Figure 15.5.1.

28^+, 30^+, 48, 48, 60, 60^+, 88^+, 94, 100^+, 108, 116^+, 116^+, 120, 126, 132.

There are two uncensored observations (failures) tied at 48 months, two censored observation tied at 116^+ months, and one uncensored and one censored observation tied at 60 months. In the latter case, it is reasonable to assume that the censored observation at 60^+ occurred just a little bit later than the uncensored observation at 60. It is easy to see that seven intervals are obtained from the survival data:

$I_1 = (0, 48]$, $I_2 = (48, 60]$, $I_3 = (60, 94]$,
$I_4 = (94, 108]$, $I_5 = (108, 120]$,
$I_6 = (120, 126]$, $I_7 = (126, 132]$.

Note that there are two censored observations in interval I_1, none in I_2, two in I_3, one in I_4, two in I_5, none in I_6 and I_7.

Table 15.5.1. Porcelain crown survival data.

i	t_i	c_i	d_i	n_i
0	$t_0 = 0$	$c_0 = 0$	$d_0 = 0$	$n_0 = 15$
1	$t_1 = 48$	$c_1 = 2$	$d_1 = 2$	$n_1 = 13$
2	$t_2 = 60$	$c_2 = 0$	$d_2 = 1$	$n_2 = 11$
3	$t_3 = 94$	$c_3 = 2$	$d_3 = 1$	$n_3 = 8$
4	$t_4 = 108$	$c_4 = 1$	$d_4 = 1$	$n_4 = 6$
5	$t_5 = 120$	$c_5 = 2$	$d_5 = 1$	$n_5 = 3$
6	$t_6 = 126$	$c_6 = 0$	$d_6 = 1$	$n_6 = 2$
7	$t_7 = 132$	$c_7 = 0$	$d_7 = 1$	$n_7 = 1$

Let
t_i = the time at which the ith failure is observed,
c_i = the number of crowns censored in the interval I_i,
d_i = the number of crowns failed at t_i,
n_i = the number of crowns at risk at instant before t_i.

It can be seen that n_i is given by a simple formula $n_i = n_{i-1} - c_i - d_{i-1}$, where $n_0 = 15$, $c_0 = 0$, and $d_0 = 0$. For example, since $n_0 = 15$, $c_1 = 2$, and $d_0 = 0$; $n_1 = n_0 - c_1 - d_0 = 15 - 2 - 0 = 13$. The values of t_i, c_i, d_i, and n_i are presented in Table 15.5.1. Let $p_i = P(\text{surviving through } I_i,$ given that crowns were functioning at the beginning of $I_i)$. Then $\hat{p}_i = \dfrac{n_{i-1} - d_{i-1}}{n_{i-1}}$. If there are no tied uncensored observations, then $d_i = 1$ for all $i = 1, 2, \cdots, k$, and $\hat{p}_i$ will be obtained by $\hat{p}_i = \dfrac{n_{i-1} - 1}{n_{i-1}}$ (Table 15.5.2). The Kaplan-Meier product limit estimator is given by

$$\hat{S}(t_i) = \hat{p}_1 \hat{p}_2 \cdots \hat{p}_i.$$

Example 15.5.1. Table 15.5.3.a and Table 15.5.3.b display implant survival data for patients whose bone height was $< 2\,\text{mm}$ or $> 4\,\text{mm}$ at the time of the implant placement. If a patient had more than two implants, one of the implants was randomly selected for the survival study. There were 41 patients with bone height $< 2\,\text{mm}$ and 56 patients with bone height $> 4\,\text{mm}$ for the

Table 15.5.2. Kaplan-Meier product limit estimates for porcelain-faced crown data.

I_i	c_i	d_i	n_i	$\widehat{p}_i$	$\widehat{S}(t_i)$
1	2	2	13	1.0	1.0
2	0	1	11	0.846	0.846
3	2	1	8	0.909	0.769
4	1	1	6	0.875	0.673
5	2	1	3	0.833	0.561
6	0	1	2	0.667	0.374
7	0	1	1	0.5	0.187

Table 15.5.4.a. Kaplan-Meier survival probability for censored data for BH < 2 mm.

I_i	c_i	d_i	n_i	$\widehat{p}_i$	$\widehat{S}(t)$
1	1	0	41	1.0	1.0
2	4	1	40	0.976	0.976
3	1	2	35	0.943	0.920
4	1	1	32	0.969	0.891
5	1	2	30	0.933	0.831
6	3	1	27	0.963	0.800
7	1	2	23	0.913	0.730
8	2	1	20	0.950	0.694
9	1	1	17	0.941	0.653
10	2	1	15	0.933	0.609
11	1	1	12	0.917	0.558
12	5	3	10	0.700	0.391

study. As usual, " $+$ " sign indicates the censored observation.

Figures 15.5.1 and 15.5.2 exhibit Kaplan-Meier product limit estimator for the survival data in Table 15.5.3.a and Table 15.5.3.b. Notice there are 11 distinct failure time points in the Table 15.5.4.a, and 7 distinct failure time points in Table 15.5.4.b. Figure 15.5.3 shows that the implant survival for those patients with bone height < 2 mm is much lower than those with bone height > 4 mm. A comparison between two survival functions will be studied rigorously in Section 15.6.

Note that the largest observed survival time in Table 15.5.3.a is 60^+, which is censored, while the largest observation in Table 15.5.3.b is 58, which is uncensored. If the largest observation is uncensored, the Kaplan-Meier product limit estimator gives the survival function equal to zero (0) beyond 58 months. If the largest observation is censored as in Table 15.5.3.a, the Kaplan-Meier estimator gives the survival function equal to 0.391 for the survival time well beyond 60 months. This makes some statisticians uncomfortable as survival functions are expected to reach zero at some time in the future. The standard error S_i of the estimate of

Table 15.5.4.b. Kaplan-Meier survival probability for censored data for BH > 4 mm.

I_i	c_i	d_i	n_i	$\widehat{p}_i$	$\widehat{S}(t)$
1	24	0	56	1.0	1.0
2	3	1	32	0.969	0.969
3	7	2	28	0.929	0.900
4	3	2	19	0.895	0.801
5	0	1	14	0.929	0.744
6	4	1	13	0.923	0.687
7	5	1	8	0.875	0.601
8	0	2	2	0.0	0.0

the cumulative survival function $\widehat{S}(t_i)$ is quite similar to the standard error for an actuarial estimate discussed in Section 15.3. The standard error for the Kaplan-Meier product limit estimate is given by Greenwood [4],

$$SE(\widehat{S}(t_i)) = \widehat{S}(t_i)\sqrt{\sum \frac{d_i}{n_i\,(n_i - d_i)}}.$$

Using the standard error, confidence limits for the survival curve can be obtained. For example,

Table 15.5.3.a. Implant survival data for patients with bone height < 2 mm.

5^+	6	6^+	8^+	8^+	9^+	10	10	12^+	15	16^+
18	18	21^+	23	25^+	26^+	26^+	28	28	34^+	35
35^+	36^+	42	45^+	46	47^+	50^+	52	56^+	58	58
58	60^+	60^+	60^+	60^+	60^+	60^+	60^+			

Table 15.5.3.b. Implant survival data for patients with bone height > 4 mm.

6^+	6^+	6^+	6^+	6^+	8^+	9^+	9^+	9^+	9^+	12^+	12^+
12^+	12^+	18^+	18^+	18^+	18^+	18^+	18^+	22^+	22^+	22^+	22^+
24	26^+	28^+	28^+	33	33	35^+	36^+	38^+	38^+	39^+	40^+
40^+	44	44	47^+	47^+	47^+	48	50	50^+	54^+	54^+	54^+
56	56^+	56^+	56^+	56^+	56^+	58	58				

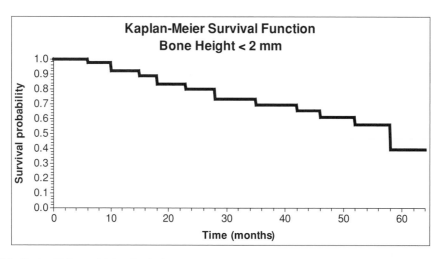

Figure 15.5.1 Kaplan-Meier survial function for impant data with BH ≤ 2 mm.

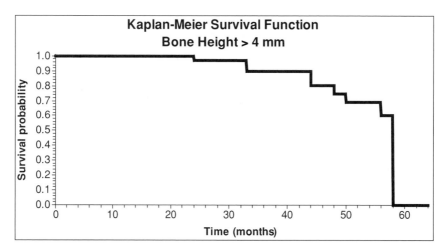

Figure 15.5.2 Kaplan-Meier survival function for implant data with BH ≥ 4 mm.

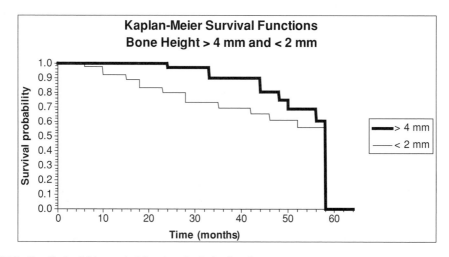

Figure 15.5.3 Two Kaplan-Meier survival functions for the implant data.

Table 15.5.5. Necessary calculations for 95% confidence bands for Kaplan-Meier survival curve for the implant data in Table 15.5.3.a.

I_i	n_i	d_i	$\widehat{S}(t_i)$	$\dfrac{d_i}{n_i(n_i-d_i)}$	$\sum \dfrac{d_i}{n_i(n_i-d_i)}$	$\widehat{S}(t_i)\sqrt{\sum \dfrac{d_i}{n_i(n_i-d_i)}}$	$\pm 1.96 \cdot SE(\widehat{S}(t_i))$
1	41	0	1.0	0.0	0.0	0.0	±0.0
2	40	1	.976	.0006	.0006	.0239	±0.0468
3	35	2	.920	.0017	.0023	.0441	±0.0864
4	32	1	.891	.0010	.0033	.0512	±0.1004
5	30	2	.831	.0024	.0057	.0627	±0.1229
6	27	1	.800	.0014	.0071	.0674	±0.1321
7	23	2	.730	.0041	.0112	.0773	±0.1515
8	20	1	.694	.0026	.0138	.0815	±0.1597
9	17	1	.653	.0037	.0175	.0864	±0.1693
10	15	1	.609	.0048	.0223	.0909	±0.1782
11	12	1	.558	.0076	.0299	.0965	±0.1891
12	10	3	.391	.0429	.0728	.1055	±0.2068

95% confidence limits for the survival function are given by

$$\widehat{S}(t_i) \pm z_{0.975} \cdot SE(\widehat{S}(t_i)) \text{ or } \widehat{S}(t_i) \pm 1.96 \cdot SE(\widehat{S}(t_i)).$$

The confidence limits for the survival function are often referred to as the confidence bands. Similarly, the 90% confidence bands for the Kaplan-Meier product limit estimates are obtained by $\widehat{S}(t_i) \pm z_{0.95} \cdot SE(\widehat{S}(t_i))$ or $\widehat{S}(t_i) \pm 1.645 \cdot SE(\widehat{S}(t_i))$. The above table (Table 15.5.5) shows the necessary calculations for the construction of 95% confidence bands for the Kaplan-Meier survival curve for the implant data presented in Table 15.5.3.a. The corresponding 95% confidence bands are depicted in Figure 15.5.4.

15.6 COMPARING SURVIVAL FUNCTIONS

The statistical problem of comparing survival functions arises often in biomedical sciences. Oncology researchers may be interested in comparing the effectiveness of two or more treatments in prolonging life or the remission period of metastatic breast cancer patients. Implant dentists may want to compare a pure titanium threaded implant with a hydroxyapatite-coated threaded implant in the canine mandible. Survival times of the different treatment groups will always vary. The differences can be illustrated by drawing graphs of the Kaplan-Meier survival curves, but this will only give a

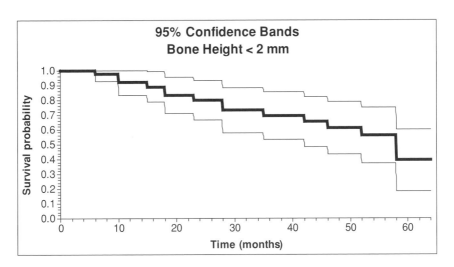

Figure 15.5.4 95% confidence bands for Kaplan-Meier survival curve for data in Table 15.5.3.a.

crude idea of the difference between the treatments. The graphs do not reveal whether the differences are statistically significant or due to chance variations. In this section, a few of the most popular non-parametric methods for comparing survival functions will be discussed. Let $S_1(t)$ and $S_2(t)$ denote the survival functions of the two treatment groups. Then the hypotheses to be considered can be stated:

$H_0 : S_1(t) = S_2(t)$ (two treatments are equally effective) against

$H_1 : S_1(t) \neq S_2(t)$ (two treatments are not equally effective), or

$H_1 : S_1(t) < S_2(t)$ (treatment 2 is more effective than treatment 1), or

$H_1 : S_1(t) > S_2(t)$ (treatment 1 is more effective than treatment 2)

If there are no censored observations in the survival data, non-parametric test procedures for two independent samples can be applied. In some situations, it may be tempting to use the two-sample t test, but keep in mind that unless the two samples are normally distributed, the t test is not appropriate. In the following discussions, the presence of censored observations in the survival data is assumed.

15.6.1 Gehan Generalized Wilcoxon Test

The Gehan generalized Wilcoxon test is an extension of the Wilcoxon rank sum test introduced in Section 14.3. It is designed to compare two independent treatment groups when the survival times are censored. In the Gehen test, every observation X_i or X_i^+ (censored or uncensored) in treatment group 1 is compared with every observation Y_i or Y_i^+ (censored or uncensored) in treatment group 2. Let n_1 be the number of samples in group 1 and n_2 be the number of samples in group 2. A test statistic is defined by

$$W = \sum_{i=1}^{n_1} \sum_{j=1}^{n_2} U_{ij} \text{ where}$$

$$U_{ij} = \begin{cases} +1 & \text{if } X_i > Y_j \text{ or } X_i^+ \geq Y_j \\ 0 & \text{if } X_i = Y_j \text{ or } X_i^+ < Y_j \text{ or} \\ & \quad Y_j^+ < X_i \text{ or } (X_i^+, Y_j^+) \\ -1 & \text{if } X_i < Y_j \text{ or } X_i \leq Y_j^+ \end{cases}$$

The value of the test statistic W would be small (a negative value) if $H_1 : S_1(t) < S_2(t)$ is true. The value of W would be large (a large positive value) if $H_1 : S_1(t) > S_2(t)$ is true. If the null hypothesis $H_0 : S_1(t) = S_2(t)$ were true, the value of W would be close to zero (0). Let's compare the implant survival data in Table 15.5.3.a with the survival data in Table 15.5.3.b. Figure 15.5.3 indicates that the implants placed in the patients with bone height > 4 mm have greater survival probabilities than those with bone height < 2 mm. The Gehen test will show if the difference between the two groups is statistically significant. Since $X_1 = 5^+$ and $Y_1 = 6^+$, it is difficult to determine which is larger or smaller, or if they are the same. Thus, it is easy to see that $U_{11} = 0$. Since $X_2 = 6$, and $Y_1 = 6^+$, it is clear that $X_2 < Y_1$. Hence, $U_{21} = -1$. Repeating the process for $n_1 n_2$ times, the value of the test statistic is obtained.

$$W = \sum_{i=1}^{n} \sum_{j=1}^{m} U_{ij} = -288$$

The calculation of W can be time consuming and laborious when the sample sizes, n_1 and n_2, are large. An alternative method suggested by Mantel [5] combines the two samples to form a single pooled sample of $n_1 + n_2$ observations. Arrange the observations in the pooled sample in ascending order. Let

$U_i =$ (no. of observations definitely greater than the ith observation)

$\quad -$ (no. of observations definitely less than the ith observation),

where $i = 1, 2, \cdots, n_1 + n_2$.

Example 15.6.1. Consider two sets of data:

(i) Sample 1: $6, 8^+, 12, 12, 23^+$
    Sample 2: $7, 7^+, 14^+, 20$
(ii) Pooled sample: $6, 8^+, 12, 12, 23^+, 7, 7^+, 14^+,$
    20
(iii) Arranging the data in ascending order:
    $6, 7, 7^+, 8^+, 12, 12, 14^+, 20, 23^+$

Then

$U_1 =$ (no. of observations definitely greater than 6)
    $-$(no. definitely less than 6) $= 8 - 0 = 8$
$U_2 =$ (no. of observations definitely greater than 7)
    $-$(no. definitely less than 7) $= 7 - 1 = 6$

$U_3 =$ (no. of observations definitely greater than 7^+)
$\quad -$(no. definitely less than 7^+) $= 0 - 2 = -2$

.

.

$U_9 =$ (no. of observations definitely greater than 23^+)
$\quad -$(no. definitely less than 23^+) $= 0 - 5 = -5$

The variance of the test statistic is given by

$$\sigma^2(W) = \frac{n_1 n_2 \sum_{i=1}^{n_1+n_2} U_i^2}{(n_1 + n_2)(n_1 + n_2 - 1)}.$$

The statistic W under H_0 can be considered approximately normally distributed with mean zero and variance $\sigma^2(W)$:

$$Z = \frac{W}{\sqrt{\sigma^2(W)}} \overset{\circ}{\sim} N(0, 1).$$

Example 15.6.2. Using the Gehan generalized Wilcoxon test, determine if there is any statistically significant difference between the two sets of survival data presented in Table 15.5.3.a and Table 15.5.3.b.

Calculations yield $W = \sum_{i=1}^{n} \sum_{j=1}^{m} U_{ij} = -288$ and following the steps described above, $\sum_{i=1}^{n_1+n_2} U_i^2 = 64,617$.

So the variance of the statistic W is obtained as follows:

$$\sigma^2(W) = \frac{n_1 n_2 \sum_{i=1}^{n_1+n_2} U_i^2}{(n_1 + n_2)(n_1 + n_2 - 1)}$$
$$= \frac{(41)(56)(64,617)}{(41 + 56)(41 + 56 - 1)} = 15,932.$$

By substituting W and $\sigma^2(W)$, the test statistic is

$$Z = \frac{W}{\sqrt{\sigma^2(W)}} = \frac{-288}{\sqrt{15932}} = -2.2817.$$

Since $Z = -2.2817 < z_{0.05} = -1.645$, the null hypothesis is rejected. The conclusion is that the survival function for treatment group 2 (Table 15.5.3.b) is statistically significantly higher, with $p = 0.0113$.

15.6.2 The Log Rank Test

The log rank test is another method that is widely used to compare two independent survival functions in the presence of censored observations. Several statisticians contributed to the development of the test procedure (Mantel, Cox, Peto and Peto), and thus there are different names associated

with the method and different versions are available to illustrate the test. Often, the procedure is simply called the log rank test. The log rank test statistic can be shown to be the sum of the differences between the observed failures (uncensored) and the expected failures in one of the treatment groups. Hence, one version of the log rank test is a χ^2 test, since the test statistic has approximately a χ^2 distribution. This is the version that is discussed in this section. Let O_1 and O_2 be the observed numbers and E_1 and E_2 the expected numbers of failures or deaths in the two treatment groups. To compute E_1 and E_2, all the uncensored observations are arranged in ascending order. Compute the number of expected failures at each observed uncensored time point and sum them. Suppose d_t denotes the number of failed observations at time t, and n_{1t} and n_{2t} be the numbers of implants still exposed to risk of failure at time t in treatment group 1 and group 2, respectively. The expected failures for the two treatment groups are expressed

$$e_{1t} = \frac{n_{1t}}{n_{1t} + n_{2t}} \times d_t, \text{ and } e_{2t} = \frac{n_{2t}}{n_{1t} + n_{2t}} \times d_t$$

Then E_1 and E_2 are given by $E_1 = \sum e_{1t}$ and $E_2 = \sum e_{1t}$. Note that E_2 is the total number of failures minus E_1. So in practice, it is sufficient to compute E_1. The test statistic

$$\chi^2 = \frac{(O_1 - E_1)^2}{E_1} + \frac{(O_1 - E_2)^2}{E_2} \overset{\circ}{\sim} \chi^2_{(1)}$$

has approximately the χ^2 distribution with one degree of freedom. A χ^2 value larger than $\chi^2_{(1, 0.95)} = 3.84$ would lead to the rejection of the null hypothesis in favor of the alternative hypothesis.

Example 15.6.3. A study was done to compare the survival of dental implants in diabetic patients with that in non-diabetic patients. The 60-month follow-up data is presented.

| Group A: (diabetic subjects) | 6, | 6^+, | 12, | 12^+, |
| | 18, | 18, | 36, | 42^+ |

| Group B: (non-diabetic subjects) | 12^+, | 24^+, | 36^+, | 48, |
| | 54^+, | 60, | 60^+ | |

Let's perform a significance test by using the log rank test at the significance level of $\alpha = 0.05$. That is, we need to test $H_0 : S_1(t) = S_2(t)$ (survival functions of the two groups are not different) vs. $H_1 : S_1(t) < S_2(t)$ (Group B has higher survival rate).

The necessary values for the test statistic are calculated and presented in the following table.

Failure Time t	d_t	n_{1t}	n_{2t}	$n_{1t} + n_{2t}$	e_{1t}	e_{2t}
6	1	8	7	15	0.5333	0.4667
12	1	6	7	13	0.4615	0.5385
18	2	4	6	10	0.8	1.2
36	1	2	5	7	0.2857	0.7143
48	1	0	4	4	0	1.0
60	1	0	2	2	0	1.0

From the above table, E_1 and E_2 can be obtained; $E_1 = \sum e_{1t} = 2.0805$ and $E_2 = \sum e_{1t} = 4.9195$. Hence, the test statistic is

$$\chi^2 = \frac{(5 - 2.0805)^2}{2.0805} + \frac{(2 - 4.9195)^2}{4.9195}$$
$$= 5.8294 > \chi^2_{(1, 0.95)} = 3.84$$

Therefore, the null hypothesis H_0 is rejected. The survival function for the implants placed in non-diabetic subjects is statistically significantly higher.

15.6.3 The Mantel-Haenszel Test

The Mantel-Haenszel test has proven extremely useful in biomedical research and epidemiologic studies where the effects of confounding variables need to be controlled. For example:

1. In comparing two treatment options for cancerous tumor, it would be important to consider prognostic factors such as stage of the tumor.
2. In studying the association between drinking and lung cancer, the investigators want to control the effects of smoking habit.
3. In studying the relationship between implant survival time and type of loading (immediate or delayed), adjustments for the effects of bone height is required.

To apply the Mantel-Haenszel test, the data have to be stratified by the confounding variable and 2×2 contingency tables are to be formed, one for each stratum. To describe the test procedure, consider the following case: A retrospective research was conducted with 493 implants to study the association between survival time and type of loading. Two 2×2 contingency tables were constructed to control the effects of bone height.

Bone height < 2 mm			
Type of Loading	No. of Failures within 5 Years	No. Surviving 5 Years	
Immediate	$d_{11} = 22$	86	$n_{11} = 108$
Delayed	$d_{12} = 23$	97	$n_{12} = 120$
	$f_1 = 45$	$s_1 = 183$	$N_1 = 228$

Bone height > 4 mm			
Type of Loading	No. of Failures within 5 Years	No. Surviving 5 Years	
Immediate	$d_{21} = 18$	107	$n_{21} = 125$
Delayed	$d_{22} = 17$	123	$n_{22} = 140$
	$f_2 = 35$	$s_2 = 230$	$N_2 = 265$

Among the samples under study, 80 implants were known to have failed within 5 years of placement, and 413 survived at least 5 years. To investigate if the type of loading is significantly associated with the implant survival rate, it was decided to control the effects of bone height, dividing the samples into those with bone height < 2 mm and those with bone height > 4 mm. The test statistic has approximate χ^2 distribution with 1 degree of freedom:

$$\chi^2 = \frac{[(d_{11} + d_{21}) - (E(d_{11}) + E(d_{21}))]^2}{\sigma^2(d_{11}) + \sigma^2(d_{21})} \overset{\circ}{\sim} \chi^2_{(1)}$$

where $E(d_{11})$, $E(d_{21})$, $\sigma^2(d_{11})$, and $\sigma^2(d_{21})$ are mean and variance of d_{11} and d_{21}.

The mean and variance of d_{11} and d_{21} can be obtained as follows:

$$E(d_{11}) = \frac{(n_{11})(f_1)}{N_1} = \frac{(108)(45)}{228} = 21.32,$$

$$E(d_{21}) = \frac{(n_{21})(f_2)}{N_2} = \frac{(125)(35)}{265} = 16.51$$

$$\sigma^2(d_{11}) = \frac{(n_{11})(n_{12})(f_1)(s_1)}{N_1^2(N_1 - 1)}$$
$$= \frac{(108)(120)(45)(183)}{228^2(228 - 1)} = 9.044$$

$$\sigma^2(d_{21}) = \frac{(n_{21})(n_{22})(f_2)(s_2)}{N_2^2(N_2 - 1)}$$
$$= \frac{(125)(140)(35)(230)}{265^2(265 - 1)} = 7.599$$

The computed χ^2 value is

$$\chi^2 = \frac{[(22 + 18) - (21.32 + 16.51)]^2}{9.044 + 7.599}$$
$$= 0.283 < \chi^2_{(1,\,0.95)} = 3.84.$$

The null hypothesis is accepted at the significance level $\alpha = 0.05$, and the test is not significant. Thus, the type of loading is not significantly associated with the implant survival time after adjusting for the effects of bone height. A different version of the test called Cochran-Mantel-Haenszel test is discussed in other statistics textbooks [6].

In Section 15.5, the well-known Kaplan-Meier product limit estimator of survival functions for censored data was introduced. The next section is devoted to an alternative estimator known as the piecewise exponential estimator which has certain advantages. Interested readers are referred to Kim and Proschan [7] for detailed discussions on the alternative estimator.

15.7 PIECEWISE EXPONENTIAL ESTIMATOR (PEXE)

A method for estimating a survival function of a life distribution for a set of censored data, called the **piecewise exponential estimator** (**PEXE**), will be discussed. PEXE is an alternative estimator to the Kaplan-Meier product limit estimator. We will illustrate the method and explain how to

Table 15.7.1. Censored data on time at cessation of observation.

Order of Observation	Time at Cessation of Observation	Cause of Cessation	Notation
1	2.0	Death	z_1
2	3.5	Withdrawal	w_1
3	4.5	Withdrawal	w_2
4	6.2	Death	z_2
5	8.0	Withdrawal	w_3
6	8.8	Death	z_3
7	11.3	Death	z_4

calculate the survival function when a data set contains censored observations.

15.7.1 Small Sample Illustration

Suppose that at time 0, seven patients have joined a clinical trial that is designed to test the effectiveness of a new treatment for hairy cell leukemia. These seven subjects are not bone marrow transplant patients. Each patient is observed until death (failure) or withdrawal from the study, whichever occurs first. The observed data on the seven patients is presented in Table 15.7.1 in the order of occurrence. The survival data in Table 15.7.1 is displayed in Figure 15.7.1.

Definition 15.7.1. Total time on test is the total amount of time spent on observing the subjects who are in study.

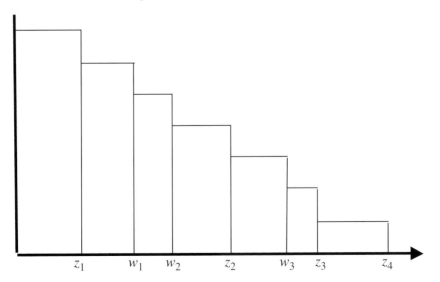

Figure 15.7.1 Number of patients remaining in the study at time t.

For example, there are 7 patients under observation during $[0, 2.0]$ and 6 patients under observation for 1.5 years during $[2.0, 3.5]$; therefore, the total time on test during $[0, w_1]$ is $(7 \times 2) + 6 \times (3.5 - 2.0) = 23.0$. The key steps to estimating the survival function from the data are as follows.

1. Estimate the average failure rate separately on each interval between successive failures.
2. Fit an exponential survival function separately for each such interval whose failure rate is the value obtained in step 1.
3. Join the separate exponential pieces (one piece per failure interval) to form a continuous piecewise exponential estimator.
4. The estimated survival function stops at the last observed failure time z_4 in the above example. Beyond z_4, all we can say is that the survival function continues to decrease.

To implement step 1, estimate the unknown average failure rate r_1 on the interval $[0, z_1]$ from

$$\hat{r}_1 = \frac{\text{Number of deaths observed during } [0, \ z_1]}{\text{Total time on test observed during } [0, \ z_1]}$$

$$= \frac{1}{7 \cdot z_1} = \frac{1}{7 \cdot 2} = \frac{1}{14} = 0.0714.$$

One death (or failure) was observed at z_1 during $[0, z_1]$, which accounts for the numerator. Seven patients each contributed z_1 years toward the total time on test observed during $[0, z_1]$, which accounts for the denominator. The resulting value of $\hat{r}_1 = 0.0714$ is the maximum likelihood estimate (MLE) of the exponential piece to be used on $[0, z_1]$, conditional on the observed withdrawal times. The concept of the maximum likelihood estimator is not discussed in this book. Interested readers are referred to Hogg and Craig [8]. On the interval $(z_1, z_2]$ (the interval of time following the first observed death and ending in the second observed death), estimate the unknown average failure rate r_2 on $(z_1, z_2]$ from

$$\hat{r}_2 = \frac{\text{Number of deaths observed during } [z_1, z_2]}{\text{Total time on test observed during } [z_1, z_2]}$$

$$= \frac{1}{6(w_1 - z_1) + 5(w_2 - w_1) + 4(z_2 - z_1)}$$

$$= \frac{1}{6(3.5 - 2.0) + 5(4.5 - 3.5) + 4(6.2 - 4.5)}$$

$$= 0.0481.$$

One death occurred at time z_2, yielding the numerator as for the denominator, 6 patients were under observation during the interval $[z_1, w_1]$, 5 patients were under observation during the interval $[w_1, w_2]$, and 4 patients were under observation during the interval $[w_2, z_2]$. Use these facts to obtain the total time on test shown in the denominator. Similarly, $\hat{r}_3$ the estimator of the average failure rate on $(z_2, z_3]$, is given by

$$\hat{r}_3 = \frac{\text{Number of deaths observed during } [z_2, \ z_3]}{\text{Total time on test observed during } [z_2, \ z_3]}$$

$$= \frac{1}{3(w_3 - z_2) + 2(z_3 - w_3)}$$

$$= \frac{1}{3(8.0 - 6.2) + 2(8.8 - 8.0)} = 0.1429.$$

Finally, we estimate the average failure rate r_4 on the last interval $(z_3, z_4]$ between the successive deaths occurred at z_3 and z_4:

$$\hat{r}_4 = \frac{1}{(z_4 - z_3)} = \frac{1}{(11.3 - 8.8)} = 0.4000.$$

To implement steps 3 and 4, compute a piecewise exponential survival function $\hat{S}(t)$ with the failure rate

$$\hat{r}(t) = \begin{cases} \hat{r}_1 = 0.0714, & \text{for } 0 \le t \le z_1 = 2.0 \\ \hat{r}_2 = 0.0481, & \text{for } z_1 \le t \le z_2 = 6.2 \\ \hat{r}_3 = 0.1429, & \text{for } z_2 \le t \le z_3 = 8.8 \\ \hat{r}_4 = 0.4000, & \text{for } z_3 \le t \le z_4 = 11.3 \end{cases}$$

For $t > z_4$, we do not attempt to obtain an estimator $\hat{S}(t)$. All one can say is that the survival function $\hat{S}(t)$ decreases with $t > z_4 = 11.3$.

15.7.2 General Description of PEXE

In this section we present a more precise and general description of the PEXE of the survival function based on censored data. For each subject, we assume the time that observation ends is the minimum of 2 statistically independent random variables X and Y; X is governed by a continuous life distribution function $F(t)$ and Y by a continuous life distribution function $G(t)$. The random variable X represents the time to death (or failure) and the random variable Y represents the time to withdrawal. Let $f(t)$ and $g(t)$ be the corresponding probability density functions. Then the each subject in the study is observed to

- death at time t with likelihood $f(t)[1 - G(t)]$,
- be withdrawn at time t with likelihood $g(t)[1 - F(t)]$, or
- experience neither death nor withdrawal during $[0, t]$ with likelihood $[1 - F(t)][1 - G(t)]$.

Suppose n new patients joined a clinical trial at time 0. We observe each patient until death due to the illness that is under study or withdrawal from further observation, whichever occurs first. The observed outcomes are listed in order of occurrence as follows:

$$0 < w_{11} < \cdots < w_{1k_1} < z_1 < w_{21} < \cdots < w_{2k_2}$$
$$< z_2 < \cdots < z_{m-1} < w_{m1} < \cdots < w_{mk_m}$$
$$< z_m < w_{m+1,1} < \cdots < w_{m+1,k_{m+1}}$$

We take $z_0 = 0$, $z_{m+1} = \infty$, and $k_i = 0$ when no withdrawals occur in (z_{i-1}, z_i). In the above expression, strict inequality occurs between successive observed values. This is a consequence of the assumption that the life distribution functions F and G are continuous. There are m observed deaths and $\sum_{i=1}^{m+1} k_i$ withdrawals. Because the total number of observations is n, we must have $m + \sum_{i=1}^{m+1} k_i = n$. Based on the ordered observations displayed above, we describe the PEXE for survival function $S(t)$. On the first failure interval $[0, z_1]$, we estimate the failure rate of the exponential survival function that best fits the data observed during $[0, z_1]$; "best" in the sense of the MLE. We are operating as if the unknown survival function $S(t)$ is exponential on $[0, z_1]$. It is well known that the MLE of the failure rate of an exponential distribution is of the following form:

$$\frac{\text{Observed number of deaths}}{\text{Observed total time on test}}.$$

Applying this principle, we obtain the failure rate estimator $\hat{r}_1$ on $[0, z_1]$,

$$\hat{r}_1 = \frac{1}{\sum_{i=1}^{k_1} w_{1i} + z_1 + (n - k_1 - 1)z_1}$$

The value 1 in the numerator is simply the number of deaths observed during $[0, z_1]$. The denominator represents the total time on test observed during $[0, z_1]$: One patient was observed until he withdrew from the study at time w_{11}. A second was observed until he withdrew at time w_{12}, etc., until

the last patient withdrew during $[0, z_1]$, contributing w_{1k_1} years to total time on test observed during $[0, z_1]$. In addition, the patient who died at time z_1 was observed for z_1 years. Finally, at time z_1, there were $n - k_1 - 1$ patients still remaining in the study that had been observed for z_1 years each. Thus, on the first failure interval, an estimator of survival function is:

$$S(t) = e^{-\hat{r}_1 t} \qquad \text{for } 0 \le t \le z_1.$$

In the similar fashion, we estimate $\hat{r}_2$ the MLE of the failure rate of the exponential distribution that fits the data on $(z_1, z_2]$:

$$\hat{r}_2 = \frac{1}{\sum_{i=1}^{k_2} (w_{2i} - z_1) + (z_2 - z_1) + (n - k_1 - k_2 - 2)(z_2 - z_1)}$$

The exponential estimator of the survival function on the second failure interval $(z_1, z_2]$ is

$$S(t) = \exp\{-\hat{r}_1 z_1 - \hat{r}_2 (t - z_2)\} \quad \text{for } z_1 \le t \le z_2$$

At $t = z_1$, the two expressions $\hat{r}_1$ and $\hat{r}_2$ agree; that is, the exponential pieces on successive intervals between deaths are joined to form a continuous survival function curve. From the two survival functions, one can see that this is accomplished for the first two exponential pieces on $[0, z_1]$ and $(z_1, z_2]$ by inserting the term $-\hat{r}_1 z_1$ in the exponent of e in $\hat{r}_2$. We continue in this fashion obtaining in succession $\hat{r}_3, \cdots, \hat{r}_m$. We can now express the survival function estimator in general over the interval $[0, z_m]$:

$$\hat{S}(t) = \begin{cases} e^{-\hat{r}_1 t} & \text{for } 0 \le t \le z_1 \\ \exp\{-[\hat{r}_1 z_1 + \cdots + \hat{r}_i(z_i - z_{i-1}) \\ \quad + \hat{r}_{i+1}(t - z_i)]\} \\ & \text{for } z_i \le t \le z_{i+1}, \\ & i = 1, 2, \cdots, m - 1 \\ \text{No estimator,} & \text{for } t \ge z \end{cases}$$

15.7.3 An Example

We will use the implant survival data in Table 15.5.3.a and Table 15.5.3.b to illustrate the PEXE. First, let's consider the data in Table 15.5.3.a, which contains 16 failures (or deaths) and 25 withdrawals. In other words, there are 16 uncensored

Table 15.7.2. Failure rate estimates for implant–bone height < 2 mm.

Failure Interval	$\hat{r}_i$
$[0, z_1] = [0, 6]$	$\hat{r}_1 = \dfrac{1}{5 + 6 + 39(6)} = \dfrac{1}{245} = 0.0041$
$(z_1, z_2] = (6, 10]$	$\hat{r}_2 = \dfrac{2}{0 + 4 + 3 + 8 + 33(4)} = \dfrac{2}{147} = 0.0136$
$(z_2, z_3] = (10, 15]$	$\hat{r}_3 = \dfrac{1}{2 + 5 + 31(5)} = \dfrac{1}{162} = 0.0062$
$(z_3, z_4] = (15, 18]$	$\hat{r}_4 = \dfrac{2}{1 + 6 + 28(3)} = \dfrac{1}{91} = 0.0220$
$(z_4, z_5] = (18, 23]$	$\hat{r}_5 = \dfrac{1}{3 + 5 + 26(5)} = \dfrac{1}{138} = 0.0072$
$(z_5, z_6] = (23, 28]$	$\hat{r}_6 = \dfrac{2}{2 + 6 + 10 + 21(5)} = \dfrac{1}{123} = 0.0163$
$(z_6, z_7] = (28, 35]$	$\hat{r}_7 = \dfrac{1}{6 + 7 + 19(7)} = \dfrac{1}{146} = 0.0068$
$(z_7, z_8] = (35, 42]$	$\hat{r}_8 = \dfrac{1}{0 + 1 + 7 + 16(7)} = \dfrac{1}{120} = 0.0083$
$(z_8, z_9] = (42, 46]$	$\hat{r}_9 = \dfrac{1}{3 + 4 + 14(4)} = \dfrac{1}{63} = 0.0159$
$(z_9, z_{10}] = (46, 52]$	$\hat{r}_{10} = \dfrac{1}{1 + 4 + 6 + 11(6)} = \dfrac{1}{77} = 0.0130$
$(z_{10}, z_{11}] = (52, 58]$	$\hat{r}_{11} = \dfrac{3}{4 + 18 + 7(6)} = \dfrac{3}{64} = 0.0469$

and 25 censored observations. Notice that these 16 failures occur at 11 distinct time points. In terms of the notation used in Section 15.7.2, the data in Table 15.5.3.a can be presented as follows:

Two uncensored observations are tied at $z_2 = 10$, $z_4 = 18$, $z_6 = 28$, and three at $z_{11} = 58$. Applying the failure rate estimator discussed in the

w_{11}	z_1	w_{21}	w_{22}	w_{23}	z_2	w_{31}	z_3	w_{41}	z_4
5^+	6	6^+	$8^+, 8^+$	9^+	10, 10	12^+	15	16^+	18, 18

w_{51}	z_5	w_{61}	w_{62}	z_6	w_{71}	z_7	w_{81}	w_{82}	z_8
21^+	23	25^+	$26^+, 26^+$	28, 28	34^+	35	35^+	36^+	42

w_{91}	z_9	$w_{10,1}$	$w_{10,2}$	z_{10}	$w_{11,1}$	z_{11}	$w_{12,1}$		
45^+	46	47^+	50^+	52	56^+	58, 58, 58	60^+ 60^+ 60^+ 60^+ 60^+ 60^+ 60^+		

Notice that there are many tied observations in the implant survival data, both censored and uncensored. For example, two censored observations are tied at $w_{22} = 8^+$, $w_{62} = 26^+$, and seven censored observations are tied at $w_{12,1} = 60^+$.

previous section, we can obtain $\hat{r}_1, \hat{r}_2, \cdots, \hat{r}_{11}$ shown in Table 15.7.2. (See also Fig. 15.7.2) Thus, the exponential estimator of the survival function $S(t)$ is obtained by:

$$
\hat{S}(t) = \begin{cases}
e^{-\hat{r}_1 t} = e^{-(0.0041)t} & \text{for } 0 \le t \le 6 \\
\exp\{-\hat{r}_1 \cdot z_1 - \hat{r}_2(t - z_1)\} = \exp\{-(0.0041)6 - (0.0136)((t - 6)\} & \text{for } 6 \le t \le 10 \\
\cdots\cdots & \\
\exp\{-[\hat{r}_1 \cdot z_1 + \cdots + \hat{r}_{10}(z_{10} - z_9) + \hat{r}_{11}(t - z_{10})]\} & \\
\quad = \exp\{-[(0.0041)6 + \cdots + (0.0130)(6) + (0.0469)(t - 52)\} & \text{for } 52 \le t \le 58 \\
\text{No estimator,} & \text{for } 58 \le t
\end{cases}
$$

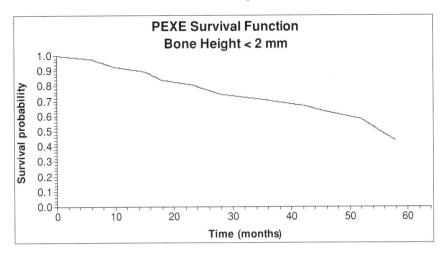

Figure 15.7.2 PEXE survival function for implant data with bone height < 2 mm.

Similarly, we can obtain the failure rate estimators for the corresponding failure intervals and the exponential survival function for the implant survival data in Table 15.5.3.b for the patients with bone height > 4 mm. (See Figure 15.7.3.)

As we saw in the Kaplan-Meier product limit estimators, the PEXE survival function for patients with bone height > 4 mm lies above that for patients with bone height < 2 mm (see Figure 15.7.4). This means that the implant survival probability for the patients with bone height > 4 mm is greater than that for the patients with bone height < 2 mm.

15.7.4 Properties of PEXE and Comparisons with Kaplan-Meier Estimator

The standard estimator widely used for the survival function when data is randomly censored is the well-known Kaplan-Meier product limit estimator (KME). In this section, some statistical properties of PEXE and comparisons of the two survival function estimators will be discussed. The PEXE and the KME are known to be asymptotically equivalent [7]. That is, both estimators would yield the unknown true survival function as the sample size

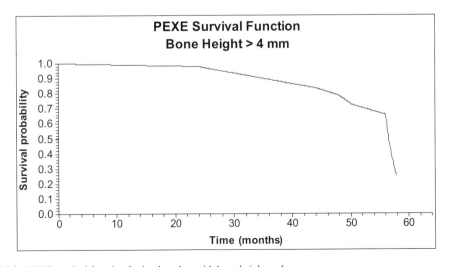

Figure 15.7.3 PEXE survival function for implant data with bone height > 4 mm.

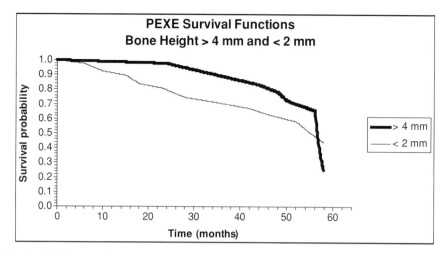

Figure 15.7.4   Two PEXE survival functions for the implant survival data.

increases without limit. For finite sample size, little is known theoretically about either estimator except that the KME has been studied when survival functions of the life distribution and the censoring distribution have proportional hazards [9]. Monte Carlo simulation has shown that for certain well-known life and censoring distributions, the mean squared error of estimation is smaller for the PEXE than for the KME. Some advantages of the PEXE are as follows.

1. The PEXE estimator has the great practical advantage that it is a continuous survival function, whereas the KME is a step function with

discontinuities at the observed failure times, as can be seen in Figure 15.7.5 and Figure 15.7.6. Many investigators in biomedical sciences would prefer to estimate a survival function known to be continuous from clinical prior knowledge or from experience with similar diseases by a continuous survival function estimator.

2. Investigators might consider counterintuitive a survival function estimator (KME) that, in effect, states that there is no chance of failure (or death) during $[0, z_1)$, then suddenly at z_1 the failure rate becomes infinite, then for another interval $(z_1, z_2]$ there is no chance of failure,

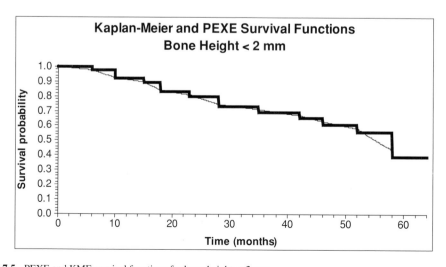

Figure 15.7.5   PEXE and KME survival functions for bone height < 2 mm.

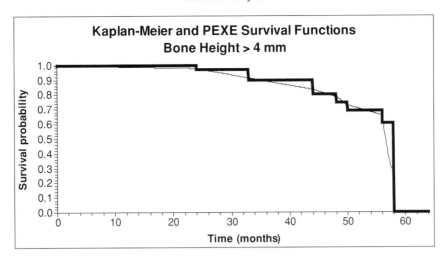

Figure 15.7.6 PEXE and KME survival functions for bone height > 4 mm.

then at z_2 the failure rate again instantly becomes infinite, and so on until z_m. In the case that no censored observations occur beyond z_m, the KME states that the patient has no probability of surviving beyond z_m. This is a startling conclusion, especially since z_m itself is random and would very likely increase if we were to increase sample size.

3. Another attractive feature of the PEXE as compared with the KME is that as the location of a censored observation changes within a given failure interval, the PEXE changes whereas the KME does not. That is, the KME is insensitive to changes in information as to the exact location of the censored observations so long as they stay within their original failure interval, whereas the PEXE is responsive to such changes. For example, in Figure 15.7.5, if each censored observation were shifted as far as possible to the left (or right) within its failure interval, the KME would remain unaffected throughout the entire time domain $[0, z_{11}]$. The PEXE would change correspondingly. In this sense, the PEXE is more sensitive to the information contained in the censored data.

4. If there are many ties among the uncensored observations, particularly in a small sample, the KME has only a few large steps and consequently appears unrealistic as an estimator for a survival function. The PEXE, in contrast, reflects the continuity inherent in a great majority of the clinical situations by decreasing at every

Table 15.7.3. Percentiles of KME and PEXE.

	$\xi_{.995}$	$\xi_{.990}$	$\xi_{.975}$	$\xi_{.950}$	$\xi_{.920}$	$\xi_{.9000}$	$\xi_{.850}$	$\xi_{.800}$	$\xi_{.750}$
KME	3.0	3.0	6.0	9.0	10.0	10.0	16.0	22.0	30.0
PEXE	1.2	2.3	4.4	7.2	9.5	10.1	13.3	20.5	25.9

possible failure time, not only at the observed failure time. The survival function is anticipated to decrease smoothly over time, therefore, in this respect alone, the PEXE is the more appealing estimator of a survival function.

5. The step function form of the KME is known to be responsible for a statistical deficiency, that is, the KME tends to overestimate the underlying survival function and its percentiles. Figure 15.7.5 and Figure 15.7.6 show that most of the time the PEXE lies below the KME. We present a few percentile points, ξ_p, where $S(\xi_p) = p$ for both estimators from the implant survival data with bone height < 2 mm. (See Table 15.7.3.)

For a given p, the percentile points ξ_p for the KME are larger than those for the PEXE, except for $p = 0.90$. This is due to KME's tendency to overestimate the underlying survival function.

15.8 EXERCISES

1 A 10-year implant survival study was conducted with 24 patients who had undergone connective tissue grafting to enhance implant esthetics. The investigators collected the following implant failure times in months.

a. Present a life table analysis of the implant survival data.
b. Calculate the hazard rate.
c. What is the mean survival time?

68.1	98.0^+	28.6	118.0^+	66.2^+	143.0	106.8	132.0^+
76.8^+	114.0^+	35.6	168.0	78.4	114.0	28.3	112.5^+
54.8	168.0	48.5	97.8^+	142.5^+	79.4^+	121.0	72.7

2 The following data represent implant survival times (in months) for 15 smokers with low bone density (less than 65%). Construct the Kaplan-Meier product limit estimator.

55.4^+	89.0	112.5^+	84.7	98.4	23.5^+	62.0	98.4^+
102.5	68.0	46.8^+	68.0	23.5^+	112.0	92.1^+	

3 What is the standard error for the Kaplan-Meier product limit estimator in Exercise 2?

4 A new treatment for acute viral hepatitis was compared with a conventional treatment. A group of 16 patients, who signed a consent form, was chosen. These subjects were randomly assigned to either the experimental group or the control group. Their survival time (in months) was carefully recorded as shown below. Is the new treatment more effective than the conventional treatment? Perform an appropriate test at the significance level of $\alpha = 0.05$.

Experimental group:	45.6^+	68.2	68.2	98.0^+
	106.4	105.5	114.8	123.8^+
Control group:	22.8	55.0	55.0^+	77.3^+
	80.2	80.2^+	92.4^+	116.4

5 Smoking is believed to be a significant risk factor for the lifetime of implants. As part of a class project, a team of three dental students examined 21 patient charts and obtained the following data.

Perform a log rank test at the significance level of $\alpha = 0.05$ to confirm if the claim is justified.

Smokers:	45.3^+	98.5	74.0^+	68.2	32.6
	103.0^+	87.2	110.4		
Non-smokers:	72.0^+	48.4^+	113.5	95.0	82.9^+
	78.6^+	125.0	110.0	95.0^+	72.0^+
	132.8	52.8^+	106.5		

6 Acidulated fluoride preparations may corrode the surface of titanium implants. Thus, patients with this type of implant are generally recommended to avoid fluoride use. The 10-year follow-up investigation of the patients with titanium implants placed in the maxillary anterior region obtained the survival data shown below.

a. Construct the piecewise exponential estimator of the implant survival function.
b. Compare the piecewise exponential estimator and the Kaplan-Meier product limit estimator with respect to their percentiles.

14.5^+	21.4^+	33.0	40.8	58.5	58.5^+
69.8	70.2	77.5^+	85.0	89.5	94.0
94.0^+	94.0^+	97.0	99.5	103.8	105.5^+
105.5^+	108.4	110.0	115.8^+	118.0	

15.9 REFERENCES

1. Altman, D. G. Statistics in medical journals: Developments in the 1980's. *Stat Med*; 1991, 10, 1897–1913.
2. Kalbfleisch, J. D., and Prentice, R. L. *The Statistical Analysis of Failure Time Data.* John Wiley and Sons. 1980.
3. Kaplan, E. L., and Meier, P. Nonparametric estimation from incomplete observations. *J. of American Stat. Assoc.*; 1958, 53, 457–481.
4. Greenwood, M. The natural duration of cancer. Report of Public Health and Medical Subjects; Vol. 33. London: Her Majesty's Stationery Office. 1926.
5. Mantel, N. Ranking procedures for arbitrarily restricted observations. *Biometrics*; 1967, 23, 65–78.
6. Lee, E. T. *Statistical Methods for Survival Data Analysis.* Wiley. 1992.
7. Kim, J. S., and Proschan, F. Piecewise exponential estimator of the survivor function. *IEEE Transactions on Reliability*; 1991, 40: 134–139.
8. Hogg, R. V., and Craig, A. T. *Introduction to Mathematical Statistics.* Third edition. The Macmillan Co. 1970.
9. Chen, Y. Y., Hollander, M., and Langberg, N. Small-sample results for the Kaplan-Meier estimator. *J. Amer. Statistical Assn.* 1982, 77, 141–144.

Appendix

SOLUTIONS TO SELECTED EXERCISES

Chapter 2

3

a. qualitative
c. quantitative, continuous
d. quantitative, continuous
f. quantitative, discrete
h. qualitative
i. quantitative, continuous
j. quantitative, discrete
l. qualitative

4

a. ratio   c. nominal
d. interval   e. ratio
f. ratio   g. nominal
l. ordinal   q. nominal
r. nomial

Chapter 3

1 a. the value of the ith observation
b. the sample mean
c. the sum of the first four observations, X_1, X_2, X_3, and X_4
d. the population mean

2 We expect to obtain different sample means due to the sample-to-sample variability.

5 a. 9, b. 5.

6 $X_1 = \$6.45$, $X_2 = \$7.25$, $X_3 = \$5.98$, and the corresponding weights are $w_1 = 0.20$, $w_2 = 0.30$, $w_3 = 0.50$.

$6.45(0.20) + 7.25(0.30) + 5.98(0.50) = 6.455$.
The weighted average is about \$6.46.

8 The mean $= \overline{X}$
$$= \frac{39.5 + 44.5 + 42.0 + 39.0}{4}$$
$$= 41.25,$$
$$\text{median} = \frac{39.5 + 42.0}{2} = 40.75.$$
The mean is 0.5 mm larger than the median.

12 There are two modes, 3.5 mm and 5.5 mm.

14 When the measurements are all equal to 1.

15 $\overline{X}_H = \dfrac{1}{\frac{1}{4}\left(\frac{1}{200} + \frac{1}{125} + \frac{1}{100} + \frac{1}{80}\right)} = 112.68$.

16 The mean of the grouped data, $\overline{X} =$
$$\frac{(16)(4.5) + (26)(7.5) + (17)(10.5)}{(16 + 26 + 17)} = 7.551$$

18 $6.0 + \frac{30-16}{26}(9.0 - 6.0) = 7.62$.

19 Midrange $= \dfrac{17.5 + 65.4}{2} = 41.45$.
Midrange is larger than the sample mean ($\overline{X} = 33.22$) and median ($\overline{X}_M = 29.1$).

20
$$\overline{X}_W = \frac{5(93.1) + 7(79.6) + 10(82.2) + 9(71.4)}{5 + 7 + 10 + 9}$$
$$= 80.235.$$

22 Mode $= 2.6$ and range $= 3.7$.

24 78.6^{th} percentile.

27 a. Mean.

30 $S^2 = 50.16$, $S = 7.08$, and $IQR = Q_3 - Q_1 = 12.5$.

32 Brand A: $\overline{X} = 50.9$, $S^2 = 53.1$, $S = 7.3$, $CV = (7.3/50.9) \times 100 = 14.3\%$.
Brand B: $\overline{X} = 51.3$, $S^2 = 107.5$, $S = 10.4$, $CV = (10.4/51.3) \times 100 = 20.3\%$.

33 Lab A: $\overline{X} = 60.8$, $S = 9.5$, $CV = (9.5/60.8) \times 100 = 15.6\%$.

Lab B: $\overline{X} = 4.7$, $S = 0.6$, $CV = (0.6/4.7) \times 100 = 12.8\%$.

Lab C: $\overline{X} = 12.1$, $S = 1.1$, $CV = (1.1/12.1) \times 100 = 9.1\%$.

Need to consider CV because the measuring units are different.

Chapter 4

2 There are 36 possible outcomes: $\{(1, 1), (1, 2), (1, 3), (1, 4), (1, 5), (1, 6), (2, 1), (2, 2), (2, 3), (2, 4), (2, 5), (2, 6), \cdots, (6, 1), (6, 2), (6, 3), (6, 4), (6, 5), (6, 6)\}$.

4 a. 1/12, b. 1/6.

5. $C \cup D = \{$erythema multiforme, lichen planus, pemphigoid, viral disease$\}$,

$C \cap D = \{$lichen planus$\}$,

$C^c = \{$erythema multiforme, pemphigoid, pemphigus vulgaris$\}$, and

$D^c = \{$pemphigus vulgaris, viral disease$\}$.

6. $P(C \cup D) = P(C) + P(D) - P(C \cap D) = 0.42 + 0.68 - 0.26 = 0.84$.

7. $P(A \cap B) = P(A) + P(B) - P(A \cup B) = 0.76 + 0.15 - 0.84 = 0.07$.

$P(B \cup C) = P(B) + P(C) - P(B \cap C) = 0.15 + 0.47 - 0.12 = 0.50$.

8. $P(A) = 0.49$ and $P(B) = 0.57$. By independence, $P(AB) = P(A) \cdot P(B) = (0.49)(0.57) = 0.2793$.

10. $P(A) \cdot P(B) = (0.10)(0.20) = 0.02 = P(AB)$. Thus, A and B are statistically independent.

12. a. We need to check if $P(A) \cdot P(B) = P(AB)$. $P(A) \cdot P(B) = (0.55)(0.40) = 0.42 \neq P(AB)$. Thus, A and B are not statistically independent.

b. $P(A) + P(B) + P(C) = 0.55 + 0.40 + 0.75 = 1.70 > 1.0$. Since the sum of the probabilities exceeds 1.0, at least two events must share common outcomes. The events A, B and C are not mutually exclusive.

c. $P(B|A) = \dfrac{P(BA)}{P(A)} = \dfrac{P(AB)}{P(A)} = \dfrac{0.25}{0.55}$
$= 0.455$.

d. $P(BC) = 0.30$. $P(C|B) = \dfrac{P(BC)}{P(B)} = \dfrac{0.30}{0.40}$
$= 0.75$.

e. Because $P(AB) = 0.25$, A and B can not be mutually exclusive.

15. $P(A \text{ or } B) = P(A) + P(B) - P(AB) = P(A) + P(B) - P(A) \cdot P(B)$, by independence $= 0.15 + 0.24 - (0.15)(0.24) = 0.354$.

16. P(a patient is referred for further examination)
$= P$(at least one of the doctors makes a positive diagnosis)
$= P(A^+ \text{ or } B^+) = P(A^+) + P(B^+)$
$- P(A^+ B^+) = 0.24 + 0.29 - 0.18 = 0.35$.

17. Let E_1, E_2, E_3, E_4, and E_5 denote the five age categories. We need to compute the conditional probability $P(E_5|A)$. Using Bayes theorem, we have

$$P(E_5|A) = \frac{P(A|E_5) \cdot P(E_5)}{P(A|E_1) \cdot P(E_1) + P(A|E_2) \cdot P(E_2) + \cdots + P(A|E_5) \cdot P(E_5)}$$
$$= \frac{(0.45)(0.10)}{(0.05)(0.20) + (0.10)(0.15) + (0.18)(0.25) + (0.23)(0.30) + (0.45)(0.10)} = 0.2446.$$

22. $P(E_1 \text{ or } E_2) = P(E_1) + P(E_2) - P(E_1 E_2) = 0.34 + 0.54 - 0.25 = 0.63$.

23. Let A_i be the event of the ith person having hypodontia. Then $P(A_i) = 0.05$.

P(all 4 persons in a family having hypodontia) $= P(A_1 A_2 A_3 A_4)$
$= P(A_1) P(A_2) P(A_3) P(A_4)$ by independence,
$= (0.05)(0.05)(0.05)(0.05) = 6.25 \times 10^{-6}$.

25. P(at most one carious tooth) $= 1 - P$(at least 2 carious teeth) $= 1 - \dfrac{428}{568} = 0.2465$.

28. Since the events A, B, and C are mutually exclusive, P(observing at least one of the events) $= P(A \text{ or } B \text{ or } C) = P(A) + P(B) + P(C) = 0.35 + 0.10 + 0.25 = 0.70$.

30. It is given that $P(A|B) = 0.89$, $P(A|B^c) = 0.08$, and $P(B) = 0.47$. $P(B^c) = 1 - 0.47 = 0.53$.

$P(A) = P(AB) + P(AB^c) = P(A|B)P(B) + P(A|B^c)P(B^c) = (0.89)(0.47) + (0.08)(0.53) = 0.4607$.

31. a. $P(D^c|S^+) = \dfrac{P(D^c S^+)}{P(S^+)} = \dfrac{0.03}{0.20} = 0.15$.

b. $P(D|S^-) = \dfrac{P(DS^-)}{P(S^-)} = \dfrac{0.016}{0.80} = 0.02$.

35. Prevalence rate at the end of June, 2001 $= \dfrac{185}{1825 - 75} = 0.1057$.

Incidence rate $= \dfrac{60}{(1825 + 1750)/2}$

$= 3.3566 \times 10^{-2}$.

37. Sensitivity rate $= \dfrac{74}{82} = 0.9024$, and

specificity rate $= \dfrac{169}{181} = 0.9337$.

38.

Relative risk

$= \dfrac{P(\text{dental caries} \mid \text{drinking water is not fluoridated})}{P(\text{dental caries} \mid \text{drinking water is fluoridated})}$

$= \dfrac{0.48}{0.08} = 6.0$.

Those individuals whose drinking water is not fluoridated are 6 times more likely to get dental caries than those living in a fluoridated communities.

Chapter 5

1. e.

2. a. 495, b. 1, c. 1, d. 720.

4. b. $n = 126$, and $p = 0.12$.

5. $P(X = 3) = 0.0819$.

7. $P(5 \le X \le 8) = P(X = 5) + P(X = 6) + P(X = 7) + P(X = 8) = \dfrac{12!}{5!7!}(0.32)^5(0.68)^7$

$+ \dfrac{12!}{6!6!}(0.32)^6(0.68)^6 + \dfrac{12!}{7!5!}(0.32)^7(0.68)^5$

$+ \dfrac{12!}{8!4!}(0.32)^8(0.68)^4 = 0.3275$.

9. a. Using the Poisson approximation to the binomial with $\mu = 6.5$, we get the probability

$P(X = 10) = \dfrac{(6.5)^{10}e^{-6.5}}{10!} = 0.0558$.

b. $P(\text{at least } 3) = 1 - \{P(X = 0) + P(X = 1) + P(X = 2)\} = 0.9570$.

c. $P(2 \text{ or fewer}) = P(X = 0) + P(X = 1) + P(X = 2) = 0.0430$.

11. $\mu = \lambda s = (3.5)(8) = 28.0$.

$P(X = 30) = \dfrac{(28)^{30}e^{-28}}{30!} = 6.7738 \times 10^{-2}$

$= 0.0677$.

13. $\mu = \lambda s = (0.04)(1000) = 40$.

$P(X = 45) = \dfrac{(40)^{45}e^{-40}}{45!} = 4.3965 \times 10^{-2}$

$= 0.0440$.

15. $Z = \dfrac{X - \mu}{\sigma} = \dfrac{5.7 - 3.2}{1.5} = 1.6667$.

16. a. $Z = \dfrac{X - 5.4}{1.8}$,

d. $P(7.0 < X) = P\left(\dfrac{7.0 - 5.4}{1.8} < \dfrac{X - \mu}{\sigma}\right)$

$= P(0.89 < Z)$

$= 1 - P(Z \le 0.89)$

$= 1 - 0.8133$

$= 0.1867$.

e. $P(8.0 < X) = P\left(\dfrac{8.0 - 5.4}{1.8} < \dfrac{X - \mu}{\sigma}\right)$

$= P(1.44 < Z)$

$= 1 - P(Z \le 1.44)$

$= 1 - 0.9251$

$= 0.0749$. About 7.5%.

17. Let X be a random variable representing the national board exam score. $X \sim N(77.8, 19.4)$,

$\sigma = \sqrt{19.4} = 4.4$. $P(75 \le X)$

$= P\left(\dfrac{75 - 77.8}{4.4} \le Z\right) = P(-0.64 \le Z)$

$= 0.7389$. About 73.9% of the students passed.

18. a. -1.282, b. 0.674, c. 1.037, d. 1.96.

19. Let $X = $ test scores. $X \sim N(66.3, 64.6)$, $\sigma = 8.04$.

a. 25th percentile: $P(X \le x) = 0.25$.

$P\left(\dfrac{X - \mu}{\sigma} \le \dfrac{x - 66.3}{8.04}\right) = P(Z \le z_{0.25})$.

Let $\frac{x - 66.3}{8.04} = z_{0.25} = -0.675$
(from Table D). Solving the equation for x, we get $x = 66.3 - (0.675)(8.04) = 60.87$.

b. 50th percentile = median = mean = 66.3.

c. 90th percentile: $P\left(\frac{X - \mu}{\sigma} \leq \frac{x - 66.3}{8.04}\right) =$

$P(Z \leq z_{0.90}) = 0.90$. $\frac{x - 66.3}{8.04} = z_{0.90} = 1.282$.
$x = 66.3 + (1.282)(8.04) = 76.61$.

d. 95th percentile: $P\left(\frac{X - \mu}{\sigma} \leq \frac{x - 66.3}{8.04}\right) =$

$P(Z \leq z_{0.95}) = 0.95$. $\frac{x - 66.3}{8.04} = z_{0.95} = 1.645$.
$x = 79.53$.

e. 99th percentile: $x = 85.03$.

21. $P(X \leq 30) = P\left(Z \leq \frac{30 - 20}{5}\right) =$
$P(Z \leq 2.0) = 0.9773$.

22. $X \sim N(20, 25)$, $\sigma = 5$.
P(Dr. Johnny spends less than 15 min. or more than 25 min.) $= P(X < 15 \text{ or } X > 25)$

$$= P(X < 15) + P(X > 25)$$
$$= P\left(\frac{X - \mu}{\sigma} < \frac{15 - 20}{5}\right)$$
$$+ P\left(\frac{X - \mu}{\sigma} > \frac{25 - 20}{5}\right)$$
$$= P(Z < -1.0) + P(Z > 1.0)$$
$$= [1 - P(Z < 1.0)] + [1 - P(Z < 1.0)]$$
$$= 0.3174.$$

23. $P(75 \leq X \leq 85)$
$$= P\left(\frac{75 - 78}{5.29} \leq Z \leq \frac{85 - 78}{5.29}\right)$$
$$= P(-0.57 \leq Z \leq 1.32)$$
$$= P(Z \leq 1.32) - P(Z \leq -0.57)$$
$$= 0.9066 - (1 - 0.7157)$$
$$= 0.6223.$$

24. Let $X =$ dental and medical expenditure. $X \sim N(11, 450, \sigma^2)$, $\sigma = 2,750$.

$P(10,000 \leq X \leq 13,000) =$

$P\left(\frac{10,000 - 11,450}{2,750} \leq Z \leq \frac{13,000 - 11,450}{2,750}\right)$

$= P(-0.53 \leq Z \leq 0.56)$
$= P(Z \leq 0.56) - P(Z \leq -0.53)$
$= 0.4142$.

25. $p = P(X \leq 1.0) = P\left(Z \leq \frac{1.0 - 1.2}{0.486}\right)$
$= P(Z \leq -0.67) = 1 - 0.7486$
$= 0.2514$.

$\binom{9}{3}(0.2514)^3(0.7486)^6$
$= \frac{9!}{3!6!}(0.2514)^3(0.7486)^6$
$= 0.2351$.

27. $p = P(X \leq 20,000) = 0.16$.
$np = 150(0.16) = 24.0$,
$\sqrt{npq} = \sqrt{20.16} = 4.49$.

Using the normal approximation to the binomial distribution,

$P(25 \leq X \leq 35) \simeq$
$P\left(\frac{(25 - 0.5) - 24}{4.49} \leq Z \leq \frac{(35 - 0.5) - 24}{4.49}\right)$

$= P(0.11 \leq Z \leq 2.56)$

$= P(Z \leq 2.56) - P(Z \leq 0.11) = 0.4510$.

31. $p = P(X \leq 50) = P\left(Z \leq \frac{50 - 58}{7.07}\right) =$
$P(Z \leq -1.13) = 0.1292$.
$P(X = 9) + P(X = 10) + P(X = 11)$
$+ P(X = 12) = \binom{12}{9}(0.1292)^9(0.8708)^3$
$+ \binom{12}{10}(0.1292)^{10}(0.8708)^2$
$+ \binom{12}{11}(0.1292)^{11}(0.8708)^1$
$+ \binom{12}{12}(0.1292)^{12}(0.8708)^0 \simeq 0$.
The chance that she will be able to complete prophylaxis in 50 min. for at least 9 of her 12 patients is nearly 0.

33. Use the normal approximation to obtain the probability 0.0015.

34. $P(7 \leq X) \simeq 0.6331$.

Chapter 6

1. Variance of $\overline{X}$ is $\frac{\sigma^2}{n} = 4.32$ and the standard error is $\frac{\sigma}{\sqrt{n}} = 2.0785$.

5. $P(84 \leq \overline{X} \leq 87)$
$$= P\left(\frac{84 - 84.5}{1.42} \leq Z \leq \frac{87 - 84.5}{1.42}\right)$$
$$= P(-0.35 \leq Z \leq 1.76)$$

$$= P(Z \le 1.76) - P(Z \le -0.35)$$
$$= 0.9608 - (1 - 0.6368) = 0.5976.$$

6. $P(15 \le \overline{X}) \approx P\left(\dfrac{15.0 - 17.8}{6.5/\sqrt{32}} \le Z\right)$
$$= P(-2.437 \le Z) = 0.9926.$$

8. Lower limit $= 183.14$ and upper limit $= 196.86$.

10. a. 0.65, b. 0.10, c. 0.75, d. 0.23, e. 0.20.

12. a. 0.85, b. 0.025, c. 0.70, d. 0.15.

Chapter 7

2. (73.54, 75.86).

3. $\left(7.24 - 2.58\dfrac{1.73}{\sqrt{15}}, 7.24 + 2.58\dfrac{1.73}{\sqrt{15}}\right)$
$= (6.09, 8.39)$.

6. $n = 24$.

7. The maximum error of estimate of the mean μ is about 5.89 min.

9. $E = t_{(n-1,1-\alpha/2)}\dfrac{S}{\sqrt{n}} = 2.093\dfrac{2.4}{\sqrt{20}} = 1.1232$.

10. About 60 more children are required to reduce the maximum error by 50%.

12. (0.7981, 0.8619).

18. A 90% confidence interval for σ^2 is given by (782.97, 1911.87).

Chapter 8

2. a. $H_0 : \mu = 30$ vs. $H_1 : \mu \neq 30$. b. A type II error can be committed by accepting the null hypothesis when it is not true. That is, accepting H_0 that the children spend 30 seconds in brushing their teeth when actually they don't spend 30 seconds.

4. $Z = \dfrac{25 - 20}{(5.2/\sqrt{35})} = 5.6885 > Z_{1-\alpha/2} = 1.96$.
Reject their speculation and conclude that vitamin E intake of the adult Americans is significantly higher than 20 IU per day.

6. a. $H_0 : \mu = 25$ vs. $H_1 : \mu < 25$.
b. We have $n = 12, \overline{X} = 23.3$, and $\sigma = \sqrt{4.2} = 2.05$. This is a one-tailed test. The value of

the test statistic is $Z = \dfrac{23.3 - 25}{(2.05/\sqrt{12})} = -2.87$.
The p value $= P(Z < -2.87) = 0.0020 < 0.05$. Thus reject H_0.

c. The average weight of the rice bags labeled 25 kg is statistically significantly lower at the significance level $\alpha = 0.05$.

9. The hypothesis to be tested is $H_0 : \mu = 3.2$ vs. $H_1 : \mu > 3.2$. We have $n = 28$, $\overline{X} = 3.8$, and $\sigma = 1.52$. Since $Z = \dfrac{3.8 - 3.2}{(1.52/\sqrt{28})} = 2.09 > 1.645$, we reject the null hypothesis. The p value $= P(2.09 < Z) = 1 - 0.9817 = 0.0183$.

11. The hypothesis we need to test is $H_0 : \mu < 10.0$ vs. $H_1 : \mu > 10.0$. We have $n = 27$, $\overline{X} = 11.26$, and $\sigma = 2.13$. Since $Z = \dfrac{11.26 - 10.0}{(2.13/\sqrt{27})} = 3.0738 > 1.645$, reject the null hypothesis at the significance level $\alpha = 0.05$. Dr. Quinn may wish to give them a 10-year guarantee.

13. The test statistics $t = \dfrac{154 - 150}{(4.52/\sqrt{20})} = 3.9576 > t_{(19,0.975)} = 2.093$. The experimental dental material has significantly larger mean bonding strength than the control at $\alpha = 0.05$. The p value is $P(3.9576 < t_{(19)}) < P(3.8834 < t_{(19)}) = 0.0005$.

18. d.

21. a. $H_0 : p = 0.43$ vs. $H_1 : p \neq 0.43$
b. $Z = \dfrac{0.38 - 0.43}{\sqrt{(0.43)(0.57)/118}} = -1.0971$. Since $Z_{(0.025)} = -1.96 < -1.0971 < Z_{(0.975)} = 1.96$, we accept H_0 and conclude that there is no significant difference.

Chapter 9

2. a. $H_0 : \mu_1 = \mu_2$ vs. $H_1 : \mu_1 \neq \mu_2$.
b. The value of the test statistic is given by

$$Z = \dfrac{\overline{X}_1 - \overline{X}_2}{\sqrt{\dfrac{\sigma_1^2}{n_1} + \dfrac{\sigma_2^2}{n_2}}} = \dfrac{3.4 - 4.2}{\sqrt{\dfrac{1.86}{18} + \dfrac{2.02}{24}}} = -1.8475.$$

Because $-1.96 < Z = -1.8475 < 1.96$, the null hypothesis is not rejected and the mean pocket depth of the two groups is not statistically significantly different at the significance level $\alpha = 0.05$.

3. a. $H_0: \mu_1 = \mu_2$ vs. $H_1: \mu_1 \neq \mu_2$.

b. The pooled estimate

$$S_p^2 = \frac{(16-1)(1,223.6) + (16-1)(2,304.8)}{16+16-2}$$
$$= 1,764.2,$$

and $S_p = 42.0$. We now can calculate the test statistic

$$t = \frac{\overline{X}_1 - \overline{X}_2}{S_p\sqrt{\dfrac{1}{n_1} + \dfrac{1}{n_2}}} = \frac{81.2 - 110.4}{(42.0024)\sqrt{\dfrac{1}{16} + \dfrac{1}{16}}}$$
$$= -1.9663.$$

Since $t = -1.9663 < t_{(30, 0.025)} = -2.042$, the null hypothesis can not be rejected. The contraction efficacy of epinephrine is not significantly different from that of bonding agent at the significance level $\alpha = 0.05$.

c. p value $= 2P(t_{(30)} < -1.9963) > 2P(t_{(30)} < -2.042) = 0.05$.

4. We need to test $H_0: \mu_1 = \mu_2$ vs. $H_1: \mu_1 \neq \mu_2$. The pooled estimate $S_p^2 = \dfrac{(12-1)(0.57) + (11-1)(0.21)}{12+11-2} = 0.3986$ and $S_p = 0.6313$. We now can calculate the test statistic

$$t = \frac{\overline{X}_1 - \overline{X}_2}{S_p\sqrt{\dfrac{1}{n_1} + \dfrac{1}{n_2}}} = \frac{4.28 - 2.65}{(0.6313)\sqrt{\dfrac{1}{12} + \dfrac{1}{11}}}$$
$$= 6.1855.$$

Since $t = 6.1855 > t_{(21, 0.925)} = 2.080$, the null hypothesis is rejected. The EMD with open flap debridement is significantly better than treatment without EMD at the significance level $\alpha = 0.05$. p value $= 2P(6.1855 < t_{(21)}) < 2P(3.819 < t_{(21)}) = 2(0.0005) = 0.0010$.

6. This is a two-sample t test problem with unequal variances. Since $n_1 = 47$, and $n_2 = 25$, the test statistic is given by

$$t = \frac{\overline{X}_1 - \overline{X}_2}{\sqrt{\dfrac{S_1^2}{n_1} + \dfrac{S_2^2}{n_2}}}$$
$$= \frac{209.1 - 213.3}{\sqrt{\dfrac{1260.25}{47} + \dfrac{1413.76}{25}}} = -0.460$$

The approximate degrees of freedom δ^* is obtained by

$$\delta^* = \frac{\left(S_1^2/n_1 + S_2^2/n_2\right)^2}{\left(S_1^2/n_1\right)^2/(n_1-1) + \left(S_2^2/n_2\right)^2/(n_2-1)}$$
$$= \frac{6949.5898}{15.6300 + 133.2478} = 46.68$$

The approximate degrees of freedom $\delta^* = 46$. From Table E, $t_{(46, 0.025)} = -2.0125$. Because $t = -0.46 > t_{(46, 0.025)} = -2.0125$, we conclude there is no statistically significant difference in mean cholesterol between smokers and non-smokers. The p value is $2P(t_{(46)} < -0.460) > 2P(t_{(46)} < -0.5286) = 0.60$.

8. We want to test $H_0: p_1 = p_2$ vs. $H_1: p_1 \neq p_2$. $\widehat{p}_1 = \dfrac{24}{68} = 0.353$ and $\widehat{p}_2 = \dfrac{14}{46} = 0.304$.
$$\widehat{p} = \frac{X_1 + X_2}{n_1 + n_2} = \frac{24 + 14}{68 + 46} = 0.333, \quad \widehat{q} = 1 - 0.333 = 0.667.$$
By the normal approximation, the test statistic is

$$Z = \frac{\widehat{p}_1 - \widehat{p}_2}{\sqrt{pq\left(\dfrac{1}{n_1} + \dfrac{1}{n_2}\right)}}$$
$$= \frac{0.353 - 0.304}{\sqrt{(0.333)(0.667)\left(\dfrac{1}{68} + \dfrac{1}{46}\right)}} = 0.5446.$$

Thus, the null hypothesis is accepted. We conclude that there is no statistically significant difference between OHI and no OHI at the significance level $\alpha = 0.05$. Based on the data, the OHI is not effective in helping patients reduce plaque scores.

10. Need to test $H_0: p_1 = p_2$ vs. $H_1: p_1 \neq p_2$. $\widehat{p}_1 = \dfrac{9}{75} = 0.120$ and $\widehat{p}_2 = \dfrac{16}{98} = 0.163$.
$$\widehat{p} = \frac{X_1 + X_2}{n_1 + n_2} = 0.1445, \quad \widehat{q} = 1 - 0.1445 = 0.8555.$$
By the normal approximation, the test statistic is

$$Z = \frac{\widehat{p}_1 - \widehat{p}_2}{\sqrt{pq\left(\dfrac{1}{n_1} + \dfrac{1}{n_2}\right)}}$$
$$= \frac{0.120 - 0.163}{\sqrt{(0.1445)(0.8555)\left(\dfrac{1}{75} + \dfrac{1}{98}\right)}}$$
$$= -0.7978.$$

The null hypothesis is accepted at the significance level $\alpha = 0.05$. There is no statistically significant difference in the proportion.

11. $n = \dfrac{(62.5 + 60.2) \cdot (1.96 + 1.03)^2}{(51.3 - 55.6)^2}$
$= 59.327$. The required sample size is 60.

14. Power

$$= P\left(Z \le -1.96 + \frac{|68.4 - 55.9| \cdot \sqrt{31/36}}{\sqrt{(75.5/31) - (80.7/36)}}\right)$$
$$= P(Z \le 3.017) = 0.9987.$$

17. $F = \dfrac{(64.8)^2}{(74.9)^2} = 0.7485 < F_{(30,25;0.975)} =$
$2.182.$ The null hypothesis is accepted. There is no statistically significant difference in the variance.

Chapter 10

1. a. H_0: There is no association between flu vaccine and contraction of the flu.

H_1: There is an association between flu vaccine and contraction of the flu.

b. $E_{11} = \dfrac{235 \cdot 94}{423} = 52.222,$

$E_{12} = \dfrac{235 \cdot 329}{423} = 182.78$

$E_{21} = \dfrac{94 \cdot 188}{423} = 41.778,$

$E_{22} = \dfrac{329 \cdot 188}{423} = 146.22.$

c. $\chi^2 = \dfrac{(|43 - 52.222| - 0.5)^2}{52.222}$

$+ \dfrac{(|192 - 182.78| - 0.5)^2}{182.78}$

$+ \dfrac{(|51 - 41.778| - 0.5)^2}{41.778}$

$+ \dfrac{(|137 - 146.22| - 0.5)^2}{146.22} = 4.2136$

d. p value $= P\left(4.2136 < \chi^2_{(1)}\right) <$
$P\left(3.84 < \chi^2_{(1)}\right) = 0.05.$

e. We reject the null hypothesis and conclude that there is a statistically significant association between flu vaccine and contraction of the flu at the significance level $\alpha = 0.05$.

2. H_0: There is no association between alcohol consumption and severity of periodontal disease.

H_1: There is an association between alcohol consumption and severity of periodontal disease.

The expected cell frequecies are

$$E_{11} = \frac{68 \cdot 108}{154} = 47.688,$$

$$E_{12} = \frac{68 \cdot 46}{154} = 20.312$$

$$E_{21} = \frac{86 \cdot 108}{154} = 60.312,$$

$$E_{22} = \frac{86 \cdot 46}{154} = 25.688$$

The value of the test statistic is

$$\chi^2 = \frac{(|44 - 47.688| - 0.5)^2}{47.688}$$

$$+ \frac{(|24 - 20.312| - 0.5)^2}{20.312}$$

$$+ \frac{(|64 - 60.312| - 0.5)^2}{60.312}$$

$$+ \frac{(|22 - 25.688| - 0.5)^2}{25.688}$$

$$= 1.2776 < \chi^2_{(1,0.95)} = 3.841.$$

The null hypothesis is not rejected. Based on the data, the test result indicates that there is no statistically significant association between alcohol consumption and severity of periodontal disease at the significance level $\alpha = 0.05$.

4. a. One may construct a 2×2 contingency table:

	Osteogenesis Imperfecta		
	Affected	Unaffected	
First born	16	24	40
Second born	10	30	40
	26	54	80

b. The χ^2 test procedure can be used in the above 2×2 contingency table, because the two samples are not independent. Each matched pair of the first born and the second born children within the same family is similar in clinical conditions. The matched pair constitutes the basic unit for the experiment so the sample size is 40, not 80. Apply the McNemar test to the following 2×2 contingency table.

Second Born	First born		
	Affected	Unaffected	
Affected	4	6	10
Unaffected	12	18	30
	16	24	40

7. a. $H_0: p_{11} = p_{12} = p_{13} = p_{14}, \ p_{21} = p_{22} = p_{23} = p_{24}, \ p_{31} = p_{32} = p_{33} = p_{34}.$

b. $\chi^2 = \sum_{j=1}^{c} \sum_{i}^{r} \dfrac{(O_{ij} - E_{ij})^2}{E_{ij}}$

$= 55.19 > \chi^2_{((r-1)(c-1),1-\alpha)} = \chi^2_{(6,0.95)}$
$= 12.592.$

The null hypothesis is rejected.

c. $p = P\left(\chi^2 < \chi^2_{(6)}\right) = P\left(55.19 < \chi^2_{(6)}\right) < 0.005.$

11. Let "Yes = 75% or better" and "No = less than 75%." We can have the following 2×2 contingency table.

Universal system	FDI System		
	Y	N	
Y	55	22	77
N	31	24	55
	86	46	132

Use the McNemar test for matched pairs. The value of the test statistic is

$$\chi^2_M = \frac{(|b - c| - 1)^2}{b + c} = \frac{(|22 - 31| - 1)^2}{22 + 31}$$

$$= 1.2075 < \chi^2_{(1,0.95)} = 3.841.$$

Thus, the null hypothesis is accepted. There is no significant association between tooth-numbering systems and learning ability of dental students at the significance level $\alpha = 0.05$.

12. The observed and expected concordance rates are:

$$P_o = \frac{O_{11} + O_{22}}{n} = \frac{41 + 29}{83} = 0.8434, \text{ and}$$

$$P_E = \frac{r_1}{n} \cdot \frac{c_1}{n} + \frac{r_2}{n} \cdot \frac{c_2}{n} = \frac{46}{83} \cdot \frac{49}{83} + \frac{37}{83} \cdot \frac{34}{83}$$

$$= 0.5098$$

$$\kappa = \frac{P_o - P_E}{1 - P_E} = \frac{0.8434 - 0.5098}{1 - 0.5098} = 0.6805$$

14. 0.5313.

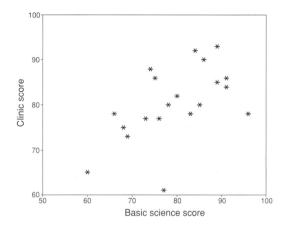

Figure A.1 Relationship between basic science and clinic performance.

Chapter 11

1. Refer to Figure A.1. Except for one individual whose basic science score is 77 and clinic score is 61, there appears to be a linear relationship between two variables. The higher the score in basic science courses, the better the clinic performance.

3. b. $\sum_{i=1}^{15} X_i = 2,101.78,$

$\sum_{i=1}^{15} X_i^2 = 295,345.52,$

$\sum_{i=1}^{15} Y_i = 191.53,$

$\sum_{i=1}^{15} X_i \cdot Y_i = 27,002.84.$

c. $\hat{Y}_i = -14.68 + 0.196 \cdot X_i.$

d. 13.74

5. $\hat{Y}_i = 72.54 - 2.16 \cdot X_i.$

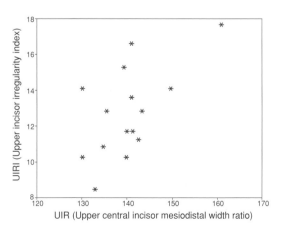

Figure A.2 Relationship between UIR and UIRI.

9. Pearson correlation coefficient $r = 0.810$ ($p = 0.008$).

13. $r^2 = 0.727$ and $r = 0.853$.

Chapter 12

2. See Section 12.6. Multiple Comparisons Procedures.

5. a.

Source of Variation	df	Sum of Squares	Mean Square	F Value
Between	4	1080.59	270.15	20.16
Within	60	803.86	13.40	
Total	64	1884.45		

b. p value $< P(F_{(4,60)} > 20.16) < 0.001$.

Chapter 13

1. The populatons from which the samples are taken are normally distributed.

The populations must be statistically independent.

The variances of the populations are equal.

3. b. If the interaction effects of the two factors exist, the curves of the mean responses in a graph are not parallel. If no interaction effects exist, the curves are essentially parallel.

7. Two.

9. a.

Source of Variation	df	SS	MS	F	p Value
Factor A (Light cure)	1	0.075	0.075	0.055	$p > 0.50$
Factor B (Time)	2	45.603	22.802	16.766	$p < 0.001$
Light*Time interaction	2	3.336	1.668	1.226	$p > 0.10$
Error (Residual)	18	24.480	1.360		
Total	23	73.494			

Chapter 14

1. The sample size is $n = 30$ (why?). We obtain $\mu = np = 15$ and $\sigma^2 = npq = 7.5$. $\sigma = 2.7386$. The test statistic T = total number of plus signs $= 21$. Using a normal approximation,

$$Z = \frac{(21 - 0.5) - 15}{2.7386} \approx 2.01$$

The p value $= P(2.01 < Z) = 0.0222 < 0.05$. We conclude that chlorhexidine is statistically significantly effective in reducing the salivary SM at the significance level $\alpha = 5\%$.

3. The sum of the ranks for Y's is $W_Y = 374$. $\mu_W = (17)(17 + 17 + 1)/2 = 297.5$ and $\sigma_W = \sqrt{(17 \cdot 17)(17 + 17 + 1)/12} = 29.03$. The test statistics is $Z = (W_Y - \mu_W)/\sigma_W = 2.6352$.

Since $Z = 2.6352 > 1.96$, the null hypothesis is rejected at the significance level $\alpha = 5\%$.

5. The median of the combined sample ($N = 26$) is 75. From a 2×2 contingency table, we obtain $\chi^2 = 0.5758$, $< \chi^2_{(1,0.95)} = 3.841$. We accept the null hypothesis and conclude there is no statistically significant difference in median between the two treatments.

7. The number of matched samples is $N = 11$, and the number of treatments is $k = 4$. The rank sums are $R_1 = 23.5$, $R_2 = 19$, $R_3 = 32.5$, and $R_4 = 35$. There are 2 sets of ties in groups 2 and 6 so $\tau = 2$ for each tied pair. By applying the Friedman test, we obtain

$$F_r = \frac{12[(23.5)^2 + (19)^2 + (32.5)^2 + (35)^2] - 3 \cdot 11^2 \cdot 4(4 + 1)^2}{11 \cdot 4(4 + 1) + \left[\dfrac{11 \cdot 4 - (40 + 2^3 + 2^3)}{4 - 1}\right]} = 9.4167$$

Since the critical value $\chi^2_{(3,0.95)} = 7.81 < F_r = 9.4167$, the test is significant. We conclude that there are statistically significant differences in patient preference among the four flavorings.

9. $\sum R(U_i)^2 = 3,494$, $\sum R(V_i)^2 = 1,402.50$, $\overline{R^2} = 4,896.5/24 = 204.0208$. $\sum_{i=1}^{N} R_i^4 = \sum_{i=1}^{n_1}[R(U_i)]^4 + \sum_{i=1}^{n_2}[R(V_i)]^4 = 1,474,070 + 288,171.38 = 1,762,241.38$. Compute the test statistic T,

$$T = \frac{3,494 - (11)(204.0208)}{\sqrt{\frac{11 \cdot 13}{24 \cdot 23}(1,762,241.38) - \frac{11 \cdot 13}{23}(204.0208)^2}}$$

$$= 2.8106 > z_{0.975} = 1.96$$

Thus, the null hypothesis is rejected. There is a statistically significant difference in the variance between manual and computerized device.

Table A. Table of Random Numbers.

03948	16937	32505	61245	34354	03151	68637	09160	77627	59716	21230
21363	91444	97097	46988	94234	18137	78243	42624	89835	18126	51551
95981	74524	97486	13560	20666	04317	46647	79424	76143	48415	46632
49061	97473	90178	64870	63680	53990	42055	64455	40290	66139	79795
13843	71385	56614	28351	07778	71963	48641	86740	96902	11514	31854
71072	31474	01147	40814	93389	37096	44071	53963	90558	17130	72535
48853	81449	34111	23782	85891	84054	84486	99960	97181	48042	77999
42074	76843	22128	31828	14858	91247	57420	45029	21301	00928	43466
21210	83388	67189	38462	66709	48433	78970	11289	46542	46072	59348
45289	26016	23322	62967	45670	62806	20128	00262	31360	25892	00382
31884	03321	60604	26893	69307	80931	17044	64707	27699	37600	39004
57349	84097	77727	82897	98369	74685	93047	04592	45126	84570	85009
42043	21335	39697	05647	70396	86310	00718	04100	60002	63963	40325
31126	06728	55622	43674	83187	36730	78370	47977	78761	12058	21658
00399	08824	52781	67192	10295	95597	66519	29761	42228	45030	44348
98581	88738	80773	17038	90731	67143	17291	05885	33128	77547	36885
72548	57216	55540	23632	49615	69200	34000	00940	94472	15784	08085
58649	92854	18416	28092	57594	53995	04488	03659	46696	45433	29044
12580	74674	48948	16432	35904	15285	40431	72348	15195	78663	38660
40521	58505	68461	62845	74999	72011	63632	98449	42442	57512	72530
36073	10563	95593	75151	15297	96004	60663	31531	89460	11422	16747
31776	52823	66757	20965	92727	26942	81622	03625	05135	62312	89865
28363	05022	01411	05876	04184	74234	21252	97931	70773	45485	30564
46195	88502	45197	87735	96000	11791	32322	87512	51563	00723	67086
90795	47274	12553	17713	86227	63727	57007	19412	70794	99612	78108
75973	46220	97916	43726	56141	53647	59749	25301	96633	63658	96788
92774	64784	39075	57974	42914	04602	19559	58763	69048	18136	14006
23973	38851	11313	99610	86995	02666	10913	45667	69021	21620	05861
93230	22448	04062	74881	50778	85063	84863	97482	40875	60326	34481
75933	73581	79648	51851	05055	18241	49978	75860	50184	16688	65693
15845	94437	33769	10003	11978	36917	70737	34351	38952	39470	21456
83054	46887	08507	55364	18062	94589	85664	11143	53762	36527	76585
61543	43300	68040	73710	64086	57436	91971	63972	93683	97414	25068
10546	03602	52902	06812	56592	75122	57208	11965	08644	16790	25481
94214	94910	65044	90684	90583	47733	50275	97852	55180	30232	58091
86859	46660	00596	50915	98263	89750	40177	95075	78806	59392	49640
29696	35150	35568	53546	92628	27749	26006	57583	80870	81755	92535
63722	26988	79368	23285	26262	66837	14797	45577	99963	33695	94399
35922	13238	50916	65558	31841	47916	93600	51487	34638	46029	73478
39745	02144	38275	68724	91200	68222	97089	21966	41810	79072	58937

Appendix

Table B. Binomial Probabilities $P(X = k)$.

n	k	.05	.10	.15	.20	.25	.30	.35	.40	.45	.50
2	0	.9025	.8100	.7225	.6400	.5625	.4900	.4225	.3600	.3025	.2500
	1	.0950	.1800	.2550	.3200	.3750	.4200	.4550	.4800	.4950	.5000
	2	.0025	.0100	.0225	.0400	.0625	.0900	.1225	.1600	.2025	.2500
3	0	.8574	.7290	.6141	.5120	.4219	.3430	.2746	.2160	.1664	.1250
	1	.1354	.2430	.3251	.3840	.4219	.4410	.4436	.4320	.4084	.3750
	2	.0071	.0270	.0574	.0960	.1406	.1890	.2389	.2880	.3341	.3750
	3	.0001	.0010	.0034	.0080	.0156	.0270	.0429	.0640	.0911	.1250
4	0	.8145	.6561	.5220	.4096	.3164	.2401	.1785	.1296	.0915	.0625
	1	.1715	.2916	.3685	.40%	.4219	.4116	.3845	.3456	.2995	.2500
	2	.0135	.0486	.0975	.1536	.2109	.2646	.3105	.3456	.3675	.3750
	3	.0005	.0036	.0115	.0256	.0469	.0756	.1115	.1536	.2005	.2500
	4	.0000	.0001	.0005	.0016	.0039	.0081	.0150	.0256	.0410	.0625
5	0	.7738	.5905	.4437	.3277	.2373	.1681	.1160	.0778	.0503	.0313
	1	.2036	.3280	.3915	.4096	.3955	.3601	.3124	.2592	.2059	.1563
	2	.0214	.0729	.1382	.2048	.2637	.3087	.3364	.3456	.3369	.3125
	3	.0011	.0081	.0244	.0512	.0879	.1323	.1811	.2304	.2757	.3125
	4	.0000	.0005	.0022	.0064	.0146	.0284	.0488	.0768	.1128	.1563
	5	.0000	.0000	.0001	.0003	.0010	.0024	.0053	.0102	.0185	.0313
6	0	.7351	.5314	.3771	.2621	.1780	.1176	.0754	.0467	.0277	.0156
	1	.2321	.3543	.3993	.3932	.3560	.3025	.2437	.1866	.1359	.0938
	2	.0305	.0984	.1762	.2458	.2966	.3241	.3280	.3110	.2780	.2344
	3	.0021	.0146	.0415	.0819	.1318	.1852	.2355	.2765	.3032	.3125
	4	.0001	.0012	.0055	.0154	.0330	.0595	.0951	.1382	.1861	.2344
	5	.0000	.0001	.0004	.0015	.0044	.0102	.0205	.0369	.0609	.0938
	6	.0000	.0000	.0000	.0001	.0002	.0007	.0018	.0041	.0083	.0156
7	0	.6983	.4783	.3206	.2097	.1335	.0824	.0490	.0280	.0152	.0078
	1	.2573	.3720	.3960	.3670	.3115	.2471	.1848	.1306	.0872	.0547
	2	.0406	.1240	.2097	.2753	.3115	.3177	.2985	.2613	.2140	.1641
	3	.0036	.0230	.0617	.1147	.1730	.2269	.2679	.2903	.2918	.2734
	4	.0002	.0026	.0109	.0287	.0577	.0972	.1442	.1935	.2388	.2734
	5	.0000	.0002	.0012	.0043	.0115	.0250	.0466	.0774	.1172	.1641
	6	.0000	.0000	.0001	.0004	.0013	.0036	.0084	.0172	.0320	.0547
	7	.0000	.0000	.0000	.0000	.0001	.0002	.0006	.0016	.0037	.0078
8	0	.6634	.4305	.2725	.1678	.1001	.0576	.0319	.0168	.0084	.0039
	1	.2793	.3826	.3847	.3355	.2670	.1977	.1373	.0896	.0548	.0313
	2	.0515	.1488	.2376	.2936	.3115	.2965	.2587	.2090	.1569	.1094
	3	.0054	.0331	.0839	.1468	.2076	.2541	.2786	.2787	.2568	.2188
	4	.0004	.0046	.0185	.0459	.0865	.1361	.1875	.2322	.2627	.2734
	5	.0000	.0004	.0026	.0092	.0231	.0467	.0808	.1239	.1719	.2188
	6	.0000	.0000	.0002	.0011	.0038	.0100	.0217	.0413	.0703	.1094
	7	.0000	.0000	.0000	.0001	.0004	.0012	.0033	.0079	.0164	.0313
	8	.0000	.0000	.0000	.0000	.0000	.0001	.0002	.0007	.0017	.0039
9	0	.6302	.3874	.2316	.1342	.0751	.0404	.0207	.0101	.0046	.0020
	1	.2985	.3874	.3679	.3020	.2253	.1556	.1004	.0605	.0339	.0176
	2	.0629	.1722	.2597	.3020	.3003	.2668	.2162	.1612	.1110	.0703
	3	.0077	.0446	.1069	.1762	.2336	.2668	.2716	.2508	.2119	.1641
	4	.0006	.0074	.0283	.0661	.1168	.1715	.2194	.2508	.2600	.2461
	5	.0000	.0008	.0050	.0165	.0389	.0735	.1181	.1672	.2128	.2461
	6	.0000	.0001	.0006	.0028	.0087	.0210	.0424	.0743	.1160	.1641
	7	.0000	.0000	.0000	.0003	.0012	.0039	.0098	.0212	.0407	.0703
	8	.0000	.0000	.0000	.0000	.0001	.0004	.0013	.0035	.0083	.0176
	9	.0000	.0000	.0000	.0000	.0000	.0000	.0001	.0003	.0008	.0020

Table B.   Binomial Probabilities $P(X = k)$ (*continued*).

n	k	.05	.10	.15	.20	.25	.30	.35	.40	.45	.50
10	0	.5987	.3487	.1969	.1074	.0563	.0282	.0135	.0060	.0025	.0010
	1	.3151	.3874	.3474	.2684	.1877	.1211	.0725	.0403	.0207	.0098
	2	.0746	.1937	.2759	.3020	.2816	.2335	.1757	.1209	.0763	.0439
	3	.0105	.0574	.1298	.2013	.2503	.2668	.2522	.2150	.1665	.1172
	4	.0010	.0112	.0401	.0881	.1460	.2001	.2377	.2508	.2384	.2051
	5	.0001	.0015	.0085	.0264	.0584	.1029	.1536	.2007	.2340	.2461
	6	.0000	.0001	.0012	.0055	.0162	.0368	.0689	.1115	.1596	.2051
	7	.0000	.0000	.0001	.0008	.0031	.0090	.0212	.0425	.0746	.1172
	8	.0000	.0000	.0000	.0001	.0004	.0014	.0043	.0106	.0229	.0439
	9	.0000	.0000	.0000	.0000	.0000	.0001	.0005	.0016	.0042	.0098
	10	.0000	.0000	.0000	.0000	.0000	.0000	.0000	.0001	.0003	.0010
11	0	.5688	.3138	.1673	.0859	.0422	.0198	.0088	.0036	.0014	.0005
	1	.3293	.3835	.3248	.2362	.1549	.0932	.0518	.0266	.0125	.0054
	2	.0867	.2131	.2866	.2953	.2581	.1998	.1395	.0887	.0513	.0269
	3	.0137	.0710	.1517	.2215	.2581	.2568	.2254	.1774	.1259	.0806
	4	.0014	.0158	.0536	.1107	.1721	.2201	.2428	.2365	.2060	.1611
	5	.0001	.0025	.0132	.0388	.0803	.1321	.1830	.2207	.2360	.2256
	6	.0000	.0003	.0023	.0097	.0268	.0566	.0985	.1471	.1931	.2256
	7	.0000	.0000	.0003	.0017	.0064	.0173	.0379	.0701	.1128	.1611
	8	.0000	.0000	.0000	.0002	.0011	.0037	.0102	.0234	.0462	.0806
	9	.0000	.0000	.0000	.0000	.0001	.0005	.0018	.0052	.0126	.0269
	10	.0000	.0000	.0000	.0000	.0000	.0000	.0002	.0007	.0021	.0054
	11	.0000	.0000	.0000	.0000	.0000	.0000	.0000	.0000	.0002	.0005
12	0	.5404	.2824	.1422	.0687	.0317	.0138	.0057	.0022	.0008	.0002
	1	.3413	.3766	.3012	.2062	.1267	.0712	.0368	.0174	.0075	.0029
	2	.0988	.2301	.2924	.2835	.2323	.1678	.1088	.0639	.0339	.0161
	3	.0173	.0852	.1720	.2362	.2581	.2397	.1954	.1419	.0923	.0537
	4	.0021	.0213	.0683	.1329	.1936	.2311	.2367	.2128	.1700	.1208
	5	.0002	.0038	.0193	.0532	.1032	.1585	.2039	.2270	.2225	.1934
	6	.0000	.0005	.0040	.0155	.0401	.0792	.1281	.1766	.2124	.2256
	7	.0000	.0000	.0006	.0033	.0115	.0291	.0591	.1009	.1489	.1934
	8	.0000	.0000	.0001	.0005	.0024	.0078	.0199	.0420	.0762	.1208
	9	.0000	.0000	.0000	.0001	.0004	.0015	.0048	.0125	.0277	.0537
	10	.0000	.0000	.0000	.0000	.0000	.0002	.0008	.0025	.0068	.0161
	11	.0000	.0000	.0000	.0000	.0000	.0000	.0001	.0003	.0010	.0029
	12	.0000	.0000	.0000	.0000	.0000	.0000	.0000	.0000	.0001	.0002
13	0	.5133	.2542	.1209	.0550	.0238	.0097	.0037	.0013	.0004	.0001
	1	.3512	.3672	.2774	.1787	.1029	.0540	.0259	.0113	.0045	.0016
	2	.1109	.2448	.2937	.2680	.2059	.1388	.0836	.0453	.0220	.0095
	3	.0214	.0997	.1900	.2457	.2517	.2181	.1651	.1107	.0660	.0349
	4	.0028	.0277	.0838	.1535	.2097	.2337	.2222	.1845	.1350	.0873
	5	.0003	.0055	.0266	.0691	.1258	.1803	.2154	.2214	.1989	.1571
	6	.0000	.0008	.0063	.0230	.0559	.1030	.1546	.1968	.2169	.2095
	7	.0000	.0001	.0011	.0058	.0186	.0442	.0833	.1312	.1775	.2095
	8	.0000	.0000	.0001	.0011	.0047	.0142	.0336	.0656	.1089	.1571
	9	.0000	.0000	.0000	.0001	.0009	.0034	.0101	.0243	.0495	.0873
	10	.0000	.0000	.0000	.0000	.0001	.0006	.0022	.0065	.0162	.0349
	11	.0000	.0000	.0000	.0000	.0000	.0001	.0003	.0012	.0036	.0095
	12	.0000	.0000	.0000	.0000	.0000	.0000	.0000	.0001	.0005	.0016
	13	.0000	.0000	.0000	.0000	.0000	.0000	.0000	.0000	.0000	.0001

(*cont.*)

Table B. Binomial Probabilities $P(X = k)$ (*continued*).

n	k	.05	.10	.15	.20	.25	.30	.35	.40	.45	.50
14	0	.4877	.2288	.1028	.0440	.0178	.0068	.0024	.0008	.0002	.0001
	1	.3593	.3559	.2539	.1539	.0832	.0407	.0181	.0073	.0027	.0009
	2	.1229	.2570	.2912	.2501	.1802	.1134	.0634	.0317	.0141	.0056
	3	.0259	.1142	.2056	.2501	.2402	.1943	.1366	.0845	.0462	.0222
	4	.0037	.0349	.0998	.1720	.2202	.2290	.2022	.1549	.1040	.0611
	5	.0004	.0078	.0352	.0860	.1468	.1963	.2178	.2066	.1701	.1222
	6	.0000	.0013	.0093	.0322	.0734	.1262	.1759	.2066	.2088	.1833
	7	.0000	.0002	.0019	.0092	.0280	.0618	.1082	.1574	.1952	.2095
	8	.0000	.0000	.0003	.0020	.0082	.0232	.0510	.0918	.1398	.1833
	9	.0000	.0000	.0000	.0003	.0018	.0066	.0183	.0408	.0762	.1222
	10	.0000	.0000	.0000	.0000	.0003	.0014	.0049	.0136	.0312	.0611
	11	.0000	.0000	.0000	.0000	.0000	.0002	.0010	.0033	.0093	.0222
	12	.0000	.0000	.0000	.0000	.0000	.0000	.0001	.0005	.0019	.0056
	13	.0000	.0000	.0000	.0000	.0000	.0000	.0000	.0001	.0002	.0009
	14	.0000	.0000	.0000	.0000	.0000	.0000	.0000	.0000	.0000	.0001
15	0	.4633	.2059	.0874	.0352	.0134	.0047	.0016	.0005	.0001	.0000
	1	.3658	.3432	.2312	.1319	.0668	.0305	.0126	.0047	.0016	.0005
	2	.1348	.2669	.2856	.2309	.1559	.0916	.0476	.0219	.0090	.0032
	3	.0307	.1285	.2184	.2501	.2252	.1700	.1110	.0634	.0318	.0139
	4	.0049	.0428	.1156	.1876	.2252	.2186	.1792	.1268	.0780	.0417
	5	.0006	.0105	.0449	.1032	.1651	.2061	.2123	.1859	.1404	.0916
	6	.0000	.0019	.0132	.0430	.0917	.1472	.1906	.2066	.1914	.1527
	7	.0000	.0003	.0030	.0138	.0393	.0811	.1319	.1771	.2013	.1964
	8	.0000	.0000	.0005	.0035	.0131	.0348	.0710	.1181	.1647	.1964
	9	.0000	.0000	.0001	.0007	.0034	.0116	.0298	.0612	.1048	.1527
	10	.0000	.0000	.0000	.0001	.0007	.0030	.0096	.0245	.0515	.0916
	11	.0000	.0000	.0000	.0000	.0001	.0006	.0024	.0074	.0191	.0417
	12	.0000	.0000	.0000	.0000	.0000	.0001	.0004	.0016	.0052	.0139
	13	.0000	.0000	.0000	.0000	.0000	.0000	.0001	.0003	.0010	.0032
	14	.0000	.0000	.0000	.0000	.0000	.0000	.0000	.0000	.0001	.0005
	15	.0000	.0000	.0000	.0000	.0000	.0000	.0000	.0000	.0000	.0000
16	0	.4401	.1853	.0743	.0281	.0100	.0033	.0010	.0003	.0001	.0000
	1	.3706	.3294	.2097	.1126	.0535	.0228	.0087	.0030	.0009	.0002
	2	.1463	.2745	.2775	.2111	.1336	.0732	.0353	.0150	.0056	.0018
	3	.0359	.1423	.2285	.2463	.2079	.1465	.0888	.0468	.0215	.0085
	4	.0061	.0514	.1311	.2001	.2252	.2040	.1553	.1014	.0572	.0278
	5	.0008	.0137	.0555	.1201	.1802	.2099	.2008	.1623	.1123	.0667
	6	.0001	.0028	.0180	.0550	.1101	.1649	.1982	.1983	.1684	.1222
	7	.0000	.0004	.0045	.0197	.0524	.1010	.1524	.1889	.1969	.1746
	8	.0000	.0001	.0009	.0055	.0197	.0487	.0923	.1417	.1812	.1964
	9	.0000	.0000	.0001	.0012	.0058	.0185	.0442	.0840	.1318	.1746
	10	.0000	.0000	.0000	.0002	.0014	.0056	.0167	.0392	.0755	.1222
	11	.0000	.0000	.0000	.0000	.0002	.0013	.0049	.0142	.0337	.0667
	12	.0000	.0000	.0000	.0000	.0000	.0002	.0011	.0040	.0115	.0278
	13	.0000	.0000	.0000	.0000	.0000	.0000	.0002	.0008	.0029	.0085
	14	.0000	.0000	.0000	.0000	.0000	.0000	.0000	.0001	.0005	.0018
	15	.0000	.0000	.0000	.0000	.0000	.0000	.0000	.0000	.0001	.0002
	16	.0000	.0000	.0000	.0000	.0000	.0000	.0000	.0000	.0000	.0000

Table B. Binomial Probabilities $P(X = k)$ (*continued*).

n	k	.05	.10	.15	.20	.25	.30	.35	.40	.45	.50
17	0	.4181	.1668	.0631	.0225	.0075	.0023	.0007	.0002	.0000	.0000
	1	.3741	.3150	.1893	.0957	.0426	.0169	.0060	.0019	.0005	.0001
	2	.1575	.2800	.2673	.1914	.1136	.0581	.0260	.0102	.0035	.0010
	3	.0415	.1556	.2359	.2393	.1893	.1245	.0701	.0341	.0144	.0052
	4	.0076	.0605	.1457	.2093	.2209	.1868	.1320	.0796	.0411	.0182
	5	.0010	.0175	.0668	.1361	.1914	.2081	.1849	.1379	.0875	.0472
	6	.0001	.0039	.0236	.0680	.1276	.1784	.1991	.1839	.1432	.0944
	7	.0000	.0007	.0065	.0267	.0668	.1201	.1685	.1927	.1841	.1484
	8	.0000	.0001	.0014	.0084	.0279	.0644	.1134	.1606	.1883	.1855
	9	.0000	.0000	.0003	.0021	.0093	.0276	.0611	.1070	.1540	.1855
	10	.0000	.0000	.0000	.0004	.0025	.0095	.0263	.0571	.1008	.1484
	11	.0000	.0000	.0000	.0001	.0005	.0026	.0090	.0242	.0525	.0944
	12	.0000	.0000	.0000	.0000	.0001	.0006	.0024	.0081	.0215	.0472
	13	.0000	.0000	.0000	.0000	.0000	.0001	.0005	.0021	.0068	.0182
	14	.0000	.0000	.0000	.0000	.0000	.0000	.0001	.0004	.0016	.0052
	15	.0000	.0000	.0000	.0000	.0000	.0000	.0000	.0001	.0003	.0010
	16	.0000	.0000	.0000	.0000	.0000	.0000	.0000	.0000	.0000	.0001
	17	.0000	.0000	.0000	.0000	.0000	.0000	.0000	.0000	.0000	.0000
18	0	.3972	.1501	.0536	.0180	.0056	.0016	.0004	.0001	.0000	.0000
	1	.3763	.3002	.1704	.0811	.0338	.0126	.0042	.0012	.0003	.0001
	2	.1683	.2835	.2556	.1723	.0958	.0458	.0190	.0069	.0022	.0006
	3	.0473	.1680	.2406	.2297	.1704	.1046	.0547	.0246	.0095	.0031
	4	.0093	.0700	.1592	.2153	.2130	.1681	.1104	.0614	.0291	.0117
	5	.0014	.0218	.0787	.1507	.1988	.2017	.1664	.1146	.0666	.0327
	6	.0002	.0052	.0301	.0816	.1436	.1873	.1941	.1655	.1181	.0708
	7	.0000	.0010	.0091	.0350	.0820	.1376	.1792	.1892	.1657	.1214
	8	.0000	.0002	.0022	.0120	.0376	.0811	.1327	.1734	.1864	.1669
	9	.0000	.0000	.0004	.0033	.0139	.0386	.0794	.1284	.1694	.1855
	10	.0000	.0000	.0001	.0008	.0042	.0149	.0385	.0771	.1248	.1669
	11	.0000	.0000	.0000	.0001	.0010	.0046	.0151	.0374	.0742	.1214
	12	.0000	.0000	.0000	.0000	.0002	.0012	.0047	.0145	.0354	.0708
	13	.0000	.0000	.0000	.0000	.0000	.0002	.0012	.0045	.0134	.0327
	14	.0000	.0000	.0000	.0000	.0000	.0000	.0002	.0011	.0039	.0117
	15	.0000	.0000	.0000	.0000	.0000	.0000	.0000	.0002	.0009	.0031
	16	.0000	.0000	.0000	.0000	.0000	.0000	.0000	.0000	.0001	.0006
	17	.0000	.0000	.0000	.0000	.0000	.0000	.0000	.0000	.0000	.0001
	18	.0000	.0000	.0000	.0000	.0000	.0000	.0000	.0000	.0000	.0000
19	0	.3774	.1351	.0456	.0144	.0042	.0011	.0003	.0001	.0000	.0000
	1	.3774	.2852	.1529	.0685	.0268	.0093	.0029	.0008	.0002	.0000
	2	.1787	.2852	.2428	.1540	.0803	.0358	.0138	.0046	.0013	.0003
	3	.0533	.1796	.2428	.2182	.1517	.0869	.0422	.0175	.0062	.0018
	4	.0112	.0798	.1714	.2182	.2023	.1491	.0909	.0467	.0203	.0074
	5	.0018	.0266	.0907	.1636	.2023	.1916	.1468	.0933	.0497	.0222
	6	.0002	.0069	.0374	.0955	.1574	.1916	.1844	.1451	.0949	.0518
	7	.0000	.0014	.0122	.0443	.0974	.1525	.1844	.1797	.1443	.0961
	8	.0000	.0002	.0032	.0166	.0487	.0981	.1489	.1797	.1771	.1442
	9	.0000	.0000	.0007	.0051	.0198	.0514	.0980	.1464	.1771	.1762
	10	.0000	.0000	.0001	.0013	.0066	.0220	.0528	.0976	.1449	.1762
	11	.0000	.0000	.0000	.0003	.0018	.0077	.0233	.0532	.0970	.1442
	12	.0000	.0000	.0000	.0000	.0004	.0022	.0083	.0237	.0529	.0961
	13	.0000	.0000	.0000	.0000	.0001	.0005	.0024	.0085	.0233	.0518
	14	.0000	.0000	.0000	.0000	.0000	.0001	.0006	.0024	.0082	.0222
	15	.0000	.0000	.0000	.0000	.0000	.0000	.0001	.0005	.0022	.0074
	16	.0000	.0000	.0000	.0000	.0000	.0000	.0000	.0001	.0005	.0018
	17	.0000	.0000	.0000	.0000	.0000	.0000	.0000	.0000	.0001	.0003
	18	.0000	.0000	.0000	.0000	.0000	.0000	.0000	.0000	.0000	.0000
	19	.0000	.0000	.0000	.0000	.0000	.0000	.0000	.0000	.0000	.0000

(*cont.*)

Table B. Binomial Probabilities $P(X = k)$ (*continued*).

n	k	.05	.10	.15	.20	.25	.30	.35	.40	.45	.50
20	0	.3585	.1216	.0388	.0115	.0032	.0008	.0002	.0000	.0000	.0000
	1	.3774	.2702	.1368	.0576	.0211	.0068	.0020	.0005	.0001	.0000
	2	.1887	.2852	.2293	.1369	.0669	.0278	.0100	.0031	.0008	.0002
	3	.0596	.1901	.2428	.2054	.1339	.0716	.0323	.0123	.0040	.0011
	4	.0133	.0898	.1821	.2182	.1897	.1304	.0738	.0350	.0139	.0046
	5	.0022	.0319	.1028	.1746	.2023	.1789	.1272	.0746	.0365	.0148
	6	.0003	.0089	.0454	.1091	.1686	.1916	.1712	.1244	.0746	.0370
	7	.0000	.0020	.0160	.0545	.1124	.1643	.1844	.1659	.1221	.0739
	8	.0000	.0004	.0046	.0222	.0609	.1144	.1614	.1797	.1623	.1201
	9	.0000	.0001	.0011	.0074	.0271	.0654	.1158	.1597	.1771	.1602
	10	.0000	.0000	.0002	.0020	.0099	.0308	.0686	.1171	.1593	.1762
	11	.0000	.0000	.0000	.0005	.0030	.0120	.0336	.0710	.1185	.1602
	12	.0000	.0000	.0000	.0001	.0008	.0039	.0136	.0355	.0727	.1201
	13	.0000	.0000	.0000	.0000	.0002	.0010	.0045	.0146	.0366	.0739
	14	.0000	.0000	.0000	.0000	.0000	.0002	.0012	.0049	.0150	.0370
	15	.0000	.0000	.0000	.0000	.0000	.0000	.0003	.0013	.0049	.0148
	16	.0000	.0000	.0000	.0000	.0000	.0000	.0000	.0003	.0013	.0046
	17	.0000	.0000	.0000	.0000	.0000	.0000	.0000	.0000	.0002	.0011
	18	.0000	.0000	[1] .0000	.0000	.0000	.0000	.0000	.0000	.0000	.0002
	19	.0000	.0000	.0000	.0000	.0000	.0000	.0000	.0000	.0000	.0000
	20	.0000	.0000	.0000	.0000	.0000	.0000	.0000	.0000	.0000	.0000
25	0	.2774	.0718	.0172	.0038	.0008	.0001	.0000	.0000	.0000	.0000
	1	.3650	.1994	.0759	.0236	.0063	.0014	.0003	.0000	.0000	.0000
	2	.2305	.2659	.1607	.0708	.0251	.0074	.0018	.0004	.0001	.0000
	3	.0930	.2265	.2174	.1358	.0641	.0243	.0076	.0019	.0004	.0001
	4	.0269	.1384	.2110	.1867	.1175	.0572	.0224	.0071	.0018	.0004
	5	.0060	.0646	.1564	.1960	.1645	.1030	.0506	.0199	.0063	.0016
	6	.0010	.0239	.0920	.1633	.1828	.1472	.0908	.0442	.0172	.0053
	7	.0001	.0072	.0441	.1108	.1654	.1712	.1327	.0800	.0381	.0143
	8	.0000	.0018	.0175	.0623	.1241	.1651	.1607	.1200	.0701	.0322
	9	.0000	.0004	.0058	.0294	.0781	.1336	.1635	.1511	.1084	.0609
	10	.0000	.0001	.0016	.0118	.0417	.0916	.1409	.1612	.1419	.0974
	11	.0000	.0000	.0004	.0040	.0189	.0536	.1034	.1465	.1583	.1328
	12	.0000	.0000	.0001	.0012	.0074	.0268	.0650	.1140	.1511	.1550
	13	.0000	.0000	.0000	.0003	.0025	.0115	.0350	.0760	.1236	.1550
	14	.0000	.0000	.0000	.0001	.0007	.0042	.0161	.0434	.0867	.1328
	15	.0000	.0000	.0000	.0000	.0002	.0013	.0064	.0212	.0520	.0974
	16	.0000	.0000	.0000	.0000	.0000	.0004	.0021	.0088	.0266	.0609
	17	.0000	.0000	.0000	.0000	.0000	.0001	.0006	.0031	.0115	.0322
	18	.0000	.0000	.0000	.0000	.0000	.0000	.0001	.0009	.0042	.0143
	19	.0000	.0000	.0000	.0000	.0000	.0000	.0000	.0002	.0013	.0053
	20	.0000	.0000	.0000	.0000	.0000	.0000	.0000	.0000	.0003	.0016
	21	.0000	.0000	.0000	.0000	.0000	.0000	.0000	.0000	.0001	.0004
	22	.0000	.0000	.0000	.0000	.0000	.0000	.0000	.0000	.0000	.0001
	23	.0000	.0000	.0000	.0000	.0000	.0000	.0000	.0000	.0000	.0000
	24	.0000	.0000	.0000	.0000	.0000	.0000	.0000	.0000	.0000	.0000
	25	.0000	.0000	.0000	.0000	.0000	.0000	.0000	.0000	.0000	.0000

Table B. Binomial Probabilities $P(X = k)$ (*continued*).

n	k	.05	.10	.15	.20	.25	.30	.35	.40	.45	.50
30	0	.2146	.0424	.0076	.0012	.0002	.0000	.0000	.0000	.0000	.0000
	1	.3389	.1413	.0404	.0093	.0018	.0003	.0000	.0000	.0000	.0000
	2	.2586	.2277	.1034	.0337	.0086	.0018	.0003	.0000	.0000	.0000
	3	.1270	.2361	.1703	.0785	.0269	.0072	.0015	.0003	.0000	.0000
	4	.0451	.1771	.2028	.1325	.0604	.0208	.0056	.0012	.0002	.0000
	5	.0124	.1023	.1861	.1723	.1047	.0464	.0157	.0041	.0008	.0001
	6	.0027	.0474	.1368	.1795	.1455	.0829	.0353	.0115	.0029	.0006
	7	.0005	.0180	.0828	.1538	.1662	.1219	.0652	.0263	.0081	.0019
	8	.0001	.0058	.0420	.1106	.1593	.1501	.1009	.0505	.0191	.0055
	9	.0000	.0016	.0181	.0676	.1298	.1573	.1328	.0823	.0382	.0133
	10	.0000	.0004	.0067	.0355	.0909	.1416	.1502	.1152	.0656	.0280
	11	.0000	.0001	.0022	.0161	.0551	.1103	.1471	.1396	.0976	.0509
	12	.0000	.0000	.0006	.0064	.0291	.0749	.1254	.1474	.1265	.0806
	13	.0000	.0000	.0001	.0022	.0134	.0444	.0935	.1360	.1433	.1115
	14	.0000	.0000	.0000	.0007	.0054	.0231	.0611	.1101	.1424	.1354
	15	.0000	.0000	.0000	.0002	.0019	.0106	.0351	.0783	.1242	.1445
	16	.0000	.0000	.0000	.0000	.0006	.0042	.0177	.0489	.0953	.1354
	17	.0000	.0000	.0000	.0000	.0002	.0015	.0079	.0269	.0642	.1115
	18	.0000	.0000	.0000	.0000	.0000	.0005	.0031	.0129	.0379	.0806
	19	.0000	.0000	.0000	.0000	.0000	.0001	.0010	.0054	.0196	.0509
	20	.0000	.0000	.0000	.0000	.0000	.0000	.0003	.0020	.0088	.0280
	21	.0000	.0000	.0000	.0000	.0000	.0000	.0001	.0006	.0034	.0133
	22	.0000	.0000	.0000	.0000	.0000	.0000	.0000	.0002	.0012	.0055
	23	.0000	.0000	.0000	.0000	.0000	.0000	.0000	.0000	.0003	.0019
	24	.0000	.0000	.0000	.0000	.0000	.0000	.0000	.0000	.0001	.0006
	25	.0000	.0000	.0000	.0000	.0000	.0000	.0000	.0000	.0000	.0001
	26	.0000	.0000	.0000	.0000	.0000	.0000	.0000	.0000	.0000	.0000
	27	.0000	.0000	.0000	.0000	.0000	.0000	.0000	.0000	.0000	.0000
	28	.0000	.0000	.0000	.0000	.0000	.0000	.0000	.0000	.0000	.0000
	29	.0000	.0000	.0000	.0000	.0000	.0000	.0000	.0000	.0000	.0000
	30	.0000	.0000	.0000	.0000	.0000	.0000	.0000	.0000	.0000	.0000

Table C. Poisson Probabilities $P(X = k)$.

k	$\mu = .5$	1.0	1.5	2.0	2.5	3.0	3.5	4.0	4.5	5.0
0	.6065	.3679	.2231	.1353	.0821	.0498	.0302	.0183	.0111	.0067
1	.3033	.3679	.3347	.2707	.2052	.1494	.1057	.0733	.0500	.0337
2	.0758	.1839	.2510	.2707	.2565	.2240	.1850	.1465	.1125	.0842
3	.0126	.0613	.1255	.1804	.2138	.2240	.2158	.1954	.1687	.1404
4	.0016	.0153	.0471	.0902	.1336	.1680	.1888	.1954	.1898	.1755
5	.0002	.0031	.0141	.0361	.0668	.1008	.1322	.1563	.1708	.1755
6	—	.0005	.0035	.0120	.0278	.0504	.0771	.1042	.1281	.1462
7	—	.0001	.0008	.0034	.0099	.0216	.0385	.0595	.0824	.1044
8	—	—	.0001	.0009	.0031	.0081	.0169	.0298	.0463	.0653
9	—	—	—	.0002	.0009	.0027	.0066	.0132	.0232	.0363
10	—	—	—	—	.0002	.0008	.0023	.0053	.0104	.0181
11	—	—	—	—	—	.0002	.0007	.0019	.0043	.0082
12	—	—	—	—	—	.0001	.0002	.0006	.0016	.0034
13	—	—	—	—	—	—	.0001	.0002	.0006	.0013
14	—	—	—	—	—	—	—	.0001	.0002	.0005
15	—	—	—	—	—	—	—	—	.0001	.0002
16	—	—	—	—	—	—	—	—	—	—

k	$\mu = 5.5$	6.0	6.5	7.0	7.5	8.0	8.5	9.0	9.5	10.0
0	.0041	.0025	.0015	.0009	.0006	.0003	.0002	.0001	.0001	—
1	.0225	.0149	.0098	.0064	.0041	.0027	.0017	.0011	.0007	.0005
2	.0618	.0446	.0318	.0223	.0156	.0107	.0074	.0050	.0034	.0023
3	.1133	.0892	.0688	.0521	.0389	.0286	.0208	.0150	.0107	.0076
4	.1558	.1339	.1118	.0912	.0729	.0573	.0443	.0337	.0254	.0189
5	.1714	.1606	.1454	.1277	.1094	.0916	.0752	.0607	.0483	.0378
6	.1571	.1606	.1575	.1490	.1367	.1221	.1066	.0911	.0764	.0631
7	.1234	.1377	.1462	.1490	.1465	.1396	.1294	.1171	.1037	.0901
8	.0849	.1033	.1188	.1304	.1373	.1396	.1375	.1318	.1232	.1126
9	.0519	.0688	.0858	.1014	.1144	.1241	.1299	.1318	.1300	.1251
10	.0285	.0413	.0558	.0710	.0858	.0993	.1104	.1186	.1235	.1251
11	.0143	.0225	.0330	.0452	.0585	.0722	.0853	.0970	.1067	.1137
12	.0065	.0113	.0179	.0263	.0366	.0481	.0604	.0728	.0844	.0948
13	.0028	.0052	.0089	.0142	.0211	.0296	.0395	.0504	.0617	.0729
14	.0011	.0022	.0041	.0071	.0113	.0169	.0240	.0324	.0419	.0521
15	.0004	.0009	.0018	.0033	.0057	.0090	.0136	.0194	.0265	.0347
16	.0001	.0003	.0007	.0014	.0026	.0045	.0072	.0109	.0157	.0217
17	—	.0001	.0003	.0006	.0012	.0021	.0036	.0058	.0088	.0128
18	—	—	.0001	.0002	.0005	.0009	.0017	.0029	.0046	.0071
19	—	—	—	.0001	.0002	.0004	.0008	.0014	.0023	.0037
20	—	—	—	—	.0001	.0002	.0003	.0006	.0011	.0019
21	—	—	—	—	—	.0001	.0001	.0003	.0005	.0009
22	—	—	—	—	—	—	.0001	.0001	.0002	.0004
23	—	—	—	—	—	—	—	—	.0001	.0002
24	—	—	—	—	—	—	—	—	—	.0001
25	—	—	—	—	—	—	—	—	—	—

Table C **317**

Table C. Poisson Probabilities $P(X = k)$ (*continued*).

k	$\mu = 10.5$	11.0	11.5	12.0	12.5	13.0	13.5	14.0	14.5	15.0
0	—	—	—	—	—	—	—	—	—	—
1	.0003	.0002	.0001	.0001	—	—	—	—	—	—
2	.0015	.0010	.0007	.0004	.0003	.0002	.0001	.0001	.0001	—
3	.0053	.0037	.0026	.0018	.0012	.0008	.0006	.0004	.0003	.0002
4	.0139	.0102	.0074	.0053	.0038	.0027	.0019	.0013	.0009	.0006
5	.0293	.0224	.0170	.0127	.0095	.0070	.0051	.0037	.0027	.0019
6	.0513	.0411	.0325	.0255	.0197	.0152	.0115	.0087	.0065	.0048
7	.0769	.0646	.0535	.0437	.0353	.0281	.0222	.0174	.0135	.0104
8	.1009	.0888	.0769	.0655	.0551	.0457	.0375	.0304	.0244	.0194
9	.1177	.1085	.0982	.0874	.0765	.0661	.0563	.0473	.0394	.0324
10	.1236	.1194	.1129	.1048	.0956	.0859	.0760	.0663	.0571	.0486
11	.1180	.1194	.1181	.1144	.1087	.1015	.0932	.0844	.0753	.0663
12	.1032	.1094	.1131	.1144	.1132	.1099	.1049	.0984	.0910	.0829
13	.0834	.0926	.1001	.1056	.1089	.1099	.1089	.1060	.1014	.0956
14	.0625	.0728	.0822	.0905	.0972	.1021	.1050	.1060	.1051	.1024
15	.0438	.0534	.0630	.0724	.0810	.0885	.0945	.0989	.1016	.1024
16	.0287	.0367	.0453	.0543	.0633	.0719	.0798	.0866	.0920	.0960
17	.0177	.0237	.0306	.0383	.0465	.0550	.0633	.0713	.0785	.0847
18	.0104	.0145	.0196	.0255	.0323	.0397	.0475	.0554	.0632	.0706
19	.0057	.0084	.0119	.0161	.0213	.0272	.0337	.0409	.0483	.0557
20	.0030	.0046	.0068	.0097	.0133	.0177	.0228	.0286	.0350	.0418
21	.0015	.0024	.0037	.0055	.0079	.0109	.0146	.0191	.0242	.0299
22	.0007	.0012	.0020	.0030	.0045	.0065	.0090	.0121	.0159	.0204
23	.0003	.0006	.0010	.0016	.0024	.0037	.0053	.0074	.0100	.0133
24	.0001	.0003	.0005	.0008	.0013	.0020	.0030	.0043	.0061	.0083
25	.0001	.0001	.0002	.0004	.0006	.0010	.0016	.0024	.0035	.0050
26	—	—	.0001	.0002	.0003	.0005	.0008	.0013	.0020	.0029
27	—	—	—	.0001	.0001	.0002	.0004	.0007	.0011	.0016
28	—	—	—	—	.0001	.0001	.0002	.0003	.0005	.0009
29	—	—	—	—	—	.0001	.0001	.0002	.0003	.0004
30	—	—	—	—	—	—	—	.0001	.0001	.0002
31	—	—	—	—	—	—	—	—	.0001	.0001
32	—	—	—	—	—	—	—	—	—	.0001
33	—	—	—	—	—	—	—	—	—	—

(*cont.*)

Table C. Poisson Probabilities $P(X = k)$ (*continued*).

k	$\mu = 15.5$	16.0	16.5	17.0	17.5	18.0	18.5	19.0	19.5	20.0
0	—	—	—	—	—	—	—	—	—	—
1	—	—	—	—	—	—	—	—	—	—
2	—	—	—	—	—	—	—	—	—	—
3	.0001	.0001	.0001	—	—	—	—	—	—	—
4	.0004	.0003	.0002	.0001	.0001	.0001	—	—	—	—
5	.0014	.0010	.0007	.0005	.0003	.0002	.0002	.0001	.0001	.0001
6	.0036	.0026	.0019	.0014	.0010	.0007	.0005	.0004	.0003	.0002
7	.0079	.0060	.0045	.0034	.0025	.0019	.0014	.0010	.0007	.0005
8	.0153	.0120	.0093	.0072	.0055	.0042	.0031	.0024	.0018	.0013
9	.0264	.0213	.0171	.0135	.0107	.0083	.0065	.0050	.0038	.0029
10	.0409	.0341	.0281	.0230	.0186	.0150	.0120	.0095	.0074	.0058
11	.0577	.0496	.0422	.0355	.0297	.0245	.0201	.0164	.0132	.0106
12	.0745	.0661	.0580	.0504	.0432	.0368	.0310	.0259	.0214	.0176
13	.0888	.0814	.0736	.0658	.0582	.0509	.0441	.0378	.0322	.0271
14	.0983	.0930	.0868	.0800	.0728	.0655	.0583	.0514	.0448	.0387
15	.1016	.0992	.0955	.0906	.0849	.0786	.0719	.0650	.0582	.0516
16	.0984	.0992	.0985	.0963	.0929	.0884	.0831	.0772	.0710	.0646
17	.0897	.0934	.0956	.0963	.0956	.0936	.0904	.0863	.0814	.0760
18	.0773	.0830	.0876	.0909	.0929	.0936	.0930	.0911	.0882	.0844
19	.0630	.0699	.0761	.0814	.0856	.0887	.0905	.0911	.0905	.0888
20	.0489	.0559	.0628	.0692	.0749	.0798	.0837	.0866	.0883	.0888
21	.0361	.0426	.0493	.0560	.0624	.0684	.0738	.0783	.0820	.0846
22	.0254	.0310	.0370	.0433	.0496	.0560	.0620	.0676	.0727	.0769
23	.0171	.0216	.0265	.0320	.0378	.0438	.0499	.0559	.0616	.0669
24	.0111	.0144	.0182	.0226	.0275	.0328	.0385	.0442	.0500	.0557
25	.0069	.0092	.0120	.0154	.0193	.0237	.0285	.0336	.0390	.0446
26	.0041	.0057	.0076	.0101	.0130	.0164	.0202	.0246	.0293	.0343
27	.0023	.0034	.0047	.0063	.0084	.0109	.0139	.0173	.0211	.0254
28	.0013	.0019	.0028	.0038	.0053	.0070	.0092	.0117	.0147	.0181
29	.0007	.0011	.0016	.0023	.0032	.0044	.0058	.0077	.0099	.0125
30	.0004	.0006	.0009	.0013	.0019	.0026	.0036	.0049	.0064	.0083
31	.0002	.0003	.0005	.0007	.0010	.0015	.0022	.0030	.0040	.0054
32	.0001	.0001	.0002	.0004	.0006	.0009	.0012	.0018	.0025	.0034
33	—	.0001	.0001	.0002	.0003	.0005	.0007	.0010	.0015	.0020
34	—	—	.0001	.0001	.0002	.0002	.0004	.0006	.0008	.0012
35	—	—	—	—	.0001	.0001	.0002	.0003	.0005	.0007
36	—	—	—	—	—	.0001	.0001	.0002	.0003	.0004
37	—	—	—	—	—	—	.0001	.0001	.0001	.0002
38	—	—	—	—	—	—	—	—	.0001	.0001
39	—	—	—	—	—	—	—	—	—	.0001
40	—	—	—	—	—	—	—	—	—	—

Table D. Standard Normal Probabilities $P(Z < z)$.

Z	.00	.01	.02	.03	.04	.05	.06	.07	.08	.09
0.00	.5000	.5040	.5080	.5120	.5160	.5199	.5239	.5279	.5319	.5359
0.10	.5398	.5438	.5478	.5517	.5557	.5596	.5636	.5675	.5714	.5753
0.20	.5793	.5832	.5871	.5910	.5948	.5987	.6026	.6064	.6103	.6141
0.30	.6179	.6217	.6255	.6293	.6331	.6368	.6406	.6443	.6480	.6517
0.40	.6554	.6591	.6628	.6664	.6700	.6736	.6772	.6808	.6844	.6879
0.50	.6915	.6950	.6985	.7019	.7054	.7088	.7123	.7157	.7190	.7224
0.60	.7257	.7291	.7324	.7357	.7389	.7422	.7454	.7486	.7517	.7549
0.70	.7580	.7611	.7642	.7673	.7704	.7734	.7764	.7794	.7823	.7852
0.80	.7881	.7910	.7939	.7967	.7995	.8023	.8051	.8078	.8106	.8133
0.90	.8159	.8186	.8212	.8238	.8264	.8289	.8315	.8340	.8365	.8389
1.00	.8413	.8438	.8461	.8485	.8508	.8531	.8554	.8577	.8599	.8621
1.10	.8643	.8665	.8686	.8708	.8729	.8749	.8770	.8790	.8810	.8830
1.20	.8849	.8869	.8888	.8907	.8925	.8944	.8962	.8980	.8997	.9015
1.30	.9032	.9049	.9066	.9082	.9099	.9115	.9131	.9147	.9162	.9177
1.40	.9192	.9207	.9222	.9236	.9251	.9265	.9279	.9292	.9306	.9319
1.50	.9332	.9345	.9357	.9370	.9382	.9394	.9406	.9418	.9429	.9441
1.60	.9452	.9463	.9474	.9484	.9495	.9505	.9515	.9525	.9535	.9545
1.70	.9554	.9564	.9573	.9582	.9591	.9599	.9608	.9616	.9625	.9633
1.80	.9641	.9649	.9656	.9664	.9671	.9678	.9686	.9693	.9699	.9706
1.90	.9713	.9719	.9726	.9732	.9738	.9744	.9750	.9756	.9761	.9767
2.00	.9772	.9778	.9783	.9788	.9793	.9798	.9803	.9808	.9812	.9817
2.10	.9821	.9826	.9830	.9834	.9838	.9842	.9846	.9850	.9854	.9857
2.20	.9861	.9864	.9868	.9871	.9875	.9878	.9881	.9884	.9887	.9890
2.30	.9893	.9896	.9898	.9901	.9904	.9906	.9909	.9911	.9913	.9916
2.40	.9918	.9920	.9922	.9925	.9927	.9929	.9931	.9932	.9934	.9936
2.50	.9938	.9940	.9941	.9943	.9945	.9946	.9948	.9949	.9951	.9952
2.60	.9953	.9955	.9956	.9957	.9959	.9960	.9961	.9962	.9963	.9964
2.70	.9965	.9966	.9967	.9968	.9969	.9970	.9971	.9972	.9973	.9974
2.80	.9974	.9975	.9976	.9977	.9977	.9978	.9979	.9979	.9980	.9981
2.90	.9981	.9982	.9982	.9983	.9984	.9984	.9985	.9985	.9986	.9986
3.00	.9987	.9987	.9987	.9988	.9988	.9989	.9989	.9989	.9990	.9990
3.10	.9990	.9991	.9991	.9991	.9992	.9992	.9992	.9992	.9993	.9993
3.20	.9993	.9993	.9994	.9994	.9994	.9994	.9994	.9995	.9995	.9995
3.30	.9995	.9995	.9995	.9996	.9996	.9996	.9996	.9996	.9996	.9997
3.40	.9997	.9997	.9997	.9997	.9997	.9997	.9997	.9997	.9997	.9998
3.50	.9998	.9998	.9998	.9998	.9998	.9998	.9998	.9998	.9998	.9998
3.60	.9998	.9998	.9999	.9999	.9999	.9999	.9999	.9999	.9999	.9999
3.70	.9999	.9999	.9999	.9999	.9999	.9999	.9999	.9999	.9999	.9999
3.80	.9999	.9999	.9999	.9999	.9999	.9999	.9999	.9999	.9999	.9999
3.90	.9999	.9999	.9999	.9999	.9999	.9999	.9999	.9999	.9999	.9999

Table E. Percentiles of the t Distribution $P(t_{(\delta)} < t)$.

df	.55	.60	.65	.70	.75	.80	.85	.90	.95
1	0.1584	0.3249	0.5095	0.7265	1.0000	1.3764	1.9626	3.0777	6.3138
2	0.1421	0.2887	0.4447	0.6172	0.8165	1.0607	1.3862	1.8856	2.9200
3	0.1366	0.2767	0.4242	0.5844	0.7649	0.9785	1.2498	1.6377	2.3534
4	0.1338	0.2707	0.4142	0.5686	0.7407	0.9410	1.1896	1.5332	2.1318
5	0.1322	0.2672	0.4082	0.5594	0.7267	0.9195	1.1558	1.4759	2.0150
6	0.1311	0.2648	0.4043	0.5534	0.7176	0.9057	1.1342	1.4398	1.9432
7	0.1303	0.2632	0.4015	0.5491	0.7111	0.8960	1.1192	1.4149	1.8946
8	0.1297	0.2619	0.3995	0.5459	0.7064	0.8889	1.1081	1.3968	1.8595
9	0.1293	0.2610	0.3979	0.5435	0.7027	0.8834	1.0997	1.3830	1.8331
10	0.1289	0.2602	0.3966	0.5415	0.6998	0.8791	1.0931	1.3722	1.8125
11	0.1286	0.2596	0.3956	0.5399	0.6974	0.8755	1.0877	1.3634	1.7959
12	0.1283	0.2590	0.3947	0.5386	0.6955	0.8726	1.0832	1.3562	1.7823
13	0.1281	0.2586	0.3940	0.5375	0.6938	0.8702	1.0795	1.3502	1.7709
14	0.1280	0.2582	0.3933	0.5366	0.6924	0.8681	1.0763	1.3450	1.7613
15	0.1278	0.2579	0.3928	0.5357	0.6912	0.8662	1.0735	1.3406	1.7531
16	0.1277	0.2576	0.3923	0.5350	0.6901	0.8647	1.0711	1.3368	1.7459
17	0.1276	0.2573	0.3919	0.5344	0.6892	0.8633	1.0690	1.3334	1.7396
18	0.1274	0.2571	0.3915	0.5338	0.6884	0.8620	1.0672	1.3304	1.7341
19	0.1274	0.2569	0.3912	0.5333	0.6876	0.8610	1.0655	1.3277	1.7291
20	0.1273	0.2567	0.3909	0.5329	0.6870	0.8600	1.0640	1.3253	1.7247
21	0.1272	0.2566	0.3906	0.5325	0.6864	0.8591	1.0627	1.3232	1.7207
22	0.1271	0.2564	0.3904	0.5321	0.6858	0.8583	1.0614	1.3212	1.7171
23	0.1271	0.2563	0.3902	0.5317	0.6853	0.8575	1.0603	1.3195	1.7139
24	0.1270	0.2562	0.3900	0.5314	0.6848	0.8569	1.0593	1.3178	1.7109
25	0.1269	0.2561	0.3898	0.5312	0.6844	0.8562	1.0584	1.3163	1.7081
26	0.1269	0.2560	0.3896	0.5309	0.6840	0.8557	1.0575	1.3150	1.7056
27	0.1268	0.2559	0.3894	0.5306	0.6837	0.8551	1.0567	1.3137	1.7033
28	0.1268	0.2558	0.3893	0.5304	0.6834	0.8546	1.0560	1.3125	1.7011
29	0.1268	0.2557	0.3892	0.5302	0.6830	0.8542	1.0553	1.3114	1.6991
30	0.1267	0.2556	0.3890	0.5300	0.6828	0.8538	1.0547	1.3104	1.6973
40	0.1265	0.2550	0.3881	0.5286	0.6807	0.8507	1.0500	1.3031	1.6839
50	0.1263	0.2547	0.3875	0.5278	0.6794	0.8489	1.0473	1.2987	1.6759
60	0.1262	0.2545	0.3872	0.5272	0.6786	0.8477	1.0455	1.2958	1.6706
70	0.1261	0.2543	0.3869	0.5268	0.6780	0.8468	1.0442	1.2938	1.6669
80	0.1261	0.2542	0.3867	0.5265	0.6776	0.8461	1.0432	1.2922	1.6641
90	0.1260	0.2541	0.3866	0.5263	0.6772	0.8456	1.0424	1.2910	1.6620
100	0.1260	0.2540	0.3864	0.5261	0.6770	0.8452	1.0418	1.2901	1.6602
110	0.1260	0.2540	0.3863	0.5259	0.6767	0.8449	1.0413	1.2893	1.6588
120	0.1259	0.2539	0.3862	0.5258	0.6765	0.8446	1.0409	1.2886	1.6577
inf	0.1257	0.2533	0.3853	0.5244	0.6745	0.8416	1.0364	1.2816	1.6449

Table E.   Percentiles of the t Distribution $P(t_{(\delta)} < t)$ (continued).

df	.975	.980	.985	.990	.9925	01 .9950	.9975	.999	.9995
1	12.706	15.895	21.205	31.821	42.433	63.657	127.32	318.31	636.62
2	4.3027	4.8487	5.6428	6.9646	8.0728	9.9248	14.089	22.327	31.599
3	3.1824	3.4819	3.8960	4.5407	5.0473	5.8409	7.4533	10.215	12.924
4	2.7764	2.9985	3.2976	3.7469	4.0880	4.6041	5.5976	7.1732	8.6103
5	2.5706	2.7565	3.0029	3.3649	3.6338	4.0321	4.7733	5.8934	6.8688
6	2.4469	2.6122	2.8289	3.1427	3.3723	3.7074	4.3168	5.2076	5.9588
7	2.3646	2.5168	2.7146	2.9980	3.2032	3.4995	4.0293	4.7853	5.4079
8	2.3060	2.4490	2.6338	2.8965	3.0851	3.3554	3.8325	4.5008	5.0413
9	2.2622	2.3984	2.5738	2.8214	2.9982	3.2498	3.6897	4.2968	4.7809
10	2.2281	2.3593	2.5275	2.7638	2.9316	3.1693	3.5814	4.1437	4.5869
11	2.2010	2.3281	2.4907	2.7181	2.8789	3.1058	3.4966	4.0247	4.4370
12	2.1788	2.3027	2.4607	2.6810	2.8363	3.0545	3.4284	3.9296	4.3178
13	2.1604	2.2816	2.4358	2.6503	2.8010	3.0123	3.3725	3.8520	4.2208
14	2.1448	2.2638	2.4149	2.6245	2.7714	2.9768	3.3257	3.7874	4.1405
15	2.1314	2.2485	2.3970	2.6025	2.7462	2.9467	3.2860	3.7328	4.0728
16	2.1199	2.2354	2.3815	2.5835	2.7245	2.9208	3.2520	3.6862	4.0150
17	2.1098	2.2238	2.3681	2.5669	2.7056	2.8982	3.2224	3.6458	3.9651
18	2.1009	2.2137	2.3562	2.5524	2.6889	2.8784	3.1966	3.6105	3.9216
19	2.0930	2.2047	2.3456	2.5395	2.6742	2.8609	3.1737	3.5794	3.8834
20	2.0860	2.1967	2.3362	2.5280	2.6611	2.8453	3.1534	3.5518	3.8495
21	2.0796	2.1894	2.3278	2.5176	2.6493	2.8314	3.1352	3.5272	3.8193
22	2.0739	2.1829	2.3202	2.5083	2.6387	2.8188	3.1188	3.5050	3.7921
23	2.0687	2.1770	2.3132	2.4999	2.6290	2.8073	3.1040	3.4850	3.7676
24	2.0639	2.1715	2.3069	2.4922	2.6203	2.7969	3.0905	3.4668	3.7454
25	2.0595	2.1666	2.3011	2.4851	2.6122	2.7874	3.0782	3.4502	3.7251
26	2.0555	2.1620	2.2958	2.4786	2.6049	2.7787	3.0669	3.4350	3.7066
27	2.0518	2.1578	2.2909	2.4727	2.5981	2.7707	3.0565	3.4210	3.6896
28	2.0484	2.1539	2.2864	2.4671	2.5918	2.7633	3.0469	3.4082	3.6739
29	2.0452	2.1503	2.2822	2.4620	2.5860	2.7564	3.0380	3.3962	3.6594
30	2.0423	2.1470	2.2783	2.4573	2.5806	2.7500	3.0298	3.3852	3.6460
40	2.0211	2.1229	2.2503	2.4233	2.5420	2.7045	2.9712	3.3069	3.5510
50	2.0086	2.1087	2.2338	2.4033	2.5193	2.6778	2.9370	3.2614	3.4960
60	2.0003	2.0994	2.2229	2.3901	2.5044	2.6603	2.9146	3.2317	3.4602
70	1.9944	2.0927	2.2152	2.3808	2.4939	2.6479	2.8987	3.2108	3.4350
80	1.9901	2.0878	2.2095	2.3739	2.4860	2.6387	2.8870	3.1953	3.4163
90	1.9867	2.0839	2.2050	2.3685	2.4800	2.6316	2.8779	3.1833	3.4019
100	1.9840	2.0809	2.2015	2.3642	2.4751	2.6259	2.8707	3.1737	3.3905
110	1.9818	2.0784	2.1986	2.3607	2.4712	2.6213	2.8648	3.1660	3.3812
120	1.9799	2.0763	2.1962	2.3578	2.4679	2.6174	2.8599	3.1595	3.3735
inf	1.9600	2.0537	2.1701	2.3263	2.4324	2.5758	2.8070	3.0902	3.2905

Table F.   Percentiles of the χ^2 Distribution $P(\chi^2_{(\delta)} < \chi^2)$.

df	.005	.010	.025	.050	.100	.900	.950	.975	.990	.995
1	0.000	0.000	0.001	0.004	0.016	2.706	3.841	5.024	6.635	7.879
2	0.010	0.020	0.051	0.103	0.211	4.605	5.991	7.378	9.210	10.597
3	0.072	0.115	0.216	0.352	0.584	6.251	7.815	9.348	11.345	12.838
4	0.207	0.297	0.484	0.711	1.064	7.779	9.488	11.143	13.277	14.860
5	0.412	0.554	0.831	1.145	1.610	9.236	11.070	12.833	15.086	16.750
6	0.676	0.872	1.237	1.635	2.204	10.645	12.592	14.449	16.812	18.548
7	0.989	1.239	1.690	2.167	2.833	12.017	14.067	16.013	18.475	20.278
8	1.344	1.646	2.180	2.733	3.490	13.362	15.507	17.535	20.090	21.955
9	1.735	2.088	2.700	3.325	4.168	14.684	16.919	19.023	21.666	23.589
10	2.156	2.558	3.247	3.940	4.865	15.987	18.307	20.483	23.209	25.188
11	2.603	3.053	3.816	4.575	5.578	17.275	19.675	21.920	24.725	26.757
12	3.074	3.571	4.404	5.226	6.304	18.549	21.026	23.337	26.217	28.300
13	3.565	4.107	5.009	5.892	7.042	19.812	22.362	24.736	27.688	29.819
14	4.075	4.660	5.629	6.571	7.790	21.064	23.685	26.119	29.141	31.319
15	4.601	5.229	6.262	7.261	8.547	22.307	24.996	27.488	30.578	32.801
16	5.142	5.812	6.908	7.962	9.312	23.542	26.296	28.845	32.000	34.267
17	5.697	6.408	7.564	8.672	10.085	24.769	27.587	30.191	33.409	35.718
18	6.265	7.015	8.231	9.390	10.865	25.989	28.869	31.526	34.805	37.156
19	6.844	7.633	8.907	10.117	11.651	27.204	30.144	32.852	36.191	38.582
20	7.434	8.260	9.591	10.851	12.443	28.412	31.410	34.170	37.566	39.997
21	8.034	8.897	10.283	11.591	13.240	29.615	32.671	35.479	38.932	41.401
22	8.643	9.542	10.982	12.338	14.041	30.813	33.924	36.781	40.289	42.796
23	9.260	10.196	11.689	13.091	14.848	32.007	35.172	38.076	41.638	44.181
24	9.886	10.856	12.401	13.848	15.659	33.196	36.415	39.364	42.980	45.559
25	10.520	11.524	13.120	14.611	16.473	34.382	37.652	40.646	44.314	46.928
26	11.160	12.198	13.844	15.379	17.292	35.563	38.885	41.923	45.642	48.290
27	11.808	12.879	14.573	16.151	18.114	36.741	40.113	43.195	46.963	49.645
28	12.461	13.565	15.308	16.928	18.939	37.916	41.337	44.461	48.278	50.993
29	13.121	14.256	16.047	17.708	19.768	39.087	42.557	45.722	49.588	52.336
30	13.787	14.953	16.791	18.493	20.599	40.256	43.773	46.979	50.892	53.672
40	20.707	22.164	24.433	26.509	29.051	51.805	55.758	59.342	63.691	66.766
50	27.991	29.707	32.357	34.764	37.689	63.167	67.505	71.420	76.154	79.490
60	35.534	37.485	40.482	43.188	46.459	74.397	79.082	83.298	88.379	91.952
70	43.275	45.442	48.758	51.739	55.329	85.527	90.531	95.023	100.425	104.215
80	51.172	53.540	57.153	60.391	64.278	96.578	101.879	106.629	112.329	116.321
90	59.196	61.754	65.647	69.126	73.291	107.565	113.145	118.136	124.116	128.299
100	67.328	70.065	74.222	77.929	82.358	118.498	124.342	129.561	135.807	140.169

Table G. Percentiles of the *F* Distribution.

Denominator df	p	Numerator df																				
		1	2	3	4	5	6	7	8	9	10	12	14	16	18	20	25	30	60	90	120	inf
1	.50	1.00	1.50	1.71	1.82	1.89	1.94	1.98	2.00	2.03	2.04	2.07	2.09	2.10	2.11	2.12	2.13	2.15	2.17	2.18	2.18	2.2
	.90	39.86	49.50	53.59	55.83	57.24	58.20	58.91	59.44	59.86	60.19	60.71	61.07	61.35	61.57	61.74	j.62.05	62.26	62.79	62.97	63.06	63.3
	.95	161.45	199.50	215.71	224.58	230.16	233.99	236.77	238.88	240.54	241.88	243.91	245.36	246.46	247.32	248.01	249.26	250.10	252.20	252.90	253.25	254.3
	.975	647.79	799.50	864.16	899.58	921.85	937.11	948.22	956.66	963.28	968.63	976.71	982.53	986.92	990.35	993.10	998.08	1001.4	1009.8	1012. 6	1014. 0	1018.
	.99	4052.2	4999.5	5403.4	5624.6	5763.6	5859.0	5928.4	5981.1	6022.5	6055.8	6106.3	6142.7	6170.1	6191.5	6208.7	6239.8	6260.6	6313.0	6330.6	6339.4	6365.
	.995	16211	19999	21615	22500	23056	23437	23715	23925	24091	24224	24426	24572	24681	24767	24836	24960	25044	25253	25323	25359	2546
	.999	405284	499999	540379	562500	576405	585937	592873	598144	602284	605621	610668	614303	617045	619188	620908	624017	626099	631337	633093	633972	63664
2	.SO	0.67	1.00	1.13	1.21	1.25	1.28	1.30	1.32	1.33	1.35	1.36	1.37	1.38	1.39	1.39	1.40	1.41	1.43	1.43	1.43	1.4
	.90	8.53	9.00	9.16	9.24	9.29	9.33	9.35	9.37	9.38	9.39	9.41	9.42	9.43	9.44	9.44	9.45	9.46	9.47	9.48	9.48	9.4
	.95	18.51	19.00	19.16	19.25	19.30	19.33	19.35	19.37	19.38	19.40	19.41	19.42	19.43	19.44	19.45	19.46	19.46	19.48	19.48	19.49	19.5
	.975	38.51	39.00	39.17	39.25	39.30	39.33	39.36	39.37	39.39	39.40	39.41	39.43	39.44	39.44	39.45	39.46	39.46	39.48	39.49	39.49	39.5
	.99	98.50	99.00	99.17	99.25	99.30	99.33	99.36	99.37	99.39	99.40	99.42	99.43	99.44	99.44	99.45	99.46	99.47	99.48	99.49	99.49	99.5
	.995	198.50	199.00	199.17	199.25	199.30	199.33	199.36	199.37	199.39	199.40	199.42	199.43	199.44	199.44	199.45	199.46	199.47	199.48	199.49	199.49	199.5
	.999	998.50	999.00	999.17	999.25	999.30	999.33	999.36	999.37	999.39	999.40	999.42	999.43	999.44	999.44	999.45	999.46	999.47	999.48	999.49	999.49	999.5
3	.50	0.59	0.88	1.00	1.06	1.10	1.13	1.15	1.16	1.17	1.18	1.20	1.21	1.21	1.22	1.23	1.23	1.24	1.25	1.26	1.26	1.2
	.90	5.54	5.46	5.39	5.34	5.31	5.28	5.27	5.25	5.24	5.23	5.22	5.20	5.20	5.19	5.18	5.17	5.17	5.15	5.15	5.14	5.1
	.95	10.13	9.55	9.28	9.12	9.01	8.94	8.89	8.85	8.81	8.79	8.74	8.71	8.69	8.67	8.66	8.63	8.62	8.57	8.56	8.55	8.5
	.975	17.44	16.04	15.44	15.10	14.88	14.73	14.62	14.54	14.47	14.42	14.34	14.28	14.23	14.20	14.17	14.12	14.08	13. 99	13.96	13.95	13.9
	.99	34.12	30.82	29.46	28.71	28.24	27.91	27.67	27.49	27.35	27.23	27.05	26.92	26.83	26.75	26.69	26.58	26.50	26.32	26.25	26.22	26.1
	.995	55.55	49.80	47.47	46.19	45.39	44.84	44.43	44.13	43.88	43.69	43.39	43.17	43.01	42.88	42.78	42.59	42.47	42.15	42.04	41.99	41.8
	.999	167.03	148.50	141.11	137.10	134.58	132.85	131.58	130.62	129.86	129.25	128.32	127.64	127.14	126.74	126.42	125.84	125.45	124.47	124.14	123.97	123.4
4	.50	0.55	0.83	0.94	1.00	1.04	1.06	1.08	1.09	1.10	1.11	1.13	1.13	1.14	1.15	1.15	1.16	1.16	1.18	1.18	1.18	1.1
	.90	4.54	4.32	4.19	4.11	4.05	4.01	3.98	3.95	3.94	3.92	3.90	3.88	3.86	3.85	3.84	3.83	3.82	3.79	3.78	3.78	3.7
	.95	7.71	6.94	6.59	6.39	6.26	6.16	6.09	6.04	6.00	5.96	5.91	5.87	5.84	5.82	5.80	5.77	5.75	5.69	5.67	5.66	5.6
	.975	12.22	10.65	9.98	9.60	9.36	9.20	9.07	8.98	8.90	8.84	8.75	8.68	8.63	8.59	8.56	8.50	8.46	8.36	8.33	8.31	8.2
	.99	21.20	18.00	16.69	15.98	15.52	15.21	14.98	14.80	14.66	14.55	14.37	14.25	14.15	14.08	14.02	13.91	13.84	13.65	13.59	13.56	13.4
	.995	31.33	26.28	24.26	23.15	22.46	21.97	21.62	21.35	21.14	20.97	20.70	20.51	20.37	20.26	20.17	20.00	19.89	19.61	19.52	19.47	19.3
	.999	74.14	61.25	56.18	53.44	51.71	50.53	49.66	49.00	48.47	48.05	47.41	46.95	46.60	46.32	46.10	45.70	45.43	44.75	44.52	44.40	44.0
5	.50	0.53	0.80	0.91	0.96	1.00	1.02	1.04	1.05	1.06	1.07	1.09	1.09	1.10	1.11	1.11	1.12	1.12	1.14	1.14	1.14	1.1
	.90	4.06	3.78	3.62	3.52	3.45	3.40	3.37	3.34	3.32	3.30	3.27	3.25	3.23	3.22	3.21	3.19	3.17	3.14	3.13	3.12	3.1
	.95	6.61	5.79	5.41	5.19	5.05	4.95	4.88	4.82	4.77	4.74	4.68	4.64	4.60	4.58	4.56	4.52	4.50	4.43	4.41	4.40	4.3
	.975	10.01	8.43	7.76	7.39	7.15	6.98	6.85	6.76	6.68	6.62	6.52	6.46	6.40	6.36	6.33	6.27	6.23	6.12	6.09	6.07	6.0
	.99	16.26	13.27	12.06	11.39	10.97	10.67	10.46	10.29	10.16	10.05	9.89	9.77	9.68	9.61	9.55	9.45	9.38	9.20	9.14	9.11	9.0
	.995	22.78	18.31	16.53	15.56	14.94	14.51	14.20	13.96	13.77	13.62	13.38	13.21	13.09	12.98	12.90	12.76	12.66	12.40	12.32	12.27	12.1
	.999	47.18	37.12	33.20	31.09	29.75	28.83	28.16	27.65	27.24	26.92	26.42	26.06	25.78	25.57	25.39	25.08	24.87	24.33	24.15	24.06	23.7

Table G. Percentiles of the *F* Distribution (*continued*).

Denominator df	p	Numerator df

Denominator df	p	1	2	3	4	5	6	7	8	9	10	12	14	16	18	20	25	30	60	90	120	inf
6	.50	0.51	0.78	0.89	0.94	0.98	1.00	1.02	1.03	1.04	1.05	1.06	1.07	1.08	1.08	1.08	1.09	1.10	1.11	1.11	1.12	1.1
	.90	3.78	3.46	3.29	3.18	3.11	3.05	3.01	2.98	2.96	2.94	2.90	2.88	2.86	2.85	2.84	2.81	2.80	2.76	2.75	2.74	2.7
	.95	5.99	5.14	4.76	4.53	4.39	4.28	4.21	4.15	4.10	4.06	4.00	3.96	3.92	3.90	3.87	3.83	3.81	3.74	3.72	3.70	3.6
	.975	8.81	7.26	6.60	6.23	5.99	5.82	5.70	5.60	5.52	5.46	5.37	5.30	5.24	5.20	5.17	5.11	5.07	4.96	4.92	4.90	4.8
	.99	13.75	10.92	9.78	9.15	8.75	8.47	8.26	8.10	7.98	7.87	7.72	7.60	7.52	7.45	7.40	7.30	7.23	7.06	7.00	6.97	6.8
	.995	18.63	14.54	12.92	12.03	11.46	11.07	10.79	10.57	10.39	10.25	10.03	9.88	9.76	9.66	9.59	9.45	9.36	9.12	9.04	9.00	8.8
	.999	35.51	27.00	23.70	21.92	20.80	20.03	19.46	19.03	18.69	18.41	17.99	17.68	17.45	17.27	17.12	16.85	16.67	16.21	16.06	15.98	15.7
7	.50	0.51	0.77	0.87	0.93	0.96	0.98	1.00	1.01	1.02	1.03	1.04	1.05	1.06	1.06	1.07	1.07	1.08	1.09	1.09	1.10	1.1
	.90	3.59	3.26	3.07	2.96	2.88	2.83	2.78	2.75	2.72	2.70	2.67	2.64	2.62	2.61	2.59	2.57	2.56	2.51	2.50	2.49	2.4
	.95	5.59	4.74	4.35	4.12	3.97	3.87	3.79	3.73	3.68	3.64	3.57	3.53	3.49	3.47	3.44	3.40	3.38	3.30	3.28	3.27	3.2
	.975	8.07	6.54	5.89	5.52	5.29	5.12	4.99	4.90	4.82	4.76	4.67	4.60	4.54	4.50	4.47	4.40	4.36	4.25	4.22	4.20	4.1
	.99	12.25	9.55	8.45	7.85	7.46	7.19	6.99	6.84	6.72	6.62	6.47	6.36	6.28	6.21	6.16	6.06	5.99	5.82	5.77	5.74	5.6
	.995	16.24	12.40	10.88	10.05	9.52	9.16	8.89	8.68	8.51	8.38	8.18	8.03	7.91	7.83	7.75	7.62	7.53	7.31	7.23	7.19	7.0
	.999	29.25	21.69	18.77	17.20	16.21	15.52	15.02	14.63	14.33	14.08	13.71	13.43	13.23	13.06	12.93	12.69	12.53	12.12	11.98	11.91	11.7
8	.50	0.50	0.76	0.86	0.91	0.95	0.97	1.00	1.00	1.01	1.02	1.03	1.04	1.04	1.05	1.05	1.06	1.07	1.08	1.08	1.08	1.0
	.90	3.46	3.11	2.92	2.81	2.73	2.67	2.62	2.59	2.56	2.54	2.50	2.48	2.45	2.44	2.42	2.40	2.38	2.34	2.32	2.32	2.2
	.95	5.32	4.46	4.07	3.84	3.69	3.58	3.50	3.44	3.39	3.35	3.28	3.24	3.20	3.17	3.15	3.11	3.08	3.01	2.98	2.97	2.9
	.975	7.57	6.06	5.42	5.05	4.82	4.65	4.53	4.43	4.36	4.30	4.20	4.13	4.08	4.03	4.00	3.94	3.89	3.78	3.75	3.73	3.6
	.99	11.26	8.65	7.59	7.01	6.63	6.37	6.18	6.03	5.91	5.81	5.67	5.56	5.48	5.41	5.36	5.26	5.20	5.03	4.97	4.95	4.8
	.995	14.69	11.04	9.60	8.81	8.30	7.95	7.69	7.50	7.34	7.21	7.01	6.87	6.76	6.68	6.61	6.48	6.40	6.18	6.10	6.06	5.9
	.999	25.41	18.49	15.83	14.39	13.48	12.86	12.40	12.05	11.77	11.54	11.19	10.94	10.75	10.60	10.48	10.26	10.11	9.73	9.60	9.53	9.3
9	.50	0.49	0.75	0.85	0.91	0.94	0.96	0.98	0.99	1.00	1.01	1.02	1.03	1.03	1.04	1.04	1.05	1.05	1.07	1.07	1.07	1.0
	.90	3.36	3.01	2.81	2.69	2.61	2.55	2.51	2.47	2.44	2.42	2.38	2.35	2.33	2.31	2.30	2.27	2.25	2.21	2.19	2.18	2.1
	.95	5.12	4.26	3.86	3.63	3.48	3.37	3.29	3.23	3.18	3.14	3.07	3.03	2.99	2.96	2.94	2.89	2.86	2.79	2.76	2.75	2.7
	.975	7.21	5.71	5.08	4.72	4.48	4.32	4.20	4.10	4.03	3.96	3.87	3.80	3.74	3.70	3.67	3.60	3.56	3.45	3.41	3.39	3.3
	.99	10.56	8.02	6.99	6.42	6.06	5.80	5.61	5.47	5.35	5.26	5.11	5.01	4.92	4.86	4.81	4.71	4.65	4.48	4.43	4.40	4.3
	.995	13.61	10.11	8.72	7.96	7.47	7.13	6.88	6.69	6.54	6.42	6.23	6.09	5.98	5.90	5.83	5.71	5.62	5.41	5.34	5.30	5.1
	.999	22.86	16.39	13.90	12.56	11.71	11.13	10.70	10.37	10.11	9.89	9.57	9.33	9.15	9.01	8.90	8.69	8.55	8.19	8.06	8.00	7.8
10	.50	0.49	0.74	0.85	0.90	0.93	0.95	0.97	0.98	0.99	1.00	1.01	1.02	1.03	1.03	1.03	1.04	1.05	1.06	1.06	1.06	1.0
	.90	3.29	2.92	2.73	2.61	2.52	2.46	2.41	2.38	2.35	2.32	2.28	2.26	2.23	2.22	2.20	2.17	2.16	2.11	2.09	2.08	2.0
	.95	4.96	4.10	3.71	3.48	3.33	3.22	3.14	3.07	3.02	2.98	2.91	2.86	2.83	2.80	2.77	2.73	2.70	2.62	2.59	2.58	2.5
	.975	6.94	5.46	4.83	4.47	4.24	4.07	3.95	3.85	3.78	3.72	3.62	3.55	3.50	3.45	3.42	3.35	3.31	3.20	3.16	3.14	3.0
	.99	10.04	7.56	6.55	5.99	5.64	5.39	5.20	5.06	4.94	4.85	4.71	4.60	4.52	4.46	4.41	4.31	4.25	4.08	4.03	4.00	3.9
	.995	12.83	9.43	8.08	7.34	6.87	6.54	6.30	6.12	5.97	5.85	5.66	5.53	5.42	5.34	5.27	5.15	5.07	4.86	4.79	4.75	4.6
	.999	21.04	14.91	12.55	11.28	10.48	9.93	9.52	9.20	8.96	8.75	8.45	8.22	8.05	7.91	7.80	7.60	7.47	7.12	7.00	6.94	6.7

df	P																					
12	.50	1.0	1.05	1.05	1.05	1.03	1.03	1.02	1.02	1.01	1.01	1.00	0.99	0.98	0.97	0.96	0.94	0.92	0.89	0.84	0.73	0.48
	.90	1.9	1.93	1.94	1.96	2.01	2.03	2.06	2.08	2.09	2.12	2.15	2.19	2.21	2.24	2.28	2.33	2.39	2.48	2.61	2.81	3.18
	.95	2.3	2.34	2.36	2.38	2.47	2.50	2.54	2.57	2.60	2.64	2.69	2.75	2.80	2.85	2.91	3.00	3.11	3.26	3.49	3.89	4.75
	.975	2.7	2.79	2.81	2.85	2.96	3.01	3.07	3.11	3.15	3.21	3.28	3.37	3.44	3.51	3.61	3.73	3.89	4.12	4.47	5.10	6.55
	.99	3.3	3.45	3.48	3.54	3.70	3.76	3.86	3.91	3.97	4.05	4.16	4.30	4.39	4.50	4.64	4.82	5.06	5.41	5.95	6.93	9.33
	.995	3.9	4.01	4.05	4.12	4.33	4.41	4.53	4.59	4.67	4.77	4.91	5.09	5.20	5.35	5.52	5.76	6.07	6.52	7.23	8.51	11.75
	.999	5.4	5.59	5.65	5.76	6.09	6.22	6.40	6.51	6.63	6.79	7.00	7.29	7.48	7.71	8.00	8.38	8.89	9.63	10.80	12.97	18.64
14	.50	1.0	1.04	1.04	1.04	1.03	1.02	1.01	1.01	1.01	1.00	0.99	0.98	0.97	0.96	0.95	0.94	0.91	0.88	0.83	0.73	0.48
	.90	1.8	1.83	1.84	1.86	1.91	1.93	1.96	1.98	2.00	2.02	2.05	2.10	2.12	2.15	2.19	2.24	2.31	2.39	2.52	2.73	3.10
	.95	2.1	2.18	2.19	2.22	2.31	2.34	2.39	2.41	2.44	2.48	2.53	2.60	2.65	2.70	2.76	2.85	2.96	3.11	3.34	3.74	4.60
	.975	2.4	2.55	2.57	2.61	2.73	2.78	2.84	2.88	2.92	2.98	3.05	3.15	3.21	3.29	3.38	3.50	3.66	3.89	4.24	4.86	6.30
	.99	3.0	3.09	3.12	3.18	3.35	3.41	3.51	3.56	3.62	3.70	3.80	3.94	4.03	4.14	4.28	4.46	4.69	5.04	5.56	6.51	8.86
	.995	3.4	3.55	3.58	3.66	3.86	3.94	4.06	4.12	4.20	4.30	4.43	4.60	4.72	4.86	5.03	5.26	5.56	6.00	6.68	7.92	11.06
	.999	4.6	4.77	4.83	4.94	5.25	5.38	5.56	5.66	5.78	5.93	6.13	6.40	6.58	6.80	7.08	7.44	7.92	8.62	9.73	11.78	17.14
16	.50	1.0	1.04	1.04	1.03	1.02	1.02	1.01	1.01	1.00	0.99	0.99	0.97	0.97	0.96	0.95	0.93	0.91	0.88	0.82	0.72	0.48
	.90	1.7	1.75	1.76	1.78	1.84	1.86	1.89	1.91	1.93	1.95	1.99	2.03	2.06	2.09	2.13	2.18	2.24	2.33	2.46	2.67	3.05
	.95	2.0	2.06	2.07	2.11	2.19	2.23	2.28	2.30	2.33	2.37	2.42	2.49	2.54	2.59	2.66	2.74	2.85	3.01	3.24	3.63	4.49
	.975	2.3	2.38	2.40	2.45	2.57	2.61	2.68	2.72	2.76	2.82	2.89	2.99	3.05	3.12	3.22	3.34	3.50	3.73	4.08	4.69	6.12
	.99	2.7	2.84	2.87	2.93	3.10	3.16	3.26	3.31	3.37	3.45	3.55	3.69	3.78	3.89	4.03	4.20	4.44	4.77	5.29	6.23	8.53
	.995	3.1	3.22	3.26	3.33	3.54	3.62	3.73	3.80	3.87	3.97	4.10	4.27	4.38	4.52	4.69	4.91	5.21	5.64	6.30	7.51	10.58
	.999	4.0	4.23	4.28	4.39	4.70	4.82	4.99	5.09	5.20	5.35	5.55	5.81	5.98	6.19	6.46	6.80	7.27	7.94	9.01	10.97	16.12
18	.50	1.0	1.03	1.03	1.03	1.02	1.01	1.00	1.00	1.00	0.99	0.98	0.97	0.96	0.95	0.94	0.93	0.90	0.87	0.82	0.72	0.47
	.90	1.6	1.69	1.70	1.72	1.78	1.80	1.84	1.85	1.87	1.90	1.93	1.98	2.00	2.04	2.08	2.13	2.20	2.29	2.42	2.62	3.01
	.95	1.9	1.97	1.98	2.02	2.11	2.14	2.19	2.22	2.25	2.29	2.34	2.41	2.46	2.51	2.58	2.66	2.77	2.93	3.16	3.55	4.41
	.975	2.1	2.26	2.28	2.32	2.44	2.49	2.56	2.60	2.64	2.70	2.77	2.87	2.93	3.01	3.10	3.22	3.38	3.61	3.95	4.56	5.98
	.99	2.5	2.66	2.69	2.75	2.92	2.98	3.08	3.13	3.19	3.27	3.37	3.51	3.60	3.71	3.84	4.01	4.25	4.58	5.09	6.01	8.29
	.995	2.8	2.99	3.02	3.10	3.30	3.38	3.50	3.56	3.64	3.73	3.86	4.03	4.14	4.28	4.44	4.66	4.96	5.37	6.03	7.21	10.22
	.999	3.6	3.84	3.89	4.00	4.30	4.42	4.59	4.68	4.80	4.94	5.13	5.39	5.56	5.76	6.02	6.35	6.81	7.46	8.49	10.39	15.38
20	.50	1.0	1.03	1.03	1.02	1.01	1.01	1.00	1.00	0.99	0.99	0.98	0.97	0.96	0.95	0.94	0.92	0.90	0.87	0.82	0.72	0.47
	.30	1.6	1.64	1.65	1.68	1.74	1.76	1.79	1.81	1.83	1.86	1.89	1.94	1.96	2.00	2.04	2.09	2.16	2.25	2.38	2.59	2.97
	.95	1.8	1.90	1.91	1.95	2.04	2.07	2.12	2.15	2.18	2.22	2.28	2.35	2.39	2.45	2.51	2.60	2.71	2.87	3.10	3.49	4.35
	.975	2.0	2.16	2.18	2.22	2.35	2.40	2.46	2.50	2.55	2.60	2.68	2.77	2.84	2.91	3.01	3.13	3.29	3.51	3.86	4.46	5.87
	.99	2.4	2.52	2.55	2.61	2.78	2.84	2.94	2.99	3.05	3.13	3.23	3.37	3.46	3.56	3.70	3.87	4.10	4.43	4.94	5.85	8.10
	.995	2.6	2.81	2.84	2.92	3.12	3.20	3.32	3.38	3.46	3.55	3.68	3.85	3.96	4.09	4.26	4.47	4.76	5.17	5.82	6.99	9.94
	.999	3.3	3.54	3.60	3.70	4.00	4.12	4.38	4.49	4.64	4.82	5.08	5.24	5.44	5.69	6.02	6.46	7.10	8.10	9.95	14.82	

Table G. Percentiles of the *F* Distribution (*continued*).

Denominator df	p	1	2	3	4	5	6	7	8	9	10	12	14	16	18	20	25	30	60	90	120	inf
25	.50	0.47	0.71	0.81	0.86	0.89	0.92	0.93	0.94	0.95	0.96	0.97	0.98	0.98	0.99	0.99	1.00	1.00	1.02	1.02	1.02	1.0
	.90	2.92	2.53	2.32	2.18	2.09	2.02	1.97	1.93	1.89	1.87	1.82	1.79	1.76	1.74	1.72	1.68	1.66	1.59	1.57	1.56	1.5
	.95	4.24	3.39	2.99	2.76	2.60	2.49	2.40	2.34	2.28	2.24	2.16	2.11	2.07	2.04	2.01	1.96	1.92	1.82	1.79	1.77	1.7
	.975	5.69	4.29	3.69	3.35	3.13	2.97	2.85	2.75	2.68	2.61	2.51	2.44	2.38	2.34	2.30	2.23	2.18	2.05	2.01	1.98	1.9
	.99	7.77	5.57	4.68	4.18	3.85	3.63	3.46	3.32	3.22	3.13	2.99	2.89	2.81	2.75	2.70	2.60	2.54	2.36	2.30	2.27	2.1
	.995	9.48	6.60	5.46	4.84	4.43	4.15	3.94	3.78	3.64	3.54	3.37	3.25	3.15	3.08	3.01	2.90	2.82	2.61	2.53	2.50	2.3
	.999	13.88	9.22	7.45	6.49	5.89	5.46	5.15	4.91	4.71	4.56	4.31	4.13	3.99	3.88	3.79	3.63	3.52	3.22	3.11	3.06	2.8
30	.50	0.47	0.71	0.81	0.86	0.89	0.91	0.93	0.94	0.95	0.96	0.97	0.97	0.98	0.99	0.99	1.00	1.00	1.01	1.02	1.02	1.0
	.90	2.88	2.49	2.28	2.14	2.05	1.98	1.93	1.88	1.85	1.82	1.77	1.74	1.71	1.69	1.67	1.63	1.61	1.54	1.51	1.50	1.4
	.95	4.17	3.32	2.92	2.69	2.53	2.42	2.33	2.27	2.21	2.16	2.09	2.04	1.99	1.96	1.93	1.88	1.84	1.74	1.70	1.68	1.6
	.975	5.57	4.18	3.59	3.25	3.03	2.87	2.75	2.65	2.57	2.51	2.41	2.34	2.28	2.23	2.20	2.12	2.07	1.94	1.89	1.87	1.7
	.99	7.56	5.39	4.51	4.02	3.70	3.47	3.30	3.17	3.07	2.98	2.84	2.74	2.66	2.60	2.55	2.45	2.39	2.21	2.14	2.11	2.0
	.995	9.18	6.35	5.24	4.62	4.23	3.95	3.74	3.58	3.45	3.34	3.18	3.06	2.96	2.89	2.82	2.71	2.63	2.42	2.34	2.30	2.1
	.999	13.29	8.77	7.05	6.12	5.53	5.12	4.82	4.58	4.39	4.24	4.00	3.82	3.69	3.58	3.49	3.33	3.22	2.92	2.81	2.76	2.5
60	.50	0.46	0.70	0.80	0.85	0.88	0.90	0.92	0.93	0.94	0.94	0.96	0.96	0.97	0.97	0.98	0.98	0.99	1.00	1.00	1.01	1.0
	.90	2.79	2.39	2.18	2.04	1.95	1.87	1.82	1.77	1.74	1.71	1.66	1.62	1.59	1.56	1.54	1.50	1.48	1.40	1.36	1.35	1.2
	.95	4.00	3.15	2.76	2.53	2.37	2.25	2.17	2.10	2.04	1.99	1.92	1.86	1.82	1.78	1.75	1.69	1.65	1.53	1.49	1.47	1.3
	.975	5.29	3.93	3.34	3.01	2.79	2.63	2.51	2.41	2.33	2.27	2.17	2.09	2.03	1.98	1.94	1.87	1.82	1.67	1.61	1.58	1.4
	.99	7.08	4.98	4.13	3.65	3.34	3.12	2.95	2.82	2.72	2.63	2.50	2.39	2.31	2.25	2.20	2.10	2.03	1.84	1.76	1.73	1.6
	.995	8.49	5.79	4.73	4.14	3.76	3.49	3.29	3.13	3.01	2.90	2.74	2.62	2.53	2.45	2.39	2.27	2.19	1.96	1.88	1.83	1.6
	.999	11.97	7.77	6.17	5.31	4.76	4.37	4.09	3.86	3.69	3.54	3.32	3.15	3.02	2.91	2.83	2.67	2.55	2.25	2.14	2.08	1.8
90	.50	0.46	0.70	0.79	0.85	0.88	0.90	0.91	0.92	0.93	0.94	0.95	0.96	0.97	0.97	0.97	0.98	0.99	1.00	1.00	1.00	1.0
	.90	2.76	2.36	2.15	2.01	1.91	1.84	1.78	1.74	1.70	1.67	1.62	1.58	1.55	1.52	1.50	1.46	1.43	1.35	1.31	1.29	1.2
	.95	3.95	3.10	2.71	2.47	2.32	2.20	2.11	2.04	1.99	1.94	1.86	1.80	1.76	1.72	1.69	1.63	1.59	1.46	1.42	1.39	1.3
	.975	5.20	3.84	3.26	2.93	2.71	2.55	2.43	2.34	2.26	2.19	2.09	2.02	1.95	1.91	1.86	1.79	1.73	1.58	1.52	1.48	1.3
	.99	6.93	4.85	4.01	3.53	3.23	3.01	2.84	2.72	2.61	2.52	2.39	2.29	2.21	2.14	2.09	1.99	1.92	1.72	1.64	1.60	1.4
	.995	8.28	5.62	4.57	3.99	3.62	3.35	3.15	3.00	2.87	2.77	2.61	2.49	2.39	2.32	2.25	2.13	2.05	1.82	1.73	1.68	1.5
	.999	11.57	7.47	5.91	5.06	4.53	4.15	3.87	3.65	3.48	3.34	3.11	2.95	2.82	2.71	2.63	2.47	2.36	2.05	1.93	1.87	1.6

Numerator df

120	.50	0.46	0.70	0.79	0.84	0.88	0.90	0.91	0.92	0.93	0.94	0.95	0.96	0.96	0.97	0.97	0.98	0.98	0.99	1.00	1.00	1.0
	.90	2.75	2.35	2.13	1.99	1.90	1.82	1.77	1.72	1.68	1.65	1.60	1.56	1.53	1.50	1.48	1.44	1.41	1.32	1.28	1.26	1.1
	.95	3.92	3.07	2.68	2.45	2.29	2.18	2.09	2.02	1.96	1.91	1.83	1.78	1.73	1.69	1.66	1.60	1.55	1.43	1.38	1.35	1.2
	.975	5.15	3.80	3.23	2.89	2.67	2.52	2.39	2.30	2.22	2.16	2.05	1.98	1.92	1.87	1.82	1.75	1.69	1.53	1.47	1.43	1.3
	.99	6.85	4.79	3.95	3.48	3.17	2.96	2.79	2.66	2.56	2.47	2.34	2.23	2.15	2.09	2.03	1.93	1.86	1.66	1.58	1.53	1.3
	.995	8.18	5.54	4.50	3.92	3.55	3.28	3.09	2.93	2.81	2.71	2.54	2.42	2.33	2.25	2.19	2.07	1.98	1.75	1.66	1.61	1.4
	.999	11.38	7.32	5.78	4.95	4.42	4.04	3.77	3.55	3.38	3.24	3.02	2.85	2.72	2.62	2.53	2.37	2.26	1.95	1.83	1.77	1.5
inf	.50	0.45	0.69	0.79	0.84	0.87	0.89	0.91	0.92	0.93	0.93	0.95	0.95	0.96	0.96	0.97	0.97	0.98	0.99	0.99	0.99	1.0
	.90	2.71	2.30	2.08	1.94	1.85	1.77	1.72	1.67	1.63	1.60	1.55	1.50	1.47	1.44	1.42	1.38	1.34	1.24	1.20	1.17	1.0
	.95	3.84	3.00	2.60	2.37	2.21	2.10	2.01	1.94	1.88	1.83	1.75	1.69	1.64	1.60	1.57	1.51	1.46	1.32	1.26	1.22	1.0
	.975	5.02	3.69	3.12	2.79	2.57	2.41	2.29	2.19	2.11	2.05	1.94	1.87	1.80	1.75	1.71	1.63	1.57	1.39	1.31	1.27	1.0
	.99	6.63	4.61	3.78	3.32	3.02	2.80	2.64	2.51	2.41	2.32	2.18	2.08	2.00	1.93	1.88	1.77	1.70	1.47	1.38	1.32	1.0
	.995	7.88	5.30	4.28	3.72	3.35	3.09	2.90	2.74	2.62	2.52	2.36	2.24	2.14	2.06	2.00	1.88	1.79	1.53	1.43	1.36	1.0
	.999	10.83	6.91	5.42	4.62	4.10	3.74	3.47	3.27	3.10	2.96	2.74	2.58	2.45	2.35	2.27	2.10	1.99	1.66	1.52	1.45	1.0

Table H. A Guide to Methods of Statistical Inference.

This guide to the statistical methods is designed as an aid in the choice of appropriate methods in given situations. The techniques are arranged according to the statistical problem which they were designed to address. Because some methods are useful in a variety of situation, they appear more than one place in the table. The conditions under which the methods may be used are left somewhat vague (e.g., "large sample") to give a general indication of the range of applicability of the methods. Relevant sections in the textbook are given in parentheses. Methods not covered in the textbook are not given. (Abbreviation, CI = confidence interval)

Analysis of One Variable in One Sample			
Data Type	Conditions	Estimation and Confidence Intervals	Hypothesis Testing
Ratio	Large sample or normal population with known σ^2	CI for μ based on normal probability table (7.2)	One-sample Z test for μ (8.3, 8.4)
	Small sample, normal population with known σ^2	CI for μ based on normal table (7.2)	One-sample Z test for μ (8.3, 8.4)
	Small sample, normal population with unknown σ^2	CI for μ based on t distribution (7.3)	One-sample t test for μ (8.5)
	Small sample, normal population	CI for σ^2 based on χ^2 table (7.5)	One-sample χ^2 test for σ^2 (8.8)
Binary	Large sample	CI for proportion (7.4)	One-sample test for proportion (8.7)
Binary	Small sample	—	Exact one-sample test for proportion

Analysis of One Variable in Two Paired Samples		
Data Type	Conditions	Hypothesis Testing
Ratio	Small sample, normal population of differences Small sample, normal population with unknown σ Small sample, non-normal population of differences	One-sample Z test for μ (8.3, 8.4) Paired t test (9.5) Sign test (14.2), Wilcoxon signed rank test (14.4)
Ordinal	Large sample (for use of normal table)	Sign test (14.2), Wilcoxon signed rank test (14.4)
Binary	Large sample (for use of normal table)	McNemar test (10.5)

Analysis of One Variable in Two Independent Samples		
Data Type	Conditions	Hypothesis Testing
Ratio	Large samples Small samples, normal populations with known variances	Two-sample Z test for means (9.2) Two-sample Z test for means 9.2)
	Small samples, normal populations with unknown, but equal variances	Two-sample t test 9.3)
	Small samples, normal populations with unknown, and unequal variances	Two-sample t test, sing Satherthwaite approximation (9.4)
	Non-normal populations	Wilcoxon rank sum test (14.3)
Ordinal	Large sample (for use of normal probability table)	Wilcoxon rank sum test (14.3)
Binary	Large sample	Two-sample test for proportions using normal approximation (9.6) χ test for 2×2 table (10.2)
Binary	Small sample	Fisher's exact test (10.2)

Analysis of One Variable in Three or More Independent Samples		
Ratio	Normal populations with equal variances Non-normal populations	Analysis of variance (12.5) Kruskal-Wallis rank test (14.6)

Index